VETERI...

for the B... ...rse

interest

Horse and ...*agement*
Third ...ion
Jeremy Houghton ... owell-Smith
and
0 6 ...

Equine Nutrition and Feeding
Second Edition
David Frape
0 632 04105 6

Horse Nutrition and Feeding
Second Edition
Sarah Pilliner
0 632 05016 0

Equine Injury, Therapy and Rehabilitation
Second Edition
Mary Bromiley
0 632 03608 7

Coaching the Rider
Jane Houghton Brown
0 632 03931 0

Horse Business Management
Second Edition
Jeremy Houghton Brown and Vincent Powell-Smith
0 632 03821 7

Teaching Jumping
Jane Houghton Brown
0 632 04127 7

Equine Medical Disorders
Second Edition
A. M. Johnston
0 632 03841 1

VETERINARY MANUAL
for the Performance Horse

Nancy S. Loving
DVM

with A. M. Johnston
BVM & S, D Vet Med, MRCVS
Royal Veterinary College
University of London

Blackwell
Science

© Equine Research Inc, 1993
This edition © Blackwell Science 1995

Blackwell Science, Ltd, a Blackwell Publishing
Company
Editorial Offices:
9600 Garsington Rd, OX4 2DQ, UK
Tel: +44 (0)1865 776868
Blackwell Science, Inc., 350 Main Street,
Malden, MA 02148-5018, USA
Tel: +1 781 388 8250
Iowa State Press, a Blackwell Publishing
Company, 2121 State Avenue, Ames, Iowa
50014-8300, USA
Tel: +1 515 292 0140
Blackwell Science Asia Pty, 54 University Street,
Carlton, Victoria 3053, Australia
Tel: +61 (0)3 9347 0300
Blackwell Wissenschafts Verlag,
Kurfürstendamm 57, 10707 Berlin, Germany
Tel: +49 (0)30 32 79 060

First published in North America by Equina
Research Inc. 1993
This edition first published in Great Britain by
Blackwell Science 1995
Reprinted 1996
Reissued in paperback 1997
Reprinted 1998, 2002, 2003

Library of Congress
Cataloging-in-Publication Data

Loving, Nancy S.
  Veterinary manual for the
performance horse/Nancy S. Loving,
with A. M. Johnston.
    p. cm.
  Originally published: Grand Prairie,
Tex.: Equine Research, c1993.
  Includes bibliographical references
(p.   ) and index.
  ISBN 0-632-04166-8 (paperback.
alk. paper)
  1. Equine sports medicine —
Handbooks, manuals, etc.
2. Competition horses — Wounds
and injuries — Handbooks, manuals,
etc. 3. Competition horses —
Health — Handbooks, manuals etc.
I. Johnston, A. M., MRCVS.
II. Title
[SF956.L68 1996]
836.1′08971027–dc20   95-658
                                CIP

ISBN 0-632-04166-8

A catalogue record for this title is available from
the British Library

Set by Setrite Typesetters Ltd, Hong Kong
Printed and bound in India by
Replika Press Pvt. Ltd. Kundli 131 028

For further information on
Blackwell Publishing, visit our website:
www.blackwellpublishing.com

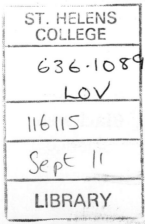

Contents

15

20

21

Disclaimer

Every effort has been made in the writing of this book to present scientifically accurate and up-to-date information based on the best available and reliable sources. However, the results of caring for horses depend upon a variety of factors not under the control of the authors or publishers of this book. Therefore, neither the authors nor the publishers assume any responsibility for, nor make any warranty with respect to, results that may be obtained from the procedures described or ingredients discussed herein. Neither the publishers nor the authors shall be liable to anyone for damages resulting from reliance on any information contained in this book whether with respect to feeding, care, treatment procedures, drug usages and dosages, or by reason of any misstatement or inadvertent error contained herein.

Also, it must be remembered that neither the publishers nor the authors manufacture any of the drugs, feeds, supplements or products discussed in this book. Accordingly, neither the publishers nor the authors offer any guarantees of any kind on such items – nor will they be held responsible for the results that may be obtained from the use of those items.

The reader is encouraged to read and follow the directions published by the manufacturer of each product, feed, supplement or drug which may be mentioned herein. And, if there is a conflict with information in this book, the instructions of the manufacturer – or of the reader's veterinarian – should, of course, be followed.

To ensure the reader's understanding of some technical descriptions offered in this book, brand names have occasionally been used as examples of particular substances or equipment. However, the use of a particular trademark or brand name is not intended to imply an endorsement of that particular product, nor to suggest that similar products offered by others under different names may be inferior. Also, nothing contained in *Veterinary Manual for the Performance Horse* is to be construed as a suggestion to violate any trademark laws.

1

CONFORMATION FOR PERFORMANCE

ANATOMY AND FUNCTION

The *ideal* horse is an image with which we compare all others. There is no such thing as a perfect horse, but a horse with good conformation makes a durable athlete. Excellent conformation does not always guarantee excellence in performance; other talents such as temperament and trained abilities are usually needed to create a superior competitor. Each horse has strengths and weaknesses in different areas, both physical and mental.

A discussion of conformation is a study in anatomy and its relation to the function of each structure. Although various parts of a horse are isolated, scrutinized, and analysed for their individual contributions to the abilities of that animal, each part influences the others as an interactive system.

(Anatomy, bone and muscle diagrams are located in the Appendix.)

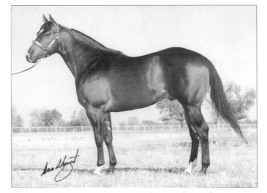

Fig. 1.1 Quarter Horse with good conformation.

1

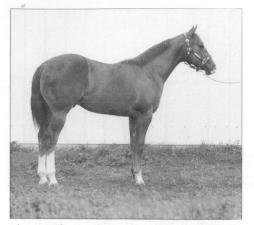

Fig. 1.2 The conformation of a yearling tells a lot about its potential for future athletic performance.

The way the skeleton is put together, *conformation*, determines the strength and coordination of individual muscles. Muscles and tendons are responsible for motion. Think of the muscles as little levers and pulleys, moving different parts of the skeleton. Muscle coordination is important for good performance. While different sports capitalize on strengthening some parts of a horse's body more than others, basic principles apply in creating any equine athlete.

To begin a conformation analysis, place the horse on a flat, level surface, and square it up. Stand back and survey the whole horse to gain an overall impression of its appearance and stance. Examine the horse's overall symmetry from front, back and side. An asymmetric area such as an atrophied leg muscle may hint at an old injury or limb disuse due to lameness.

Balance

A balanced horse makes a better athlete. Balance depends on the location of a horse's centre of mass. As a rule of thumb, a horse with optimum balance is visually proportional into thirds:

• the neck, from the poll to the withers
• the back, from the withers to the point of the hip
• the hindquarters

Of course, no horse can be divided exactly into thirds, but a horse that comes close to these guidelines will be

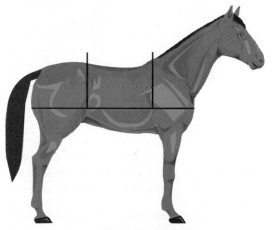

Fig. 1.3 The horse divided into thirds.

well balanced.

Another way to visualize the balance of a horse is with a box. The height at the withers, the height at the hip, and the length of the body should be *approximately* the same. There are variations among breeds, for example, some Arabians have one less thoracic vertebra than other breeds. Thoroughbreds come closest to meeting the 'box' guidelines.

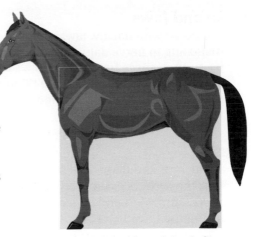

Fig. 1.4 An imaginary 'box' for judging balance.

Whichever method is used, the imaginary dividing lines place the centre of gravity of the well-balanced horse directly under a mounted rider, with 60 – 65% of the horse's weight falling on the forelegs. If a horse's head is too big or the neck is too long, it is difficult for the hindquarters to effectively counteract the extra weight up front. If the hindquarters are too small, there is no power to push the heavier front end.

Head

The head should be proportionate to the rest of the body, with ample length to provide room for strong teeth and the nasal passages. A head that is too large can create a heavy load on the front end, especially if attached to a relatively short neck.

Nostrils

The nostrils should be generous in size so the horse can breathe plenty of oxygen to fuel performance. A deeply dished face pinches the nostrils and nasal passages, and limits the performance of a speed or endurance horse.

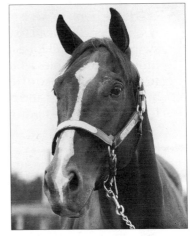

Fig. 1.5 Quarter Horse with a well shaped head.

Nose and Jaws

A horse with narrow jaws may also have a narrow throatlatch, predisposing to nerve damage, which can lead to *roaring*. There should be enough space between the jaws to allow for an active and open airway. The nasal passages are filled with many blood vessels to cool or to warm incoming air to body temperature, preventing shock to the respiratory system.

Eyes

The eyes should be well placed for good vision. The ideal location is at the corners of the forehead. The eyes should have a nice soft expression, alert and interested. Poor eyesight may pose behavioural problems.

Neck

As a biomechanical structure, a horse's neck is the ultimate in design. The triangular shape enhances its function as a cantilever beam to evenly distribute the weight of the head. There is more variety in the necks of horses than in other species due to changes in breed and conformational characteristics developed through centuries of controlled breeding.

Neck Function

For the horse, a neck of proper length is necessary for survival. The neck lowers the head for grazing and drinking, and assists vision by swinging the head for accurate eye focus. The neck's large range of motion also enables a horse to shift and fine tune its centre of gravity to maintain balance of its massive body. A horse with well-formed and coupled limbs and back can only achieve fine athletic potential if it can balance the body while in motion.

Neck as a Balance

What do all equine athletes have in common? Each uses its neck to shift the centre of gravity in the necessary direction to maintain balance and manoeuvrability. Consider the following examples:

- A racehorse at full gallop with neck and head extended to increase the length of stride and speed. This simple shift in the centre of gravity enhances speed and also reduces fatigue.
- A dressage horse with an arched neck, as it executes precision movements of pirouette or piaffe which require collection and engagement of the hindquarters.

- A long distance riding horse with head and neck extended, manoeuvring up a steep embankment. As it descends a hillside, it raises the neck and head to lighten the front end, allowing the hindquarters to sink down for better stability on irregular footing.
- A roping horse (used in catching cattle with a lasso) as it slides to an abrupt stop, the neck raised as it sinks onto the haunches.

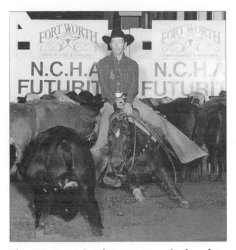

Fig. 1.6 A cutting horse moves its head to facilitate shifts in direction.

- A cutting horse (used to separate out cattle) quickly shifting side to side to follow a cow's manoeuvres, moving its head to facilitate shifts in direction.

Bascule

A jumping horse must arch its neck into a *bascule*, which is an arc created by moving one end which is then counterbalanced by the other. This principle is the same as the seesaw. The bascule involves a series of steps: extending and lowering the head, arching the back, flexing the *lumbosacral joint* (L-S joint), and finally engaging the hindquarters. In this way, a horse translates horizontal forward movement into vertical motion up and over a jump.

Neck As A Counterbalance

Analysis of a horse's forward motion illustrates that the downswing of the head and neck is accompanied by a forward pull of the back muscles. As

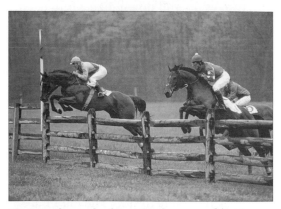

Fig. 1.7 The neck of jumping horses arching to function as a bascule.

the body moves forward, propelled from the hind legs to the forelegs, the hindquarters lift from the ground to advance to the next forward stride. As the horse steps under itself, the neck and head continue to work as a counterbalance. With the hind legs supporting the horse, the head and neck rise, followed by elevation of the forequarters and a forward swing of the forelegs to further advance the stride.

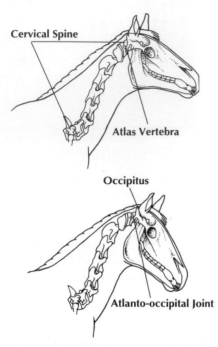

Fig. 1.8 The 'Yes' joint showing flexion of the horse at the poll.

Neck Structure

The bony spine is buried within the muscular structure of the neck. It provides a scaffold for attachment of all other ligamentous and muscular parts.

'Yes' Joint

The *cervical spine* is connected to the *occipitus*, or base of the skull, by the *atlas vertebra*, which is the first cervical vertebra after the skull. The joint formed at their connection, the *atlanto-occipital joint*, moves up and down, like a hinge, earning it the name of the 'yes' joint.

The head moves up and down without moving the rest of the neck or body, but the protrusions of the atlas vertebra restrict lateral, side to side movement of this joint. For riding purposes, the yes joint enables flexion at the poll to complete the stretch through the topline that aids self-carriage and can advance a horse to higher levels of performance.

'No' Joint

The *atlas vertebra* joins the *axis* (second) *vertebra* at the *atlanto-axial joint*, also called the 'no' joint, because it rotates the head and neck from side to side. The joint barely extends due to pressure against the atlas vertebra of another bony piece, the *dens*. (*The dens is the part of the axis vertebra which hooks under the atlas vertebra*

*and cannot be seen in the il-
lustrations.)*

Other Cervical Joints

The other cervical joints in
the neck are similar to each
other in shape and range of
motion. They are capable of
flexion, extension and *lateral*
movement. Throughout a
horse's life, the flexion and
extension capabilities of
these joints remain relatively
constant. However, there is
an age-related reduction in axial rotation in the middle section of the
neck, leading to reduced suppleness in later years.

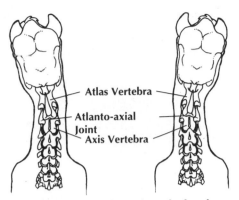

Fig. 1.9 The 'No' joint swings the head
from side to side.

Neck Length and Shape

Every horse has seven cervical vertebrae, and it is the length of each
of these which determines if a neck is long or short. A horse's neck
can be compared to a gymnast's balancing pole as it moves to accommodate shifts in equilibrium of the body.

Short Neck

A short neck limits the range of
flexibility of the head and neck,
and is less able to adjust rapidly, which is necessary to
fine tune balance. Often, a
short neck is also thick
and muscular, which not
only reduces the neck's
suppleness, but also adds
substantial weight. A
thick throatlatch, often
associated with a thick
neck, limits airflow through
the windpipe. It can also
limit flexion of the head
when a rider asks the horse to go 'on-the-bit'.

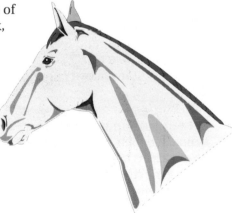

Fig. 1.10 A thick throatlatch limits air flow.

Neck Muscles and Stride Length

Neck muscles enable all body structures to work together to
achieve balance. Interconnecting muscles between neck and

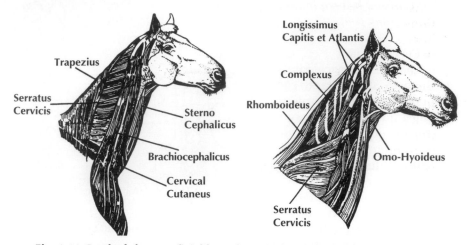

Fig. 1.11 On the left, superficial lateral cervical muscles. On the right, deep lateral cervical muscles.

shoulders swing a horse's forelegs through each stride. Neck muscles can contract and expand two-thirds of their natural length and in so doing advance the shoulder and forelegs through a stride. For the hindquarters to propel a horse forwards, the shoulders and forelegs must swing freely.

The length of a horse's stride is closely correlated to neck length: in extended gaits the forelegs can never reach past the point of the nose. Hence, a short neck limits the range of foreleg movement, and can increase wear and tear on the legs, because more steps are required to move a certain distance across the ground. Short, choppy strides result in wasted energy for movement and cause limb fatigue.

Long Neck

A horse performing at rapid speeds, such as a racehorse, eventer or jumper, benefits from a moderately long and finely muscled neck. Too long a neck is a disadvantage as it adds extra weight to the front end, shifting the centre of gravity forwards. This shift forces a horse to travel on the forehand (front third in front of the shoulders), creating excess stress on the forelegs.

Muscles in a neck that is too long may have greater difficulty developing strength and are prone to fatigue. The neck and head might droop, forcing the horse on to the forehand and reducing efficiency of movement. If a horse does not have the strength to support its own head and neck, it tends to pull on a rider's hands, depending on them for support.

As an example of the relationship of form to function, horses with very long, slender necks may be predisposed to *roaring* syndrome, or *laryngeal hemiplegia*. To breathe efficiently, the larynx at the top of the trachea must be able to fully open with inspiration. The muscles that open the *arytenoid cartilages* are

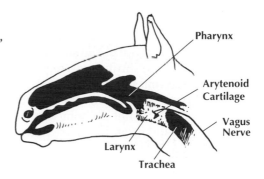

Fig. 1.12 Side view of the throat.

innervated by the two recurrent laryngeal branches of the *vagus nerve* on either side.

A longer neck is thought to increase tension on the vagus nerve, in most cases the left branch, leading to nerve damage and paralysing the laryngeal muscle that opens the airway for breathing. The arytenoid cartilage controlled by this muscle then collapses into the airway on the left side. As air passes through the restricted opening it produces turbulence and creates a 'roaring' sound. Exercise tolerance and stamina are compromised. *(See more information in Chapters 5 and 6.)*

Low-Set Neck

Ideally, the neck should join the chest just above the point of the shoulder. A low-set neck throws a horse on to the forehand by shifting the centre of gravity forwards and down, restricting shoulder movement and mobility as well as stride length. For a show hunter or western riding horse, travelling 'long and level' is ideal for competi-

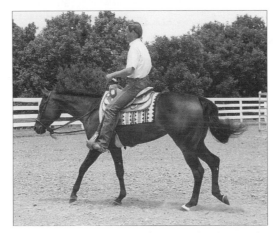

Fig. 1.13 A western riding horse with a low and level neck.

tion, but it can seriously compromise the performance and coordination of a jumper, eventer or dressage candidate.

Even in sports where a level neck is desirable, training a horse to carry its neck too low is dangerous to both horse and rider. The horse falls heavily on the forehand, increasing concussion to the forelegs. A low neck set reduces the shoulder's freedom of movement, so the horse tends to shuffle and frequently stumbles.

The external shape of the neck depicts the internal configuration of the cervical spine. Over time, training methods build individual muscle groups, but the bony vertebral scaffold is unchangeable. The neck's actual *shape* has more influence on the way a horse travels than does its length.

Neck Influence on Head Carriage

The shape of the neck and its connection to the head and withers determine normal head carriage in a horse. Normal head carriage at a 45° angle to the ground optimizes a horse's field of vision while allowing the head and neck the mobility necessary to retain body balance. In this position, the larynx is open to promote efficient breathing. The bit falls on the bars of the mouth rather than sliding into the cheeks so the rider has more control.

Carrying the head at this natural angle enables the neck muscles connected to the shoulder to lift the shoulder so the forearm can freely swing, increasing limb advancement across the ground.

Ewe-Neck

A horse with a *ewe-neck* is predisposed to high head carriage, result-

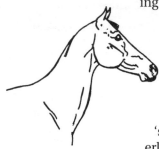

ing in a hollow back and an inability to engage the hindquarters or move forward on to the bit. A horse with its head in the air is unable to move effectively because its rear end is poorly connected to its front end. Therefore, it is unbalanced. Such a ride is uncomfortable to both horse and rider. With the head in a 'star gazing' position, the bit does not properly contact the bars of the mouth. The situation is further aggravated as the horse throws its head higher to escape the irritating bit pressure.

Fig. 1.14 Ewe neck.

Arched Neck

If the neck is arched, the head is in a vertical position which limits the horse's range of vision. The cervical vertebrae in the neck assume an 'S' curve that functionally shortens neck length. These factors are important to advanced levels of dressage. A collected head carriage benefits performance of lateral precision movements. Shortening the neck length moves the centre of gravity towards the hind end. Shifting the centre of gravity backwards frees the head and neck to move up and down. Therefore, suppleness increases from side to side. The shoulders and forelegs also move with greater freedom.

Withers

The withers are formed by the top portions of the 3rd through 8th thoracic vertebrae of the spine.

Stretch Through the Topline

For many equine athletic endeavours, the aim is to achieve longitudinal flexion (arching of the spine) through the entire back and topline. Stretched muscles are relaxed muscles. Consequently, they are less prone to fatigue and injury. Interactive use of muscle groups adds strength to a horse's movements. Stretch through the entire topline and neck starts at the withers.

The Role of the Withers

The *scalenus muscles* of the neck connect to the first rib. As these muscles raise the base of the neck, an increase in the lever arm at the withers improves stretch through the topline. As the first rib is pulled

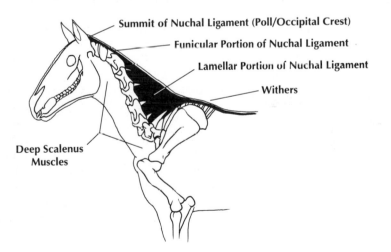

Fig. 1.15 The nuchal ligament supports the head and neck.

forwards, the rib cage expands and increases respiratory capacity for speed and stamina.

The fibroelastic *nuchal ligament,* an extensive fan-like structure forming the crest of the neck, extends from the base of the skull and anchors onto the withers where it is directly continuous with the lumbo-sacral part of the supraspinatus ligament. The nuchal ligament passively supports the head and neck to distribute the mechanical load, and assists extensor muscles of the head and neck. Additional neck muscles that raise the head and neck, or move them from side to side, anchor to the withers. Muscle groups that elevate the shoulder and extend the spine also anchor here.

A proper crest of the neck that carries well back over the withers enhances the fulcrum effect of the withers. As the withers rise when a horse stretches through its neck, the back and spine arch, engaging the hindquarters with hocks and stifles moving well underneath the body.

This specific arching movement is important not only to dressage horses, but also to jumping and long distance horses. Such flexibility and suppleness are not only dependent upon conformational structure, but also require conditioning.

High Withers

The withers should sit about 1 inch higher than the horse's croup. A high withers allows a greater range of movement for the neck and back muscles that attach to it. Like a seesaw, the higher the fulcrum point (withers), the more freedom both sides of the seesaw (neck and back) have to move up and down. A high, broad withers provides greater flexibility through the back and spine. As a horse lowers and extends the neck, the back rises. If the withers are too high, there can be problem with the fit of a saddle.

Low Withers

If the withers are too low, the saddle and rider slide forwards, shifting the centre of gravity forward and increasing impact to the forelegs. The saddle and rider may also injure poorly muscled withers.

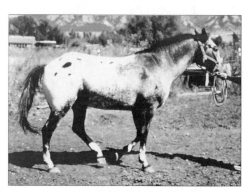

Fig. 1.16 An example of low withers.

Chest

A good chest is deep and well-defined to allow for a large respiratory capacity and a well developed heart. The depth of a horse's chest is more important than width. The ribs should have ample space between them and project backwards. Such ribs improve chest depth and allow for excellent lung expansion during athletic pursuits.

Proper Width and Depth of Chest

A chest that is too wide does not allow good clearance for the elbows, and the horse is prone to girth gall. The greatest width of the barrel should lie behind the

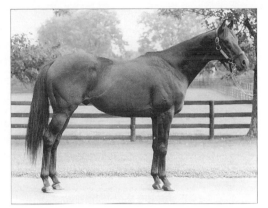

Fig. 1.17 Thoroughbred showing good withers and chest depth.

girth so shoulder movement is not restricted. A narrow chest can result in limb interference such as *plaiting,* which is crossing one foot over the other while in motion, or striking the inside of a leg with the opposite foot.

For example, a horse with *base-narrow,* toed-out conformation where the hooves are closer together than the shoulders, will wing with its feet as it moves. (If it was pigeon-toed, it would paddle instead.) Winging results in limb interference, potentially injuring the splint bones. The base-narrow stance also creates pressure on the inside of the knee joints and inside splint bones, increasing the chance of developing *splints.*

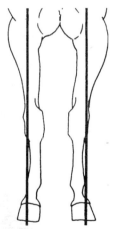

Fig. 1.18 Base-narrow and toed-out.

Shoulder

Bones that are located higher in the leg have greater influence on the freedom of limb swing. It is actually the relationship of the shoulder bone *(scapula)* to the arm bone *(humerus)*

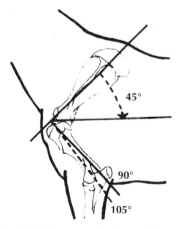

Fig. 1.19 The scapulo-humeral angle should be greater than 90°.

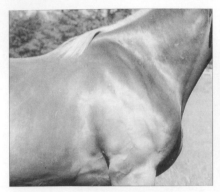

Fig. 1.20 A sloping shoulder.

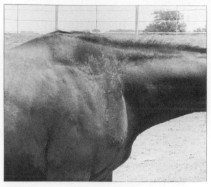

Fig. 1.21 A vertical shoulder.

that has the most influence on arm swing and stride length. Ideally, the angle between the scapula and humerus should be greater than 90°, preferably nearing a more open angle of 105°.

Stride Length

A horse's stride length depends on the conformational angles of its shoulder and foreleg. The longer a horse's stride, the faster it can cover ground, and the fewer steps the horse takes to get from point to point. If the number of steps is greater, the horse fatigues faster, and experiences more stress and strain on the limbs. Therefore, a shorter stride length increases the possibility of lameness since the forelegs absorb up to 65% of the weight-bearing impact.

Sloping Shoulder

A sloping shoulder at an angle of 45° to the ground anatomically moves the withers further back to relieve the shock of impact for the rider. A sloping shoulder distributes the attachment of muscles and ligaments over a greater area, diffusing the impact on the horse's musculoskeletal system.

Vertical Shoulder

If the shoulder is vertical and upright, a horse will have greater knee action. The knees will be lifted high with each step, creating a rough, inelastic ride that transfers concussion to the rider while the horse covers less ground with each stride. Again, the greater the number of steps taken, the faster the onset of fatigue.

Forelegs

Viewed from the side, the foreleg should be a straight column from the elbow to the fetlock. Straightness of this column promotes equal loading, or axial compression forces moving down the leg with weight-bearing, across the joints and bones.

Looking at the side of a horse, a plumb line dropped from the middle of the shoulder blade and bisecting the fetlock should fall directly behind the heel. Any deviation from the straightness of the column predisposes to degenerative joint disease (DJD), known as arthritis. Abnormalities in bone growth plates lead to *angular limb deformities.* These deformities also predispose to DJD because of abnormal

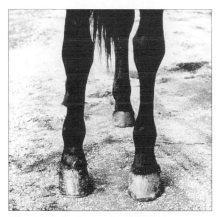

Fig. 1.23 A pigeon-toed horse.

Fig. 1.22 A plumb line intersecting all parts of the foreleg.

loading forces on the joint. Examples of these syndromes are: knock-knee *(carpus valgus),* bowlegged *(carpus varus),* splayfooted *(fetlock valgus),* and pigeon-toed *(fetlock varus).* The pigeon-toed horse is often afflicted with ringbone, a DJD of the pastern or coffin joint.

Upper Arm

The humerus should be at least half as long as the scapula. If the point of the shoulder is high, the humerus is long and steep, creating a more open shoulder angle. The longer the humerus, the greater a horse's ability to move the elbow away from the body. If a horse can move the elbow forwards with greater freedom, it improves things such as better racing stride, jumping, and crouching low to head a calf.

If a horse can move the elbow sideways, it can execute lateral movements important to dressage, polo and cutting.

A horse with a short humerus has short, choppy strides, and does not easily perform speed or lateral work. If the humerus lies in a horizontal plane, the *scapulo-humeral* angle closes. The limbs cannot fold tightly, and the horse has difficulty with sports such as cutting, jumping or polo.

The elbow should be in front of the peak of the withers so the humerus does not fall horizontally. A horizontal humerus produces a pigeon-breasted horse that stands with the forelegs too far under the body. It is hard for a pigeon-breasted horse to move in balance.

Forearm

The muscles in the forearm extend the limb forwards and absorb the shock of impact. It is preferable to have strong, well developed muscles. A long forearm increases the length of a horse's stride. A long forearm coupled with a short cannon bone and a medium length pastern creates structural stability in the limb, while achieving optimal leverage and strength of the *musculotendinous* attachments.

Knees

Normally a horse's knee *(carpus)* is slightly sprung and not entirely straight due to the normal curvature of the forearm bone *(radius)*. The front contours of the knees should be flat and shield-shaped, with well defined corners.

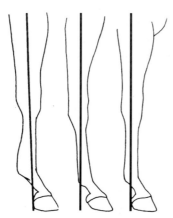

Fig. 1.24 From left to right: tied in behind the knee, calf knee, normal limb.

Problem Knees
Bucked Knees

Excessive curvature of the radius leads to bucked knees or *over at the knee*, and places strain on the flexor tendons. An enlarged and thickened tendon, or *bowed tendon* can result as it prematurely flexes with each weight-bearing stride.

Calf Knee

A knee that is set too far back is called a *calf knee*, a major flaw that often leads to fractured knee bones in the racehorse, and degenerative joint disease in other athletes. An upright pastern and a long-toe – low-heel foot configuration create a functional calf knee, stressing the knee joints and flexor tendons and delaying *breakover* of the foot.

Other Knee Problems

Knock-knee *(carpus valgus)* occurs when the knees deviate towards each other. Bowlegged *(carpus varus)* horses have knees which deviate away from each other. Both of these abnormalities predispose to DJD.

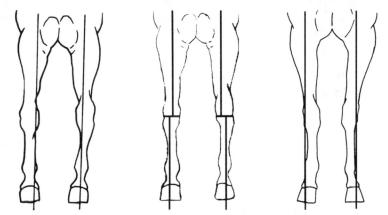

Fig. 1.25 From left to right: bow-legged, bench knees, knock-knee.

Cannon Bone

If the measurement at the top of the cannon bone is less than at the bottom of the cannon bone, the horse is *tied in* behind the knees. The width of the flexor tendons and suspensory ligaments is smaller at the top of the cannon area, predisposing them to strain and injury.

When the cannon bone is offset to the outside of the forelegs, known as a *bench knee*, greater stress is placed on the inside of the knee joint.

Pasterns

The angle of the pastern's slope to the ground is important to the stability of the joints in the lower legs and smoothness of stride. In general, the relationship of the angles of the hoof, pastern and shoulder to the ground should be the same. The pasterns should be of medium length. A short pastern is upright, while a long pastern tends to slope towards the ground.

Short Pastern

A short pastern acts as a poor shock absorber. Not only does this configuration result in an uncomfortable ride, but the horse receives added concussion to the middle third of its feet, predisposing it to navicular disease.

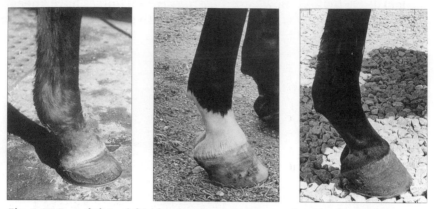

Fig. 1.26 From left to right: short pastern, medium pastern, long pastern.

Long Pastern

A long pastern provides a comfortable ride, but it predisposes to tendon injury because the fetlock drops further with each weight-bearing stride. Excessive fetlock drop increases the pull on the flexor tendons. A horse with a long pastern often develops *windgalls* which are swellings of the fetlock joint capsule (articular windgalls) or of the flexor tendon sheath (tendinous windgalls). It also increases the risk of a bowed tendon, *sesamoiditis* (inflammation of the fetlock sesamoid bones), or *suspensory desmitis* (inflammation of the suspensory ligament).

Back

The sixth, last, lumbar vertebra joins the sacrum, the dorsal part of the pelvis, at the lumbar-sacral joint. The longissimus dorsi muscle, the largest and longest in the body, extends from the sacrum and ileum to the neck, filling the space between the lumbar transverse processes and the upper ends of the ribs. This gives the muscle a three-sided prism shape. How the muscles of the hindquarters connect to the back at the lumbosacral joint is called *coupling*. To achieve the greatest strength and flexibility, hindquarter muscles should be carried well forwards into the back. The loin is unable to flex from side to side, therefore a long lumbar span creates a weak back. A short back limits the range that a horse can move the legs and elbows vertically, or *scope*. Scope is important in events such as racing, jumping and hunting.

A back that is too long may eventually develop a *sway back* as muscular attachments weaken with age and use. A swaybacked horse is often plagued with chronic back pain. A long back also prevents a horse from executing lateral movements with ease. Ribs and interlocking facets of lumbar vertebrae prevent a horse from rotating sideways in the area in front of the ninth thoracic vertebra. Maximum bending and rotation lie behind the area under the saddle and behind the rider's legs.

Loins

Ideal loins are short and only encompass a handspan, or about 8 inches, between the last rib and the point of the hip. The horse that uses its loins well also has rounded *gluteal* muscles for upward thrust of the leg off the ground, and developed *quadriceps* muscles on the thigh that pull the hind leg forward. A weak loin that is too long results in a lack of drive in the hindquarters, with underdeveloped gluteals and quadriceps.

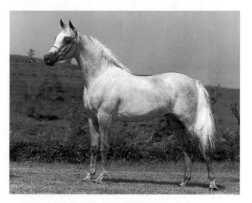

Fig. 1.27 This Arabian has a slightly long topline, but the well-rounded gluteal muscles in the hindquarters indicate a strong back and loin.

Loins and Body Carriage

As the horse carries its head and neck in the correct position for bit contact, it engages the hindquarters to relax and round the back, allowing the forelegs to be used most efficiently. Weight is distributed evenly fore and aft, and a horse in this frame is balanced and agile. A balanced frame permits shoulders to extend and flex to their full potential, not only lengthening the stride but adding to suspension and smoothness of the stride.

Hindquarters

Many equine sports require quick turns, sudden stops and perfect balance. A horse normally carries as much as 65% of its weight on the front end. Events such as dressage, jumping, polo and long distance riding have at least one similar characteristic. These sports transfer a horse's centre of gravity towards the rear end. Without strong hindquarters, it cannot perform well. The propulsive muscles of the body

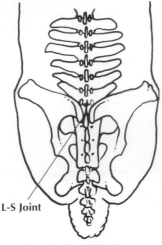

L-S Joint

Fig. 1.28 The L-S joint pivots and rotates the hindquarters.

originate on the pelvis, so a strong hind end means greater power and drive.

Effects of Exercise on Hindquarters

Just as callisthenic exercises for people strengthen the attendant muscle groups, a horse in training improves muscle condition to retain balance through gait transitions and various movements.

Collection of a horse starts in the hindquarters, specifically at the lumbosacral joint (L-S joint) at the top of the croup, and is carried on through the back, withers and neck to the poll. If a horse's hindquarters are likened to an engine because they propel the horse into motion, then the L-S joint at the top of the croup is the transmission. The L-S joint pivots and rotates the hindquarters and pelvis forward under the body. The abdominal muscles help pull the pelvis forwards to engage the hindquarters.

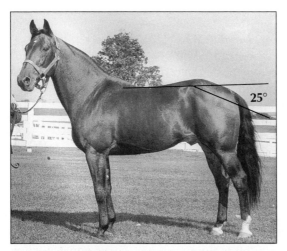

Fig. 1.29 Standardbred with nice conformation showing a good croup angle.

Angle of Croup and Pelvis

The slope of the pelvis bone from the point of the hip to the point of the buttocks determines the slope of a horse's croup. The more slope and length to the pelvis, the greater the horse's *power*. A horse with a very steep pelvis generates a greater upward thrust, although its steps are small. Consider the slope

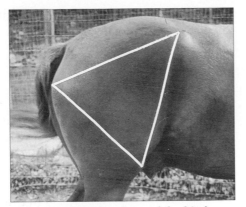

Fig. 1.30 Triangular shape of the hind-quarters.

and width of a working draft horse that is the essence of power and push from the hindquarters.

On the other hand, a pelvis that inclines towards the horizontal enhances *speed*, especially at the trot. A more horizontal pelvis allows the hip joint to lengthen when the hind leg is extended. Therefore, a horizontal pelvis results in a greater push forward. This configuration gives a fluid, ground-covering stride.

The ideal croup inclines about 25° and is relatively long in proportion to the body. Long muscles over the croup have a greater range of muscle contraction across the skeleton, improving speed, which is important to the racehorse. A shorter croup decreases leverage and muscle power.

The hindquarters should have ample vertical depth as defined by a triangle formed by the point of the hip, the point of the buttock, and the stifle joint. For the athletic horse, the best results are obtained by a long, perpendicular thigh and a gaskin that is a bit shorter than the length of the thigh.

The Stifle

The stifle should sit at the same height as the elbow. The stifle is turned slightly out so a horse can move forwards freely without physical interference from the flank. This preferred position of the stifle causes many horses to slightly toe out on the hind legs.

A long thigh and short gaskin with good muscling are advantageous in any athletic endeavour except for the racehorse. For racehorses, especially sprinters, a long hip, gaskin and thigh increase the muscle leverage for optimal stride length power and speed during a sprint effort.

A relatively straight hind leg is more efficient at thrusting at the ground for pushoff. This characteristic can be helpful for events such as jumping, Quarter Horse racing, etc. However, if the limb is too straight, excess stress on both stifle and hock joints can lead to arthritis. These horses are also prone to *upward fixation of the patella*

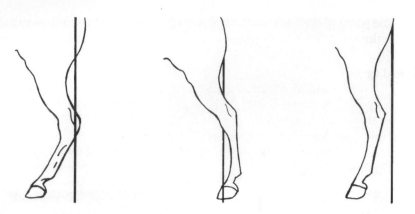

Fig. 1.31 Poor hind leg conformations, from left to right: sickle hocked, camped out, and camped under.

where a ligament of the stifle locks over the kneecap, and *thorough-pin,* which is a windgall of the Achilles tendon behind the hock.

In contrast, a longer, angled hind leg helps the horse bring the hocks under the body which is important for dressage. Stride length increases with a more angled hind leg. When this characteristic is extreme, the horse may be *camped out,* where the hind legs stick out behind, or *sickle hocked,* where the hind legs angle beneath the horse.

Horses with these conformation problems are prone to:

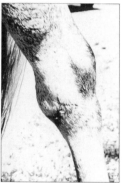

- *bog spavin*—excess joint fluid in the hock from inflammation
- *bone spavin*—DJD of the hock
- *curb*—strain of the plantar ligament on the back of the hock

If the limb is too long and angled, the croup may rise higher than the withers with each stride, resulting in a rough, uncomfortable ride.

More than 80% of hind leg lameness develops in the hock or stifle joints, therefore conforma-

Fig. 1.32 Bog spavin.

tion of these structures is very important to continuing soundness in the performance horse. Any athletic pursuit that moves the horse's weight towards the hindquarters, for example, dressage, amplifies the stress on these joints.

Hind Legs

From the side, a plumb line dropped from the point of the buttocks to the point of the hock should fall along the back of the tendons to the fetlock.

Post-Legged

A horse with hind legs that are too straight is *post-legged* (straight-legged). This conformational flaw increases concussion and loading of the joints. The tendon sheaths therefore have a tendency to puff from poor circulation. A straight-legged horse is predisposed to upward fixation of the patella, DJD, thoroughpin, and bone spavin in the hocks.

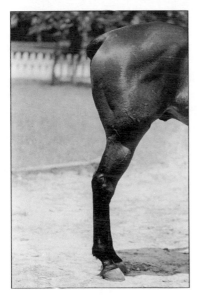 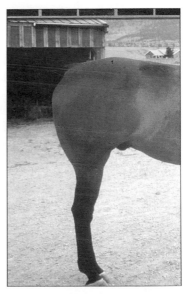

Fig. 1.33 On the left, a normal hind leg. On the right, a post-legged horse.

The Hocks

The hocks alternately flex and swing and then support and push the limbs to produce drive. A 'low-set hocked' horse (which results from a relatively short cannon bone) has more power for pushing and quick turns. This power is important in all sprint efforts. It is also desirable to have open angles on the front face of the hind legs approximating 160°.

Cowhocks

A horse with **true** *cowhocks* has limbs very different from the normal toed-out conformation seen with Arabians . As seen from behind, the cowhocked horse has fetlocks that reach much further apart than do the point of the hocks. A toed-out horse has fetlocks placed underneath the hocks, yet the toes turn out from below the

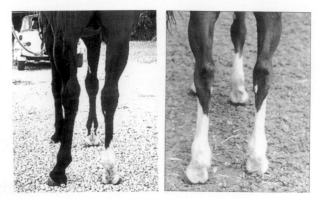

Fig. 1.34 On the left, true cowhocks of a Thoroughbred. On the right, the hind leg stance of an Arabian.

fetlocks. Cowhocks place excessive strain on the insides of the hocks and stifles, predisposing to DJD.

Similar characteristics for the lower part of the forelegs apply to the hind legs for mechanical efficiency. As in the foreleg, it is preferable to have short cannon bones in the hind leg so that tendons can effectively pull on the point of the hock to create drive. The fetlocks should be clean and tight, without bumps or nicks, and the pasterns should be strong, well defined and of medium length.

2

DEVELOPING STRONG BONES

Bones provide a mechanical scaffold from which muscles, ligaments and tendons are supported. Efficiency of movement depends on how the skeleton is conformed. The muscles work like levers and pulleys as they are superimposed on the skeleton. The visible size, shape and structure of bone in each horse are the subject of much debate regarding conformation and its relation to performance. Yet there is no question that the internal architecture of bone is important to a horse's ability to absorb impact without developing lameness. *(See anatomy, bone and muscle diagrams in the Appendix.)*

BONE STRENGTH
Internal Remodelling

Lameness is the primary cause of poor performance in the equine athlete. Prematurely subjecting a horse's bones to stressful exertions can permanently affect its potential.

Bone, as a dynamic organ, continually alters its shape and mass according to the stresses placed upon it. By understanding a little about the microscopic changes that occur, an owner or trainer can

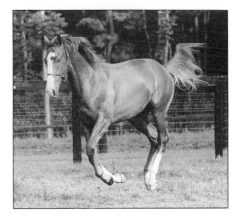

Fig. 2.1 Bone continually alters shape and mass according to the stresses placed upon it.

modify bone strength with conditioning. Bone changes itself, conforming to stress by increasing or decreasing its mass accordingly. Cells that form new bone are called *osteoblasts*. New bone is produced in weaker areas. Bone is one of the few tissues in the body capable of *regeneration* rather than repairing with a scar. *Resorption,* or removal of bone by cells called *osteoclasts,* occurs in areas that no longer need to respond to stress.

These active processes are called *remodelling*. Bone has abundant blood vessels that supply nutrients and oxygen to support remodelling and mineralization in adapting to physical stress.

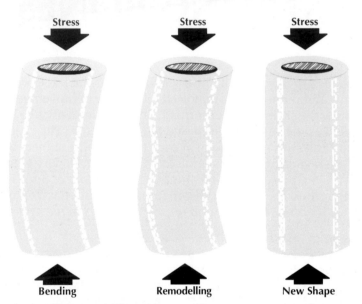

Fig. 2.2 The remodelling response of bone to stress. Bone becomes stronger and no longer bends when stressed.

Bone is also a storage reservoir for calcium and phosphorus. The deposition or removal of these minerals is controlled by:

- physical stress on the bone
- hormonal influences from the endocrine glands
- nutrition

Bone responds to stress by changing the arrangement, type and amount of bone. Age determines which hormones are more active; for example, a growing skeleton is affected by hormones that encourage the deposition of minerals into bone.

As bone matures, minerals (calcium and phosphorus) are deposited into the bone at the expense of *cellular fluid* to occupy up to

65% of the space. By the time a horse is fully mature, the minerals make up 95% of the bone. The amount of these minerals in a bone determines its *bone mineral content* (BMC).

Internal remodelling proceeds without changing the observable shape of the skeleton. However, these invisible changes in the bones greatly affect intrinsic strength and skeletal maturity of a horse.

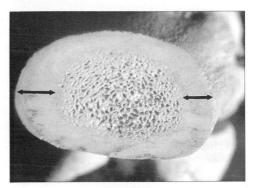

Fig. 2.3 Cross section of a cannon bone. Greater bone deposition on the left shows effects of internal remodelling.

Bone Strength Indicators

At one time the skeletal maturity of a horse was estimated by radiographic assessment of closure of the growth plates, and by subjective evaluation of body growth and development. Recent research on athletic stress of young racehorses indicates that bone strength depends on more than growth plate closure. Bone strength depends on its cross-sectional area and bone mineral content.

Cross-sectional area increases with skeletal maturity, especially if coupled with intelligent conditioning methods for a young horse. An increase in cross-sectional area logarithmically increases bone strength so it can ultimately sustain more stress.

Measuring the cannon bone just below the knee helps determine the horse's current structural strength. For optimal strength, the measurement of the cannon bone should yield *at least* 7 inches circumference for every 1000 lb of body weight. Using these figures as guidelines, the ideal circumference of an individual horse's cannon bone can be determined. The formula looks like this:

$$\frac{\text{7 inches}}{\text{1000 lb}} \times \text{body weight of horse} = \text{ideal circumference}$$

For example, if a horse weighs 750 lb the formula would be:

$$\frac{\text{7 inches}}{\text{1000 lbs}} \times 750\,\text{lb} = \text{ideal circumference}$$

Then,   **0.007 × 750 = 5.25 inches**

Therefore, the ideal circumference of the cannon bone of a 750-lb horse is 5¼ inches. This formula may help a trainer to determine the bone strength of an individual athlete. If the result is more than the actual circumference, the trainer may modify his or her expectations, or attempt to increase bone mineralization by implementing a careful exercise programme. Both cross-sectional area and bone mineral content are also influenced by the horse's age and physical maturity. These factors determine the ability of the bones to withstand stress.

How can the body and mind of a young horse be strengthened without overtaxing the musculoskeletal system? Nutritional manipulation or exercise regimens cannot hasten growth and maturation. Genetics and breed determine skeletal maturity, and these factors are dictated by time. Yet, conditioning programmes can improve ultimate bone strength and build a durable athlete. **Taking time to properly condition** the young athlete will pay high dividends in future soundness. Failure to take care of an immature, and incoordinate, youngster may lead to irreversible bone or joint damage.

Exercise and Bone Strength

The mechanical forces of exercise stimulate change in weight-bearing bones. Exercise increases bone strength by increasing mineral deposition and bone mass. The *quantity* of bone, but not necessarily the *quality*, increases with exercise. Human sports medicine studies show increases of up to 20% in bone mass of active athletes as compared with non-athletes.

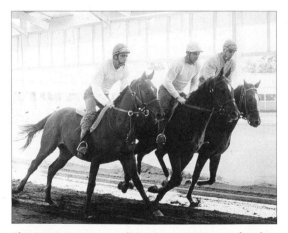

Fig. 2.4 A proper conditioning programme for the young horse builds a durable athlete.

The Importance of Consistent Exercise

Sports medicine research reveals another significant factor that is most applicable to the equine athlete. Not only does exercise enhance bone mineralization, but, more important, the *rate* at which a mechanical force is applied to the bones greatly influences the degree of bone development. For instance, consistent running with gradual increases in distance effectively increases bone mineral content, whereas occasional and sporadic exercise has little effect on bone mineral content. A *routine* of conditioning is essential to increase bone strength.

Daily exercise does not need to be excessive or prolonged. There is a threshold that stimulates deposition of minerals into the bone. Once the threshold is met, more exercise does not further increase bone mineral content. Loading bone with exercise for a short time each day (i.e. 20–30 minutes) stimulates as much new bone development as a lengthy workout. The actual time required to strengthen bone may be more or less, depending on the individual's maturity and fitness level.

Training Techniques

To most effectively increase the cross-sectional area and bone mineral content of equine bone, a vigorous, intermittent exercise of short duration is best. After a warm-up of 10 – 15 minutes, a short sprint or 20 minutes of hill work is more effective than a 3-mile slow gallop. Gradual increase in incremental exercise also strengthens the ligaments, tendons and muscles of a horse. Such a programme resembles *interval training* techniques that build, but do not overtax, the musculoskeletal system of a young horse. *(See Chapter 6 for more information on interval training.)*

Inactivity

The opposite effect, demineralization, occurs when the skeleton is subjected to weightlessness or reduced gravitational loading. The extreme case occurs in the human example of space flight and to a lesser degree with bed rest. Of course, these specific phenomena are of no concern in caring for the equine athlete. However, applying a cast or disuse of an injured limb for an

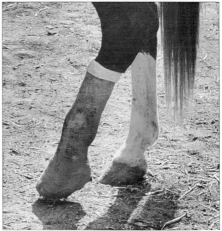

Fig. 2.5 Immobilization caused by an injury can decrease bone strength.

extended period similarly decreases bone strength. Bone mineral content diminishes: cells dissolve existing bone while bone-forming cells remain quiescent. With this caution in mind, rehabilitation of an injured horse must proceed **slowly**.

A loss of bone, or lack of development, can also result from administering excessive amounts of corticosteroids. Such problems can also result from the body's manufacture of corticosteroids when a horse is subjected to mental stress. Mental stress develops from chronic pain, overtraining, and competition.

BONE RESPONSE TO BIOMECHANICAL STRESS

The term biomechanical stress refers to all the forces applied to a bone during weight-bearing. The laws of physics define the way different forces affect the bone. *Stress* measures force per unit area; the degree to which a bone deforms to the stress is termed *strain*. Removing a stress allows a bone to return to its original shape; this is its *elasticity*. The ability of a bone to resist being deformed is defined as *stiffness*.

For example, since a horse bears more than 60% of the weight-bearing force on the forelegs, the cannon bone reflects changes in bone from consistent biomechanical stress. The cannon bone resembles a cylinder. According to the laws of physics, the total

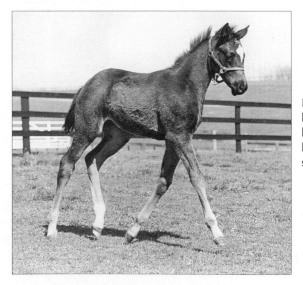

Fig. 2.6 As young horses mature, their bones become stronger by increasing in cross-sectional area.

strength of a cylinder is a function of its cross-sectional area and the elastic strength of its component materials. In a growing horse, the cross-sectional area enlarges while the elastic component essentially remains the same. As a horse increases in body weight and mass, the total weight-bearing capabilities of the bones adapt correspondingly.

Mineral Reinforcement

Mineral reinforces the connective tissue of fibrous collagen in the bone. Not only does bone *density* increase with bone mineral content, but stiffness also increases, improving a bone's resistance to deforming forces.

As a young horse matures, its bones become increasingly strong and able to withstand more axial loading down the limbs. Again, this strength is accomplished by increases in cross-sectional area and bone mineral content, and by conversion of randomly arrayed immature bone cells into highly structured mature bone cells.

Forces That Stress Bone

The impact of exercise exerts varied biomechanical stresses on bone:

- axial compression (squeezing together directly down the bone)
- axial tension (pulling apart)
- torsion (twisting)

The structural complexity and internal organization of a bone determine its ability to resist injury and microscopic damage from biomechanical stresses.

Compression and Tension

Collagen, the connective tissue of bone, accounts for tensile (stretch) strength while the mineral content determines compressive strength and stiffness. Bone mineral content provides maximal strength to a bone since it is most adept at resisting compressive forces.

Excessive and repeated concussion to a limb results in a progressive loss of stiffness and decrease in strength, inviting bone fatigue and failure. With fatigue, a horse's performance suffers, and it is prone to injury and lameness.

Torsion (twisting)

An equine limb can withstand large amounts of compressive force, but the torsional strength is only one-third as strong as the compressive strength. Torsion results from:

- abnormal conformation
- angular limb deformities
- rutted ground
- inconsistent composition of the ground surface
- lack of uniformity in the moisture content and cushioning features of the ground
- caulks or toe-grabs on horseshoes

A horse in any of these situations is particularly prone to bone injury.

Propulsive Forces

At a walk, most limb strain occurs in the swing phase when the foot is off the ground. The predominant force on the limb is the tension of tendon pull. At a gallop, reaction forces from the ground contribute to bone strain. These strains occur as the limb is loaded when the foot hits the ground.

Multiple Forces

A bone is not uniform in cross-sectional area. Its shape varies along the shaft, and *cortical walls* vary in thickness. Because of these variations, different forces are applied simultaneously within a single bone.

Stresses and strains on bone result from multiple forces at one time:

- the pull of tendons, ligaments, and muscles
- the effect of weight-bearing and the support of body mass
- the forces created from impact with the ground

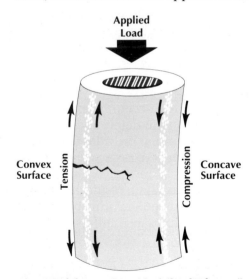

Fig. 2.7 If the tension side fails, the bone will fracture.

Bone Fracture

When simultaneous forces on a bone overcome its inherent strength, the bone fails, or fractures. A bone's ability to withstand tension (stretching) forces is only two-thirds of its ability to withstand compression. As bone is compressed, it expands, causing the compression side (concave surface) to push or bend the tension side (convex surface). As the tension side fails, it moves outwards, creating a break.

MANAGING YOUNG BONE
Dangers of Excessive Biomechanical Stress

From 3 months of age up to 1 year, equine bone increases in compressive strength due to increased bone mineral content. Compressive strength stabilizes at this level until 3 years of age. Between 4 and 5 years of age, compressive strength again improves as bone mineral content continues to increase until a horse is about 7 years old.

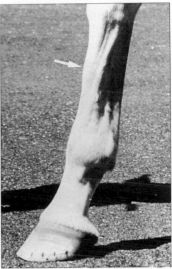

Fig. 2.8 Swelling typical of sore shins.

Bone Failure in Young Athletes

Excessive and repetitive stresses to *young* limbs cause failure. Of 3-year-old racing Thoroughbreds, 70% suffer from *bucked (sore) shins* (microfrac-tures in the cannon bone along the front and inside surfaces). In humans, a similar phenomenon called *shin splints* occurs along the lower tibia. Initially, microscopic fractures appear in the bone cortex, but with an eventual overload a total stress fracture results.

Activities That Increase Risk

Certain types of activities should be avoided or carefully controlled to protect young horses from significantly increased biomechanical stress:

- weight-bearing stress of carrying a rider
- lungeing, even in large circles, which exerts twisting forces on bones and particularly on immature joints
- jumping a young horse, which radically overloads the limbs
- long distance work, particularly at speed, which is especially detrimental to a growing skeleton

Bone Fatigue

When bone begins to lose elasticity after being deformed by load-ing and unloading cycles, it has reached its *fatigue state.*

To illustrate how differently applied loads on a limb affect strength, consider the following example. If a Thoroughbred runs at top speed on a straight line, assuming all else is normal, it can run for 19 miles before fatigue failure of the cannon bone. Yet, running through a turn dramatically increases the load per unit area. Instead of 19 miles, bones subjected to uneven loading in the turn can travel only 0.2 miles before fatigue develops. There is a level of exercise that brings bones past a fatigue state, into an overload range, with subse-quent disaster.

Skeletal Maturity

Different breeds mature at different rates. Closure of the growth plates of the long bones is not the only criterion used to determine the age at which a horse can begin competitive athletics. One long

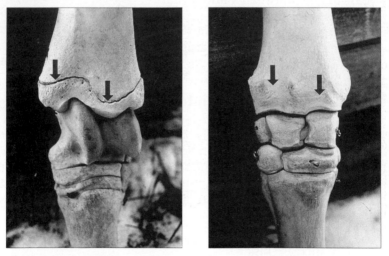

Fig. 2.9 On the left, the open growth plate on the distal tibia in a young horse. On the right, the closed growth plate of the distal radius in a mature horse.

bone, the *distal radius* above the knee, has previously served as a monitor for the entire body. In most horses, the growth plates of the long bones close by 3 years of age. For example, in a Thoroughbred or Quarter Horse the radial growth plate closes by 2–3 years. Once the growth plate closes, a bone stops growing longer. It instead con-centrates on converting to mature and more mineralized bone and on remodelling to conform to biomechanical stresses.

The AERC *(American Endurance Ride Conference)* and the NATRC *(North American Trail Ride Conference)* recognize the need for a horse to reach skeletal maturity before exposing it to the rigorous exertion of long distance riding. (Equivalent bodies in Europe are the ELDRC (Endurance and Long Distance Riding Club, part of the FEI (International Equestrian Federation)) and the clubs of each country, e.g. the UK Edurance Ride Club (ERC), the Scottish Endurance Ride Club (SERC) and the Endurance Horse and Pony Society), The AERC regulations require that a horse must be 5 years old before competing in a 50-mile endurance race, and 4 years old before attempting a 25-mile ride. **Allowing a horse to mature skeletally to at least 5 years of age before demanding severe exertion tremendously prolongs its durable athletic life.**

Dietary Requirements for Young Horses

While a young horse is growing, careful dietary management encourages young bones and joints to develop normally. Feed a proper calcium to phosphorus ratio of 1.5 : 1, and safe levels of protein and minerals. Excesses of certain minerals, energy, and protein, or a calcium to phosphorus ratio that exceeds 2 : 1, can create serious orthopaedic problems. Examples of these developmental abnormalities include:

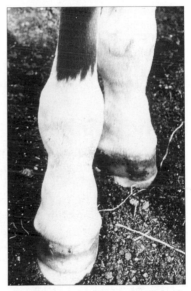

Fig. 2.10 Epiphysitis in the fetlock of a foal.

- *epiphysitis* (inflammation of the growth plate)
- *osteochondrosis* (failure of complete ossification, or bone formation, beneath the joint cartilage, leading to cystic defects or incomplete cartilage flaps)
- *contracted tendons*
- acquired *angular limb deformities*

To guarantee feeding a balanced diet, consult with a veterinarian or an equine nutritional specialist. Good nutrition promotes stronger and healthier bone development, allowing genetic potential to be achieved. More important, an erratic and unbalanced nutritional

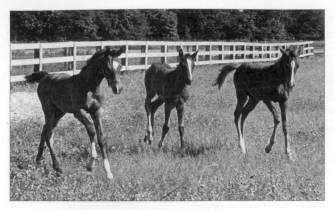

Fig. 2.11 Foals playing in a pasture build strong bones and muscles.

source adversely affects the alignment and strength of the maturing skeleton. Care must be taken to ensure that a foal or young horse is not overweight as this will increase the possibility of orthopaedic problems. *(For more dietary information see Chapter 7.)*

Early Training

A youngster can be trained without subjecting it to extreme physical stress. Penning one up and allowing it to lie fallow wastes an opportunity to build a foundation for athletic development. A young foal should be turned out to pasture and allowed to play. This activity strengthens bones and muscles, and builds reflexes. The foal learns to use its body athletically. Ponying a foal behind the mare on short rides is another way to build stronger bones.

One to Three Years

To properly prepare and also to protect yearlings to 3-year-olds for many future events, long lining and driving a light cart in harness are excellent ways to supple and strengthen a growing horse. The young horse learns discipline and obedience, and the feel of tack and equipment. From this type of work it learns voice commands, and the subtle feel of a bit and reins. As a teaching method, driving allows an equine body to grow, while exercising mental concentration and acceptance of authority.

Three to Four Years

For many breeds, weight carrying should be delayed until between 3 and 4 years of age. Leave any tight circle work for even later years. Show the young horse big, open spaces, and slowly increase the duration and distance of a ride. This method will optimize the principles of consistent exercise that build bone mass. Gradually introduce speed training over the year after a foundation has been built with long, slow distance conditioning. As the musculoskeletal system matures and adapts to increased physical demands, the cardiovascular system also matures and adapts to conditioning by increasing capillary beds and enzymatic biochemical functions. Stamina slowly develops in the whole body and mind.

Raising a young horse is a slow process, but a horse is a misleading animal to train. Because of a horse's size and brute strength it is easy to ask for more than it has to offer—long before its body and mind are capable. Prevent problems by applying an intelligent conditioning programme and quality nutrition during a horse's growing years so it can realize its full athletic potential. A little care with less haste, at this stage will be more than repaid by a significant increase in the number of years during which the horse will function and give the rider pleasure.

3

IMPROVING MUSCLE PERFORMANCE

An athletic equine body displays firm, well defined skeletal muscle. The horse depends on skeletal muscle to hold the body together, to manoeuvre, to support joints, and to convert stored food energy into mechanical motion. More than one-third of a horse's weight consists of skeletal muscle. It is a tissue capable of varied adaptation in response to training and conditioning. *(See anatomy, bone and muscle diagrams in the Appendix.)*

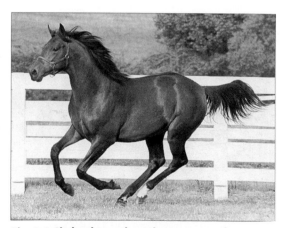

Fig. 3.1 Skeletal muscle makes up more than one-third of total body weight.

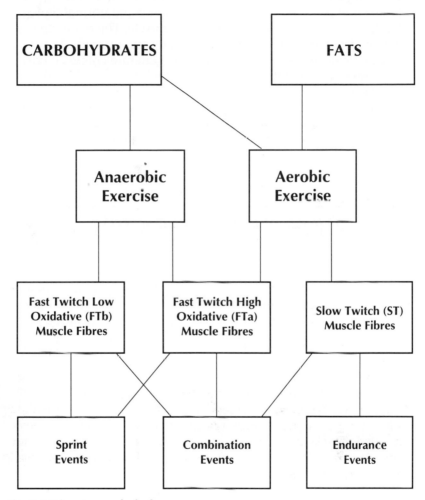

Fig. 3.2 Primary muscle fuels.

FOOD FOR ENERGY

To achieve its athletic potential, a horse involved in a rigorous conditioning and training programme must be fuelled with high-energy food. Food becomes fuel for everyday living and normal biological functions, as well as for hard-working muscle. The main types of fuel derived from food are carbohydrates, fats and proteins. Protein is a metabolically expensive food source to generate energy. It costs more energy to metabolize than other food fuels, while at the same time it creates very little energy for working muscles as compared with carbohydrates and fats. Its use as a muscle fuel therefore has limited application to the adequately fed performance athlete. Therefore, the most important fuels for working muscles are carbohydrates and fats.

Muscle Fuels

Carbohydrates are organic compounds that are composed of carbon, hydrogen, and oxygen. Fats are made up of *glycerol* and *fatty acids*. Grain, hay, and forage provide carbohydrates and fatty acids which are digested by bacterial residents of the bowel. Vegetable oil is also an important fat supplement for the performance horse. Carbohydrates and fats supply fuel for the muscle cells to produce energy for exercise. As the food travels through the intestines, *glucose* and fatty acids are absorbed into the bloodstream.

Glucose/Glycogen

Glucose is a carbohydrate obtained from digestion of grain, hay and forage. Glucose in the bloodstream is either used immediately by muscle tissue to produce energy, or it can be stored as *glycogen* in skeletal muscle and in the liver. Glucose can also be stored in fat reserves *(adipose tissue)* as *triglycerides* or fat for later use. (A triglyceride is composed of one molecule of glycerol joined to three molecules of fatty acid.) Glycogen is a connected chain of glucose sugar molecules. To be used by muscle cells, stored glycogen must broken back down into sugar molecules.

Fatty Acids

Another source of fuel, volatile fatty acids (VFAs), are produced from carbohydrates as they are fermented in the large intestine. VFAs can be used immediately to fuel muscle contraction. If they are not needed immediately, they are stored in adipose tissue as triglycerides.

Likewise, the fats in the horse's feed (or vegetable oil) are digested, and formed into triglycerides. Their fatty acid components can be used immediately as muscle fuel or stored in adipose tissue. Later, when the horse needs more fuel, the triglycerides are released from the adipose tissue into the bloodstream, and then they are called *free fatty acids. (See more about supplementing dietary fats in Chapter 7.)*

Muscles Produce Energy

For a muscle to provide locomotion, it must contract, which requires energy. Muscles cannot store enough energy for more than a few seconds of forceful contractions. With glucose and fatty acids, the muscle cells produce and consume millions of energy molecules called ATP *(adenosine triphosphate).* An ATP energy molecule consists of an amino acid attached to three phosphate molecules.

To create energy, muscle enzymes break apart the bond between two of these phosphate molecules. This action creates energy for muscle contraction. Left over is ADP (adenosine diphosphate), which is an amino acid attached to two phosphate molecules, and the unattached, free phosphate molecule.

To produce more ATP energy molecules, the above process is reversed. The muscle cells use glycogen and fatty acids as fuels to reattach a free phosphate molecule back onto an ADP, creating ATP.

These processes occur within the muscle cells thousands of times each microsecond. Without fuel, the phosphate molecule cannot be reattached. ATP would not be formed, so there would be no phosphate bond to break, and no energy for muscle contraction. (See also '*Normal Muscle Contractions*'.)

Fatty Acid Versus Glycogen

Fatty acids, both VFAs and free fatty acids, are more efficient at generating ATP energy molecules than glycogen, which is why fatty acids are the preferred fuel for muscle contraction. A diet that is supplemented with fats allows the muscles to create more energy during extended aerobic work.

ENERGY PRODUCTION

Muscle fibres contracting and relaxing consume large amounts of energy. The processes of energy production and consumption are called *metabolism.* How the muscles produce and consume energy distinguishes certain muscle fibre types from each other. There are two basic types of muscle metabolism. *Aerobic metabolism* uses oxygen to produce energy, while *anaerobic metabolism* does not.

Aerobic Metabolism

Aerobic metabolism means the muscle cell burns fuels using oxygen and enzymes to produce energy. Both of the muscle fuels, glycogen and fatty acids, can be burned aerobically. This method is the most efficient way of producing energy, because it completely burns these fuels without creating toxic by-products. The by-products of aerobic metabolism are carbon dioxide and water, which are non-toxic and are easily carried from the muscle by the circulatory system. For this reason, all performance horses, regardless of their specific event, should be involved in aerobic training.

Muscle cells that function aerobically produce energy in specialized cellular 'factories' called *mitochondria*. Mitochondria break down fatty acids and glycogen, forming energy, carbon dioxide, and water. Because these processes are so complicated, aerobic metabolism produces energy relatively slowly. With greater exertional demands on the muscles, energy must be generated more quickly. This is done by anaerobic metabolism.

Anaerobic Metabolism

Anaerobic metabolism means the muscle cell burns fuel using enzymes, but without using oxygen, to produce energy. Anaerobic metabolism produces energy faster but less efficiently than aerobic metabolism. Fatty acids cannot be burned anaerobically, but glycogen can be used either aerobically or anaerobically. There are two types of anaerobic metabolism, each using a different fuel, phosphocreatine or glycogen.

Sudden, High Intensity Work

The first type of anaerobic metabolism occurs as a horse accelerates with a burst of speed from the starting gate. At this point in the event, the muscles are fuelled by *phosphocreatine*. High energy phosphocreatine can support the high intensity work required of a sprint acceleration or jumping effort for only a few seconds. The energy is provided by breaking apart the phosphocreatine molecule's bonds and does not require oxygen. It also does not produce toxic by-products. Although great thrust and rapid speed are possible when muscles are fuelled by phosphocreatine, its supply is extremely limited.

After several seconds the phosphocreatine supply is depleted in the muscles; the muscles then depend on aerobic metabolism or the second type of anaerobic metabolism for continued sprint performance. Phosphocreatine is replenished in about 3 minutes, but by then the sprint activity is finished. Neither conditioning nor dietary strategies can increase phosphocreatine stores in the muscles.

Lack of Oxygen During Strenuous Work

The second type of anaerobic metabolism occurs when the horse cannot breathe in enough oxygen to support strenuous work. Muscle enzymes break down glycogen into energy without using oxygen. The toxic by-product of this type of anaerobic metabolism is *lactic acid*, which if produced in excessive amounts will depress enzyme systems and limit the amount of ATP that is produced. With a limited energy supply available for contraction, muscles rapidly fatigue and performance suffers. (See also '*Muscle Fatigue*'.)

USE OF ENERGY

Remember that one energy form is not used exclusively by working muscle; however, the longer the muscles can use fatty acids to fuel exercise, the more glycogen is spared for later use, and the longer fatigue is delayed. Depending on blood circulation and oxygen supply in the muscles at any given moment, fats or carbohydrates (fatty acids, glucose and glycogen) will be used as needed. Oxygen supply depends on the horse's level of fitness and the type of activity. Some sports are primarily aerobic, others are primarily anaerobic, and some depend on a balance between the two types of metabolism.

Endurance-Type Activities—Aerobic

Endurance-type sports consist of prolonged activity at steady paces of walk, trot and slow canter averaging 8–12 mph. Horses involved in these activities primarily use aerobic metabolism, relying on fatty acids and glycogen as energy sources. They include:

- long distance riding
- combined driving
- dressage
- competitive long distance events
- pleasure riding
- the roads and tracks phase of eventing

Sprint-Type Activities—Anaerobic

Sprint-type activities, for example Quarter Horse racing, demand intense efforts of short duration (up to 1 minute) at or near maximum speed. A horse depends heavily on anaerobic metabolism during a short sprint. The muscles are fuelled from sources that do not require oxygen, such as glycogen and phosphocreatine.

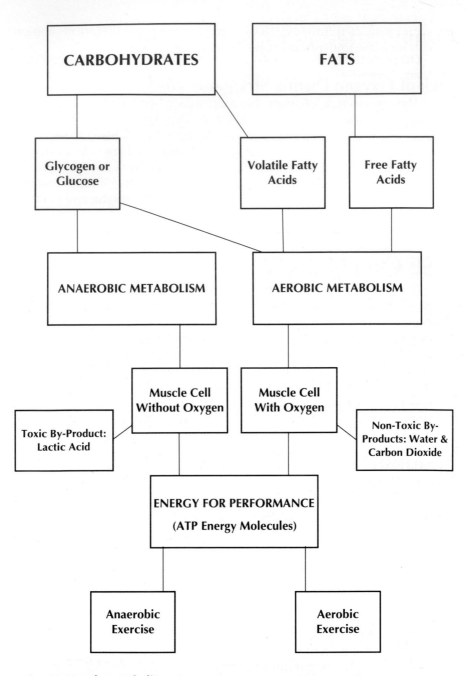

Fig. 3.3 Muscle metabolism.

Combination Activities

Other activities balance both aerobic and anaerobic metabolism. These activities include:

- steeplechasing
- Thoroughbred racing
- polo
- three-day eventing
- Standardbred racing
- jumping

In Thoroughbred and Standardbred racing, the initial sprint is

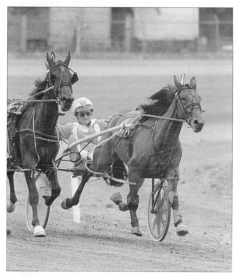

anaerobic, using the phosphocreatine method of energy production. Then the horse begins using aerobic metabolism of fatty acids and glycogen. When aerobic metabolism is no longer sufficient for the racehorse's energy needs, it again depends on anaerobic metabolism, using glycogen for fuel. Of course, these processes happen simultaneously in the muscles. At any one point in the event the horse may depend more on one type of muscle metabolism than on another type.

Fig. 3.4 Standardbred racing is a combination activity.

Muscle Fibre Types and Metabolism

The contraction and relaxation of a muscle fibre is called a *twitch*. How fast a certain fibre twitches defines its type. There are three possible muscle fibre types:

- *slow twitch* (ST)
- *fast twitch high oxidative* (FTa)
- *fast twitch low oxidative* (FTb)

Each of these three fibre types contracts at different rates and in environments varying in oxygen content. Most muscles contain a mixture of all three fibre types. Studies in equine sports physiology show how different types of muscle fibres, and their production and consumption of energy, influence athletic potential. One athlete may have a higher proportion of a certain type of muscle fibre than another athlete that is suited to a different performance effort.

For example, slow twitch muscle fibres contract at one-third the rate of fast twitch muscle fibres, and are particularly suited to endurance work. The faster contraction rates of fast twitch fibres produce the speed and power required by sprint work.

Slow Twitch Muscle Fibres

Slow twitch muscle fibres use oxygen to produce energy. Each ST fibre has a considerable blood supply and special cellular factories (mitochondria) to take in and use oxygen to burn fatty acids and glycogen. These fibres are small in cross-sectional diameter and surrounded by capillaries (tiny blood vessels) so oxygen can quickly reach them. ST fibres are the muscle type best suited for endurance sports. Up to 50% of an elite endurance athlete's muscle may be ST fibres.

Slow twitch fibres, however, produce energy so slowly that they cannot meet the intense energy demands of short, rapid bursts of speed or quick thrusts required by racing, or polo.

Fast Twitch Muscle Fibres

Fast twitch muscle fibres have high concentrations of enzymes that rapidly produce energy from glycogen in the muscle cells during exercise. The faster the twitch, the greater the muscle cell's ability to contract rapidly and forcefully to create the speed and power so important for sprint type sports. Horses with up to 80% FT muscle fibres, such as Thoroughbreds, Quarter

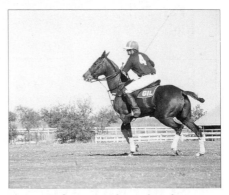

Fig. 3.5 Polo ponies depend on fast twitch muscle fibres for quick acceleration.

Horses and Standardbreds, have excellent speed potential.

Fast Twitch High Oxidative

Fast twitch fibres are further divided into two subtypes: fast twitch high oxidative (FTa) and fast twitch low oxidative (FTb). FTa fibres can use oxygen to some degree to produce energy. When at least 50% of the FT muscle fibres are FTa, the horse performs well at high speed over limited mileage (less than 5 miles), as in Thoroughbred and Standardbred racing.

Fast Twitch Low Oxidative

Fast twitch low oxidative muscle fibres work in an anaerobic muscle cell environment. FTb fibres are unable to use oxygen even if it is available because they lack certain enzymes. Quarter Horse racing competitors that sprint for less than 30 seconds are an example of horses with high proportions of FTb fibres.

OVERVIEW OF MUSCLE FIBRE TYPES		
Fibre Type	**Metabolism**	**Activity Examples**
ST— **Slow Twitch**	Aerobic—Breaks down glycogen or fatty acids to produce energy using oxygen	Competitive Long Distance Combined Driving Dressage Pleasure Riding
FTa— **Fast Twitch** **high oxidative**	Both Aerobic and Anaerobic	Three-Day Eventing Polo Jumping Thoroughbred Racing Standardbred Racing
FTb— **Fast Twitch** **low oxidative** (Can convert 7% to FTa.)	Anaerobic—Breaks down glycogen to produce energy without using oxygen	Quarter Horse Racing

Fig. 3.6

Fibre Types, Genetics and Conditioning

All three muscle fibre types exist in all horses. The ratio of ST to FT fibres is genetically determined. The horse's genetic predisposition for certain muscle fibre types is based on breed and heritable tendencies. Aerobic conditioning can slightly alter ratios among FT fibre types, with potential conversion of some to 7% of the FTb to FTa. The slower contracting ST fibres cannot be trained to contract faster.

The Process of Exercise

When a horse first begins exercising, capillaries have not yet opened to feed oxygen to the muscles. Initial muscle metabolism relies on an anaerobic fuel source, phosphocreatine, in the fast twitch muscle fibres. Within a few minutes of warm-up, circulation is active in the muscles, and aerobic sources of energy are tapped. If the horse continues at slow speeds at a heart rate less than 150–160 beats per minute (using aerobic metabolism), fatty acids initially provide the primary fuel source for the muscle.

As a horse continues to exercise, different muscle fibres are selectively recruited according to need. A certain muscle may rely on aerobic fuel supplies (fatty acids or glycogen) or anaerobic fuel supplies (glycogen) at various times in the activity, depending on the work intensity each individual muscle tissue is asked to do.

For example, endurance performance calls on slow twitch and fast twitch high oxidative fibres. With a longer or faster effort, an increasing dependency on anaerobic fuel supplies calls more FTa and FTb fibres to work. Once glycogen is depleted, the muscles run out of fuel, and fatigue sets in. As an endurance horse nears exhaustion, all three muscle fibre types have been used, with depletion of all forms of fuel.

Sprint events, such as Quarter Horse racing, recruit all three muscle fibre types at the same time throughout the effort, although these horses have a greater proportion of FT than ST fibres. Because they use more anaerobic than aerobic metabolism, lactic acid may accumulate in the working muscles of these horses, which causes fatigue.

Fibre Type Correlated With Activity

Many studies of muscle composition have tried to correlate an individual horse's abundance of one muscle fibre type with excellence in a specific event. The studies have not yielded reliable results on the individual level. However, if a breed *in general* has more ST fibres, those horses are more suitable for performance in endurance type events. Breeds with greater numbers of FT fibres are more suitable for performance in sprint-type events.

Muscle Contraction

An equine muscle is composed of thousands of individual fibres. Organized contraction of stimulated muscle fibres creates movement of a muscle. A tendon connects a muscle to a bone. Movement of a muscle moves the complementary bone and joint. Large muscle groups working together propel a horse into motion or slow it down. Muscle control and coordination improve with practice and training to produce greater precision, power and speed.

Concentric Contraction

Concentric contractions shorten the muscles. As a simple analogy of muscle contraction, think of a fully elongated extension ladder—a relaxed muscle fibre. A muscle contraction shortens the ladder as the rungs slide over one another. As parts of the ladder overlap, it thickens as it shortens; so does a muscle fibre in concentric contraction. Pulling apart the extension pieces once again lengthens (or relaxes) the ladder (or muscle fibre). Pulling a ladder apart or pushing it together requires work, as does moving a muscle to flex a joint.

Eccentric Contraction

Another common type of muscle contraction is an *eccentric* contraction that lengthens the muscle. It is used to overcome the pull of gravity as a horse's full weight is supported by a limb. If extensor muscles did not perform this protective kind of work, then joints could overflex and be damaged. A horse that travels down a steep hill uses eccentric muscle efforts to slow the descent.

Isometric Contraction

Some muscle fibres do not change length with contraction. If the length remains the same because of an opposing pull from another muscle, it is called an *isometric* contraction. Isometric contractions occur in a horse that is on the verge of moving. For example, an event horse that is tensely poised in the start box, or a racehorse poised at the gate, is using isometric contraction.

MUSCLE FATIGUE

In any equine sport, muscle fatigue develops due to several factors:

- lack of fuel, especially glycogen
- lactic acid accumulation in working muscle
- imbalances in body fluids and electrolytes
- heat build-up in working muscle

Intense speed workouts accumulate lactic acid in the muscle faster than endurance events because at speed the muscles must produce energy without oxygen. Excessive lactic acid in the muscles can lead to soreness, fatigue, exhaustion or tying-up *(myositis)* in any type of sport.

Aerobic Conditioning of Muscles

Aerobic metabolism produces energy using oxygen. Oxygen is an essential ingredient for sustained exercise of muscles. After 3 or 4

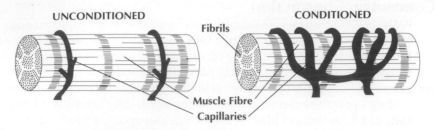

Fig. 3.7 After 3 or 4 months of steady aerobic conditioning, capillary beds expand in size and quantity.

months of steady aerobic conditioning, capillary beds expand in size and quantity to supply greater blood and oxygen circulation to the muscles. Then removal of toxic by-products such as lactic acid also improves.

The aerobic conditioning process also doubles the activity of aerobic enzyme systems for more efficient energy production in the muscles. Muscles are therefore able to function for longer periods before energy reserves are depleted. This efficiency delays the need for anaerobic metabolism and therefore delays lactic acid accumulation in the muscles.

Conserving Glycogen
Using Fatty Acids as Fuel

According to Dr. Philip Swann in his book, *Racehorse Training and Sports Medicine*, more than 30 times the energy is stored in a horse's fat depots than in all the glycogen reserves in the skeletal muscles and liver. The primary benefit of aerobic conditioning is that it promotes the use of fatty acids as an energy source. Fatty acids are released into the bloodstream from adipose tissue storage, and carried to the muscles for fuel. Using fatty acids conserves glycogen stores and delays muscle fatigue so a horse can perform for a longer time without accumulating lactic acid. An aerobically trained horse can better convert fatty acids into energy instead of using glycogen as fuel.

However, fatty acids cannot provide an exclusive energy source because their rate of uptake by muscle tissue is limited. If exercise intensity increases and oxygen supplies decrease, then the muscles must rely on glycogen as a fuel source. The depletion of glycogen reserves leads to exhaustion. This lack is what ultimately limits the endurance athlete's performance.

Increasing the fat stores in the horse by allowing it to gain weight will not improve the body's ability to use fatty acids for energy production. Only aerobic conditioning can accomplish this goal. In fact, extra body weight is detrimental because the horse uses more energy to carry the extra weight around, and a layer of stored fat prevents heat dissipation from working muscles. Both of these factors lead to fatigue.

Increased Glycogen Storage

Not only do a horse's muscles learn to more efficiently metabolize fatty acids as an energy source, but conditioning also creates more glycogen stores in the muscles. Over a 10-week conditioning period, glycogen reserves may increase by as much as 33%.

Anaerobic Conditioning of Muscles

Increased Muscle Mass

Anaerobic conditioning builds muscle mass because the cross-sectional areas of the fast twitch muscle fibres increase to improve muscle strength and power. For example, compare the heavy muscling of a Quarter Horse with the lean, flat muscling of an Arabian. The large hindquarter muscling of the Quarter Horse athlete is partly a result of anaerobic muscle conditioning, and partly a result of genetics.

Lactic Acid Tolerance

During intense bursts of exercise, anaerobic metabolism of muscle glycogen is the main source of energy. Because energy demands increase 200-fold during these intensive exertions, the high rate of energy production provided by anaerobic metabolism is essential to a sprinting horse. During most anaerobic metabolism, glycogen is broken down into energy and lactic acid.

At first, this toxic by-product is carried away from the muscle by the bloodstream. As energy demands increase, however, more lactic acid is produced than the circulation can remove. Lactic acid accumulation in the muscles slows energy production and weakens the contractions of muscle fibres. Therefore, accumulating lactic acid causes fatigue and muscle soreness.

Anaerobic Threshold

The *anaerobic threshold* is the point at which lactic acid begins to accumulate in the muscles and bloodstream. Sprint conditioning can raise the anaerobic threshold by making anaerobic energy production more efficient. It also trains specific enzyme systems to buffer or neutralize lactic acid. Raising the anaerobic threshold delays the onset of fatigue. With a higher anaerobic threshold, a racehorse can travel at faster speeds or an endurance horse can go longer distances before excessive lactic acid accumulates in the muscles.

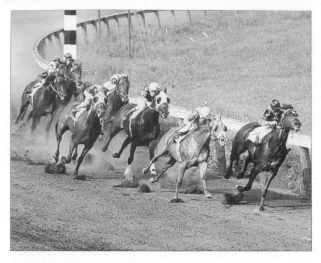

Fig. 3.8 Increasing the anaerobic threshold delays muscle fatigue in the racehorse.

Sodium Bicarbonate

Before a race, racehorses are commonly treated with a sodium bicarbonate (baking soda) drench, called a 'milkshake', in an attempt to counteract the lactic acid and enhance race performance.

Although sodium bicarbonate does seem to improve the buffering capacity of the blood, recent studies report no statistical differences in racing times of horses receiving milkshakes before racing, particularly in studies with Quarter Horse or Thoroughbred racehorses.

The use of sodium bicarbonate is still controversial. It is thought that high intensity exercise of 2 – 9 minutes, such as Standardbred racing, may be enhanced with sodium bicarbonate. Quarter Horse and Thoroughbred races are finished in less than 2 minutes, and the value of milkshakes for these horses is as yet inconclusive. Many other variables such as environmental conditions, track surface and jockey experience also influence racing results. Some milkshakes also contain electrolytes, and can actually be detrimental if the horse has no access to water before the race.

Studies with human athletes indicate that for events involving multiple bouts, performance is enhanced with sodium bicarbonate. The use of multiple bouts is an important element in Standardbred racing and training. The longer duration of exercise coupled with multiple workouts may make milkshakes beneficial to the Standardbred racehorse.

To be effective (if it is indeed effective) the horse must be drenched at a dose of 0.4 grams of sodium bicarbonate per kilogram of body weight. The maximal buffering effects are attained approximately 3 hours after drenching, so plan to drench the horse about 3 hours before race time.

Sodium bicarbonate should *never* be administered to the long distance horse, as losses of electrolytes in the sweat for several hours tend to excessively alkalinize the bloodstream.

Other Benefits

The horse evolved as a flight and flee animal able to escape from predators by fast bursts of speed. Studies confirm that training specifically for intense bursts of speed does not change the metabolism of glycogen. However, conditioning does improve nerve signals, coordinating muscle movement. The rate of muscle contraction and the removal of lactic acid are also improved by anaerobic conditioning of muscles.

MUSCLE STRENGTHENING

All forms of conditioning strengthen a horse's muscles. Along with improved oxygen use and lactic acid tolerance, the muscles learn to contract faster and with more force to enhance speed. In addition, nerve control to the muscles is fine tuned, improving muscular coordination.

General muscle strengthening is as important to a horse's performance as learning the skills of the athletic endeavour. Strength in the muscles makes the task easier. Muscle strength delays the onset of fatigue, particularly during the demands of a competition. Strong muscles reduce the risk of a misstep that could strain tendons, ligaments, or joints.

It is equally important to train for the specific athletics a horse will perform. An endurance horse must train over irregular terrain and at competition speeds. On the other hand, endurance training cannot sufficiently educate muscles to respond to the quick energy bursts required by such events as racing or jumping. If a horse is to accomplish these tasks, it must practise them.

Muscle strengthening is a process requiring many months. It is also cumulative over years. Living tissues return to fitness faster after short periods (weeks) of layoff than they did at the beginning of training. Along with the horse's genetic and psychological predisposition, the amount of effort put into the horse's training determines its durability and ability to perform.

Muscle Exercises

Aerobic Exercise

Muscles adapt to the type of stress applied to them. A horse that exclusively performs aerobic exercises does not build power or bulk in muscle. An example of the effect of aerobic exercises is the flat muscling typical of Arabian endurance horses. Aerobic exercises are low resistance but highly repetitive, like trotting down a level trail at the same rhythm and speed for miles. This exercise improves stamina, neuromuscular precision and economy of movement. The range of movement and the elasticity of muscles also improve. The slow twitch fibres benefit from aerobic conditioning by improving their use of oxygen.

Anaerobic Exercise

In contrast, anaerobic exercises are high resistance efforts with fewer repetitions, lasting up to 30 seconds. Short brisk gallops or rapid hill climbs are examples of anaerobic drills. During each intense exercise, muscles are quickly depleted of stored energy, and then rested between bouts. These exercises increase the bulk and substance of fast twitch muscle fibres.

Resistance

As an example of the effect of resistance on muscles, consider the development of a horse's neck muscles as it is trained to accept bit

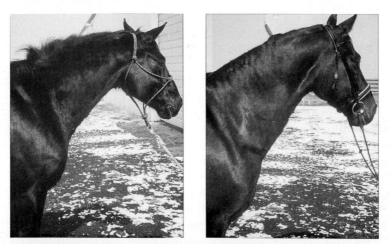

Fig. 3.9 On the left, an untrained horse's neck. On the right, the muscular neck of a trained dressage horse.

contact. With the neck in a normal, relaxed position, the nuchal ligament stretching from the poll to the withers passively assumes the load of the head. The muscles along the top of the neck are not stressed when the neck is in a relaxed position. When the horse is asked to go on bit contact, its neck and head arch and activate those muscles on the top of the neck. The head acts as a 'weight' to provide some resistance to the exercise. The horse then actively holds the head and neck with muscular effort rather than by passive support from the ligaments. Continual exercise of the neck muscles develops them over time and builds up the neck.

Faster Gait

To increase the resistance of an anaerobic exercise, add a faster gait to the muscle training period. For example, trotting up a hill places more demand on muscle tissues than walking up a hill.

Hill Work

An inclined grade or a hill challenges and strengthens body muscle. The resistance of a horse's body weight as it climbs a hill develops hind leg, forearm and shoulder muscles. Walking or trotting a hill develops independent muscles in each hind leg.

As the horse accelerates into a canter or gallop, it propels itself forwards by pushing off the ground with both hind legs at about the same time. A hill climb in a canter or gallop exercises the hind legs as a unit, with considerable strain on the rump and back muscles. These muscles strengthen accordingly.

Downhill work strengthens pectoral, shoulder and forearm

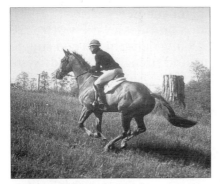

Fig. 3.10 Hill work at the canter strengthens the hind legs, rump and back muscles.

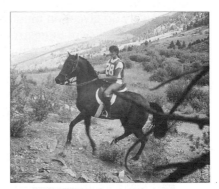

Fig. 3.11 Hill work helps prepare a horse for rocky, mountainous terrain during a competitive long distance event.

muscles, while the quadriceps muscles in the hind legs are strengthened by a braking motion.

Hill work has more advantages besides muscle strengthening. A horse gains as much training effect on the muscles and cardiovascular system doing a hill climb as it would covering three times the distance on flat ground. Also, bones and joints do not receive as great an impact stress with hill work as with flat work, which attempts to reach the same heart rate by increasing speed.

Deep Footing

Work in deep footing, such as sand, snow or a spongy meadow creates resistance in thigh and pectoral muscles. Mud is not a good medium for this type of training as it can cause tendon injuries and even bone fractures. If mud is incorporated into a training routine, work at the walk, never at the trot or canter. Slow and careful conditioning accustoms a horse to deep footing, preventing tendon strain.

Benefits of Cross Training

Sprint work benefits endurance performance by improving the efficiency of the fast twitch fibres. These fibres contribute to the staying power of a long distance horse as it eventually depletes aerobic fuel supplies and resorts to the recruitment of FT fibres.

Endurance conditioning benefits a sprint horse by improving aerobic metabolism, which reduces the horse's dependency on anaerobic energy production. Then less lactic acid is produced. In addition, aerobic conditioning develops the capillary beds, which makes removal of lactic acid more efficient. Also, aerobic conditioning increases muscle glycogen stores. A sprint horse relies almost exclusively on glycogen metabolism for energy.

The abundance of equestrian sports provides a variety of exercises to develop and strengthen muscles. Long rides stretch and supple muscles, teach balance and rhythm, and strengthen all body systems. Obstacles such as cavaletti poles teach precision through a gymnastic routine. The even footing of a track is excellent for speed workouts. Cross training builds a versatile and durable athlete.

Sports-Specific Strengthening Exercises

Dressage

Combining callisthenics (developing muscular tone) with strength training improves the back, belly and hind leg muscles in the dressage horse, making it capable of performing precision movements with ease. Work the horse on bit contact and in a dressage frame, and

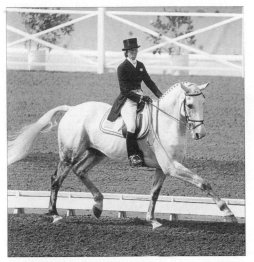

Fig. 3.12 Dressage movements create a fit and responsive horse.

then allow it to relax and stretch between difficult exercises. Repetitive practice and correct execution of advanced movements of half-pass, piaffe, passage, and pirouettes strengthen the associated muscles. Trotting cavalettis teaches rhythm and balance, and also teaches the horse to work with the hocks up and under the body. Cantering 2-foot fences spaced one stride apart encourages simultaneous hind leg use, developing croup and back muscles. Downhill walking also teaches a horse to balance with its hindquarters, an important element of collected work.

Jumping

A jumping horse propels off the ground with strong hindquarter muscles. Furthermore, landing exerts considerable force on shoulder and neck muscles. These horses particularly benefit from hill climbs at a canter, with slower downhills to rest the muscles between strengthening exercises. Cavaletti work and dressage exercises also strengthen hindquarter muscles.

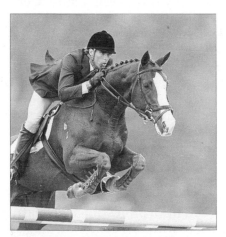

Fig. 3.13 A jumping horse requires strength in the hindquarters.

Racing

Two of the most beneficial exercises for the racehorse are hill climbs and interval training. Hill work strengthens the hindquarter muscles for acceleration and drive. It also provides aerobic conditioning, which is an important factor in racing.

Interval training consists of repeated sets of speed work and partial heart rate recovery periods. Interval training increases speed and promotes lactic acid tolerance. *(See Chapter 6 for more information on interval training.)*

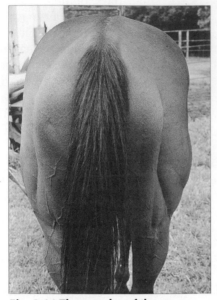

Fig. 3.14 The muscles of the rump and thighs are prone to myositis.

MYOSITIS

The hard-working performance horse is subject to a skeletal muscle disease syndrome, generally called exercise-associated *myositis*. This syndrome also goes by other names: 'tying-up', 'Monday morning disease,' exertional rhabdomyolysis, azoturia and paralytic myoglobinuria. The causes of these syndromes may be different, but their symptoms are the same and can be similarly treated. Myositis literally means 'muscle inflammation' and is a general term for all these syndromes. It is a complex disorder and the clinical signs vary considerably.

Performance can suffer in cases of myositis, even if muscle cramping is not actually seen. The symptoms may be as subtle as poor racing times or a shorter stride than normal.

Myositis is a painful condition similar to a severe cramp in a person's leg. When the large, fleshy muscles over the rump or along a horse's thigh suddenly spasm and cramp. In the more obvious form the horse assumes a stiff stilted gait in the hindquarters, and may eventually refuse to move. The muscles may feel hard as a brick, instead of having a normal pliable consistency. There may be tremors or quivers in the muscles. Some horses seem wobbly and unsteady, while others sweat, act 'colicky', and want to lie down and roll. The horse can be in obvious distress and in need of immediate veterinary attention. Keep the horse warm with a blanket, and do not move it, until professional help arrives as the pain and the obvious anxiety with this condition may be exacerbated.

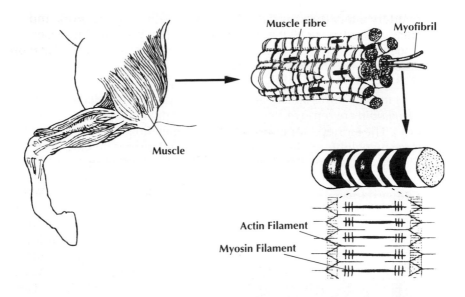

Fig. 3.15 A muscle fibre is made of thousands of filaments.

Normal Muscle Contraction

A normal contraction of a muscle fibre is caused by a series of biochemical events. A muscle fibre is made up of thousands of filaments. There are two types of filaments: *actin* filaments and *myosin* filaments, which partially overlap. The myosin filaments have 'heads' which attach to the actin filaments.

A nerve impulse from the brain releases calcium into the muscle cells. Calcium activates sites on the actin filament so that the head of the myosin filament attaches to it. Then the myosin head tilts and swivels to pull the actin filament. The head then detaches and moves to another active site on the actin filament. This cycle of head tilt, filament movement and head detachment continues to contract the muscle fibre with a ratchet-like movement.

The Role of Calcium

As long as calcium is in the cell, a fibre will continue to contract. A cellular 'calcium pump' normally removes calcium from the cell, allowing the muscle fibre to relax. ATP (adenosine triphosphate) energy molecules fuel the pump that removes calcium from the muscle cell.

If calcium channels are blocked due to lack of ATP energy molecules, the muscle cannot relax. Calcium remains in the muscle cells activating the actin filaments, and the heads of the myosin filaments remain attached. This unrelenting contraction, multiplied by many thousands of fibres, causes muscle cramps. With each spasm, more ATP is depleted and the cycle continues.

Muscle and Kidney Damage

As muscle fibres spasm and tear apart, pigment molecules called *myoglobin* are removed by the bloodstream and carried to the kidneys. The kidneys' function is to filter small molecules. The relatively large myoglobin molecules may be trapped inside the kidneys and block them. There, they may interfere with oxygen diffusion to kidney cells, and may cause kidney failure, resulting in shock or death. Kidney damage is proportionate to the amount of myoglobin trapped within the kidneys.

Coffee-coloured urine is evidence that myoglobin has reached the kidneys. Intravenous fluid therapy is sometimes necessary to flush the kidneys and improve circulation in the muscles, while prompt veterinary attention including the use of anti-inflammatory drugs stop the cycle of muscle damage and pain. It is essential to ensure that a horse with muscle damage drinks plenty of clean water to flush the kidneys.

Causes of Myositis

Some horses are taken out to exercise and show signs of discomfort within the first several minutes (Type A myositis), while others develop myositis after several hours of steady exercise (Type B myositis).

Classically the disease is seen in horses that have returned to exercise after being rested for one or more days on full rations, but other factors such as vitamin E/selenium deficiency, excitement and influenza virus have been suggested as being involved.

Type A Myositis

In Type A myositis a horse begins to experience severe muscle cramps after only a few minutes of exercise. This syndrome is caused by stress, hormonal influences or defects in energy metabolism in the muscle.

Accumulation of lactic acid in the muscles reduces the rate of energy production and the contraction of muscle fibres. Less energy produced means less energy to fuel the calcium pump, and uncontrolled muscle contraction causes the cramping of myositis. A fat or unconditioned horse stores more glycogen in the muscle and metabolizes it less efficiently than a conditioned horse. These factors increase lactic acid production.

Horses that work above the anaerobic threshold at speeds greater than 20 mph accumulate measurable lactic acid in the tissues and bloodstream. A high concentration of lactic acid in the muscles increases the risk of myositis. Lactic acid does not necessarily cause myositis, but high lactic acid concentrations worsen muscle damage.

Type B Myositis

Electrolyte Loss

Type B myositis develops after long periods of exercise, either during the exertion or within an hour after work has stopped. Endurance horses, such as long-distance riding horses and three-day-event horses, work mostly at aerobic speeds. Therefore, they develop myositis for different reasons than lactic-acid-related myositis in racehorses or jumping horses. The horse that exercises steadily for long periods can develop electrolyte (body salt) imbalances and de hydration, leading to exhaustion and myositis.

Potassium

Prolonged exercise, especially on an excessively hot and humid day, encourages loss of electrolytes, such as potassium and chloride, in the sweat. Potassium dilates small blood vessels in the muscle during exercise. With low potassium, the blood vessels do not dilate enough to deliver adequate oxygen to the muscles and fuel the slow twitch muscle fibres.

Chloride

A loss of chloride causes *metabolic alkalosis* (increased pH in the bloodstream). An increased pH in the bloodstream directly affects the ability of the muscle cells to extract oxygen from the blood.

Fluid Loss

Fluid loss from sweat dehydrates a horse and decreases the circulating blood volume. Decreasing the amount of blood also limits the amount of oxygen available to muscles.

In sum, the lack of electrolytes and fluids decreases the amount of oxygen available to the muscles. Therefore, aerobic metabolism in the slow twitch fibres cannot continue and the fast twitch fibres are recruited. Lactic acid begins to accumulate, slowing energy production and increasing the risk of myositis.

Also, working muscles generate heat. Heat build-up in the muscles increases the oxygen and energy requirements of muscles, adding to the problems of electrolyte imbalances, dehydration and energy depletion.

Candidates For Myositis

Horses in Training

A horse in training that is fed rich feed (grain or alfalfa) is a candidate for this syndrome. This is especially true if the horse remains on a generous grain supplement while rested for a day or two, and then is immediately returned to vigorous exercise. When a horse is not active on a particular day, reduce its grain intake. Rapid increases in work difficulty or demands for speed from an unconditioned horse can also cause a crisis.

Myositis is predominantly a disease of the fast twitch muscle fibres. (Slow twitch fibres are surrounded by greater numbers of capillaries, so more oxygen is readily available to them.) FT fibres that receive little or no oxygen are susceptible to impaired blood flow from constriction of blood vessels. FT fibres also produce more lactic acid than ST fibres.

The stress of training can reduce normal thyroid activity and change its control of internal body temperature and oxygen supply to working muscles. A cold day similarly constricts blood vessels in the muscle, so less blood and oxygen are supplied to the fibres. All these factors can lead to excessive lactic acid production.

Genetic Predisposition

Genetic tendencies for myositis have been observed in some breed lines. This tendency may be related to a defect in muscle metabolism in affected individuals. Heavily muscled horses with greater numbers of FT fibres are prone to the disease. Examples of these horses are Quarter Horses and Appaloosas and certain draft breeds such as the Clydesdale, Shire, Belgian and Percheron.

Nervous horses, especially mares and fillies, seem prone to myositis, possibly due to female endocrine influences.

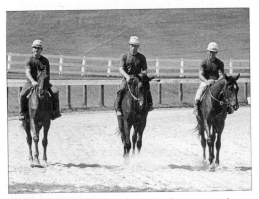

Fig. 3.16 Warming-up is a good preventative measure to help avoid myositis.

Preventing Myositis

Many factors influencing myositis are out of human control, such as climate, genetics, and skeletal muscle metabolism disorders unique to an individual. Horses that develop myositis may suffer repeated episodes and require careful management and training. Yet, strategies for prevention exist. An educated conditioning programme enables a horse to perform the athletic demands with the least stress to body and mind. Never work a horse with, or suspected of having, a viral infection.

Warm-Ups and Cool-Downs

Attention to a proper warm-up opens capillary beds in the muscles and activates enzyme systems. A warm-up actually increases muscle temperature by one or two degrees. Warmed muscles are more elastic so they contract and move more efficiently. An adequate cool-down flushes lactic acid from the muscle. A muscle massage loosens fatigued muscles and enhances circulation to the tissues. *(See Chapter 6 for more information.)*

Conditioning

As mentioned earlier the entire body of a horse benefits from conditioning. It encourages development of the heart and lungs, and of blood vessels and capillaries in the muscles, improving oxygen delivery and toxic by-product removal. Conditioning trains enzyme systems in the muscles to efficiently use energy sources, delays the build-up of lactic acid, and improves muscle tolerance of toxic by-products, to reduce the risk of myositis.

The Sprint Horse

A sprint horse depends on fast twitch muscle fibres to produce acceleration and power. Sprint training increases the anaerobic threshold so lactic acid does not accumulate as quickly and energy production can continue. Sprint training also develops enzymes which buffer the tiring effects of lactic acid.

The Endurance Horse

Training strategies for the long-distance performer improve the horse's *aerobic capacity.* Training reduces the cross-sectional area of slow twitch muscle fibres, allowing better diffusion of oxygen into the muscle cells. The longer the slow twitch fibres can function in aerobic metabolism, the longer it takes for recruitment of fast twitch muscle fibres that are more prone to developing myositis. In long-distance competitions it is possible to prevent extreme electrolyte imbalances by supplementing a horse with oral electrolytes during the event. A sufficient water supply should always be provided, and the long-distance horse given many opportunities to drink so as to prevent dehydration. This is important in hot conditions when a self-limiting form of muscle cramping develops following dehydration, electrolyte imbalances, and disturbances in thermoregulatory and circulatory function. *(See Chapter 6 for more information on dehydration.)*

Other Prevention Methods

Avoid applying water to the large buttock or back muscles of a hot horse that has just stopped working. The cool water causes blood vessels to constrict away from the skin surface, trapping heat and toxic by-products in the muscle. In addition, blood and oxygen circulation in the muscles is diminished, leading to muscle cramping.

To prevent chill and cramping of the working muscles, especially of a long-distance competitor, use a rump rug during rainy, cold or extremely windy conditions. A rump rug covering the haunches keeps the working muscles warm and supple and makes them less likely to cramp.

During periods of inactivity between events, races, or regular training schedules, grain should be reduced. The horse should be turned out for self-exercise to maintain muscle tone.

Anaemias caused by intestinal parasitism or by inadequate feed intake or nutrient absorption further reduce oxygen circulation in the blood. Consistent deworming schedules, tooth care, and attention to a horse's overall health and attitude allow it to optimally use nutrients that fuel muscles and help prevent myositis.

HYPERKALAEMIC PERIODIC PARALYSIS

Over the last decade, a condition of skeletal muscle weakness has been recognized. This syndrome, *hyperkalaemic periodic paralysis* (HYPP), has been genetically linked to a certain line of Quarter Horses.

Clinical Signs

As an episode of HYPP begins, an affected horse experiences persistent muscle twitching over the trunk, hindquarters, flanks, neck and/or shoulders. Muscles of the face also spasm, causing flared nostrils and lips that are taut and drawn. In addition, the third eyelid often drops over the eye as the muscles around the orbit spasm.

As the episode progresses, the skeletal muscles become weak, with the horse collapsing to the ground or sitting on its haunches like a dog. Mild attacks may only elicit signs of muscular weakness such as swaying and staggering, with the horse not going down completely. The horse may buckle at the knees, sag in its hocks, or be unable to raise its head and neck. Throughout a crisis the horse remains alert, although slightly depressed, and is in no pain. The overall relaxed attitude of the animal helps distinguish HYPP from similar-appearing syndromes of colic or myositis. Between episodes of HYPP, the horse appears completely normal.

Cause of HYPP

HYPP occurs due to a defect in the transport system that regulates the movement of potassium and sodium across cell membranes.

Preventing HYPP Episodes

Prevention relies mostly on feeding strategies. Recommendations suggest feeding a diet containing a maximum of 1% potassium, and avoiding alfalfa hay, rich spring pasture, molasses and sweet feed (which contains molasses). Oats, barley and maize contain less than 0.4% potassium. Grain portions should be fed in small amounts 2 – 3 times daily.

Treatment

If a horse develops early signs of an attack, walking or lungeing the horse can stimulate the circulation of adrenaline. Adrenaline drives potassium back into the muscle cells.Severe attacks require immediate veterinary attention.

Genetic Test

To detect if a horse may develop HYPP, a blood sample can be evaluated for a specific gene in the DNA. This test is available through the University of California-Davis School of Veterinary Medicine.

Not all horses of the affected lineage have the HYPP gene. If only one parent has the mutant gene, a foal has a 50% chance of being afflicted. If both parents possess the gene, a foal has a 75% chance of developing HYPP. A horse that tests negative for the mutant gene will not pass the syndrome on to future generations, and may confidently be used as breeding stock.

4

PERFORMANCE FEET

Daily care and attention to a horse's feet provide a wealth of information regarding their health. Clean the feet with a hoof pick and examine them for foul odours, stones, nails or hoof cracks. Watch a horse in motion around the paddock or pasture so lameness is recognized early.

The size of the feet should be proportionate to the body. Study the feet for balance and symmetry. Note abnormal contours in the hoof wall. Compare the front feet with each other, and back feet with each other. Study other horses' feet and

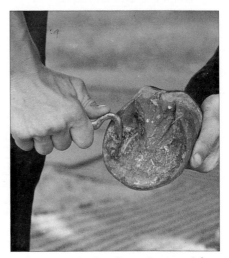

Fig. 4.1 Regular hoof care is essential for good performance.

make comparisons. Develop an eye for the normal; learn to notice oddities. Daily care may prevent a simple problem from developing into a long-term, chronic disease.

FOOT FUNCTION AND STRUCTURE

The hoof is the hard outer covering of the foot. Beneath the hoof lies a complex arrangement of bones, cartilage, ligaments, and tendons. The foot is a complex and dynamic structure, elastic and alive.

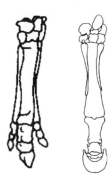

Evolution has developed a horse's front legs from rudimentary fingers. Starting with the tips of a person's middle finger, the fingernail and the small bone up to the first joint correspond to a horse's front foot. The rest of that finger back to where it joins the hand has developed into the two pastern bones. The cannon and splint bones are similar to the bones in the back of a hand. The other fingers and thumb have disappeared.

Fig. 4.2 On the left, ancient horse leg. On the right, modern leg bones and hoof.

Imagine walking on one finger. It is easy to understand why lameness develops when one considers the enormous load per square inch that a 1000-lb animal places upon each limb during performance.

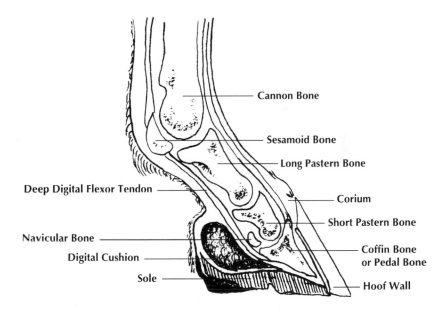

Cannon Bone

Sesamoid Bone

Long Pastern Bone

Deep Digital Flexor Tendon

Corium

Short Pastern Bone

Navicular Bone

Digital Cushion

Coffin Bone or Pedal Bone

Sole

Hoof Wall

Fig. 4.3 Internal and external structures of the foot.

The coffin bone, or pedal bone lies inside the hoof capsule. Seated beneath and behind the coffin bone is the navicular bone. It functionally increases the surface area of the coffin joint, reducing the impact of landing. The deep digital flexor tendon runs behind the navicular bone and attaches to the back of the coffin bone. The position of the navicular bone moves the deep digital flexor tendon away from the centre of the coffin joint, creating a larger range of motion of that joint. These internal structures of the foot absorb downward compressive forces by the body and gravity. As a horse strides forward, the heel contacts the ground before the toe. This impact expands the heel outward, pushing the *digital cushion,* a fibroelastic fatty pad forming the heel bulbs, against the *collateral cartilages.*

As a horse's foot impacts the ground, the frog is compressed while the short pastern bone is forced downwards. Then the digital cushion overlying the internal frog surface is compressed, further expanding the collateral cartilages. This expansion forces the network of blood vessels within the hoof wall to alternately constrict and dilate. In this way, blood and oxygen are moved around the tissues of the foot and up and down the legs.

Optimal biomechanical function of the foot is determined by the:

- balance of the foot
- conformation
- shoes that are worn
- contour of the terrain
- impact surface of the ground

Any deviation from normal has a pronounced effect on a horse's performance, because all these factors contribute to overall soundness of the limbs.

Health, Genetics and Performance

The ultimate factor dictating the response of a foot to environmental influences is the genetic predisposition of a horse. It is hard to make an anatomical structure better than its genetic potential. Exercise and good, balanced nutrition maintain foot health and restore diseased feet to normal. The conformational shape, size and hoof-wall thickness are controlled by genetics, but improper shoeing, lack of stable hygiene, and environmental dehydration can adversely alter genetic tendencies.

Hoof Colour

Many people claim that hoof colour (white versus black) affects the strength and durability of a hoof. Many believe that white feet are softer, more crumbly and more predisposed to bruising and injury than black feet. However, a scientific study (1983) on the mechanical properties of equine hooves found *no* difference in the stress and strain behaviour or ultimate strength properties between black and white hooves. Black hooves contain melanin granules, which make them feel harder on cutting.

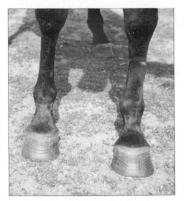

Fig. 4.4 A horse with different sized feet due to disease.

Hoof Size

Feet that are too wide are prone to bruising, collapsed heels, and dropped soles. Feet that are contracted with a narrow straight wall do not give under pressure. A small foot or one with poor conformation is prone to problems. A foot that is too large or too small lacks shock-absorptive ability. Excess concussion is absorbed in the feet and up the limb.

Not all horses have front feet that are exact mates in size and shape, and this may be normal for some individuals. However, any difference in size should be viewed with suspicion as a sign of disease.

Hoof Structure and Growth

The *coronary corium* underlying the *coronary band* where the hoof meets the skin produces new hoof wall growth. The corium is a layer of connective tissue containing an elaborate blood and nerve supply that nourishes the foot.

Hoof Wall

The hoof wall, composed of *keratin*, is a modified extension of the skin. A continuously growing structure, the hoof grows down from the coronary band. A young horse grows hoof faster than a mature horse. For example, a foal may grow ½ inch of hoof per month, but a mature horse grows hoof at the rate of about ⅜ inch per month.

The hoof also grows at different rates throughout the year, depending on season and climate. It grows fastest during periods of warm temperatures and moisture, corresponding with springtime and lengthening daylight hours.

At the rate of ⅜ inch per month, the toe—and any hoof damage— entirely grows out in about a year, while the heels replace themselves every 4 – 5 months.

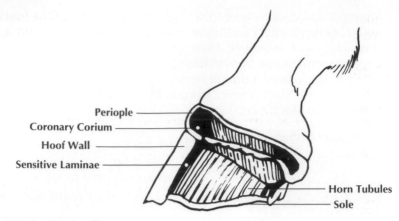

Periople

Coronary Corium

Hoof Wall

Sensitive Laminae

Horn Tubules

Sole

Fig. 4.5 The hoof wall.

Horn Tubules

Elastic *horn tubules* absorb concussion by bending and flexing and by compressing, reducing the impact on other structures in the limbs. Normal moisture content promotes elasticity of the hoof, enabling it to absorb concussion.

By the peculiar anatomy of the hoof, Mother Nature has provided a way of maintaining natural hoof moisture. Moisture in the equine hoof comes from internal water carried through the blood and lymphatic vessels to sensitive structures deep within the foot. From there it is transferred to the horn tubules that make up the hoof wall. Exercise enhances this circulatory process.

Rigid and closely packed horn tubules aligned in a vertical and parallel arrangement in the hoof wall retain moisture much as a sponge holds water. The configuration of the foot dictates the direction in which the horn tubules lie. This factor is important in moisture retention.

For example, one of the problems associated with a long-toe–low-heel configuration, and the spreading English hunter type of foot is that it loses the neat, parallel alignment of horn tubules. Spacing between tubule cells is spread apart, and moisture is quickly lost from the foot.

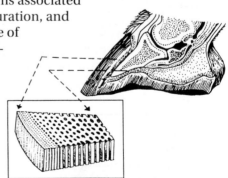

Periople

A protective, waxy covering called the *periople* delays loss of internal moisture from the

Fig. 4.6 Horn tubules within the hoof.

hoof. The periople 'hoof varnish' is a very thin layer of cells that readily wears off although it continually grows from the coronary band.

Moisture

In an adult horse, the elastic properties of the hoof wall are reduced if normal moisture levels are not maintained at about 25% water. If the hoof horn becomes dry and brittle, and is unable to absorb concussion, it will crack in small fissures. Brittle hooves also do not hold nails well so it is difficult to keep shoes on.

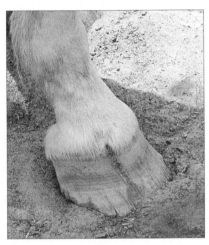

Fig. 4.7 Dry and brittle hoof due to low moisture content.

Water is Nature's moisturizer, but too much is not good for the feet. Prolonged and excessive moisture from sodden ground or urine-soaked stalls is harmful to hoof moisture. Equally harmful are excessive dryness and abrasion from coarse, sandy soil, or the overzealous use of a farrier's hoof rasp. These situations degrade the thickness and structure of the hoof wall. The hoof then loses its internal moisture retention capabilities and the waxy covering of the hoof wall dissolves. A hoof hardening and waterproofing product, Keratex Hoof Hardener®, is said to work without the problems of 'case hardening' or destruction of the horn.

Hoof Dressings

Hoof dressings of an oil or grease base, especially with the addition of rosin (pine tar) or lanolin, are helpful if the feet experience continuous wet and dry cycles. These dressings act as an artificial periople to reduce evaporation of internal moisture. Daily application is necessary so that the dressing is not worn away as was the original periople.

Some people liberally paint all manner of grease over dry hooves under the mistaken impression that it puts needed moisture back into the foot. This assumption is false because most hoof moisture comes from internal sources, and only a small amount is gradually assimilated by *osmosis* from the environment. Rather than adding moisture to the foot, damp ground slows the evaporation rate of

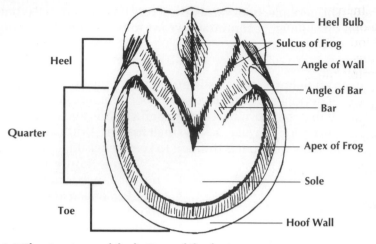

Fig. 4.8 The structures of the bottom of the foot.

internal moisture from the foot.

Many hoof dressings are astringent and dehydrate the foot. Examples of harsh dressings include those containing turpentine, bleach, formalin, or phenol. Such compounds are useful only if occasionally applied to a moist frog or sole to control bacteria that thrive in wet conditions.

Building Strong Feet

The most important ingredients to ensure strong feet are balanced nutrition, exercise, proper trimming and balancing, and basic hygiene.

Balanced nutrition provides energy, protein, vitamins and minerals for hoof growth. The rate of hoof growth corresponds to a horse's rate of weight gain. Various feed supplements and hoof dressings are also merchandised to strengthen hoof walls.

Supplements
Biotin

Other avenues have been explored to encourage hoof growth. Biotin at doses of 15 – 30 milligrams per day for up to 9 months has been reported to improve the quality of horn in studies performed on pigs. In cases of known B-complex vitamin deficits, biotin may correct cracked hooves.

In many cases of thin, brittle hooves, biotin was added to the diet along with changes in exercise and shoeing. There is no evidence that biotin alone has improved the hooves of these horses, despite related anecdotal experiences. Most foodstuffs, especially maize, provide ample biotin, but this is not always in a completely biologically available form. For example, biotin in wheat is only 10% available, 40–50% in barley, 70–80% in sorghum, with all available in maize. However, biotin supplementation is not harmful to a horse, and may be good for a sick or debilitated animal. Horses with damage to the small intestine require higher levels of biotin in the diet. Biotin is water-soluble and the body rapidly excretes excessive amounts.

DL-methionine

Another supplement said to enhance hoof growth is DL-methionine. It is speculated that the sulphur precursors of DL-methionine contribute to the growth of horn tubules. There is no evidence, however, that this compound speeds hoof growth, but inclusion in the diet after an illness may improve the quality of horn. Do not exceed the inclusion rates on the pack.

Exercise

The importance of exercise to a horse's feet cannot be overemphasized. Exercise stimulates the expandability of the hoof, increasing the surface area and reducing concussion during a performance effort. It increases blood circulation to the feet, promoting the health and elasticity of the hoof wall, and stimulates new growth of all foot structures. The sole toughens with repeated use, making it less vulnerable to bacteria and bruises. The scrubbing action of soil clods as they are flung from moving feet contributes to

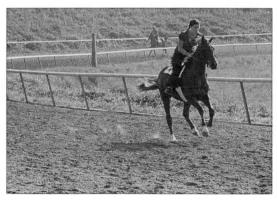

Fig. 4.9 Exercise is an important key for foot health.

foot hygiene by removing dead pieces of sole and frog. Exercise encourages the circulation of tissue nutrients throughout the limbs, and reduces the stagnation often seen as 'stocked up' legs. It strengthens ligaments and tendons that support the joints and act as shock absorbers to cushion the load on the joints.

Massage of Coronary Band

Massage of the coronary bands stimulates hoof growth. This stimulation is accomplished by applying sheepskin coverings saturated with lanolin over the coronary bands, or by daily massage with vegetable or mineral oil or products such as Cornucrecine®.

Basic Hygiene

Thrush

Reducing equine foot disease depends on care and observation. Thrush *(pododermatitis)* results from moist and unhygienic conditions. Accumulation of manure, rotten straw, or mud on the bottoms of the feet encourages growth of bacteria within the crevices *(sulci)* of the frog. Often, a thrush infection travels deep into the sensitive layers of the frog, causing considerable pain and lameness and adversely affecting the horse's performance.

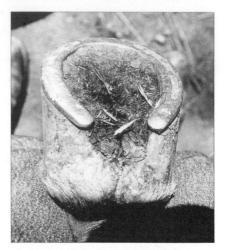

Fig. 4.10 A foot with thrush.

A foul odour is associated with thrush, and the frog becomes dark and discoloured by discharge. The sole should be concave, and the frog firm but pliable like a rubber eraser. With thrush, the frog feels spongy as it degenerates. Daily foot cleaning removes debris. For most horses, frequent trimming every 6–8 weeks removes dead tissue that traps debris. Performance horses may need trimming and shoeing every 4–6 weeks. Applying an iodine solution or copper sulphate to the bottom of the foot (frog and sulci) a couple of times each week controls thrush and canker.

Canker

Canker is a rare occurrence due to modern hygienic practices, but may develop in unusually wet and warm climates. A horse with canker develops a foul smelling, moist infection of the frog and sole. The frog tissues overdevelop *(hypertrophy)*. Affected foot structures are white and have a cottage cheese consistency, in contrast to the black, decaying appearance of thrush. Canker invades deeper into the horny tissues than does thrush, with thrush confined primarily to the frog. Veterinary atttention is required as aggressive surgical removal of all affected tissue is required to treat canker.Prompt attention in the case of both thrush and canker reduces the severity and the possible long period off work. The hoof wall normally diffuses the concussive force from the ground, while the internal structures such as the digital cushion, frog, *laminae*, and coffin bone absorb downward compressive forces by the body and gravity. The ideal weight-bearing surface of the foot is the hoof wall—not the sole. If shoes contact the sole at any point, that pressure will bruise underlying structures. If a hoof is trimmed excessively, or if a foot is worn down by harsh soil conditions, the lack of hoof wall forces a horse to walk on the soles of its feet, setting up conditions for subsolar abscesses, corns or *laminitis*.

Abscesses

Watching a horse's movements about the paddock can help an owner or trainer see other causes of lameness such as *subsolar abscesses*. Abscesses result from stone bruises or corns or from improperly trimmed and shod feet. Bruises and corns occur beneath the surface of the sole; they aren't always visible with daily cleaning and inspection.

If a shoe is left on a foot for too long (more than 8 weeks), it may pinch the heels. The pinching creates an inflammation near the *angle of the bar* (separating the frog and the sole), producing a corn and possibly an abscess.

Abscesses also occur from nail punctures, or from severe bruising and trauma to the sole. If a nail is found in the foot, always identify the site if it is removed. As the nail may have penetrated underlying structures, seek veterinary attention immediately to permit rapid treatment including possible surgery. Where a joint or bursa is penetrated, flushing and infusion of antibiotics within six hours is often critical for the success of any treatment.

The Hoof as a Visual Record of Stress

Examining the appearance of the hoof tells how concussive forces are directed across the foot, and may identify illness. Although some changes are internally subtle, over time they will produce a visual record on the face of the hoof. Flares and growth rings in the hoof wall reflect uneven stress. With more impact, the hoof wall steepens; with less, it flares.

Coronary Band Response to Uneven Stresses

A hoof responds to uneven stresses with an increased growth rate at the point of concentrated impact. The less impacted side of the foot experiences a relatively reduced circulation and therefore slower hoof growth.

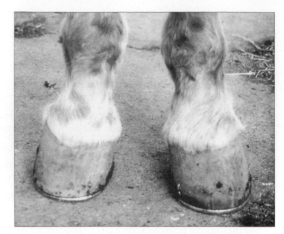

Fig. 4.11 Uneven coronary bands on both feet.

In a normal foot, the coronary band is a straight line across the front of the hoof, in a plane parallel to the ground. It gradually slopes away to the heels, equally on both sides. Alterations in the circulatory tissue nourishing the foot or uneven stresses on the foot change the alignment of the coronary band. The coronary band realigns itself and appears asymmetrical (not properly aligned). This configuration can foretell a lameness problem due to unbalanced feet. Foot imbalances occur from incorrect hoof trimming, or from uneven loading created by poor conformation.

Hoof Wall Response to Uneven Stresses

Abnormal contours and 'rings' of the hoof wall provide historical insight into the feet. For example, in chronic laminitis the heels grow faster than the toes. As the toe and heel of the hoof wall are produced at different rates, it assumes a wavy contour. Just as the growth rings of a tree chronicle seasonal and climatic variation in its development, so does the hoof reflect internal and external stresses on its face.

Ring Development

Fine longitudinal lines in the hoof running from the coronary band to the ground show the position of horn tubules as they grow down from the coronary corium. Anything that interferes with blood flow in the foot directly affects the rate of hoof wall growth. If the growth rate increases or slows in different areas of the foot, a change is visible. Rings develop in the hoof wall as the growth plates diverge between heels and toe.

Improper Shoeing

If a foot is unbalanced, or if the shoes were fitted improperly, stress lines appear on the hooves as irregularities or ridges at the points of abnormal pressure by the shoe.

Change in Diet

Not all hoof wall rings indicate disease in the foot. A change in diet or quality of nutrition can also alter the growth and chemistry of keratin, and may create ridges in the hoof wall. As the hoof grows, an abnormal ring moves towards the ground, followed by healthy and consistent hoof wall.

Seasonal Effects

Seasonal variations can produce a similar effect, when the warmth and moisture of lengthening spring days stimulate a surge of hoof growth. Such growth spurts appear as several ridged rings across the hoof wall.

Fever

A fever that lasts for several days also stimulates a growth spurt in the feet, and rings may be evident weeks later.

Inflammation

Any inflammation of the foot or coronary band creates rings in the hoof wall. Increased circulation through the coronary corium causes a rapid growth of the wall, possibly leading to divergent growth planes at the toe and heel.

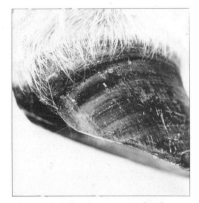

Fig. 4.12 Divergent growth planes lead to rings in the hoof wall.

Hoof Cracks

An injury or defect in the coronary band often results in a permanent crack in the hoof wall. The permanent crack is due to an interruption of horn tubule growth.

Another type of hoof crack can start at the bearing surface and work towards the coronary band. Depending on its location it is a toe crack, a quarter crack, or a heel crack, and may indicate an unbalanced foot. Improper trimming and excessively dry or thin

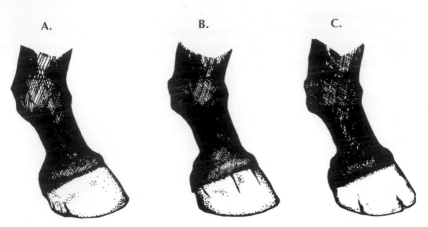

Fig. 4.13 Various cracks. (A) Quarter and heel cracks. (B) Toe, quarter and heel cracks originating at the coronary band. (C) Toe and quarter cracks.

walls can contribute to the hoof cracking. Daily inspection identifies cracks before they become a simmering problem. Hoof cracks cause pain when the sensitive tissue moves with weight-bearing. Hoof cracks also provide an avenue for infection to invade the inner structures of the foot.

Horizontal Grooves and Cracks

Horizontal grooves and cracks across the hoof wall that are parallel to the coronary band may indicate *selenium toxicity*. These cracks usually appear in more than one foot. Because selenium is substituted for sulphur in the amino acids of body proteins, kera-

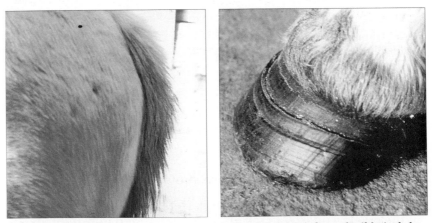

Fig. 4.14 The first symptom of chronic selenium toxicity is loss of tail hair, left. On the right, the same horse with horizontal hoof cracks, which occurs later.

tinized structures (hair and hoof) are most affected. Hair loss will occur before lameness develops. Eventually, the hoof horn will reflect the internal poisoning of the body by separating from the foot's internal components and sloughing off.

SHOES AND PADS
History of the Horseshoe

Since the earliest times that horses have been used as beasts of burden, as transportation or as war steeds, humans have searched for optimal foot protection to prevent lameness. Foot care for the horse may have begun as long ago as 1600 BC. Attention to foot care eventually encouraged the development of equine foot gear, with protective shoes dating back at least 2000 years to the first or second centuries BC.

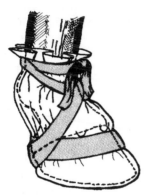

Equine hooves did not always benefit from such protection. About 330 BC, at the time of Alexander the Great, it is reported that cavalry expeditions were interrupted to allow the horses to restore hoof horn to their tender feet. Evidence of the use of horse foot coverings surfaced 200 – 300 years later. A battlepiece mosaic discovered at Pompeii, which fell in AD 79, depicts horseshoes fitted to horse feet.

Historical predecessors to a modern equine shoe assumed form as very thin plates of gold, silver, or iron that were fastened to leather and then secured by straps attached to the hoof or fetlock. Such 'hipposandals' provided some protection from abrasive ground.

Fig. 4.15 An ancient horseshoe.

A terracotta Roman tablet illustrates boot-like protective coverings extending up the legs of chariot racing horses to protect them for the brief, but traumatic, period of competition.

Shoes made of durable woven twigs and reeds were used on tender-footed mounts in the days of Julius Augustus Caesar (27 BC – AD 14). Another Roman emperor, Nero (AD 56 – 68), had his horse shod with silver while his wife, Poppea, protected the feet of her mules with gold.

By the era of the ancient Tartar and Mongolian warriors, at the time of Christ, shoes were more common. Excavation of ancient burial mounds of these warriors unearthed remains of horses still wearing shoes. These 'shoes' were circular, nailed only to the outer bearing surface of the hoof, as a 'unilateral' shoe.

The nailed horseshoe as we know it today was used in Europe by about the fifth century AD. By the eighth and ninth centuries, lists of cavalry equipment itemized crescent-shaped iron shoes and nails as part of the basic inventory. Until AD1000, shoes were primarily used on war horses or as decorative adornment for nobility. After AD1000, people began to travel further on newly constructed roads, and horseshoeing became customary.

Historic illustrations describe continual attempts by humans to 'defend the hoof' and enhance the usefulness of the horse. Just 100 years ago, the text of Mile's *Modern Practical Farriery* (1896) commented: 'Considering the apparent simplicity of the process to an ordinary observer, the method of fastening a piece of iron to a horse's foot has been the occasion of more dissertations, essays, guides, manuals, "practical" instructions, theories, disputes, and— we sorrow to write it—hard words and abuse, than any other subject we are acquainted with.'

Today we take 'modern' inventions of horseshoes for granted as these devices allow us to ride our horses over long distances and terrible terrain, to jump and gallop, and to pull heavy loads with a reduced risk of foot injury.

Despite our 20th century technology of rubber, plastic, and metal alloy, the same disputes rage over appropriate methods of horseshoeing. In ancient times the issue was simpler: to shoe or not to shoe, and how to keep a shoe affixed to the foot. Modern civilization has long since overcome such obstacles, offering anything from nails to special glues to affix a plethora of shoe designs to a hoof. Set the traditions aside, and address each horse's feet as a unique case with a unique performance purpose.

Shoeing: Injury Versus Protection

Nobody would argue the intrinsic value of a horseshoe to support the foot off the ground and minimize bruising and *contusion*. Still, a shoe may be a necessary evil: it is protective on one hand, and injurious to the foot on the other.

In an unshod foot the heel impacts the ground slightly before the toe, expanding the heel outwards. As a limb bears weight, the short pastern bone compresses against the digital cushion. The digital cushion then pushes against the collateral cartilages, and downwards against the frog that absorbs only a small degree of impact shock. Compression of the digital cushion dissipates energy as heat, transferring it to a profuse network of blood vessels in the digital cushion. The bloodstream removes the heat energy up the leg, away from the foot.

When the toe hits, an upward compressive force is relayed through the horn tubules that make up the hoof wall. These cells absorb a great deal of energy by their spiral, spring-like configuration. Laminae that 'glue' the coffin bone to the hoof wall further resist the downward forces of limb loading by holding the foot together.

The frog contributes to shock absorbance and assists as an anti-slip mechanism.

Alterations Caused by Shoeing

- Shoeing adds weight to the limb, which hastens fatigue.
- The hoof wall is weakened by nails.
- The protective periople is often removed with a rasp, interrupting the moisture retention properties of the hoof.

A shoe alters the expandability of the entire foot, causing it to absorb concussion rather than dissipate the impact through the limb. Heel bruising, sole bruising, coffin bone inflammation *(pedal osteitis)* and laminitis can develop.

Because applying a shoe alters the normal biomechanics within the hoof, it is imperative to fit and size a shoe to accommodate the foot. Long-term, improper balancing of a foot or improper fitting of a shoe leads to a sore foot, sprains, tendon injury or degenerative joint disease.

The hoof should be trimmed and the foot balanced before fitting the shoe.

Shoeing for Protection

Despite the problems mentioned above, unshod horses could not withstand the athletic exertions asked of them. Feet would become too sensitive. The hoof wall would erode so a horse would be weight-bearing on the sole, and stones and rutted ground would severely bruise the feet.

A horse, especially a performance horse, would become crippled. As we ride our horses more rigorously, the foot cannot withstand extended and abrasive wear and tear without a shoe.

Importance of Daily Care

Successful shoeing practices depend on foot care and hygiene by the farrier, and also by the daily caretaker. Picking the hooves daily removes collected wads of manure and pebbles, which may cause sole bruises and lameness. Also, hoof picking prevents overgrowth of bacteria, preventing thrush and canker. During winter in cold climates, remove snowballs from the feet so packed snow and ice won't bruise the sole. During periods of excessive wetness, check that horseshoes are firmly affixed. The sucking action of mud can loosen the nail clinches, twisting the shoe, causing corns, or removing it, causing sole bruises.

Shoes should be taken off and the hoof trimmed at intervals appropriate to each individual horse and *not* related to when the shoe is worn.

Importance of Proper Shoeing

There is no absolute correct angle of the hoof with the ground. The most important rule-of-thumb is that the hoof and pastern are aligned in the same axis angle so they act as a good shock absorber for the limb. If the heel is too low and the toe too long, the hoof–pastern angle is broken. This configuration places excess stress on the navicular apparatus and heels, and on the ligaments of the coffin joint. If the heel is too high and the toe too short, a horse may develop a club-footed appearance which can create bruising at the toe.

A shoe limits normal flexibility of the hoof wall and its spread at the ground surface. Heel expansion is possible because the hoof wall is thinner at the heels and quarters than at the toe. The heels can expand and rebound with weight-bearing. According to biomechanical stress studies, the *extent* of heel expansion is unaffected by a shoe. However, a shod foot expands *faster* than a barefoot hoof, which changes the shock absorption ability of the foot, especially the horn tubules.

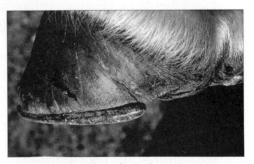

Fig. 4.16 A horizontal crack results from uneven loading across the foot due to a shoe that is too small.

The hoof wall can lose flexibility if:

- a shoe is too small for the foot
- the branches pinch inwards
- the branches do not extend far enough back under the heel to provide weight-bearing support

Stress rings appear at the heels and quarters, or hoof cracks form at the point of compressive loading. Stress rings and cracks are evidence of improper shoeing techniques or poor conformation, resulting in unequal load distribution across the foot.

An appropriately sized shoe applied wide enough at the heels encourages heel expansion. A shoe may also be slippered (bevelled) to encourage the heels to expand with impact. Nails should not be placed behind the widest bend in the quarter of the hoof or heel expansion will be limited.

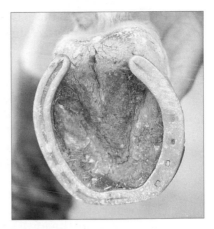

Fig. 4.17 Uneven wear of a shoe due to improper balancing of the foot. This horse also has sheared heels.

Sheared Heels

By studying each foot and its changes over several months, we can appreciate the effects of trimming and shoeing on the hoof. Just as in a barefoot hoof, flares develop on the side of an unbalanced hoof that is least loaded. The heavily loaded side grows hoof wall faster, resulting in a steeper wall. Then the heels may reveal unequal loading stresses, with one heel bulb higher than another. This syndrome is known as *sheared heels,* and can cause lameness if the heel bulbs become unstable. The presence of heels with varying degrees of

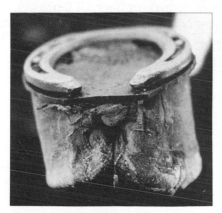

Fig. 4.18 Sheared heels after corrective shoeing.

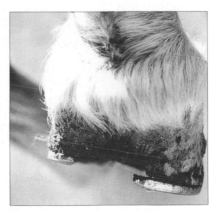

Fig. 4.19 A poorly balanced foot.

hardening, with keratin 'hanging' over the branches of the shoe, can suggest a foot trimming / shoeing problem.

Corrective Shoeing

Balancing the foot from side to side and fore and aft corrects many shoeing problems. The goal is to encourage an equal distribution of weight across all weight-bearing surfaces of the foot. With compressive forces evenly loaded across the foot, no one side of the joints or ligaments receives excess strain.

Once a horse has matured in skeletal growth, 'corrective shoeing' for poor limb conformation can only attempt to balance and level each foot as best as possible. Filing one side of a foot shorter than the other worsens an already less-than-perfect situation, adding *torque* and strain across the joints.

Treating Sole Bruises

Sole bruises are frustrating to treat. Most horses respond within a couple of weeks to soaks in warm water and Epsom salt, anti-inflammatory drugs, and rest. Others require 4–6 months to recover. Crushing of the *subsolar corium* leaks red blood cells which stain the horn. This stain is later visible as a pinkish area on the underside of the foot. Bruises are not always visible at the time of trimming, however, especially in a black foot. In a thicker-footed horse, bruising may occur deep at the level of the coffin bone so the blood pocket *(haematoma)* is not visible in the thick hoof wall.

Not all sole bruising results in overt lameness; instead, performance may suffer. A horse may race slower, or back off fences. A dressage horse may be unwilling to collect and engage the hindquarters. Or, a horse may be reluctant to make sharp, quick turns if active as polo pony.

Treating Corns

An improperly fitted or sized shoe or a foot grown too long between shoeings can result in *corns*. Corns are areas of pressure *necrosis* (tissue death) at the *angle of the wall* and the *bars*. The heel of the shoe applies abnormal pressure to this area if it contacts it. Repeated point loading at the angle of the bar causes deep bruising and blood or serum pockets beneath the sole. Abscesses may develop, and a fluid pocket in the sensitive tissues can cause lameness.

Fitting a shoe wide at the heels and long enough in the branches to eliminate pressure at the angle of the bars prevents corns.

Schedule appropriate shoeing every 4,or up to 6 weeks, and employ a competent farrier who will fit the foot with a properly sized and applied shoe.

Sole bruises or corns can put a horse out of action for a time, and then it may be advantageous to pad, encasing the entire bottom of the foot in a protective capsule. For a normal horse without temporary problems, padding can have some adverse long-term effects.

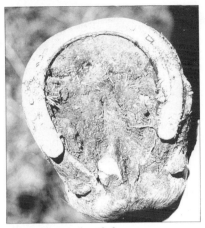

Fig. 4.20 A twisted shoe can cause corns at the angle of the wall.

Padding the Shoe

A still unresolved dilemma exists: to pad or not to pad. There is never one right way to approach a problem, so all sides of the argument should be considered. Pads limit normal expandability of the foot by adding rigidity to an already rigid shoe. On the other hand, some horses have naturally tender feet, flat feet, or low pain thresholds.

Pads as Short-Term Treatments

In some cases it is necessary to do more than just apply a standard shoe to cover the bearing surface of the hoof wall.

Pads may be a necessary therapy for short-term problems, such as healing a:

- sole abscess
- nail puncture
- serious bruise
- pedal osteitis
- corn

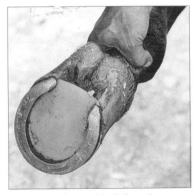

Fig. 4.21 Shoe with full pad.

Effects of Long-Term Padding
Weakened Foot

A full pad decreases focal (specific area) bruising of the subsolar corium and sensitive tissues, and slightly reduces concussion to the foot. However, there is a trade-off: padded feet become pad-dependent. The foot softens and weakens underneath the pad. If a padded foot loses a shoe, the sole is very soft and vulnerable to injury and deep bruising. Nails tend to loosen easily through a pad, so shoes are lost more often.

Sole Flattening

A padded foot softens and lacks support from the ground surface, promoting sole flattening. A foot that starts out properly cupped and concave may flatten with time under a pad. When the pads are removed, soles are susceptible to repeated trauma.

Thrush Development

Moisture under a pad promotes bacterial growth, resulting in thrush. An inadequate seal of the packing material (commonly used are silicone, oakum/pine tar or foam) allows dirt to seep in under the pad. Local pressure points of dirt or pebbles create bruises or abscesses, accompanied by lameness.

Special Cases for Padding

A horse with laminitis, navicular disease or chronic heel pain, or a horse that is prone to bruising from genetically flat feet, may need to wear pads continually. In these cases the benefits may outweigh any detriments. Use should follow discussion between your farrier and veterinary surgeon.

Alternatives to Padding

Consider alternatives before padding a horse's feet. Inactive or stall confined horses develop weak feet that are easily bruised. Turnout and regular exercise strengthen and toughen such feet.

The sole of the foot should be concave, or cupped. Beware the overzealous use of hoof nipper, knife or rasp that removes too much foot, leaving behind a very thin sole. This man-made insult to the foot is avoided with good common sense and caution by a competent farrier.

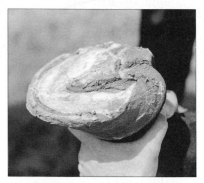

Fig. 4.22 Overzealous trimming causes flat feet where the sole is not concave.

Products with phenol, formalin or iodine are avaiable to harden the hoof. Care must be taken to prevent contact of these products with the skin as they will cause irritation. They are often helpful with sole or frog problems.

Wide-Web Shoes

Wide-web shoes increase protection to the bottom of the foot without the ill effects of a pad. Especially with wide-web shoes, the shoe should not contact the sole. The shoe support should rest only on the weight-bearing hoof wall. The sole is meant to bear only *internal* weight as a limb is loaded and advanced along the ground. Whenever the sole contacts the ground, or a shoe rests on the sole instead of the hoof wall, misapplied stresses can damage the foot.

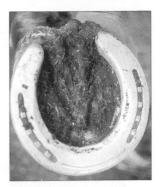

Fig. 4.23 Wide-web shoe.

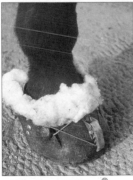

Fig. 4.24 Easy Boot®.

Easy Boots®

For a long distance riding horse, consider using Easy Boots® over the shoe and foot as added protection. These plastic boots withstand rocky terrain, and have been used successfully on 100-mile endurance competitors. The boot must fit well and not contact or abrade soft skin tissue such as the coronary band. Cut away the plastic to fit each foot. Cotton packing behind the heel bulbs prevents small stones and dirt from sifting into the boot.

Rim Pads

Some people believe that rim pads minimize the concussion transmitted by a metal shoe up the legs. A pad between the hoof wall and a shoe does not provide the same energy dissipation offered by an unshod foot. A rim pad does provide a lightweight spacer that raises the sole further from the traumatic ground surface. Rim pads do not exert negative effects on the sole as would a full pad, but remember that nails tend to loosen, and a shoe is more easily lost with any pad. This loss results in trauma and bruising if a shoe is thrown and the foot goes unprotected.

Time and Use

The hoof wall and sole can be strengthened over time. Just as bones in the body strengthen with appropriate stress, the hoof responds to external stimuli. Not only does the foot conform to internal stress, but the hoof also builds stronger horn to accommodate hard ground surfaces. Horses turned out into rocky pastures soon develop tough feet, with stronger soles and hoof walls that are resistant to bruising. These horses are less likely to need pads.

FOOT LAMENESS

Any noticeable lameness or stiffness should receive veterinary attention as soon as possible. Due to the complexity and interaction of the internal structures of the foot, inflammation or trauma of one area can cause a problem in neighbouring tissues. Pain in the feet, along with mechanical damage, adversely affects future performance capabilities.

Laminitis

Equine laminitis, also referred to as *founder*, is a complicated disease with multiple causes. It is a devastating disease deserving immediate veterinary attention. Laminitis varies in degree, from mild to severe, and can seriously jeopardize a horse's productive performance career. Hoof wall rings can signal a serious insult to the health of the foot in the form of laminitis, where the laminae in the foot die and the coffin bone detaches from the hoof wall. A veterinary examination with radiographic evaluation determines whether the source of hoof wall rings is due to laminitis, or simply to uneven concussive stresses, nutrition, fever or seasonal growth spurts.

Characteristics of Laminitis

An affected horse appears 'stiff' in the front end, or shifts its weight from foot to foot. Severe cases may not move and often show signs similar to colic. The horse is often reluctant to move, and places both hind legs well under its body to shift weight from the painful front feet to the hind legs. This weight shift is amplified as the horse is asked to turn. A mildly affected

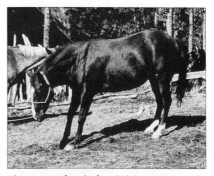

Fig. 4.25 Classic laminitis stance.

horse appears to 'walk on eggs.' Immediate damage must be attended promptly and the underlying problem corrected.

Causes of Laminitis

Understanding the anatomical relationships within the foot helps to explain the disease process. Internal parts of a horse's foot receive oxygen through a branching network of blood vessels. The main vessels run down the leg towards the foot. At the coronary band they branch into smaller divisions. The *dorsal laminar arteries* feed the front of the foot as branches of the *circumflex artery* that runs around the bottom of the coffin bone. A latticework of tissue and blood vessels called *laminae* (hence *laminitis)* support the coffin bone within the hoof wall. For blood to reach sensitive laminae in the front of the foot, it must flow *against* gravity, with blood moving upwards from the bottom of the foot.

Any *systemic* disease affecting the entire body that interrupts blood flow to the foot causes an inflammatory crisis within the laminae. Toxins which have been ingested or the result of a disease or disorders may have a similar effect. Blood and oxygen supplies are reduced to the tissues while blood pressure elevates. A pounding arterial pulse is felt in the lower limb. Constricted vessels shunt blood and oxygen away from the laminar structures in the foot. Decreasing oxygen circulation in the foot causes the laminae to die. Then there is nothing to counteract the weight of the horse and the pull of the deep digital flexor tendon that at-

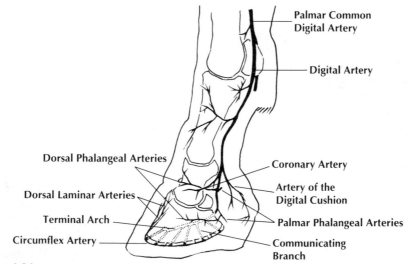

Palmar Common Digital Artery

Digital Artery

Dorsal Phalangeal Arteries

Coronary Artery

Artery of the Digital Cushion

Dorsal Laminar Arteries

Terminal Arch

Palmar Phalangeal Arteries

Circumflex Artery

Communicating Branch

Fig. 4.26

taches to the back of the coffin bone. The toe creates a lever effect, further amplifying the pull from the tendon. The coffin bone detaches from the hoof wall.

Without its supportive laminar attachments, the coffin bone can rotate or sink to the bottom of the sole. In a very severe case, the bone may perforate the bottom of the foot. If the laminitic process is halted early, rotation of the coffin bone may be prevented. However, in some cases, it can rotate as soon as 3 hours after the laminae begin to swell.

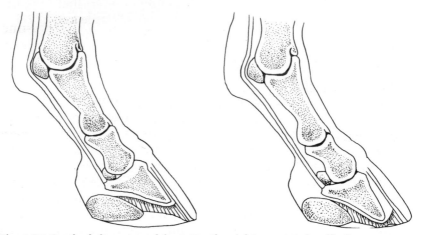

Fig. 4.27 On the left, a normal foot. On the right, a rotated coffin bone.

Metabolic Problems

Whenever normal metabolic functions are altered, laminitis can follow. Stress from transport or disease can cause laminitis. Diarrhoea, septicaemic infections (overwhelming bacterial infections) or kidney or liver diseases have noticeable effects on the amount of *endotoxins* produced. When excess amounts of these toxins circulate in the bloodstream, the liver is unable to neutralize all of it. A discussion of the gut environment will help to provide an understanding of endotoxins and their role in laminitis.

Environment of the Gut

Bacterial flora that normally reside in a horse's bowel live in a delicately balanced ecosystem. The food a horse eats influences this environment, with the bacteria slowly adapting to small dietary changes. Rapid overeating of carbohydrate-rich grains promotes overpopulation by *Lactobacillus* organisms. The pH within the intestine changes to an acid environment.

Horses that normally receive grain, such as performance horses, are particularly at risk when suddenly fed an over-generous amount. A normal population of these acid-producing microorganisms already lives in the presence of highly fermentable grain. Grain-fed horses typically already have a mild acid environment in their intestines, with conditions primed for impending disaster.

An acid environment disrupts the fragile one-cell barrier between the cavity of the bowel and the blood vessels in the intestinal wall. As the pH continues to decline, other residents of the intestines (the Gram-negative bacteria) die. The cell wall of Gram-negative organisms contains poisonous components called endotoxins. The death of these microorganisms due to the intestine's acid environment rapidly releases endotoxins into the large intestine where they are absorbed throughout the body.

Role of Endotoxins

The body is consistently exposed to endotoxins as small amounts are released into the bloodstream with the normal, daily death of small numbers of Gram-negative bacteria. Under normal circumstances, the liver detoxifies endotoxins, and local immune responses inactivate them.

Excess endotoxins exert profound effects. If a horse absorbs an overwhelming amount of endotoxins due to a carbohydrate overload or an underlying metabolic problem, and if the body is previously sensitized to endotoxins as with grain fed horses, a massive immune response results. The immune response creates havoc to the blood supply to the feet and causes founder.

Colic

Colic associated with changes in the normal movement of the intestines also stimulates bacterial overgrowth, and therefore endotoxin production. The harmful effects of endotoxin are felt throughout the horse's body; small blood vessels constrict, including those in the feet.

Occasionally, an overheated or exhausted horse experiences metabolic problems that alter normal blood flow and disrupt the laminar integrity of the foot.

Overweight Horses

Unfortunately, many in the horse-show world favour overweight horses, and these horses are predisposed to laminitis. Obese horses are prime candidates for founder. These horses suffer from metabolic problems involving a low tolerance for glucose and carbohydrate intake. If a horse consumes a carbohydrate overload in the form of excess grain or rich alfalfa, it is at high risk for founder.

Retained Placenta

A broodmare that has foaled yet retained the placenta for more than 3 – 4 hours after birth is susceptible to laminitis. Endotoxins are absorbed from the uterus into the bloodstream as the placenta decomposes and infection develops.

Pituitary Disorder

Older horses sometimes develop a tumour of the pituitary gland in the brain. *Pituitary adenomas* cause an imbalance in neurotransmitter chemicals and hormones, causing excess production of corticosteroids. Overproduction of steroids, (or too much pharmaceutical steroids) ultimately causes increased glucose in the bloodstream, which can precipitate laminitis. These horses easily go unrecognized. A coarse, shaggy coat

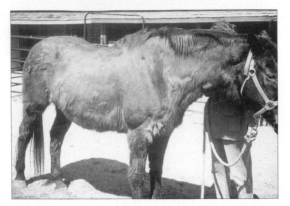

Fig. 4.28 A coarse, shaggy coat that fails to shed out may be a sign of a pituitary adenoma.

that fails to shed out, or a horse that drinks and urinates excessively, may be the only signs of this problem.

Road Founder

Laminitis is also caused by mechanical factors. 'Road founder' develops from trauma and bruising of the laminae after vigorous exercise on hard, concussive surfaces. Feet that are excessively trimmed or worn are easily traumatized. Stone bruises or nail punctures that result in infection or foot abscesses can also cause laminitis.

Support Founder

'Support founder' weight-bearing laminitis results from an injury, such as a fracture, to a leg that renders it inactive for months at a time. Blood flow stagnates in the opposite, uninjured limb, and with excessive weight-bearing the 'good' foot may founder.

Recognizing Chronic Laminitis

A dished contour to the hoof wall or 'laminitic rings' indicate that the horse has experienced prior inflammatory incidents. Horn tubules of the foot normally grow in a straight, nearly vertical line from the coronary band. When the coffin bone is compressed downwards or rotates within the hoof wall during a laminitic crisis, the horn-generating coronary corium is compressed and trapped between the hoof wall and the *extensor process*. The extensor process is a bony protrusion at the top of the coffin bone to which the extensor tendon attaches.

Horn tubules at the top of the hoof wall bend at steep angles, further crushing the sensitive coronary tissue and reducing the blood supply. Once the coronary corium is compressed and its blood supply is limited, oxygen deprivation of the tissues alters growth of the hoof wall in the front third of the foot.

Horn tubules then grow out deformed. Toe growth slows considerably due to misalignment of the horn tubules from the coronary corium. The result is divergent growth planes in the hoof wall.

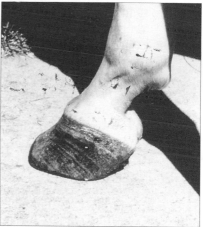

Extensive collateral circulation in the heels allows them to grow at a normal rate. Unless corrective measures are taken, the front of the hoof wall develops a dish shape, also indicating an internal deformity in the coffin bone.

A horse with chronic laminitis records the decreased circulation to the front of the foot on the hoof wall. The insensitive laminar layer excessively keratinizes as the toe grows out slowly. Thick, irregular ridges form across the wall, parallel to the

Fig. 4.29 A dished hoof wall is a sign of chronic laminitis.

coronary band. New hoof growth follows these growth planes, maintaining the telltale laminitic rings and dished wall.

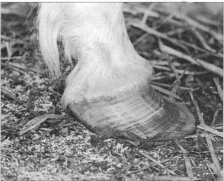

Realignment of the horn tubules along this distorted path causes dehydration of the hoof wall, and loss of its elastic properties. With laminitis, circulation to the front of the hoof is reduced. Loss of an internal source of moisture contributes to drying of the hoof wall.

Fig. 4.30 Rings are also a sign of chronic laminitis.

Altered blood flow, dehydration, and reduced weight-bearing due to pain inevitably lead to contraction of the entire foot, as well as a deformed appearance of the wall. The hoof wall tells a story of daily internal and external stresses which shape its strength and outward appearance.

Therapy for Laminitis

There is no single recipe for therapy for laminitis; each case must be tailored to the severity of the crisis and the unique metabolic problem of the horse. Many medical therapies are discussed, and tried with varying success. Basic steps can be taken upon recognition of a crisis:

- Call a veterinarian to attend to the cause.
- Eliminate rich feed (grain, alfalfa, pasture) from the diet to prevent an acidic intestinal environment.
- Put an overweight horse on a diet to reduce metabolic upset, and to reduce weight on the compromised feet.
- Non-steroidal anti-inflammatory drugs (flunixin or, phenylbutazone) counteract pain and inflammation, and flunixin is also beneficial against the effect of endotoxins.
- Provide sandy bedding, as sand provides a cushion under the sole and helps support the foot.
- Apply a circle, or a heart bar shoe, possibly with special pads or wedges under the frog to support the coffin bone.
- Confine the horse so movement does not continue to tear the laminae. Confinement may be necessary for a month or more.
- Warm or cold foot soaks are controversial. While cold soaks reduce pain, they tend to constrict blood vessels. Warm soaks enhance the inflammatory process, yet dilate the capillary beds and vessels within the foot.
- X-ray films are useful after about 24 hours to evaluate the degree of rotation of the coffin bone within the hoof, and to aid corrective hoof trimming to reduce stress on the laminae.

Treating Overconsumption of Grain

Horses that manage to enter a feed room and overindulge in grain can be treated prophylactically (a prevention) against colic or laminitis by a veterinarian if discovered within 8 – 12 hours.

Mineral Oil

Stomach tubing with mineral oil limits fermentation of grain within the intestines and minimizes development of an acid environment. Mineral oil coats the bowel to reduce absorption of endotoxins. An oil coating also protects the fragile intestinal cells from disruption by acids and endotoxins. Its laxative effect aids in rapid elimination of the rich foodstuffs.

NSAIDs

Non-steroidal anti-inflammatory drugs (NSAIDs) block the progression of the inflammation contributing to the crisis and provide pain relief. Finadyne® may also help to counteract the effects of endotoxin.

Managing Laminitis

Immediate care dramatically affects the outcome and prognosis of the disease. Because the foot grows continually, laminitis is often managed suc-

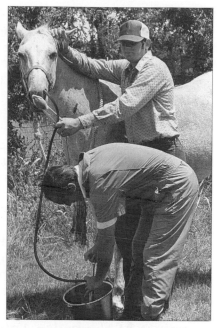

Fig. 4.31 Stomach tubing with mineral oil.

cessfully. As a foot grows out, the diseased tissue is removed in successive trimmings.

Preventing Rotation of Coffin Bone

The therapeutic goal is to prevent the bone from rotating or sinking within the hoof wall. This goal is accomplished by the following, either individually or in combination with one or more of these measures:

- vigorous medical management
- corrective trimming and shoeing
- thick wedge pads to relieve the pull from the deep digital flexor tendon
- bar shoes to provide a base of support to the foot

Feet with a rotated coffin bone are frustrating to treat and may never resume normal athletic function.

Preventing Laminitis

A well balanced ration and consistent exercise and turnout are key ingredients to a horse's health. Consult with a veterinarian about dietary management, weight control, foot hygiene and health. Good management and a general physical exam can obviate many of the causes of founder. Great care must be taken to avoid overfeeding in spring and early summer when grass is at its most nutritious. It may be necessary to restrict access to grass severely.

Navicular Disease

Any interference with normal limb function impairs a horse's performance. The athletic horse is subject to a variety of lameness problems. One disease that can develop in the actively working horse involves the *navicular apparatus* of the foot: the *navicular bone, navicular bursa*, and the deep digital flexor tendon. Conformation and the type of athletic endeavour equally contribute, but there is strong evidence that improper shoeing can predispose a horse to navicular disease. Horses that perform rigorous, concussive activities such as racing, jumping or polo absorb considerable impact in their feet. It is essential that their feet be balanced and appropriately shod.

Structure of Navicular Apparatus

The navicular bone is a shuttle-shaped bone wedged between the coffin bone and the deep digital flexor tendon in the foot. The flexor tendon passes behind the navicular bone, attaching to the back of the coffin bone. Between the navicular bone and the tendon is a bursa that provides a smooth gliding surface for the tendon. The bottom *(flexor)* surface of the navicular bone is also smooth, and enhances the gliding effect.

The top *(articular)* surface of the navicular bone increases the surface area of the coffin joint. Increasing the surface area of this joint decreases the concussive load on it as the limb impacts the ground. The top of the coffin bone is supported by ligaments that anchor to the wings of the navicular bone. These ligamentous supports, along with the deep digital flexor tendon below,

Navicular Bone

Navicular Bursa

Deep Digital
Flexor Tendon

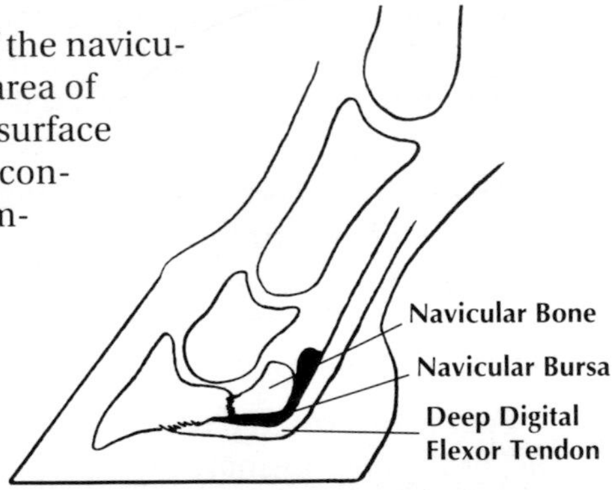

Fig. 4.32 The navicular apparatus.

maintain the position of the navicular bone within the foot.

Inflammatory changes involving the navicular apparatus, including the bone, bursa, tendons and ligaments, damage the surface of the flexor tendon that contacts the navicular bursa. This may develop from increased pressure between the bone and the tendon, or from local tendon strain. Tendon fibres may rupture and roughen. The roughened tendon erodes the flexor surface of the navicular bone, compromising the smooth gliding motion of the tendon and causing pain and lameness.

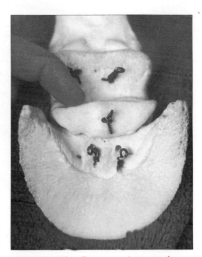

Fig. 4.33 The finger points to the navicular bone.

Characteristics of Navicular

Navicular disease commonly occurs in Thoroughbred, Standardbred and Warmblood breeds, and in Quarter Horses, although no breed is immune to the disease. It is not a genetically transmissible disease, but certain conformational traits predispose to it and bone and conformational structure are heritable traits. A horse with a straight shoulder, upright pastern and small feet is prone to develop the disease. Similarly, a flatfooted horse with a low heel is also at risk.

The disease usually surfaces between 4 and 9 years of age, but can occur in any age of horse. It typically affects both front feet, although one may be more painful than the other. Lameness may be intermittent, and may appear at different times in each foot. It develops slowly over time, and is aggravated by hard work, while rest alleviates the symptoms. An affected horse may point an aching foot in front of it, with the heel elevated slightly off the ground. It may shift its weight back and forth between sore feet. Lameness is exaggerated on hard packed surfaces or hills, and eased by soft, level ground.

Navicular disease is a typical form of lameness which sometimes shows characteristic radiographic changes in the navicular bone. However, these changes do not always correspond with the presence or symptoms of navicular disease.

Navicular Stride

The typical stride of a 'navicular horse' is short and choppy to reduce the impact upon the sore heels. The horse stumbles frequently. Some horses try to land toe first, instead of landing with the normal placement of heel first. These individuals are prone to bruised toes, and a sole abscess can develop with severe bruising.

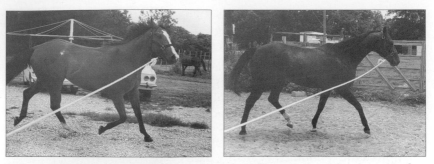

Fig. 4.34 On the left, a normal horse lands heel first. On the right, the navicular horse tries to land toe first.

Change in Foot Size

As the disease progresses, one or both forefeet may appear noticeably smaller, with the heel contracted and drawn in. The frog appears shrunken and diseased. It is sometimes hard to tell if a foot is contracted if both forefeet are affected. A contracted heel represents underlying pain in the foot that forces a horse to reduce the normal weight-bearing load on that foot.

Theories on Navicular Development

Concussion Theory

One explanation speculates that excess concussion between the navicular bone and the deep digital flexor tendon results in inflammation of the bursa, coffin joint, and associated structures. Inflammation stimulates demineralization and thinning of the navicular bone. Normally, concussion is not a problem because structures like the horn tubules, frog, and collateral cartilages dissipate energy from the foot.

The concussion theory also suggests that poor hoof conformation or trimming creates vibrations and oscillations within the structures of the foot. Friction produced between the bone and the tendon cause fraying and degeneration of both structures.

Impaired Blood Supply

A second but unsubstantiated theory blames an impaired blood supply to the navicular bone as a prime factor in navicular disease. Damage to the ligaments attached to the navicular bone may interfere with blood supply, as blood vessels enter through this region. Lack of oxygen from a reduced blood flow creates pain and furthers the disease process in the navicular bone. Experiments have attempted to prove this theory, with no success.

A Current Theory

Dr Roy Pool (University of California at Davis) has developed a 'unifying' theory that combines several previous theories to explain the events leading to navicular disease. Bone is a dynamic organ, continually remodelling in response to exercise and stress. When excess pressure is placed on the navicular bone, inflammation and microscopic swelling in the bone amplify the remodelling process.

Compression between the bone and the deep digital flexor tendon stimulates remodelling activity. Cells that demineralize the bone outstrip the ability of bone builders to produce new bone. 'Holes' form in areas where the tendon has compressed the navicular bone, and the defect is filled in with granulation tissue. Scar tissue forming between the tendon and the bone is called an *adhesion*. Adhesions limit the mechanical efficiency of the limb and create pain as they continually tear when the horse moves.

Damage to the deep digital flexor tendon where it contacts the navicular bursa develops from increased pressure between the bone and the tendon, or from local tendon strain. Some tendon fibres may tear and roughen. Roughened tendon erodes the flexor surface of the navicular bone, and compromises the smooth gliding motion of the tendon.

Joint Inflammation Theory

A further clarification of the disease progression has been proposed by Dr Paul W. Poulos of the University of Florida. He suggests that vigorous work and poor shoeing lead to inflammation of the joints next to the navicular bone. Joint inflammation causes the *synovial membrane* (the lining of the joint) to swell and infiltrate the navicular bone. The membrane remains permanently embedded in the navicular bone. Eventually, the bone and flexor tendon adhere to one another, spurs develop on the bone, and ligamentous attachments lose their flexibility. Deterioration progresses, as does lameness.

Improper Shoeing Theory

Excess concussion and trauma to the heel occur as a result of shoeing in a long-toe – low-heel (LTLH) configuration, which works to a mechanical disadvantage for a horse. Of horses with navicular disease, 77% have a low, under-run heel. A low heel increases the pressure between the navicular bone and the deep digital flexor tendon. It reduces the weight-bearing surface area, therefore the foot is less able to absorb impact. The horn tubules grow horizontally which lessens their ability to absorb energy. The centre of gravity of the foot is moved forwards, shifting an excessive amount of concussion to the heels. A low

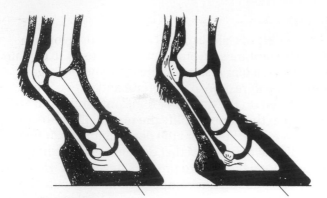

heel also places extra strain on the other ligaments and tendons in the back of the leg and foot.

A long toe lengthens the lever arm, making it more difficult for a horse to move the foot. The limb fatigues faster. Tendinitis develops from strain of the flexor support structures, especially of the deep digital flexor tendon.

Fig. 4.35 On the left, a normal foot. On the right, an LTLH foot configuration strains the flexor tendons.

In an LTLH foot, the hoof-pastern axis angle is broken. This places excess tension on the deep digital flexor tendon, further compressing the navicular bone. An unbalanced foot forces uneven stress on the joints and all internal structures of the foot. The difference between a correct angle and an incorrect angle can be subtle to the untrained

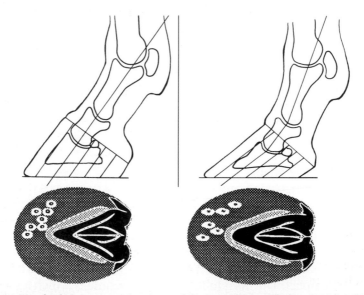

Fig. 4.36 On the left, a properly trimmed foot and horn tubules. On the right, an LTLH foot and elongated horn tubules.

eye, but over time the incorrectly shod horse will develop lameness problems. Increased and uneven loading on an unbalanced foot predisposes to navicular disease, or it worsens an already existing condition.

Diagnostic Tests for Navicular

Diagnosis of navicular disease is not a clear-cut issue. To classify a horse as truly navicular, an obvious

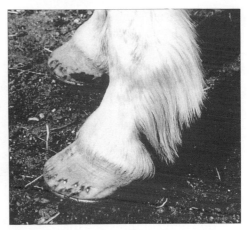

Fig. 4.37 An LTLH configuration.

lameness or stilted gait should be apparent. Many criteria are used to diagnose the disease and make a prognosis for continued athletic function. Gathering all diagnostic information enables a veterinarian to make a clinical diagnosis. A horse may be diagnosed with true navicular disease if it demonstrates some of the following symptoms:

- characteristic lameness with pottery gait
- sensitivity to hoof testers over the heel
- trotting off lame after flexion of the foot
- lameness improves with palmar digital nerve blocks, but switches to the opposite foot

A veterinarian's clinical experience may support a judgement despite lack of fulfilment of all criteria. For example, disease of the digital cushion, heel bulbs, collateral cartilages, presence of an abscess or corn, or thrush must be ruled out before claiming disease of the navicular apparatus.

Hoof Tester

Hoof testers are specially shaped 'pliers' that pinch specific areas of the foot. A horse's response to the testers allows a veterinarian to localize the source of pain, and to suggest appropriate therapy. A hoof tester applied across the heels, or between the centre of the frog and the hoof

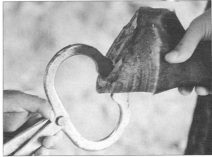

Fig. 4.38 Hoof testers help locate the source of pain.

wall, often elicits pain from a diseased horse, but not always.

Flexion Test

Another diagnostic test is called a 'flexion test'. The coffin and pastern joints are tightly flexed for 1–2 minutes, and the horse is trotted off. In a navicular horse, flexion of the coffin joint exaggerates lameness by increasing the tension on the deep digital flexor tendon and compressing the navicular bursa and bone. A similarly effective method asks a horse to stand on a block to elevate only its heel, and then the horse is trotted off the block to evaluate change in lameness.

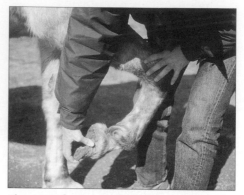

Fig. 4.39 Flexion test.

Nerve Block

As a diagnostic workup continues, local anesthetic is injected into the *palmar digital nerves* on both sides of the lower pastern to create a *nerve block*. If a lame horse improves from this particular nerve block, then the source of pain is the back one-third of the foot. However, other structures are present there besides the navicular apparatus.

With navicular disease, a nerve block of one foot often improves the gait in that limb, only to accentuate lameness in the opposite limb.

The Role of X-Ray Films in Navicular Diagnosis

Once the source of pain is localized to the navicular region, a veterinarian may pursue radiographic analysis. Multiple views of X-ray films show all contours of the navicular bone. Irregular and rough contours may support evidence for disease of the navicular apparatus. A fracture of the navicular bone can also be identified on X-ray film.

X-ray films do not always show changes in the bone typical of navicular disease. The reverse is also true: many horses show radiographic 'lesions', only to be totally sound and free of navicular disease. For example, normal wear-and-tear lesions show up on X-ray films in an ageing horse. These lesions must be distinguished from a disease process, so a horse is not unnecessarily condemned.

Too often navicular X-ray films are used to determine a 'no or go' on the purchase of a potential athlete. Keep in mind that some horses may have sore heels due to incorrect shoeing. X-ray films must only be used to corroborate the clinical picture. Occasionally, a horse meets the clinical criteria but shows no radiographic changes despite obvious evidence of navicular or coffin joint disease. Only 60% of cases with clinical lameness correlate with radiographic evidence.

Lollipop Lesions

Changes in the size, number and configuration of the blood vessel channels on the flexor surface of the navicular bone indicate disease of the coffin joint. Mushroom-shaped holes in the bone are called 'lollipop lesions' where synovial tissue (resulting from coffin joint inflammation) has infiltrated the navicular bone. Like an old scar, these lesions may reflect a current or a resolved problem. Although coffin joint disease and navicular disease are related, lollipop lesions do not necessarily indicate navicular disease.

Cystic Lesions

Cystic lesions in the navicular bone represent severe inflammatory disease accompanied by demineralization of the bone and adhesions resulting from coffin joint inflammation. The presence of large cysts in the navicular bone indicates an active degenerative process.

Bone Spurring

Spurring on the wings of the navicular bone as seen on X-ray film represents damage to ligaments due to the stress of exercise, abnormal foot conformation, or fatigue. This change is seen in older horses with many years and miles of exercise, without accompanying lameness or navicular disease. However, in a young horse bone spurring may indicate navicular disease. It is also likely to be of greater importance if present in a young horse.

Navicular Bone Thinning

Thinning of the flexor surface of the navicular bone reveals tendinous adhesions and erosion of the cartilage. This radiographic change is seen with 80% of horses with navicular disease, and may be the only radiographic image that corresponds to damage from the navicular disease.

All horses respond to pain differently. Some may experience navicular disease, yet have too much heart to quit. Other individuals cannot tolerate even small degrees of pain, and their usefulness for performance is limited.

Management Techniques For Navicular Disease

Therapy for a horse with navicular disease is aimed at *reducing pain,* and should not be misconstrued as a *cure.* The disease is a degenerative process, and will progress over time.

Corrective Shoeing

Corrective shoeing improves over 50% of affected horses, but it may take up to 4 months for results to be appreciated. Balance of the foot is essential to therapy. The foot should land flat, with a horse's weight distributed equally over all weight-bearing structures of the foot. A properly balanced foot not only relieves pain, but prevents development or progression of navicular disease.

If a rod is dropped perpendicularly through the centre of the cannon bone, it should drop just behind the heel bulbs. This area is where a horse needs the base of support. The ends of the shoe should extend past the heels of the foot, ending approximately $\frac{5}{8}$ of an inch in front of the heel bulb at most.

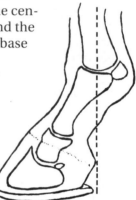

Many shoes are incorrectly affixed with the branches ending 2 inches or more before the back of the heel bulbs. Affixing a shoe this way creates a long-toe – low-heel effect and a broken hoof–pastern axis angle, which amplifies heel concussion. If a shoe is too small for the foot, as the foot hits the ground it will drop backwards with the body weight be-

Fig. 4.40 A perpendicular line lands behind the heel.

hind it, increasing tension on the deep digital flexor tendon and compressing the tendon and bone.

An appropriately sized large shoe provides ample heel extension. The shoe can be applied wide enough at the heels to encourage heel expansion. A shoe may also be slippered (bevelled) to encourage the heels to expand with impact.

Consistent trimming is important. As a foot grows, the toe lengthens faster than the heels, placing additional stress on the deep digital flexor tendon. Excess toe must be removed every 5 – 8 weeks to remove its lever arm effect.

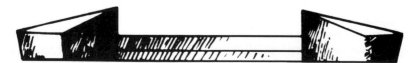

Fig. 4.41 Rear view of a slippered shoe, which encourages heel expansion.

Rolled Toe and Raised Heel

To move the centre of gravity back in line with the skeletal column, the toe is shortened and rolled to 'shorten the wheelbarrow'. Allowing the force to pass through the bony skeletal column decreases the load on the deep digital flexor tendon, and more quickly 'dumps the load' by making it easier for the foot to lift and break over.

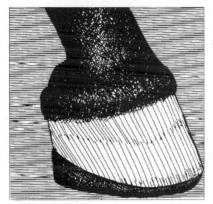

Fig. 4.42 A shoe with a rolled toe and raised heel.

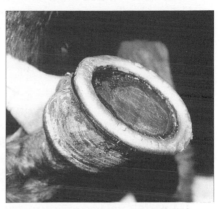

Fig. 4.43 Egg-bar shoe with full pad.

Bar Shoe

A bar shoe stabilizes the heel region and reduces trauma. Bone demineralization is reduced fivefold by applying bar shoes to a navicular horse. The shoe should be long and wide at the heels to increase the surface area of contact with the ground, and to encourage hoof expansion for enhanced circulation in the foot. A wedge pad, which is a full pad that is thicker at the heel than at the toe, reduces heel concussion, and relieves tension on the deep digital flexor tendon.

The equine foot is a sensitive gauge for exactness of technique. A slight deviation in the balance of the foot or shoe causes corrective shoeing to fail as a therapeutic aid.

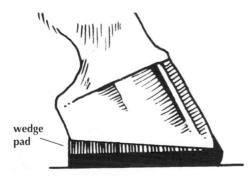

wedge pad

Fig. 4.44 A wedge pad reduces heel concussion.

Exercise Programme

Another important aspect in managing horses with navicular disease is an exercise programme of at least 2 – 4 miles a day, or 30 minutes a day, rather than applying the old theory of stall rest and confinement. Rest seems to aggravate the problem. Daily exercise reduces the formation of scar tissue and adhesions of the flexor tendon, while a horse maintains fitness, flexibility and ample foot circulation. Confinement causes affected horses to move stiffly despite efforts of corrective shoeing. In a young horse which is showing signs similar to navicular disease it is advisable to turn it away until the following year.

NSAIDs

Non-steroidal anti-inflammatory drugs relieve both pain and the inflammatory process. Low levels of phenylbutazone or Finadyne® may allow a horse to work comfortably and relatively pain-free. These medications also temporarily arrest the deterioration process.

Vasodilatory Drugs

A peripheral vasodilatory drug called *isoxsuprine hydrochloride* has been used with varying success. It appears to be most effective if administered early in the disease. This drug promotes blood supply in the lower limb to improve the blood flow in the foot, and it has mild anti-inflammatory effects. Isoxsuprine is relatively free of side effects, but it should not be used for pregnant mares.

Neurectomy

Some horses do not respond to any of the above mentioned therapies. These horses may be candidates for a *neurectomy*. This involves cutting the palmar digital nerves on both sides of the pastern. Cutting the nerve prevents the transmission of pain from the foot to the brain. The palmar digital nerve is the same nerve that is injected with local anaesthetic to arrive at a diagnosis. Whatever the degree of gait improvement achieved by the nerve block will be the maximum improvement gained by a neurectomy.

Neurectomies are not without complications, which should be seriously considered. Possible problems include:

- A *neuroma* can form at the surgical site, causing a painful lump of nerve tissue, again resulting in lameness.
- The palmar digital nerve can regenerate over time and defeat the surgery.
- Occasionally, stray nerve branches of the palmar digital nerve

provide enough sensation to the heel to prevent a complete return to soundness.
• Rarely, the deep digital flexor tendon ruptures, or circulation to
the entire foot may be disrupted, causing the hoof to slough off.

A neurectomized horse cannot feel the back third of its foot, but it
retains complete sensitivity in the
other two-thirds. The owner of a
neurectomized horse should recognize that if the horse steps on a
nail in the heel, it will be unaware
of it. It will not feel abscesses in
the back third of its foot, and a
fracture of the navicular bone will
go unnoticed. These are the risks
taken with a 'nerved' horse hence
neurectomy and should only be
done after careful consideration of
the risks.

Navicular disease continues to
be one of the more frustrating
lameness problems to manage.
Time, cost, and emotional involvement in training a performance horse are major
investments. A veterinary
prepurchase exam can steer a pro-

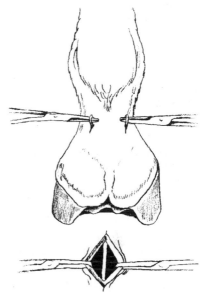

Fig. 4.45 Nerving incision site.

spective buyer away from identifiable problem horses or conformational predispositions to foot disease.

5

PROTECTING THE RESPIRATORY SYSTEM

The overall health of the equine respiratory system is as essential to optimal performance as a sound set of legs. The unique anatomy of the equine nasal cavity, pharynx, and larynx is an evolutionary structure of sophisticated aerodynamic design. It means that with each breath a horse fuels its body with vital oxygen so it can perform to its optimum athletic capabilities.

Respiratory health dictates stamina, and contributes to mental willingness. The lungs must pull in oxygen to fuel the musculoskeletal tissues, heart, liver, kidneys and intestinal tract, parts of the equine machine each of which depends on the others for optimal performance.

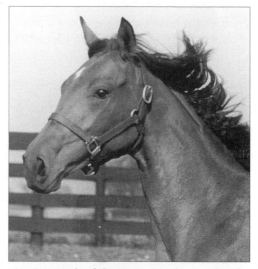

Fig. 5.1 Much of the space in a horse's head is dedicated to respiration.

The respiratory tract, or airway, is a two-part system.(Fig. 5.2.) The upper airways include all structures from the nostrils to the *thorax*. (The thorax is the part of the body between the neck and the abdomen.) These structures are the nasal passages, pharynx, larynx, and trachea. The lower airways resemble a tree, as larger *bronchi* branch over and over again into smaller *bronchioles*, ending in air saccules *(alveoli)* within the lungs.

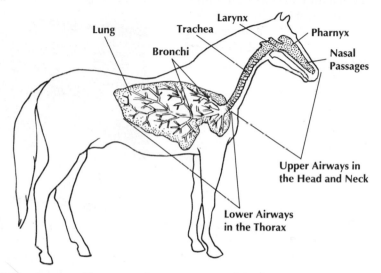

Fig. 5.2 The upper and lower respiratory systems of the horse.

ACCOMMODATING AIR FLOW

The equine body has developed special adaptations to best accommodate air flow. Air is a mixture of gases, the most important of which is oxygen. As a horse inhales, its rib cage and thorax expand to create a negative pressure, or vacuum, within the thorax. Air then flows into the nostrils, along the nasal passages, over the soft palate and through the pharynx, through the larynx, down the trachea, and into the lungs. In the alveoli, oxygen is exchanged for carbon dioxide.

Due to differences between the relatively positive atmospheric pressure outside and the negative pressure inside the thorax, twice as much energy is required for the horse to inhale as to exhale. With any suction force, structures surrounding the airway would tend to collapse. Yet the equine respiratory tract is protected from such dynamic collapse in many ways. For example, the nasal cavity is supported largely by bone. Special dilating muscles in the nostrils, the nasopharynx above the soft palate and the larynx also help to overcome the suction force of inhalation. The larynx is suspended from the base of the skull by a rigid bony scaffold called the *hyoid apparatus.*

The trachea is kept spread and open by reinforcement with rings of cartilage. A strap muscle *(sternothyrohyoideus)* extends from under the sternum (the breastbone in the chest, running between the fore-legs), up the chest and along the underside of the neck to attach onto the hyoid apparatus. Contractions of this muscle bundle keep the trachea and larynx open under athletic demand. This muscle group is visible as a bulging strap along the underside of the neck in the horse that travels with head up and back hollowed. Contractions of the diaphragm, which is a dome-shaped muscle behind and beneath the lungs, additionally enlarge the airways and keep the trachea open. The airway's inter-connected tissue framework en-ables it to operate in response to oxygen demand. Man-made im-positions of hardware in the mouth, head carriage and weight-carrying change normal breathing functions.

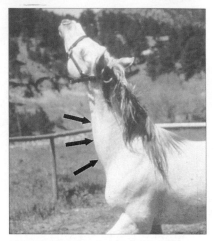

Fig. 5.3 The strap muscle is visible when the horse throws its head back.

Size of the Airways

The size of the air passages directly influences the efficiency of air flow. According to the laws of physics, air flows best down a straight, circular tube with smooth, rigid and preferably parallel walls.

Resistance to air flow is dramatically affected by the diameter of the tube. For example, if the diameter of the tube is increased to twice its original size, air flow is *sixteen times* as efficient. Therefore, if the horse's airways are as straight and smooth as possible, with minimal bends or obstructions, air flow is optimized, the oxygen demand is met, and performance is enhanced.

Inflammation of the airway with swelling or mucus, any mechani-cal obstruction (such as roaring, chronic pharyngitis, soft palate hy-pertrophy, nasal polyps, etc.), or any bend in the airway functionally creates a smaller diameter and therefore greater air flow resistance.

In a normal horse that does not suffer from respiratory disease or mechanical obstructions of the airways, the upper airway still creates more than half of the total air flow resistance.

Air Flow and Exercise

The mechanics of breathing in the exercising horse are quite different from the resting horse, because more oxygen is needed to metabolically support the body in exertion. The anatomy of the pharynx, larynx, and trachea require the exercising horse to stretch out its neck and head. For example, a horse at play that is running in the field, or a determined racehorse as it speeds down the track, extends the head and neck forwards. This position streamlines the airway, minimizing air flow resistance.

Streamlining the Airways

Certain anatomical events occur for an exercising horse to maximize air flow. The nostrils dilate to improve air intake. Erectile tissue in the nose is abundant in blood vessels that constrict, further widening the nasal passages and limiting air flow resistance down the airway.

When the horse extends its head and neck, the airway is straightened out, eliminating bends and turbulence. Also, the elastic mucosa lining the top and bottom walls of the nasopharynx and larynx is stretched, providing a smoother surface and reducing air flow resistance.

Small muscles hold the soft palate down and the roof of the nasopharynx up, but these muscles are somewhat weak and need head and neck extension to prevent fatigue.

As the larynx outwardly expands and opens, the airway into the trachea is smoothed to limit resistance. During exercise, a normal larynx expands its cross-sectional area three times wider than at rest.

Flexion at the Poll and Neck

Partial flexion of the head and neck, required by show jumping and dressage, restricts this airway streamlining by creating a bend in the airway. When a horse is asked to flex at the poll and neck to improve its balance and impulsion, it is no wonder that the horse reacts with mental resistance and evasion as it struggles to optimize its air flow. The horse attempts to maintain air flow by carrying itself 'upside down' with the neck arched towards the ground and the back hollowed. This upside-down carriage allows it to extend the head and neck, opening the airways.

When a horse is trained to go on the bit, it loses some of its airway freedom. The upper and lower walls of the nasopharynx are relaxed and flaccid. (This causes air to vibrate in the pharynx and results in noise.) If the head is maintained in this flexed position while faster and more difficult demands are asked of the horse, it may not be able to perform to its utmost due to lack of oxygen.

Meeting the Air Demand

Because the horse is strictly a nose-breathing animal, physical adaptations accommodate the demand for air at speed. In the back of the mouth, a sheet of tissue arises from the bottom of the hard palate and extends backwards and up across the nasopharynx. This sheet of tissue is called the *soft palate*, and a hole *(ostium)* at the back of it provides a 'buttonhole' through which the larynx fits.

For normal respiration, there must be a perfect air-tight fit between the soft palate and the larynx so the 'button' (larynx) fits snugly against the 'buttonhole' (ostium of the soft palate). The tongue is connected to the larynx so when one moves the other must move. Swallowing, hanging the tongue out of the mouth or pulling the tongue behind the bit causes the larynx to move in relation to tongue position. When the larynx or soft palate moves, the seal between them is broken *(laryngo-palatal dislocation)*, which creates an obstruction with partial closure of the airway.

Bit Evasion

A horse may evade a bit in the mouth by moving its tongue around. The larynx may slide backwards and separate from its snug fit with the soft palate. If the tongue is pulled over the bit, swallowing returns it to normal. Swallowing requires a complete disconnection of the larynx from the ostium of the soft palate. It closes the airway so food or saliva are not drawn into the lungs.

Other bit evasion tactics include opening the mouth. This action breaks the airtight seal of the lips. Air entering the mouth causes the soft palate to vibrate or lift up. Laryngo-palatal dislocation may result. Use of a dropped noseband or a flash or figure-eight noseband keeps the mouth shut and deters these evasion tactics. However, nostrils should not be pinched by

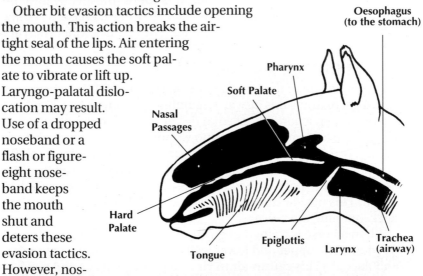

Fig. 5.4 Swallowing breaks the seal between the soft palate and the larynx.

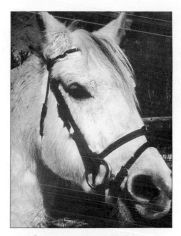

Fig. 5.5 A flash noseband keeps the mouth shut.

snugging the noseband down too tightly.

A bit that fits properly and is comfortable encourages a horse to accept it, and reduces the horse's tendency to spit it out. If a performance horse is ridden 'on to the bit', a goal is to achieve jaw flexibility and softness. Bit acceptance is often accompanied by excessive salivation, which may also stimulate swallowing with brief laryngo-palatal dislocation.

Roaring

To increase the cross-sectional area of the larynx during exercise, the two arytenoid cartilages on either side of the larynx must be opened. Opening of the arytenoid cartilages is regulated by the recurrent laryngeal nerves. Damage to one or both of these nerves or their loss of function results in a syndrome called *laryngeal hemiplegia*, which is a paralysis usually of the left side of the larynx. Air flow resistance through the greatly diminished airway results in a 'roaring' sound in an exercising horse. Such horses are subject to 'choking down' or suffocation, followed by abrupt halt of exercise. A milder form of this syndrome contributes to exercise intolerance, because the horse is unable to breathe in enough oxygen to fuel the body.

Roaring is diagnosed by passing an endoscope into the nose to the back of the throat. It may be necessary to examine the horse while it is working on a treadmill.

Surgery may return the horse to athletic performance. The most common surgical procedure to correct roaring is called a tie-back, where the cartilage is actually tied open. There are other, more controversial methods, for example nerve implants. After roaring surgery, a course of antibiotics helps prevent infection, and the horse should be stalled for 6 weeks. It must be gradually reintroduced to exercise.

Not all roaring and gurgling sounds are caused by laryngeal paralysis. Some horses just like the noise that resonates in the nostrils and purposefully allow them to flap with inhalation.

Bleeding

Another syndrome which causes exercise intolerance is exercise induced pulmonary haemorrhage (EIPH), or 'bleeding'. One theory states that respiratory disease weakens some areas of lung tissue, causing bleeding. Another theory holds that conditions of recurrent laryngeal neuropathy (RLN), including roaring, cause bleeding. RLN causes an upper airway obstruction which may exert enough pressure changes in the lungs to cause rupture of capillaries and bleeding. *(See Chapter 6 for more information on roaring, RLN and EIPH.)*

Performance and Air Flow

Exercises requiring optimal respiration are more affected by laryngo-palatal dislocation or loss of streamlining of the airways. For example, steeplechasing and cross-country events exert dramatic demands on the respiratory system.

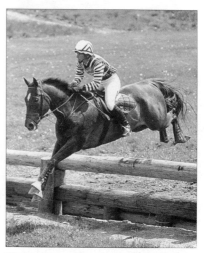

Fig. 5.6 Eventing and steeplechasing require a very hardy respiratory system.

The jumper that is lifting its body while weight-carrying needs all the oxygen it can get to fuel the muscles. An endurance horse operates best aerobically (with oxygen), and any limitation to air intake can severely compromise performance. Polo ponies and dressage horses rely on both aerobic and anaerobic (without oxygen) fuelling systems, but again, the more oxygen provided to the system, the greater the stamina. *(See Chapter 3 for more information.)* Likewise, a racehorse cannot sacrifice even the smallest amount of incoming air as it races down the track with its head and neck stretched forwards to improve airway efficiency.

Other less challenging athletics do not require the horse to operate at maximal exertion. The horse can therefore compensate for a slight loss in respiratory efficiency.

Keep the need for airway efficiency in mind when the horse seems to pull excessively on the reins while galloping. Sometimes the pulling is a credit to the horse's willingness and desire to run, but it may indicate that the horse cannot get enough air. By relaxing a little and letting go of its head and allowing it be comfortable, both rider and horse will have a better ride.

Respiration at Speed

At a gallop, respiratory rates run as high as 150 – 200 breaths per minute. The respiratory rate is directly synchronized with the stride frequency in a canter or gallop (unlike the walk or trot). When the forelimbs are forwards and not weight-bearing, the rib cage is also pulled forwards and expanded outwards and the neck is up, allowing the horse to inhale. Inertia moves the internal organs backwards, further expanding the thoracic space. As the forelimbs impact the ground, the rib cage absorbs the force and compresses inwards. Like a piston the internal organs move forwards, the neck is down, and air is forcefully exhaled.

RESPIRATORY ILLNESS

Just as good quality nutrition gives a horse the resources to build healthy tissue, so does the quality of the air around the horse determine the health of the respiratory system, and entire body.

Management greatly influences a horse's respiratory health. During winter, many horses are confined inside a stable, rather than turned out into the cold, wet or snow-laden air. The atmosphere of the barn must be evaluated. Are there noxious fumes or dust? Is there a damp, musty odour, or ammonia fumes? Are there dust particles floating in the air? Are the horses coughing?

The result of poor management is a heavily polluted environment. A stabled horse breathes this environment around the clock. It is important to understand the effects that a contained, polluted atmosphere has on the respiratory system.

Defence Against Foreign Particles

Upper Airways

Nasal Passages

During inhalation, the horse's airways filter a large percentage of particles in the air. Nasal passages filter the largest particles. Humidity in the air increases a particle's size and density, because water condenses on it. These large particles are easily trapped by the nasal passages, preventing entry to the respiratory tree. However, some large particles are so heavy that they fall out of the nasal filtration trap and are inhaled into the upper airways.

Mucociliary Apparatus

The upper airways have a clearance mechanism that is called the *mucociliary apparatus* (MCA). Particles deposited in the upper airways are cleared away from the lungs by a one-way flow of mucus that lies on top of the *epithelial cells* lining the airways. These are specialized cells with beating cilia that propel the mucous layer, with attached particles, outwards towards the throat, where it is swallowed or coughed away. The epithelial cells are damaged by infectious agents, noxious gases (ammonia or carbon monoxide), or extremes in temperature or humidity. Interference in their function severely reduces the efficiency of the MCA.

Coughing

Another airway clearance mechanism is coughing. Certain nerves in the upper airways respond to dust, ammonia and other irritants. These nerves stimulate a cough reflex to forcefully expel mucus and particles from the airways.

Excessive inflammation caused by irritants also stimulates a reflex constriction of the bronchioles in the lungs. This constricted diameter of air passages diminishes the efficiency of the coughing clearance mechanism.

Lower Airways

Combined with an effective mucociliary apparatus, specialized white blood cells called *alveolar macrophages* provide a primary line of defence against infection of the lower respiratory tract. An alveolar macrophage binds microorganisms, such as bacteria and viruses, to its cell membrane, and internalizes and inactivates each organism.

Smaller particles, and droplets of water containing bacteria and viruses *(droplet nuclei)*, may remain suspended in the inhaled air, not dropping out until they reach the bottom of the lungs. Normally, any particles that descend past the mucociliary apparatus are removed from the lungs by a fluid layer that slowly moves outwards until it reaches the MCA. Or, the particles may penetrate through the mucous layer to be consumed and destroyed by alveolar macrophages, or they are circulated with the alveolar macrophages to the MCA. Nerve endings in the smaller airways do not elicit coughing, but they will stimulate airway constriction. Interference in any of these events results in inadequate control of infection. Both the macrophage and the MCA are adversely affected by poor air quality.

Hay and Bedding Dust

Many barns have overhead hay storage that can compromise the respiratory system. As hay is thrown from the loft above, a large quantity of dust and mould spores are cast out to sift down through the atmosphere. It may take several hours for small fungal spores to settle out of the air. Also, horses moving around in their stalls kick up bedding and dust. Dust concentrations in the air can increase up to threefold, further irritating the respiratory tract.

Fungal Spores

Damp, decomposing bedding generates ammonia fumes, and promotes development of fungal spores. Warm temperatures, coupled with a high relative humidity caused by inadequate ventilation, encourage fungal growth. Fungal growth is greater in straw than in wood shavings. Horses lying in straw and mouldy bedding are subjected to massive numbers of mould spores even in the best ventilated stable.

The 'hay dust', fungal spores, and other irritants start a degenerative process in the airways by causing a hypersensitivity reaction similar to allergies in people. Horses continually exposed to these air contaminants may develop *chronic obstructive pulmonary disease* (COPD). Studies show that feed and bedding are the main sources of stable dust.

Riding Arena Dust

Many exercise and riding arenas connect to the stabling area, providing a warm enclosed space in which to ride during bad weather. Unfortunately, this practice complicates the problem of confinement in the barn. As horses and people move around these arenas, stirred dust mixes with the still air inside the barn. Not only are working horses exposed to this polluted air, but so are stalled horses.

Attempts to water the arena to hold down the dust increase the humidity in the barn. If an arena is 'moistened' with an oil mixture instead, oil particles in the air have toxic effects on the respiratory tract.

Humidity

High humidity levels contribute to respiratory infection. Adequate and effective floor drainage of water or urine is essential to limit humidity in the barn, and to remove moisture from bedding.

Carbon Monoxide

Machinery, such as tractors, is driven in and out of some barns to assist with stall cleaning or raking of the arena. Machinery contributes to build-up of carbon monoxide fumes within the stable. Appropriate ventilation is important when this equipment is in operation.

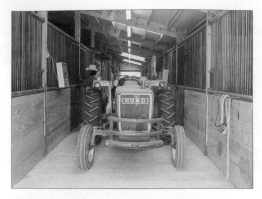

Fig. 5.7 Tractors give off air pollutants.

Respiratory Viruses

One often hears the axiom: 'No legs, no wind, no horse'. All too frequently the emphasis is placed upon the 'no legs' portion of this statement, and the health of the equine respiratory tract is taken for granted. A mild bout of influenza is explained away as '...something it will get over'. In fact a respiratory infection may require 3 weeks for a return to health.

Urbanized living congregates horses together in big barns and stables, increasing the opportunity for viral respiratory illness. More horses are housed under one roof, and are stressed by training and competition. A viral respiratory outbreak can easily grab hold and maintain itself in a concentrated equine population. Transcontinental and intercontinental transport of competition and breeding horses increases possibilities for spreading viruses on a global scale.

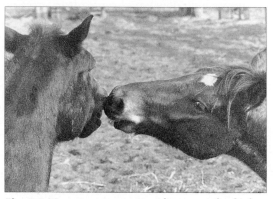

Fig. 5.8 Nose-to-nose contact is one method of spreading viruses.

Spread of infectious respiratory viruses occurs via droplet nuclei in the air, or directly from nose-to-nose contact. Viruses are also spread by indirect contact with tack, stable personnel, or in a contaminated grooming or wash stall common to all horse traffic.

Replication of a Virus

Unlike bacteria, viruses cannot duplicate themselves without inserting themselves into a host cell. There, they command the cell's replication mechanisms to reproduce the virus. Eventually, the cell is so full of new viral particles that it bursts. The cell is killed and viral particles are released to infect other cells.

The horse's immune system recognizes the viral proteins as foreign, and begins to produce antibodies. Specifically, antibodies recognize *haemagglutinin (HA) spikes* on the surface of viral particles. They attach to the virus and neutralize it. Each HA spike is made of a specific sequence of amino acids (components of proteins). Recognition of these specific amino acids on the spike is essential for the antibody to attach to it, with subsequent neutralization of the virus. In this way, antibodies disrupt viral replication by preventing viruses from entering the host cells.

Effects of Vaccination
On the Immune System
Vaccines train a horse's immune system to respond to viral particles. The initial vaccination, called *primary immunization*, primes the cells which produce antibodies. Subsequent boosters stimulate actual antibody production. A booster vaccine stimulates a rapid immune response, and the antibodies rise to high levels due to antibody 'memory', or *anamnestic response*. 'Anamnestic' is the Greek word for recollection. To invoke the anamnestic response, it is necessary to wait 4 – 6 weeks for the second booster.

Vaccination stimulates the immune system to make specialized antibodies against a specific strain of virus. Vaccine also stimulates cross-protective antibodies against variations of a strain. Antibodies developed against a specific strain are better at neutralizing that particular virus than are cross-protective antibodies. Yet, cross-protective antibodies rally when a horse is exposed to a similar but unfamiliar virus.

Because antibodies prevent the virus from invading respiratory cells, an immunized horse does not develop clinical symptoms of disease. Vaccinations are *not* completely protective, but they reduce the risk of contracting disease while minimizing symptoms. Both illness time and recovery time are shortened dramatically in a vaccinated horse.

On Herd Health
Vaccinating a herd or a large population of horses reduces the number of susceptible horses. Antibody levels are present in the entire group, preventing a viral infection from gaining a foothold. Assume, for example, that only 10% of a herd has been vaccinated. During an outbreak the virus carried by the other 90% is an overwhelming challenge to the immune systems of the vaccinated horses. Vaccination is therefore not enough to protect the vaccinated

10% against an overwhelming insult. A vaccine breakdown results, with clinical disease in epidemic proportions.

To prevent serious epidemics, at least 70% of a population should be vaccinated. When an outbreak does occur, all as yet unaffected individuals should be vaccinated to limit the spread of disease. Vaccinated horses develop a high-level immune response that 'blocks' further transmission of virus from horse to horse. There is no point in vaccinating already-sick animals.

Factors Affecting a Vaccination Programme

Aggressive immunization programmes help ensure respiratory health. However, even the most aggressive will not entirely eliminate disease if horses are stressed, overcrowded, or faced with poor stable hygiene, inadequate nutrition, or parasitism.

Age of the Horse

Each horse's immune system is unique in its ability to respond to vaccines. The age of a horse determines how frequently it should be boostered. Young horses under 2 years old are most susceptible to respiratory viruses. Because a youngster has not encountered a full spectrum of viruses or bacteria, its immune system is not fully competent to ward off all infections.

Occupation

The occupation of a horse is critical in determining a vaccination schedule. A highly competitive and mobile horse is frequently exposed to respiratory viruses, and should be vaccinated every 2 – 3 months. Although a horse may not be clinically ill, it can carry a virus home and spread it to others. Horses in livery stables or in barns have a high risk of exposure.

A horse that rarely socializes with strange horses may only need boosters twice a year. This programme may be sufficient to maintain a protective antibody level. In 6 months, antibodies do not decline so low as to prevent an anamnestic response to a booster vaccine.

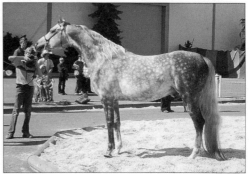

Fig. 5.9 A competitive and mobile horse is frequently exposed to viruses.

Previous Vaccinations

The number of previous vaccinations an individual has received should be considered in planning vaccination frequency. As the number of booster injections that a horse receives in its lifetime increases, the duration of an antibody response also increases. However, the level of antibody response can only increase up to a certain point.

Vaccine Types

Finally, the type of vaccine used determines booster frequency. *Inactivated* or *killed* vaccines protect for barely 3 months, whereas a *modified live* vaccine protects for 4 – 6 months depending on the product. Some killed vaccines use carrier agents, called *adjuvants*, that affect how well immunity is stimulated. (The adjuvant is the liquid carrier which contains the virus.) A 'depot' adjuvant enhances both the level and duration of antibody response by slowly releasing the vaccine over several weeks. As the foreign protein is presented to the immune system over a prolonged period, it continually stimulates antibody production.

Respiratory Virus Modification

Viruses can modify themselves so they are no longer recognized by the immune system. There are various strains or subtypes of viruses, and it is necessary to immunize against viruses that are currently prevalent, and are not out-dated. Use of vaccines with 'current reference viruses' is important for effective immunization.

Viral Shift

Viruses modify themselves in two ways. The first, called *viral shift*, is the appearance of an entirely new strain of virus due to a combination of two different strains. For example, the last major shift of equine influenza virus in the US occurred in 1963 with the outbreak of the Miami/63 strain. In the past few years, new subtypes of equine influenza virus have appeared in Europe and China. With intercontinental movement of horses, there is an increased possibility for exposure to new subtypes that horses are immunologically ill-equipped to combat.

Antigenic Drift

The second method by which a virus alters itself is *antigenic drift*. An antigen is any foreign protein presented to the immune system to stimulate antibody production. Drift is a minor change in the viral antigenic structure and makeup. If viral proteins are changed in a process of *mutation,* antigenic drift results and a horse's immune system cannot defend against it. Neutralization by antibodies is prevented, and viral infection and clinical disease develop.

Viral Duplication

Whenever a virus successfully infects a horse and begins to duplicate itself, there is an opportunity for mutation and drift. The rate of drift is relative to the number of passages through horses, so the more horses infected in a population, the greater the likelihood of antigenic drift.

Antibodies are less effective at neutralizing these different 'looking' viruses created by antigenic drift. Disease produced by a viral mutant is not necessarily more severe, but a horse's immune system is less able to defeat a mutant virus. Unvaccinated and immunologically naive horses are susceptible to illness. Sick horses are reservoirs for disease.

Reporting outbreaks of respiratory disease in a horse or herd to a veterinarian tracks epidemics, shifts in viral subtypes, and antibody response to various vaccines. This practice ensures that vaccines are up to date with the current reference viruses.

Telling others about the need and frequency of immunizations against respiratory viruses benefits the entire horse population. Limiting the number of susceptible animals that could carry viral respiratory disease promotes health within a population. Keeping current with an aggressive immunization programme prevents loss of valuable training, conditioning, and competition time.

Influenza Virus

The flu can strike rapidly and unexpectedly, usually requiring an incubation time of only 1 – 5 days. An affected horse is lethargic, depressed, unresponsive, and often uninterested in food. Rectal temperature may reach 103 – 106° F. The respiratory rate increases to 60 breaths per minute. A sick horse moves with deliberate concentration, indicating aching muscles *(myalgia)* or head. Often, a watery, nasal discharge is observed, and a dry hacking cough is heard in about 40% of affected horses.

Some horses' immune response is effective enough so they are not apparently ill, but they may still have a *subclinical infection* that allows shedding of viral particles.

Coughing is a principal means of spreading the virus from horse to horse. Respiratory secretions ejected from a coughing horse into the air contain infective doses of viral particles. If viral particles are coughed into a moist environment, such as a damp barn or shipping van, the influenza virus remains alive and infective for several days.

Infectious secretions are passed by direct nose-to-nose contact, and from contaminated housing, food, water, human hands or clothing.

The First Line of Defence

Secretory antibodies in the nasal passages are the first line of defence against influenza virus. Secretory antibodies respond to influenza virus only if previously 'trained' to do so either by a prior infection or by vaccination. If the virus is inhaled, and not neutralized by secretory antibodies, it colonizes the mucous membrane lining of the upper respiratory tissues and trachea.

Circulating Antibodies

If the flu virus penetrates this first line of defence, antibodies circulating throughout the body limit the infection. Circulating antibodies also develop in response to prior infection or vaccination.

Damage to Airways

The flu virus invades and kills the ciliated epithelial cells lining the respiratory tract. Cilia are tiny hair-like structures protruding from the cells which trap debris. At 4 days after successful invasion by an influenza virus, there is a significant degeneration of these cells. By 6 days after infection, the cells are almost entirely denuded of cilia and the respiratory tract cannot adequately clear debris, dust, viruses or bacteria from the lungs.

The mucociliary apparatus that normally moves debris out of the airways no longer functions properly. Depending on the infection's severity, it takes 3 – 6 weeks to repair once the virus is defeated and healing begins. Even in an uncomplicated case of influenza, a minimum of 3 weeks is necessary for functional recovery of the respiratory epithelium.

Because the denuded respiratory tract epithelium cannot respond to further insult, opportunistic bacterial infections can develop, possibly leading to pneumonia, long-term damage to the lungs, or death.

Resuming Exercise

Exercise can resume 7 – 10 days after body temperature returns to normal and coughing stops altogether. (Once clinical symptoms have abated, a horse is still infectious to others for 3 – 6 days.) If exercise causes coughing, wait another 4 or 5 days before resuming a training programme. To ensure full recovery, a horse with a mild illness and a cough should not return to full training for 3 – 5 weeks.

Recovery Period

Having a horse removed from training and competition for a month or more for full recovery is an emotional and economic cost to a horse owner. However, if a horse is prematurely returned to work, a relapse is possible. In rare instances, the heart is affected by the influenza virus and develops an arrhythmia. In general, the mortality rate from an influenza infection is remarkably low in uncomplicated cases.

An adult horse receiving adequate supportive care, rest, and protection from secondary complications usually recovers uneventfully with no permanent problems. Careful monitoring during both sickness and recovery are essential to success.

Only 5% of foal deaths are caused by respiratory viral infection. However, a common cause of foal death (up to 6 months of age) is bacterial pneumonia. This pneumonia is a secondary infection to a viral respiratory infection. Once the protective defence of the respiratory lining is breached, a young horse can rapidly deteriorate in as quickly as 48 hours.

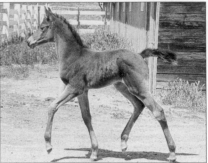

Fig. 5.10 Foals are particularly susceptible to bacterial pneumonia.

Prevention

It is best to avoid equine influenza viral infection if possible. The protective antibody response to an influenza virus infection is rapid but short-lived. By about 100 days, circulating antibodies have diminished and a horse is again susceptible to illness. (A human influenza antibody response lasts for 6 months up to years.)

New arrivals to a herd or barn should be quarantined for 2 – 3 weeks. This practice isolates horses that are incubating disease or are shedding viral particles.

Equine influenza was first identified as a subtype-A1 virus, but a more virulent form appeared in an epidemic in 1963 called the subtype-A2 flu strain, also known as the Miami/63 influenza strain. The outbreak in Europe in the late 1980s involved a drifted form of subtype-A2 virus. It is important to use a current vaccine to ensure that the horse is protected against the current strain of influenza virus.

An active performance horse is frequently exposed to respiratory viruses, and can carry these viruses home to other animals.

Current requirements by the Jockey Club (and FEI/BHS) are for a primary course of two doses at not less than 21days and not more than 90 days apart. This is followed by the primary booster at be-tween 150 and 190 days, and an annual booster at not more than 365 days apart. If overdue by even one day, the whole course must start again. No horse may be presented at a race meeting if the vaccine was given less than 10 days previously.

An influenza vaccine is now available in the UK that is said to confer immunity for up to 15 months. Vaccination does not prevent all respiratory disease. There have been reports of persistent coughing/poor performance syndrome after vaccination.

Equine Herpes Virus

Another respiratory virus for which a vaccine is available is the Equine Herpes Virus (EHV), or *rhinopneumonitis*. Often referred to as 'Rhino,' the virus has different subtypes. EHV-1 causes viral abor-tion, a neurological form of this disease, and also takes a respiratory form. EHV-4 primarily takes a respiratory form.

Abortion occurs from 14 to 120 days after exposure to the virus. A mare may show no signs of disease, but the placenta and foetus are invaded by the virus. Most EHV-1 abortions occur in the last half of pregnancy, particularly the last trimester.

EHV-4 must replicate before clinical signs appear. It has a longer in-cubation time than the influenza virus, as long as 3 weeks. Infection may not be as severe as that seen with the flu because the horse's de-fence mechanisms begin to respond to EHV during the incubation period.

Symptoms

Fevers can run as high as 106° F. Early on, a watery nasal discharge develops. This discharge often progresses to a mucopurulent dis-charge, which contains both mucus and pus, due to secondary bac-terial infection. For this reason, rhinopneumonitis is nicknamed the 'snots.'

Vaccination Schedule

Horses less than 2 years old are most susceptible to EHV, yet any stressed, mobile or competitive horse, and any pregnant mare should be vaccinated. Protection with the killed EHV1 virus vaccine is limited to less than 3 months, so pregnant mares should receive EHV-1 vaccines at 5, 7 and 9 months of pregnancy. A new aqueous inactivated vaccine against EHV1 and EHV4 has been introduced for use in healthy horses and ponies from 5 months of age. Following the primary course, booster vaccinations should be given every 6 months. Currently no vaccine protects against the neurological form. Horses that travel may contact it from horses that show no outward clinical signs.

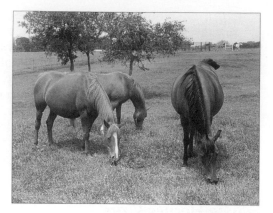

Fig. 5.11 Broodmares should be vaccinated against rhino infection, which can cause abortion.

Rhinovirus

The rhinopneumonitis virus (EHV) should not be confused with the Rhinovirus (ERV) for which there is no vaccine. ERV is associated with a fever lasting 1 or 2 days, swelling of the pharyngeal lymph nodes accompanied by a sore throat, and a watery to grey–green nasal discharge due to inflammation of the trachea and lower airways, or *tracheobronchitis*. Often, horses are infected without producing clinical signs, and serve as carriers to other, less durable individuals.

Heaves (COPD)

Chronic obstructive pulmonary disease (heaves) is a respiratory syndrome in horses similar to asthma or emphysema in humans. It is sometimes referred to as 'heaves' or 'broken wind'. COPD often occurs in stabled horses. An overwhelming concentration of organic dust allergens in the environment, particularly moulds and mould spores, initiates a hypersensitivity reaction. Some horses become allergic to alfalfa hay and exhibit a similar clinical response.

Viral invasion of the respiratory tract lining can also stimulate the development of COPD. The airways become hyperirritable, leading to spasms in the airway. Also, the destroyed ciliated epithelium lining the respiratory tract regenerates with thickened or altered cells, causing excess mucus production.

Symptoms of COPD

Large amounts of mucus or pus accumulate in the air passages. Constriction and spasm of these small airways *(bronchoconstriction)* results in their narrowing, causing obstruction. A horse has difficulty exhaling or properly ventilating the lungs. It stands depressed, with nostrils flared and with an increased respiratory rate (greater than 20 – 24 per minute). Occasionally, a wet or pus-filled nasal discharge is present. Wheezing may be audible. An increased exhaling effort is obvious with each breath. Forceful exhaling over time overdevelops abdominal muscles that labour to push air out of the lungs. This overdevelopment is visible as a *heave line* between the flank and the thorax. A severely affected horse loses its appetite, loses weight, and appears unthrifty. Chronic coughing is a key symptom of this disease, particularly if a cough persists for several weeks.

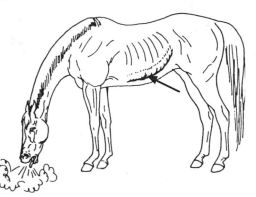

Fig. 5.12 A heave line between the flank and the thorax.

The Disease Process

The sequence of events that stimulate this condition begin with an inhaled allergen, such as mould. If hay is baled with a high moisture content, heat generated in the bale encourages the growth of mould. A horse with no symptoms may develop them within 1 or 2 hours and up to 10 hours after exposure. An allergic response proceeds rapidly, calling in specific inflammatory cells.

Mast cells release substances, such as histamines, that cause spasms and constriction of the smooth muscles of the airways, and an increase in mucus production. *Neutrophils*, a type of white blood cell, release substances that also constrict the airways and enhance mucus production. Normal airflow is interrupted by all these changes:

- thickening of epithelial cells lining the airways
- bronchoconstriction
- excess mucous congestion
- inflammatory cell infiltration

The mucociliary apparatus clearance mechanism is seriously impaired. Bronchial nerve reflexes become hyper-reactive and result in coughing.

Managing COPD

The goal for managing COPD is to reduce allergen levels below a threshold that causes clinical disease in the individual. It is not possible to remove all allergens from the environment. Each horse responds differently to similar allergens, just as people do. What may be below threshold level for one horse may still be allergenic for another.

Drugs

Many pharmacological drugs are available to deal with COPD, but have temporary effects unless management is altered. These drugs include prednisone, terbutaline, and aminophylline. Clenbutenol is a very effective drug.

Housing

A horse should be moved to the open air if possible, with constant fresh air flow into the environment. Bedding should be wood shavings, peat moss or shredded paper, but *not* straw. Housing should be located at least 50 yards upwind of any hay supply.

Feeding

The horse should be fed off the ground, not out of racks or raised feeders. By keeping its head down as it eats, normal blowing ejects particles from the nasal passages. Never feed mouldy hay, and remove alfalfa from the diet if a horse seems at all sensitive to it.

A cubed or pelleted diet is preferable, or at least wet grass hay. Even good quality grass hay contains a large amount of fungal spores. Wetting the hay may not completely prevent allergic effects due to continued exposure to the offending antigen. Opening the bale of hay and hosing down may help to remove the spores. This is often more effective than soaking in a tub of water. A pasture situation is ideal, particularly if plants are not in bloom. Tree and grass pollen have been implicated as allergens, as have straw mites.

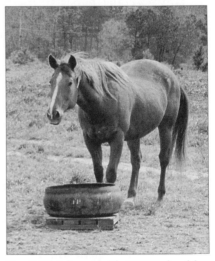

Fig. 5.13 A horse with COPD should be fed off the ground.

Vaccinations

A viral respiratory infection weakens a horse's resistance to other disease, and renders a horse more susceptible to COPD.

Once a horse has developed COPD, its respiratory immune system is weakened against further viral and bacterial insult.

A horse afflicted with COPD should be kept in as dust-free an environment as possible. To successfully manage a horse with compromised respiratory health is frustrating and requires diligent attention to detail. Prevention of the problem requires unpolluted open air and good clean living conditions.

Bacterial Infection

Secondary Infections

During a viral infection, bacteria that normally inhabit the upper airways may colonize, infect and inflame the lower airways. Normally, the mucociliary apparatus and macrophage systems clear bacteria, but viruses destroy the ciliated epithelial cells of the MCA and reduce the ability of macrophages to attach to, digest and kill bacteria.

Strangles

Strangles is a bacterial infection caused by *Streptococcus equi*. Normally the bacteria invade the upper respiratory tract, multiplying in the lymph nodes of the head.

Once the Strep bacteria have contaninated a property, they survive for months in the environment and in carrier horses that harbour the bacteria without showing clinical signs of illness, which provide a reservoir for cyclical infection.

Symptoms

Affected horses have a fever and a mucopurulent nasal discharge often accompanied by a cough. Other signs are similar to viral respiratory infections: the horse is depressed and off feed, and reluctant to swallow due to a painful throat. The most telling indication of a strangles infection is the enlargement of the lymph nodes under the jaw *(submandibular lymph nodes)* or in the throatlatch *(retropharyngeal lymph nodes)*. If the lymph nodes swell to grotesque proportions, the windpipe is so obstructed as to make breathing difficult — a horse can then 'strangle' to death for lack of air.

Lymph node action

An abscessed lymph node eventually breaks open and drains a thick creamy pus, contaminating the environment and other horses with highly infectious material. Even before the lymph node breaks, sick horses pass the infection to others through nasal discharge or coughing. Communal feeders and waters and nose-to-nose contact also spread the disease.

Any horse showing the slightest hint of impending sickness should be isolated as far from other horses as possible. An infected horse continues to shed bacteria for up to 6 weeks, despite appearing fully recovered.

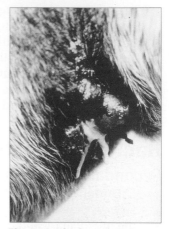

Fig. 5.14 The lymph node eventually breaks open.

Complications

Occasionally complications from a strangles infection can be serious, including:

- a bacterial pneumonia as the infection invades the lower respiratory tract
- a guttural pouch infection leading to a chronic nasal discharge
- purpura haemorrhagica
- bastard strangles, where the infection travels to the lymph nodes of the intestinal tract, abdominal organs or the brain

Young horses less than 3 years of age have a difficult time coping with infection. Mature horses usually have sufficient immunity to prevent the disease from turning into life-threatening pneumonia.

Preventing Respiratory Illness

Maintaining excellent hygiene and minimizing the horse's stress are key elements in preventing respiratory illness. To significantly reduce shedding of bacteria and viruses in the environment, aggressive respiratory vaccine programme should be implemented. A virally infected coughing horse sprays millions of viral particles into the air. Horses protected by vaccines are less likely to develop clinical viral disease or associated bacterial infections; consequently, they are less likely to shed these organisms in epidemic or infectious doses.

By keeping accurate records and a calendar, it is easy to implement an effective vaccine schedule to avoid respiratory illness. Respiratory vaccines are extremely cost-effective as insurance that a horse can train and deliver an optimal athletic performance.

Pregnant Mares

A previously vaccinated pregnant mare should receive a booster vaccination about 1 month before foaling. This practice allows enough time to develop antibodies, which will secrete into the mammary glands where they are available to the foal in the *colostrum* (the first milk).

Any mare that receives a vaccination booster before foaling will provide plenty of antibodies to the foal through the colostrum. Colostral antibodies provide passive protection to a foal until it is about 3 months of age. Until then, maternal antibodies from the colostrum block a foal's active immune response to a vaccine so a foal is unlikely to benefit from vaccination until it is 3 – 4 months old.

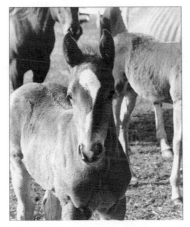

Fig. 5.15 Foals should begin vaccinations at 2 – 3 months.

Foals

The age at which foals are started on a vaccination programme depends on the vaccination status of the mare. If a mare has a cloudy history or is not current on her vaccines, it is better to start vaccination of a foal between 3 and 4 months.

The first vaccine given primes the immune system, and turns on the cells which produce protective antibodies. It is then necessary to wait 4 – 6 weeks to booster a second time and invoke the anamnestic response. After that, an optimal schedule includes influenza vaccine boosters at between 5 and 7 months later, followed by annual boosters at not more than 1 year apart and if appropriate more frequently.

Respiratory Vaccine Schedule

If a horse is less than 2 years old, highly stressed, highly mobile, or at risk of exposure to a transient population, vaccinating every 2 – 3 months may be necessary.

An effective respiratory vaccine schedule is as follows:

- Vaccinate pregnant mares at 5, 7 and 9 months of pregnancy against rhinopneumonitis viral abortions. Use approved products for pregnant mares.
- Vaccinate pregnant mares 1 month before foaling, using tetanus–influenza booster vaccine.
- Vaccinate foals at 3 months with tetanus–influenza vaccine. If an adult horse has not received vaccinations before, begin im-

munization as for foals. Vaccinate foals for EHV1 and EHV4 from 5 months of age.

- Vaccination should be completed at least 2 weeks before antici-pated exposure, travel or stress.
- With some vaccines there is a recommendation to avoid strenu-ous exercise (and here we quote from the *Veterinary Formulary*), particulary following primary vaccination, and it is normal prac-tice in the UK not to work the horse for 1 week, with only light exercise for 3–4 days, after each vaccination injection.

The immune system will have developed heightened antibody pro-tection against viruses by then.

Vaccination Reaction

Some individuals develop adverse reactions to injections. Mild influenza-like symptoms, such as fever, depression or a lack of appe-tite may occur. Lower leg swelling, or muscle soreness at the injec-tion site, are common vaccination reactions. Uncommonly, a localized abscess develops at an injection site.

Some horses react adversely to a specific adjuvant (the liquid carrier which contains the virus). Switching products and manufacturers pe-riodically may prevent these reactions. Other horses benefit from an intravenous injection of a non-steroidal anti-inflammatory drug when vaccinated to prevent ill effects. Rarely, an adverse reaction is severe enough to preclude use of a specific vaccine. An owner or trainer must weigh the benefits versus the risks of foregoing a vaccine.

Temperature-Sensitive Vaccine

To develop an influenza vaccine without adverse side effects, re-searchers are developing a temperature-sensitive vaccine given as an intranasal spray. The vaccine virus can replicate at the lower tempera-tures of the nostrils, but cannot migrate further into the warmer respi-ratory tract. Replication in the nasal passages stimulates development of secretory antibodies that are the primary line of defence against upper respiratory infections. Developing an intranasal spray inocula-tion against the subtype-A2 influenza is still in the research stages.

Genetic Engineering Research

A variety of other genetic engineering efforts are also in the infant stages of research. One such effort involves developing recombinant strains of viral vaccine by reassorting and combining genetic material from two different strains of influenza virus. Such a mutant would stimulate antibody production, yet would not produce illness or cause a horse to be infective.

Maintaining Air Quality

Poor ventilation in a barn creates an inadequate air exchange, and promotes a build-up of humidity and irritants (dust, allergens and gases), and an increase in numbers of airborne, disease-causing agents *(pathogens)* in the environment. Dust not only irritates the respiratory lining, but it also provides a vehicle for particles, increasing the *dose* of pathogens introduced into the airways.

Ammonia fumes degenerate the ciliary epithelial cells, in essence paralysing them, as well as decreasing the secretion of the mucous layer. Ammonia suppresses the ability of macrophages to kill bacteria. If a person can smell the ammonia fumes, the levels are too high.

An increase in humidity forms aerosolized droplet nuclei. These droplets enclose the bacteria or viruses, protecting them from the lethal effects of drying or temperature extremes. Protection from the elements enhances the spread of respiratory pathogens.

Benefits of Ventilation

An increase in numbers of circulating pathogens in the air presents an increased dose to a horse's respiratory tract. Under normal circumstances, the immune system may be able to inactivate a low dose level, whereas a greater dose can overwhelm and infect a horse with disease. Most infections are dose-dependent, meaning that exposure to a small quantity of a pathogen results in a milder disease or one that passes unrecognized. Frequent and rapid air turnover by a good ventilation system reduces the concentration of particles in the air (and dose).

Natural Ventilation

A natural ventilation system is achieved by holes in the walls and/or under the eaves of the roof, or by cross-ventilation created by doors open at opposite ends of the barn. Wind forces air through the building, but can create draughts if openings are inappropriately placed.

An example of good ventilation is stalls with ventilation openings with dimensions of 2 feet by 2 feet in the walls, and 1 foot by 1 foot near the roof. Larger wall openings allow a horse to put its head outside, giving it fresh air and relieving mental boredom.

Convection

If the air is still, or the holes are baffled to prevent draughts, the only means for air movement is by natural convection. Convection results from a temperature difference between the warmer air inside the stable (generated by the horses) and the cooler air outside. Hot air rises to exit from the upper holes, while cool, fresh air enters lower holes.

Effective insulation of a building increases the temperature differences between the inside and outside of the barn, maximizing natural convection. Roof insulation reduces radiant heat loss during cold winter nights, decreasing condensation (and resultant humidity) in the building.

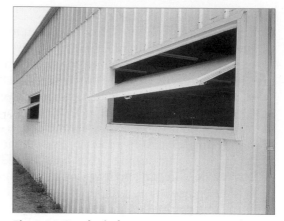

Fig. 5.16 Good windows to promote natural ventilation.

In a very large horse barn (twenty or more horses) it is difficult to maintain precise mixing of the air masses. Barns that are shut up tightly in the winter, with all doors and windows closed, have still air conditions with inadequate ventilation. Auxiliary ventilation openings along the roof allow entry of air into and out of the building, or specialized air flow systems should be installed.

Mechanical Air Flow Systems

Mechanical air flow systems should be exhaustive rather than recirculating, with a minimum air exchange of four times every hour. Anything less than two air exchanges per hour results in a dangerous build-up of mould spores. Exhaust units should be placed at a sufficient distance from the air inlets for adequate air turnover.

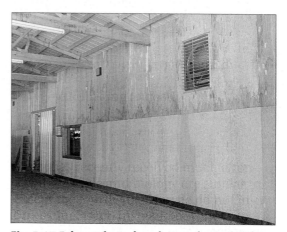

Fig. 5.17 Exhaust fans placed away from air inlets allow air turnover.

Ideal Management Practices

Optimal air quality in a barn to promote respiratory health depends on specific measures:

- Institute an ideal ventilation system in the barn to bring in fresh air, and to exhaust the old air.
- Separate riding and exercise areas from the stabling section.
- Store hay in another building. This practice reduces air pollutants, and decreases a fire hazard. Hay stored under cover from the weather develops less mould.
- Use good quality, dust-free bedding.
- Ensure adequate drainage for water and urine.
- Clean stalls frequently to reduce ammonia levels. Apply 1 or 2 pounds of hydrated lime to the stall floors after cleaning to reduce ammonia levels.

By following these practices, not only will the air quality and health of the horses improve, but humans will directly benefit from these good management procedures. (*See also Chapter 6.*)

Stress Factors

Training and Exercise

Stress increases the risk of respiratory infections. Routine training and strenuous exercise are frequent stresses to a horse. This stress results in increased *cortisol* secretion by the body, coupled with exercise-related inflammation of the lung tissues. Cortisol is a steroid hormone that inhibits the immune function of the alveolar macrophages and other white blood cells.

Cortisol depletes the number of immunoglobulins in respiratory secretions. Immunoglobulins are specialized proteins that decrease the ability of bacteria and viruses to attach to and infect epithelial cells. They also coat the organisms with a substance to enhance uptake by white blood cells. Immunoglobulins chemically attract other white blood cells to the area to help clean up infection.

Transportation

Transportation over long distances is a stressful condition that increases a horse's susceptibility to viral or bacterial infection, particularly 1 week after the trip. Horses subjected to stresses such as hard training, competition, and travel benefit from optimal air quality. Other significant stresses that adversely affect a horse's immune response include overcrowding, poor quality nutrition, fatigue and rapid changes in temperature.

Rapid Temperature Changes

It is preferable to maintain a constant temperature within a barn rather than having extreme fluctuations between hot and cold temperatures. Many stalled horses are rugged and are often body clipped. The only insulating layer of protection against cold for a clipped horse is the blanket or rug. If a horse is rugged at the beginning of the winter season, or clipped to prevent growing a winter hair coat, it is necessary to consistently rug it throughout the cold season. If the horse has a fur coat and is not used to being rugged, be careful of overheating it by rugging on a sporadic basis. Chills and draughts, or improper cooling out of an overheated horse, further compromise the immune response.

6

CONDITIONING FOR PERFORMANCE

MAXIMIZING POTENTIAL

An elite equine athlete is born with a potential to excel, and an intelligent conditioning programme maximizes that potential. Different breeds and individual horses excel in endurance-type or sprint-type sports depending on their conformation and the inherited composition of their muscle fibres. Muscles, the cardiovascular system, the respiratory system, and neuromuscular co-ordination respond favourably to conditioning programmes. The most effective conditioning programme carefully strengthens ligaments, tendons, bones, joints and muscles to avoid injury, while also developing the cardiovascular system to full capacity.

Competitive Edge

A primary goal of training is to improve a horse's *aerobic capacity*. The aerobic capacity is the ability of the horse to exercise longer and further without using anaerobic metabolism. Anaerobic metabolism produces energy without using oxygen. A more efficient method of energy production is aerobic metabolism, which produces energy using oxygen. Unlike anaerobic metabolism, aerobic metabolism does not generate toxic by-products which can cause muscle fatigue and soreness. A horse that is conditioned to perform for long periods using aerobic metabolism, where fuels (glycogen and fatty acids) are converted to energy with oxygen, often has the competitive advantage.

When either the oxygen or the fuels are depleted, the horse begins to rely on anaerobic metabolism of glycogen. At this point, the horse has reached the anaerobic threshold. Lactic acid, which is a toxic by-product of anaerobic metabolism, begins to accumulate in the muscles and bloodstream. Eventually, this accumulation results in fatigue, which is the limiting factor in performance. (See *Chapter 3 for more information on metabolism.*)

Submaximal Exercise (Endurance)

Most horses work at aerobic levels if their *heart rate* remains under 150 beats per minute (bpm). This exercise is called submaximal or endurance exercise. Examples of this level of activity include pleasure riding, competitive long distance events, endurance racing, dressage, and the roads and tracks phase of three-day eventing. At or below this heart rate, lactic acid does not accumulate in the muscles. Any small amount of lactic acid that forms is flushed from the muscles by the circulation or is aerobically metabolized.

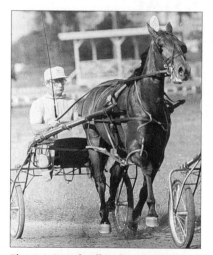

Fig. 6.1 Standardbred racing uses anaerobic and aerobic metabolism.

Maximal Exercise (Sprint)

Sprint sports require maximal exercise which in most horses occurs at heart rates above 180 – 200 bpm. These sports depend almost exclusively on anaerobic energy metabolism. Quarter Horse racing is a good example of such athletic efforts.

Combination Exercise

Examples of activities that depend on both aerobic and anaerobic metabolism are Thoroughbred and Standardbred racing, jumping, polo, and three-day eventing.

EFFECTS OF CONDITIONING
Conditioning Muscles Aerobically

The longer a horse can exercise using oxygen to produce energy, the longer fatigue is delayed. The body adapts to aerobic conditioning by increasing the ability of the cardiovascular system to supply oxygen to the muscles and improving the ability of the muscle systems to use oxygen to produce energy. These systems include improving blood circulation, improving metabolism, and converting some FTb (fast twitch low oxidative) muscle fibres to FTa (fast twitch high oxidative) muscle fibres. *(See Chapter 3 for more information on muscle fibre types.)*

Blood Circulation

Aerobic conditioning develops extensive capillary beds in the muscles and decreases the cross-sectional area of the ST (slow twitch) muscle fibres. Both factors improve blood circulation, which supplies more oxygen and helps remove toxic by-products such as lactic acid. More oxygen and less lactic acid in the muscles reduce fatigue.

Metabolism

Increasing the length of time during which muscles are fuelled by glycogen and fatty acids improves the aerobic capacity. Glycogen is a connected chain of glucose sugar molecules, and is a carbohydrate obtained from grain and forage. Fatty acids are produced by carbohydrate fermentation in the large intestine, or from fats in the feed.

With the blood circulation increased, the increased availability of oxygen promotes the use of fatty acids as a fuel rather than glycogen. The glycogen in the muscles and liver is spared, leaving more fuel in reserve for later use. Prolonging the time until glycogen reserves are depleted also delays the onset of fatigue, and reduces muscle soreness.

Each muscle cell that uses oxygen to convert fuel to energy has energy factories within it called mitochondria. The number of mitochondria increases with aerobic conditioning, improving oxygen use and energy production in the muscle cells.

Converting FTb to FTa

Aerobic conditioning improves a horse's aerobic capacity by converting up to 7% of FTb muscle fibres (low oxidative) into FTa muscle fibres (high oxidative). These FTa fibres can use oxygen to produce energy. Thoroughbreds and Standardbreds are able to compete at speed for longer distances than the Quarter Horse types (Quarter Horse, and Appaloosa) because they are genetically endowed with more FTa than FTb fibres.

Improving the blood circulation, improving metabolism, and increasing the number of FTa muscle fibres improve the horse's ability to exercise longer, faster, and further without the effects of lactic acid build-up in the muscles. However, with faster or longer exercise, the horse's aerobic capacity is exceeded and all three types of muscle fibres (FTa, FTb, and ST) are depleted of fuel. Therefore, improving the anaerobic method of energy production is also essential.

Conditioning Muscles Anaerobically

Over a period of months, sprint conditioning repetitively depletes these fuel stores. In response, the muscles 'learn' to store more fuel.

Anaerobic metabolism requires specific enzymes to convert fuel into energy without oxygen. Sprint conditioning improves anaerobic metabolism by developing the cellular systems which produce these enzymes. Body systems which remove lactic acid from the working muscles, including the cardiovascular system, also improve through sprint conditioning.

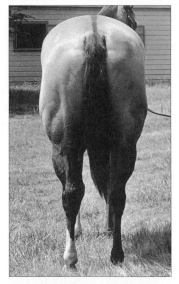

Fig. 6.2 Sprint conditioning strengthens gluteal and thigh muscles.

Increasing Muscle Mass

Sprint conditioning increases the cross-sectional area of muscle fibres. An increase in the area of each individual fibre increases muscle mass as a whole. Most affected are the gluteal and thigh muscles, the chest, and the forearm muscles. Increased cross-sectional area of muscle fibres creates strength for the fast, explosive acceleration so vital to a successful sprint horse.

Buffering Lactic Acid

Anaerobic metabolism during sprint conditioning produces lactic acid, which causes fatigue. Muscle tissue normally contains protein buffers that neutralize lactic acid. Sprint conditioning stimulates the production of these proteins, which increases the buffering capacity of muscle cells, and therefore delays fatigue. *(See Chapter 3 for more information.)*

Using Lactic Acid as Fuel

The stamina of the sprint-type horse also depends on the availability of glycogen supplies. If glycogen is depleted, the muscles run out of fuel and muscle contractions weaken. A sprint horse works so quickly and for such a brief duration that lactic acid cannot be immediately flushed from the muscles. Some of this lactic acid can be metabolized by FTa muscle fibres that use oxygen to produce energy. Any lactic acid that can be converted to energy by FTa fibres once oxygen is freely available again improves a sprint horse's stamina.

Anaerobic training helps a horse's muscles learn to tolerate the anaerobic state. They learn to store more glycogen, increase in mass, develop enzyme systems to neutralize lactic acid, and can even produce energy from lactic acid to a small degree.

General Muscle Conditioning

Some conditioning effects do not depend on the type of metabolism occurring in a muscle fibre. Efficient heat dissipation and improved neuromuscular coordination are examples of general conditioning benefits.

Improving Heat Dissipation

The biochemical reactions that burn fuels for energy also produce heat as a by-product. Conditioning improves a horse's sweating mechanisms to efficiently dissipate heat from the working muscles. Reducing heat build-up further delays the onset of fatigue. *(See Chapter 8 for more information.)*

Improving Neuromuscular Reflexes

Conditioning improves neuromuscular reflexes, which in turn improves muscle coordination and efficiency of motion. Muscles work together to prevent straining a muscle, or damaging a joint. To prevent excessive exertion and damage in early stages of conditioning, *agonist* muscles have opposing *antagonist* muscles to counteract them. For example, an agonist flexor muscle that flexes a joint is opposed by an antagonist extensor muscle. This system limits muscle action to a safe degree.

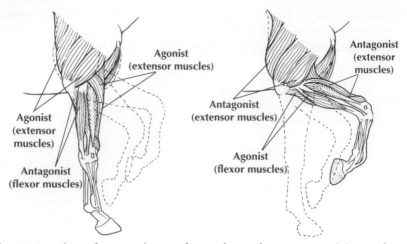

Fig. 6.3 Agonist and antagonist muscles work together to move a joint, each limiting the others' range of movement to prevent muscle and joint damage.

A young, awkward horse does not have fine-tuned coordination of the agonists working in concert with the antagonist muscles. If too much demand is placed on an undeveloped musculoskeletal system in the form of speed or distance, the unfit horse becomes muscle sore and is at risk of ligament or tendon damage as the muscle groups work against each other. Over time, reasonable repetitive exercises coordinate movement and improve neural signals to the muscles.

Conditioning the Respiratory System

The parts of the respiratory system include the larynx, trachea (windpipe), lungs and diaphragm. The respiratory system does not directly adapt to conditioning. However, as other body systems (such as the circulatory system) become stronger, the respiratory system must maintain its efficiency of oxygen intake.

The relationship of the respiratory system to the abdominal cavity helps maintain breathing efficiency at speed. At the canter and gallop, each stride is accompanied by a breath. The synchronization of breathing with the stride prevents motion from interfering with air intake.

Synchronization of Stride and Breath

When the forelegs are off the ground in the canter or gallop, they are reaching forwards. The head and neck swing upwards, and pull on connecting muscles that attach to the thorax. This action pulls the rib cage forwards and expands it outwards. The body accelerates for-

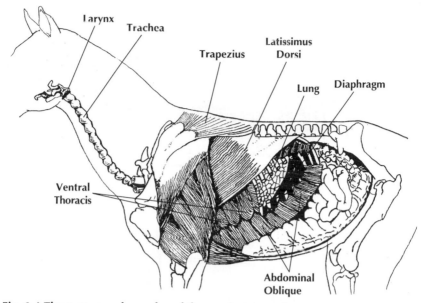

Fig. 6.4 The organs and muscles of the respiratory system.

wards as the hind legs push off the ground. At the same time, the internal organs are displaced to the rear, making more room in the chest. The combination of rib movement and internal organ displacement allows efficient inhalation.

When the leading foreleg hits the ground, the rib cage is compressed as it absorbs some of the force of impact. The fast-moving horse slightly decelerates and, like a piston, the internal organs slide forward to squeeze air from the lungs. The compression of the rib cage and forward movement of the intestines promote exhalation.

As the number of strides increases with speed, each inhalation and exhalation must move as much air as possible to fuel the tissues with oxygen. Muscles that work the respiratory system (the diaphragm, abdominal and thoracic muscles) become stronger with conditioning.

Conditioning the Cardiovascular System

If a horse is to use the aerobic method of energy production, it must have adequate oxygen. Improving a horse's aerobic capacity in the skeletal muscles therefore requires similar development of the cardiovascular system. Conditioning strengthens the heart to contract with increased power. At rest, a horse's skeletal muscles receive

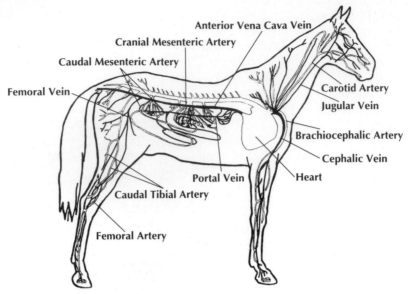

Fig. 6.5 The cardiovascular system.

only 15% of the total blood flow in the body, but during rigorous exercise 70% of the blood is circulated to the muscles, carrying oxygen to support aerobic metabolism. Blood flow to the skeletal and cardiac muscles and to the lungs increases 20-fold with conditioning.

Increased Red Blood Cells

During intense exercise, a horse increases its oxygen consumption 36-fold. Red blood cells contain *haemoglobin* which binds oxygen and carries it through the bloodstream to the organs and tissues. To accommodate the huge demand for oxygen, the bloodstream is flooded with a reserve of red blood cells. These cells are stored in the spleen for the times when more oxygen is required in the muscle tissues. With conditioning, the number of haemoglobin molecules in the body increases up to 50%. At high altitudes, a horse's body similarly compensates for the reduced oxygen by manufacturing more haemoglobin, increasing the oxygen-carrying capacity of the blood. More oxygen in the blood means more oxygen available in the muscles for aerobic metabolism.

Heart Rate

Resting Heart Rate

A horse's heart rate increases sixfold during exercise to further improve the circulation of blood and oxygen to the tissues. A horse's normal resting heart rate is between 30 and 40 bpm, but some horses may have resting heart rates in the low 20s. At maximal exertion the heart rate may be as high as 240 bpm.

Conditioning does not necessarily lower a horse's resting heart rate. The resting heart rate seems to be genetically determined. However, conditioning will lower the horse's working heart rate at a specific effort. Lowering the working heart rate decreases the energy consumption of the heart, and gives the heart more time between beats to fill with the maximum volume of blood possible. When the heart is pumping more blood per contraction, blood flow to the tissues is optimized, therefore ample oxygen reaches the muscles.

Heart Rate Recovery

Conditioning improves a horse's heart rate recovery so that, when exercise stops, the heart rate quickly returns to the resting rate. The heart rate of a well conditioned endurance horse should drop to 100 bpm within 1 minute, and to less than 60 – 70 bpm within 10 minutes of rest. A sprint horse should recover to 150 – 180 bpm after 30 seconds, and to a rate between 100 – 140 bpm after 1 minute.

If recovery exceeds the recommended time, the horse's speed should be decreased or the distance shortened. Evaluating the heart rate provides detailed information about when to push to the next level of fitness without injury.

Heart Rate Variables

Heart rate is a measure of work output and is affected by many variables. The hotter and more humid the day, the more effort is required of the horse. The difficulty of terrain and footing affect a horse's heart rate, as do distance and fatigue, fear and excitement, and the genetic predisposition of a horse's muscle fibre type. An illness such as a fever or colic will also raise the heart rate.

VALUE OF A HEART RATE MONITOR

One way to consistently evaluate the horse's working heart rate is by using a heart rate monitor. A heart rate monitor is a pocket-sized digital computer that is plugged into electrodes. These electrodes are placed on the horse's withers and beneath the girth. It is a handy, inexpensive device that enables a scientific training programme to achieve maximum results.

The monitor allows the athlete's work effort to be measured by the

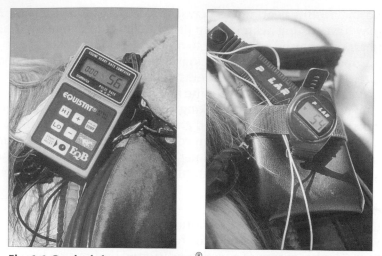

Fig. 6.6 On the left, an EqB Equistat® heart rate monitor. On the right, a V-Max heart rate monitor with wrist watch receiver. Both types are valuable conditioning tools.

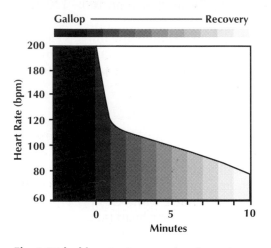

Fig. 6.7 Ideal heart rate recovery after a 1 – 2 mile gallop.

working heart rate while it is still exercising. Without the use of a heart rate monitor, by the time a rider stops the horse, dismounts, and counts the heart rate for 15 seconds, it has dropped 50 – 100 bpm.

Monitoring Working Heart Rate

With a heart rate monitor a horse can be ridden within its abilities while its level of fitness is systematically evaluated. For example, a horse in endurance-type training moves at paces of walk, trot and slow canter with a heart rate between 124 and 150 bpm. To develop the aerobic capacity, work the horse just below the level of lactic acid accumulation. (Lactic acid accumulation begins at heart rates above 150 – 160 bpm.) The time necessary to develop the aerobic capacity will vary with the individual. As the aerobic capacity improves, work the horse at 200 bpm for short periods. This training effect further improves a horse's aerobic capacity while minimizing the risk of musculoskeletal injury. It is the ability of the cardiovascular system, not the heart rate *per se*, which determines when lactic acid accumulation begins by it ability to maintain an aerobic rather than an anaerobic state.

A heart rate monitor also enables the rider to gradually increase the distance at a specified heart rate, incrementally and safely stressing the cardiovascular and musculoskeletal systems. Each progressive level of challenge created by an increase in speed *or* distance stimulates the body's adaptive response.

For example, hill climbs elevate the heart rate and lactic acid production, but once at the top of the hill, the heart rate should decrease to less than 150 bpm for muscle recovery and removal of excess lactic acid. Within 1 minute of downhill, the heart rate should be less than 110 bpm.

Another example of the use of a heart rate monitor in conditioning is the training of a racehorse. After a 1-or 2-mile gallop at 200 bpm, the heart rate should recover to less than 120 within 2 minutes, and to less than 80 within 10 minutes.

Detecting Fatigue

A monitor accurately gauges a horse's work effort to indicate the onset of fatigue. The heart rate elevates as fuel reserves are depleted. If the heart rate increases at a constant work effort, the pace should be reduced to avoid metabolic or musculoskeletal problems.

Detecting Injury

Not only does a heart rate monitor fine tune a horse's conditioning programme, but it is acutely sensitive to subtle pain created by a beginning musculoskeletal injury. If a horse's normal working heart rate at a specific task is known and there is a rise of 10 bpm over normal while the horse is attempting that task, work can be stopped immediately before a mild injury is aggravated.

Performing a Field Fitness Test

A heart rate monitor is useful to perform a *field fitness test* to evaluate a horse's aerobic capacity. This test is done by measuring the velocity at 200 bpm (V_{200}) after a warm-up period. Velocity is the distance per unit of time (miles per hour, for example). To perform the field test, measure and mark off a set distance of ¾ – 1 mile, and then record the time it takes for the horse to cover that distance with the heart rate maintained as close to 200 bpm as possible. The fitter the horse, the faster it must go to achieve a heart rate of 200 bpm, and the greater its aerobic capacity. V_{200} can be compared every month, determining improvements in fitness. Heart rate measurements only evaluate aerobic capacity, however, not structural strength.

If a horse is unfit initially, then evaluate it at 160 bpm (V_{160}). This is the rate at which lactic acid accumulates faster than it can be metabolized. The speed it can go at this heart rate while lactic acid is being formed defines the horse's aerobic capacity. V_{160} is not a perfectly accurate indicator of fitness because pain or excitement can artificially drive the heart rate up to 160 bpm without muscular work being performed. However, it is a useful rate to start with for a horse re-entering training after a long layoff, or for an older or young horse at risk of musculoskeletal injury at fast speeds.

CONDITIONING PREPARATION

Conditioning a horse does not just apply to exercise programmes. It is important also to 'condition' a horse's overall health to provide it with a solid metabolic and structural foundation.

Veterinary Evaluation

Before beginning an intensive training schedule, arrange an appointment with a veterinarian for an evaluation. A veterinarian can assess the horse's general physical condition, with nutritional planning to accommodate the level of work the horse currently sustains and the rigorous level of athletics it should reach in the months ahead.

Feet

The feet should be balanced and shod before beginning a consistent exercise schedule. As workouts accelerate, healthy feet are imperative to ensure continued soundness. Conscientious maintenance prevents bruises, torn hooves or hoof cracks. A properly balanced foot best absorbs concussion and deters lameness. *(For more information, see Chapter 4.)*

Diet

Rigorous exercise requires more food. However, be careful not to feed too much rich spring grasses, alfalfa hay, or grain as these feeds can lead to gas colic or laminitis. Horses need ample roughage in the diet to maintain a healthy intestinal tract. *(For more information, see Chapter 7.)* Check stored hay supplies to ensure that they have not become dusty and are free of mould. Dust and mould are harmful to the lungs, and can result in chronic respiratory disease.

Teeth

Only a well nourished athlete can perform to potential. A horse's teeth should be examined and rasped, if necessary, to encourage efficient digestion of food. Teeth should be in good condition so feed is adequately ground and can be processed by the digestive tract, decreasing the possibility of gaseous or impaction colics.

Rasping the teeth also eliminates sharp edges, preventing painful ulcers in the mouth that might interfere with bitting or response to bit contact. If *wolf teeth* are present, and are to be removed, do so before beginning the conditioning schedule so healing can proceed with minimal interference to performance.

Immunizations

The athlete should be on a thorough immunization programme before and during a conditioning regimen. Protection against viral respiratory diseases is critical because a performance horse is exposed to other horses as it competes. The body is mildly stressed by exercise workouts, and the immune system is further challenged by contact with other horses and new areas. There has been much research work recently on suppression of the immune response in human athletes. This shows that it is important to minimize stress by, for example, planning to complete vaccination programmes in advance of bringing the horse to competition fitness. Each horse must be considered as an individual when drawing up the plan.

In areas where diseases such as Venezuelan Encephalitis, *equine viral arteritis* or rabies are prevalent, include vaccines to build immunity to these threats. *(For more information, see Chapter 5.)*

Deworming

An aggressive deworming schedule every 6 – 8 weeks reduces the damage caused by intestinal parasites. Intestinal worms also cause colic by interrupting normal intestinal movement and altering the blood supply to the intestines. Clean the manure from the paddock twice a week to limit reinfection with parasite eggs. *(For more information, see Chapter 14.)*

Stall Hygiene

If a horse is confined to a stall, careful attention should be paid to daily stall cleaning and hygiene. Removing faecal matter and soiled bedding prevents reinfection by parasite eggs, and controls the conditions that favour thrush. Removing urine-soaked bedding also reduces ammonia fumes, promoting respiratory health.

TRAINING METHODS

Ultimately each athlete is trained for a specific task. However, the performance horse must have a strong foundation on which to build for each phase of the conditioning process. A strategically planned conditioning programme means a commitment to pursue it for many months.

Consistency of workouts is an important ingredient to increasing biomechanical strength. 'Progressive training' methods include a recovery period for the body to adapt to training and stress. In this way, a horse continues to build strength with less risk of strain or fatigue, and develops into a fit athlete.

Humans typically require about 10 weeks to increase muscular strength by 50%, because neuromuscular coordination is required for 'neural learning' and control. Similar biophysical processes occur in horses, and all body tissues must respond to incremental challenges. Tissue with a generous blood supply responds quickest: muscle tissue

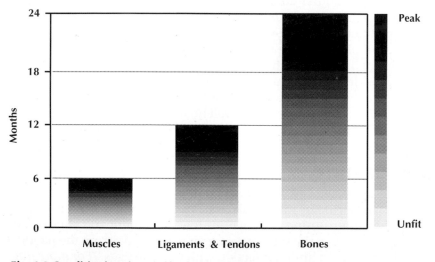

Fig. 6.8 Conditioning times of body structures.

is the fastest to respond (about 3 – 6 months), ligaments and tendons take longer to condition (6 – 12 months), and bone takes the longest time to fully condition (1 – 2 years). To advance a horse to absolute peak condition may require as long as *2 years.*

Once a horse has been well conditioned, it does not rapidly lose fitness. While people lose fitness in only 2 weeks, a horse retains condition for a month or more and is able to return quickly to previous levels of conditioning. Once a foundation has been built, only 3 – 6 months is necessary to return a horse to peak condition after a long layoff.

Value of Repetition

Progressive increases in speed or distance over time (conditioning) enhance strength and durability. Once a conditioning programme is begun, commit to it. To condition a horse, it must be *repeatedly and consistently* stressed before the tissues have a chance to fully recover from a prior workout. This method promotes adaptation and strengthening of body structures to build a solid foundation. Bone, cartilage, ligaments and tendons must be slowly trained over time to meet the demands of added exertion. Sudden speed bursts on unconditioned support structures in the limbs can overload these living components, resulting in damage and lameness. Progressive stresses, however, challenge the tissues and result in *strength* training of muscles, ligaments and bone.

Value of Walking

Do not underestimate the value of walking. Walking improves condition by slowly stimulating ligaments, tendons, and muscles to accept a slight increase in load. Walking loads a horse's ankle with 2½ times its weight. The stifle and hip are loaded with 1½ times the horse's weight. Walking increases the heart rate to 90 bpm. Blood vessels dilate and become elastic, allowing blood to flow with less resistance. An adequate warm-up of 10 minutes of walking enhances delivery of blood and oxygen to working muscles. Only a small

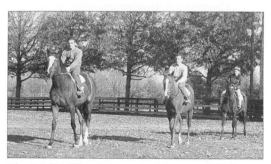

Fig. 6.9 Walking is important for conditioning.

percentage of muscle fibres are recruited at a walk, primarily the slow twitch and a few of the fast twitch high oxidative muscle fibres. These muscle tissues learn to improve oxygen delivery and removal of toxic by-products. Walking alone does not adequately stress the tissues to train them to higher levels of effort. However, it is an excellent starting point to build on, and is useful for a relaxed exercise.

Value of Swimming

Swimming can be added to a routine conditioning programme of flat and hill work to provide cardiovascular and respiratory conditioning without concussive stress on the limbs. It is also a useful form of training that can be applied to a young horse or while rehabilitating an injured horse. For the young horse, swimming strengthens the cardiovascular system without straining growing bone, and develops joints, tendons and ligaments. The exercise of swimming maintains cardiovascular and respiratory fitness of an injured horse without any loading stress placed on the injured limb. The movement of the limbs through the water passively stretches healing joints and tendons, and the water massages the tissue to improve circulation.

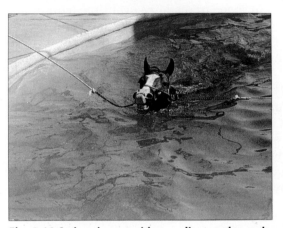

Fig. 6.10 Swimming provides cardiovascular and respiratory conditioning without weight-bearing.

However, using swimming as the sole means of exercise while rehabilitating a horse will not provide the cyclic loading stress on bones, joints, tendons, ligaments, and hooves that is part of a normal conditioning process. The horse will also require the weight-bearing stresses of adequate land preparation before beginning or returning to competitive athletics.

Phase 1: Long Slow Distance Training

Long slow distance (LSD) is used to build a foundation for further training for any equine sport. As an initial conditioning technique it slowly develops the structural strength of bone, muscle, ligaments, joint cartilage, and hooves with minimum risk of injury. All LSD work is performed below the anaerobic threshold so minimum lactic acid accumulates. LSD develops muscle fibres that use oxygen to burn fuel for maximum stamina.

An intelligent conditioning programme starts with long, slow mileage, and speed is then increased gradually as the months go by. As a horse is incrementally challenged, speed and distance are *never* increased at once. One or the other is increased, but never both together.

The first month of conditioning is different for a young horse or for a horse recovering from an injury or illness than for a mature and

PHASE I — YOUNG OR INJURED HORSE	
Long Slow Distance Training	
FIRST MONTH **Week 1**	15 – 20 minutes, every other day or 3 days per week Alternate between ⅔ walk and ⅓ trot
Week 2	30 minutes, 3 – 4 days per week Alternate between walk and trot
Week 3	30 – 60 minutes, 4 – 5 days per week Increase distance but keep speed same as first two weeks Lengthen trot duration Mild inclines at the walk
Week 4	Add canter intervals for 1 – 2 minutes Change leads intermittently
SECOND MONTH (Same as Mature, Sound Horse)	Build to 10 miles per day at walk and trot, 3 – 4 days per week Increase mileage not speed
THIRD MONTH (Same as Mature, Sound Horse)	Add speed for HR 120 – 150 bpm for 1 hour: 4 – 7 m.p.h. in hilly terrain *or* 8 – 12 m.p.h. on level ground

Fig. 6.11

sound horse. Young or injured horses need a lower intensity schedule so as not to overtax their systems. The second and third months of conditioning are the same for either level of fitness; however, these exercises are recommendations only. Every horse is different and trainers or owners will need to make adjustments. Tailor the conditioning programme to the athlete. Veterinary advice is recommended for all phases of conditioning.

LSD Training for the Young or Injured Horse

During the first month of LSD training for the young or injured horse, it is best to start working on flat, even, and forgiving footing, preferably in straight lines. Lungeing strains underconditioned joints and tendons, but has the advantage of not adding additional weight to the horse. A start can be on long-lining which includes circles to promote flexibility and avoid back pains.

The First Month

Spend the first 2 weeks of the programme alternating between the walk and trot, while spending two-thirds of the overall time at a walk. Start with 15 – 20 minutes for each exercise period, working up to an hour by the end of 2 weeks. Initially it is best to exercise a horse every other day, or 3 – 4 days a week, as this schedule allows time for some tissue recovery and adaptation between stress efforts.

The third week, add a day of exercise and increase the distance but work at speeds similar to those used in the first 2 weeks. The duration of trot intervals can be lengthened to several minutes at a time. Very mild inclines can be added for the walk interval.

The fourth week, add canter intervals of 1 – 2 minutes but don't forget to ask intermittently for both leads so both sides of the body are exercised equally. Within a month the horse should be consistently working for 60 minutes, 5 days a week, at an average of 4 – 5 m.p.h.

LSD Training For the Mature and Sound Horse

The First Month

LSD training for a mature, uninjured horse can be slightly more demanding than the programme outlined above. Initial workouts can begin with 20 – 30 minutes of walking and slow trotting. After 1 week, workouts should last a minimum of 30 minutes, 4 days a week. By the end of the second week, the horse can work for 30 – 60 minutes to stimulate an aerobic training effect. During the third and fourth weeks, a horse can walk and slow trot 4 – 6 miles a day, about 5 days a week. Several minutes of canter intervals can be introduced at the beginning of the fourth week.

Vary the types of exercise performed, not only to supple and strengthen different muscle groups, but also to keep a horse's mind interested and active. Variety can include arena work, cavalletti poles, and long distance riding. Race training could include off-track walking, or riding, and hand-grazing when *(and where)* possible provides a change of scene on a scheduled rest day.

PHASE I — MATURE AND SOUND HORSE	
Long Slow Distance Training	
FIRST MONTH **Week 1**	20 – 30 minutes, 3 days per week Alternate between walk and slow trot
Week 2	30 – 60 minutes, 4 days per week
Week 3	60 – 90 minutes, 5 days per week Walk and slow trot 4 – 6 miles per day
Week 4	Add canter intervals for 3 – 5 minutes
SECOND MONTH	Build to 10 miles per day, at walk and trot, 3 – 4 days per week Increase mileage not speed
THIRD MONTH	Add speed for HR 120 – 150 bpm for 1 hour: 4 – 7 m.p.h. in hilly terrain *or* 8 – 12 m.p.h. on level ground

Fig. 6.12

The Next Two Months

During the second month of workouts increase mileage, not speed, building to 10 miles a day of walk and trot, 3 – 4 days a week. The third month add speed. The conditioning goal is to work at a heart rate of 120 – 150 bpm for at least 1 hour. To achieve this goal, work the horse at 4 – 7 m.p.h. in hilly terrain, or 8 – 12 m.p.h. on level ground such as a track.

PHASE II — ALL HORSES
Cardiovascular Training

FOURTH MONTH	• Warm up 20 – 30 minutes at an extended trot on flat ground • Add speed play workouts including short, fast gallops or uphill canters once or twice per week • Increase duration *or* speed of hill work • Slow downhill work at the walk and some trot

Fig. 6.13

Phase 2: Cardiovascular Conditioning
The Fourth Month

The second phase of conditioning improves a horse's cardiovascular fitness to increase oxygen delivery to the tissues and delay the onset of fatigue. Hill training is an excellent way to improve both the musculoskeletal and cardiovascular systems. Working a horse on hills is similar to weightlifting; it develops shoulder muscles, hip extensors, and the quadriceps muscles which swing the hind leg forwards. As muscles become more powerful, locomotion is less tiring and the whole body operates more efficiently. Perform downhill work slowly to reduce wear and tear on the forelegs. A slow downhill trot helps a horse learn balance, but it should not be overdone.

Once the horse has successfully come through the first 3 months of LSD, 20 – 30 minutes of extended trot on flat ground warms the muscles and increases circulation, preparing the horse for a slightly greater intensity of exercise. Then a gradual increase in duration or speed of hill work can be incorporated into the training periods.

During the fourth month, add speed workouts once or twice a week to stimulate the fast twitch high oxidative muscle fibres. *Fartleks*, or speed plays, include short, fast gallops or uphill canters interspersed between walk, trot and canter paces. Both high intensity, short duration exercises and low intensity, long duration exercises improve a horse's aerobic capacity with a short period between them so that the heart rate stays elevated.

Once the musculoskeletal system is strengthened through LSD and the cardiovascular system is similarly strengthened, customize the training programme towards the specific tasks of the intended competitive athletics through *interval training*.

Phase 3: Interval Training for Speed and Anaerobic Tolerance

Interval training teaches a horse's body to tolerate the anaerobic state, and it develops a horse's inborn potential for speed. These goals are accomplished by performing repeated bouts of high intensity exercise for a set distance or time, followed by a walk or trot recovery period between each high intensity effort. This technique conditions horses for maximal exertions up to 3 minutes, reducing the risk of structural damage.

Training Effects

The effects of interval training (IT) include:

- strengthening of the heart, with increased blood pumped with each contraction
- expansion of blood vessels
- increased blood vessel elasticity to improve blood flow

Optimizing Oxygen Use

With interval training, fast twitch high oxidative muscle cells produce mitochondria. Having more mitochondria increases the use of available oxygen and produces more energy.

Interval training also encourages the spleen to increase the storage capacity for red blood cells. These red cells should enter the circulation about twice a week by sprinting the horse about ¼mile. If this does not occur, inactive red blood cells are destroyed by the spleen because they distort with age and lose their oxygen carrying capacity.

Reduced Lactic Acid

Interval training creates less lactic acid, delaying fatigue. Lactic acid fatigues muscles because it generates an acid environment (low pH) in the muscles. It takes about 30 minutes to clear lactic acid from the muscles and bloodstream after hard or prolonged exercise. Walking or slow trotting maintains blood flow to the muscles and flushes away lactic acid.

The intermittent recovery periods during IT promote *partial* lactic acid clearance from the muscles. Initially, recovery periods of 5 – 10 minutes flush enough lactic acid from the muscles to prevent rapid fatigue. Yet the fast intervals of IT challenge muscle cells to adapt to a low oxygen environment and to increase the anaerobic threshold. Eventually, with improved condition, the recovery periods can be shortened to 5 minutes, and the high intensity work can be sustained for slightly longer.

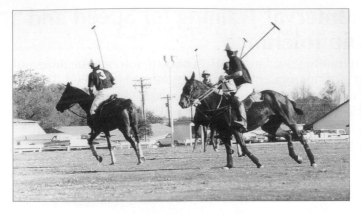

Fig. 6.14 Polo ponies benefit from interval training.

The Fifth Month

By the fifth month, add interval training to the conditioning programme about twice a week. IT is particularly useful for the racehorse, event horse or polo pony because it improves lactic acid tolerance. It enables a horse's heart, lungs and muscles to accommodate speed work for a competitive advantage. An endurance horse can also benefit from sessions of interval training. IT provides resources for when the endurance athlete lapses into anaerobic work due to difficult mountainous climbs, an excessively fast pace, or the onset of fatigue.

Challenge Without Risk

Over each exercise session of interval training the horse is cumulatively worked at greater distances and higher speeds than it would normally encounter if it were asked to gallop continuously. A horse can tolerate such training stress if it is not maintained for long periods. For example, the horse may be exercised at a heart rate of 180 – 200 bpm for at least 2 minutes. A trot recovery period of 4 – 5 minutes brings the heart rate down towards 100 bpm. Because the high intensity periods are of limited duration, musculoskeletal injury is reduced yet the horse is challenged at intense conditions similar to or greater than competition.

It is necessary to incrementally challenge the equine athlete. Without some 'moderate' stress to the system, the system will remain at current strength. A heart rate monitor enables the trainer to find a level of safe stress by working the horse between 180 and 200 bpm. The heart rate should drop to 110 bpm or below before embarking on the next high intensity interval. The heart rate recovery takes up to 10 minutes in an unfit horse and 4 – 5 minutes in a fit horse.

PHASE III — ALL HORSES	
Interval Training	
FIFTH MONTH	**Twice a week, repeated sets of high intensity work with walk or trot recovery between:** **Exercise at HR of 180 – 200 bpm for 2 min.** **Trot recovery period:** • **4 – 5 min. for a fit horse** • **Up to 10 min. for an unfit horse *or* until HR drops to 110 bpm or below**

Fig. 6.15

Long Fast Distance Training

Long fast distance training methods often lead to failure. Prolonged speed creates breakdown injuries or exhaustion. This training method does not allow the body to repair, much less strengthen, between efforts. The horse continually disintegrates and cannot improve past a certain performance level.

CAUSES OF POOR PERFORMANCE

To have the winning edge, an equine athlete must be able to summon all its resources to maximize performance. Some days everything clicks into place, and the horse just cannot be beat. But occasionally a horse reaches a period of crisis where performance begins to wane, imperceptibly at first, and then more consistently with each workout.

Overtraining

A common reason for poor performance is a phenomenon known as *overtraining*. A horse is ridden too often at too high a level of demand without a sufficient recovery period. Muscles exhaust their energy supplies during strenuous exercise, and they need time to restore energy and enzymes to drive biochemical reactions. Usually, complete recovery only takes 12 – 24 hours. After extreme exertion, such as a competition or hours of very hard work, several days of rest may be necessary to replenish the stores. If a horse is continually pushed past the body's limit, all its reserves are depleted. The horse cannot compensate for the lack of muscle fuel needed to drive performance, and fatigue results.

Without rest and replenishment of carbohydrates, the depleted muscle cells of the overtrained horse will consume each other in an attempt to metabolize protein into glycogen. The bright bursts of brilliant performance typical of that individual fail to appear.

Initial Indications

Initial indications that a horse is stressed from an excessively intense training schedule include:

- elevated resting pulse
- abnormal sweating
- muscle tremors
- elevated working pulse
- poor heart rate recovery
- diarrhoea

Symptoms of Overtraining

The overtrained horse is recognized by:

- failure to gain weight
- stiff and sore muscles
- stance becoming less alert
- weight loss
- dull eyes
- picking at food

Rest and Relaxation

If a horse starts to fail in performance, try backing off to an every other day training schedule rather than a daily workout, or consider walking for an hour on one of the days scheduled for a rigorous training period. Once the horse's fatigued body starts to recuperate, appetite will improve. The horse will facilitate its own rehabilitation by consuming needed nutrients and energy. Often trainers and riders attempt to supplement a horse with food additives and vitamins to restore lustre, when what it really needs is rest and relaxation. To determine whether a horse is suffering from muscle damage or nutritional deficiencies, blood chemistry profiles can be analysed before and after exercise. Such profiles can be helpful in monitoring the progress of the training programme.

Inability to Perform

Not all horses have the ability to be a premier athlete. It is sometimes puzzling that a horse that has everything in its favour is unable to meet an expected level of performance, especially when compared with other similarly endowed horses. Sometimes a horse does not have the combination of attributes to drive it to a pinnacle of excellence. Many times a horse's genetic capabilities are not properly suited to the assigned career. In other instances there is a physiological reason for failure to perform to expectations.

Exercise Intolerance: Musculoskeletal Pain

A primary cause of exercise intolerance is injury or pain in the musculoskeletal system. If a horse hurts while exercising, it will try to avoid any movement that stimulates pain. Behavioural changes are a tip-off that something is wrong. The horse may swish its tail, pull its ears back, menace when saddled, or refuse the task at hand.

A practical and inexpensive method of detecting very subtle pain is to consistently ride the horse with a heart rate monitor. After many readings of the normal heart rate response to a given exertion, it is possible to identify beginning signs of discomfort. The heart rate rises during exercise that normally would not cause heart rate elevation.

Examples of Musculoskeletal Pain

Back pain results from improper conditioning, overexertion, forced head sets, or poor saddle fit. A heavy rider mismatched to a small horse also causes the horse back pain, as does an unbalanced or inexperienced rider. Poor conformation in

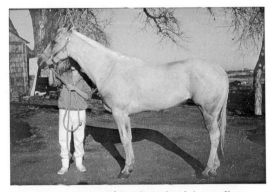

Fig. 6.16 A horse with a long back is predisposed to chronic back pain.

the form of a long back exaggerates all of these factors. A horse with a sore back communicates displeasure by humping the back, kicking, bucking, wringing the tail, or gnashing the teeth.

A jumping horse with back pain may refuse or rush a jump, jump too flat, or twist the hind legs when clearing the jump. An event horse may demonstrate similar problems: the horse's speed may slow, and enthusiasm wanes as it fatigues faster than normal. Standardbred racehorses are also prone to back pain, as are dressage horses that are asked for continuous efforts of collection and engagement of the hindquarters.

A horse with muscle problems in any part of the body quickly stiffens and tires with exertion, leading to poor performance. Tying-up *(myositis)* can cause a horse to stop work because of severe pain. *(See Chapter 3 for more information.)*

A horse with chronic arthritis often experiences days when the pain is sufficient to affect performance. A horse with sore feet is especially prone to poor performance as its stride shortens, and muscles become restricted and tight as the horse tries to guard against the pain.

Hoof Imbalance

A frequent reason for musculoskeletal pain is hoof imbalance. Because the lower joints of the limb primarily move in flexion and extension with little rotation or sideways motion, defects in conformation or unbalanced shoeing create abnormal sideways stress on the lower joints. One side of the hoof contacts the ground before the other, placing strain on joint ligaments and cartilage. The hoof records this stress with an uneven coronary band, along with flares and ridges in the hoof wall.

A long-toe – low-heel foot configuration creates extreme and prolonged fetlock drop, resulting in excessive pull on the deep digital flexor tendon and coffin joint. This poor type of foot alignment creates low grade chronic pain which reduces performance. A treadmill gait analysis effectively analyses dynamic placement of the foot in motion. This analysis may be important because 'balance' of the static foot does not always produce optimal results for the moving limb.

Diagnostic Lameness Exam

A veterinarian can identify the source of the pain with a lameness workup. A diagnostic lameness exam includes:

- careful evaluation of the horse at the walk and trot on different ground surfaces (hard or soft), with or without a rider's weight, and on different inclined planes (this includes trotting in circles)
- hoof testers to check for a specific painful area
- careful palpation and manipulation of all structures in the limb to test for a pained response
- flexion tests of the affected limb to stress different joints
- diagnostic nerve blocks to anaesthetize parts of the limb starting from the ground and working up the limb in a process of elimination

- radiographic evaluation of the painful area that has been isolated through the clinical exam and the above described diagnostic procedures.
- ultrasound, and nuclear scintigraphy (see below), may also be helpful.

New Techniques

Sophisticated technology is also incorporated into an exam of the musculoskeletal system if the source of the problem is not readily apparent. Video technology enables the veterinarian to analyse a horse's gait in slow motion for an accurate measure of foot fall, stride length and imbalance to diagnose an obscure lameness. Detailed gait analysis on a treadmill helps a veterinarian recommend shoeing changes that might improve the horse's movement.

Diagnostic ultrasound is useful for assessing the health and integrity of tendons and ligaments. *(See Chapter 9 for more information.)*

Nuclear scintigraphy is a technique that involves injecting a radio-pharmaceutical into the bloodstream. This compound concentrates in areas of increased circulation and emits gamma rays. Then a camera converts the gamma rays to light and exposes film to produce an image. Nuclear scintigraphy is used to identity abnormalities or areas of inflammation (also called 'hot spots') in the bones, joints, and muscles.

Infrared thermography is a tool to measure the temperature differences within tissues to similarly identify pockets of inflammation.

Lameness Classification

To facilitate communication with a veterinarian when discussing an injury, the American Association of Equine Practitioners (AAEP) provides terminology classifying lameness relative to the degree of severity. This is on a scale of 1 to 10 in the UK. Lameness is best seen at the two-beat gait of a trot. As the affected limb hits the ground, the horse lifts the head in an effort to quickly remove the weight off that leg. As the sound limb hits the ground, the head drops because the horse is willing to assume weight on the good leg.

Grade 1 lameness is difficult to observe because it is inconsistent, but may appear while circling, weight-carrying, or on hard surfaces. A visually apparent head nod or bob occurs with each stride in a circle in a Grade 2 or greater lameness. Any lameness that persists as a Grade 3 (visible at every stride) or more should quickly receive veterinary care.

LAMENESS CLASSIFICATION	
Grade	**Observable Signs**
Grade 1	Difficult to observe, not consistently apparent with weight-carrying, circling, inclines, or hard surfaces.
Grade 2	Difficult to observe at walk or trot in straight line. Apparent with weight-carrying, circling, inclines, and hard surfaces.
Grade 3	Consistent at trot under all circumstances.
Grade 4	Obvious lameness with marked head nodding, hitching, or a shortened stride. Visible at walk.
Grade 5	Minimal weight-carrying in motion and/or at rest, or the inability to move.

Fig. 6.17

Exercise Intolerance: Respiratory Problems

Another common cause of exercise intolerance is a failure of the respiratory tract to meet the demands of performance. The respiratory tract is divided into two sections: upper and lower.

Upper Respiratory System

The upper respiratory system includes the nostrils, nasal passages, pharynx larynx, and trachea up to the thorax.

A horse may make a noise on exercise which does not affect performance.

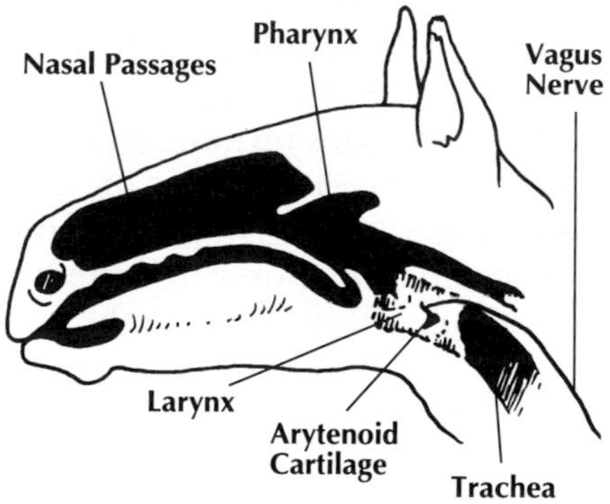

Fig. 6.18 The upper respiratory system.

Roaring

Racehorses, steeplechasers, eventers and jumpers are often asked to perform at peak speeds, and the tiniest impairment to respiratory ability can quickly turn a potential winner into a loser. At least 5% of Thoroughbred racehorses suffer from *laryngeal hemiplegia* (also called recur-

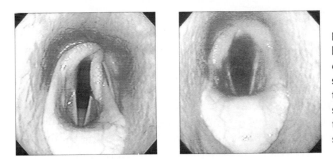

Fig. 6.19 On the left, the arytenoid cartilage before surgery, seen through an endoscope. On the right, the airway after surgery.

rent laryngeal neuropathy, or RLN) which causes a *roaring* condition.

The muscle which opens the arytenoid cartilage of the larynx is stimulated by the recurrent laryngeal nerve (a branch of the vagus nerve). If the nerve is damaged, the muscle is paralysed. The cartilage then collapses into the airway. As air passes through the diminished opening, air turbulence creates a roaring noise with each breath. A horse with this condition is unable to breathe enough oxygen to fuel the demanding muscles, therefore speed and performance are severely compromised.

Dr W. Robert Cook has linked a narrow jaw width with RLN. The average Thoroughbred has a normal jaw width equivalent to at least 4 fingers (7.2 centimetres). To measure the jaw width, fold the fingers at the joint below the knuckles with the back of the hand resting against the underside of the horse's neck. The fingers are placed between the lower jaw bones at the level of the throatlatch. The narrower this measurement, the greater the likelihood the horse will be afflicted with some degree of RLN.

Roaring is also diagnosed by passing an *endoscope* into the horse's nose to the back of the throat. Use of the 'slap test' during endoscopy helps in making a diagnosis of roaring. To determine the extent of the laryngeal paralysis, it is sometimes necessary to examine the horse while it is working on a treadmill. Surgery is moderately successful in returning affected horses to top performance.

Other Throat Problems

Other throat problems can lead to a diminished opening of the larynx and airway obstruction and can be identified with an endoscope. These problems include:

- *dorsal displacement of the soft palate*
- *epiglottic entrapment*
- *pharyngeal lymphoid hyperplasia*
- *arytenoid chondritis*

165

The first two syndromes interfere with the seal created by the soft palate and the larynx that maintains air pressure in the airways. The other two syndromes involve inflammation and distortion of the back of the throat that may obstruct normal air flow.

Lower Respiratory System

The lower respiratory organs include the branches of the trachea, bronchi, and the left and right lungs. Problems relating to the lower respiratory system usually result from viral or bacterial infection, or allergic reactions. Viral respiratory infections can predispose to:

- bacterial pneumonia or pleuropneumonia
- lung abscesses
- chronic obstructive pulmonary disease (COPD, or heaves)
- parasitic or fungal infection

These problems may produce lasting conditions that permanently interfere with a horse's respiratory capacity and performance. On rare occasions, cancer in the thorax may slowly compromise a horse's lung capacity.

Bleeding

Exercise-induced pulmonary haemorrhage (EIPH) is a condition seen primarily in racehorses; affected animals are called *bleeders*. Blood accumulates in the airways, and occasionally flows from the nose. It is not always easy to diagnose a horse affected by EIPH. Sometimes the horse coughs, or swallows excessively. On occasion, a horse may have trouble breathing. Difficulty in breathing may cause it to pull up suddenly during a race. The best way to identify a bleeder is to examine a suspect horse with an endoscope within 2 hours after exercise.

Vigorous Activity

Researchers are still trying to understand what actually causes EIPH. It seems to be a syndrome of horses that exercise strenuously, as with racing or steeplechasing. As many as 50–70% of horses participating in these sports have some degree of EIPH.

Lung Damage

EIPH may be the result of altered blood flow in areas of the lungs that have suffered previous inflammation. Inflammation in the airways increases blood flow in the walls of small airways, making them susceptible to rupture.

With maximal exertion the lungs are inflated to full capacity at rates greater than 150 breaths per minute. If a previously damaged region of the lung fails to inflate, the adjacent good lung tissue that has inflated may distort the diseased area. Altered pressure differences develop between the good and bad lung tissue. Pressure changes and tissue tearing may rupture fragile capillary walls in the diseased lung area, causing bleeding.

The uninflatable area of the diseased lung can be a result of:

- prior infection or inflammation that has grown scar tissue
- mucus or debris in the airways following an attack of influenza or pneumonia, which reduces the opening of the airway, creating uneven pressures in the lungs
- allergies which constrict the airways with spasms, and functionally reduce the opening of the small airways
- bronchiectasis following patent stage of lungworm infection

Upper Airway Obstruction

Although lower airway disease is the currently accepted theory to explain EIPH, Dr W. Robert Cook maintains that RLN creates pressure changes in the lungs by obstructing airflow through the upper respiratory tract. As a horse with RLN inhales, the collapsed arytenoid cartilage obstructs airflow. This obstruction creates above normal pressure changes in the lungs that are strong enough to damage blood vessels in the lungs and cause bleeding.

Predisposition to EIPH

A horse may be predisposed to EIPH due to the following conditions:

- lung tissue has been damaged from inflammation due to viral, bacterial, parasitic infection, or allergic reactions
- blood pressure increases due to tremendous heart pumping during strenuous exertions
- a genetic predisposition to weak blood vessels lining the lungs
- recurrent laryngeal neuropathy

Lasix®

The impact of isolated incidents of EIPH on performance is not very well understood. Pre-race prevention using a diuretic called frusemide (Lasix®) has improved racing times in horses afflicted with EIPH. Because it is a diuretic, Lasix® causes urination within minutes. There is no doubt that chronic bleeding permanently alters lung tissue with an adverse effect on performance.

Prevention of EIPH

Prevention is difficult to define for a disease which is not entirely understood. However, any management procedures that can be used to minimize disease of the small airways may prevent EIPH. These techniques include:

- improved ventilation in barns
- relatively dust-free bedding
- high quality, dust-free and mould-free hay
- ample recovery time (3 weeks) for respiratory infections
- an aggressive viral vaccination programme
- deworming at 6 – 8 week intervals to minimize damage from worms migrating through the lungs

Horses should be screened for RLN by an endoscopic exam, and the jaw width evaluated using techniques developed by Dr W. Robert Cook.

Exercise Intolerance: Cardiac Problems

Heart Irregularities

Heart disease is uncommon in horses. Heart murmurs or irregularities in heart rate (arrhythmias) can be evaluated by ultrasound and an ECG (electrocardiogram). *Degenerative myocardial disease* is unusual, but does occur. Chronic respiratory disease places strain on the heart, and can create arrhythmias. Viral, bacterial or protozoal infections can injure the heart valves. Electrolyte imbalances in the exercising horse have profound effects on heart contraction and cardiac output. Any condition that creates anaemia or interferes with blood flow to the heart muscle also compromises the heart's effectiveness as a pump to supply blood and oxygen to the tissues. Certain drugs, toxins or electrolyte imbalances can mimic heart disease symptoms, including:

- rapid heart rates
- poor recovery rates
- irregular heart rates
- acute fatigue
- fainting

Anaemia

Red blood cells (RBCs) contain haemoglobin, which carries oxygen to the tissues as the blood circulates through the body. Any condition that results in blood loss or a failure of the body to manufacture red blood cells leads to *anaemia*. A large intestinal parasite load, a chronic infection or an inflammatory condition can result in loss of RBCs. Nutrient deficiencies of iron, copper, protein, and B vitamins can impair the body's ability to manufacture sufficient RBCs. A blood sample can be evaluated for anaemia.

Packed Cell Volume

The *packed cell volume* (PCV) measures the percentage of circulating red blood cells in the bloodstream. Normally a horse has a PCV of around 40%. A highly fit individual may store up to one-third of its RBCs in the spleen. Because the RBCs are present but hiding in the spleen, a fit horse may have a PCV of about 30%. A horse with a PCV of less than 30% should be investigated for anaemia.

Ulcers

A competitive horse is a stressed horse and may be prone to bleeding gastric ulcers. Often a horse with stomach ulcers has episodes of colic. If this condition is suspected, the stomach can be examined with an endoscope. Faeces can be evaluated in the lab for the presence of digested blood that may indicate a bleeding intestinal ulcer.

WARM-UPS AND COOL-DOWNS

The horse is naturally designed for short bursts of speed to flee from predators. In the wild it does not have to sustain this flight or fight response for more than a few moments. Today, horses are asked to perform for extended periods at a maximal level of work. Many equine sports require fast bursts of speed combined with abrupt stops and turns, or jumping over obstacles while carrying a rider. Other sports involve long hours of steady work under saddle with infrequent rest periods. Just as with human athletes, a horse needs to limber up and stretch before beginning a workout.

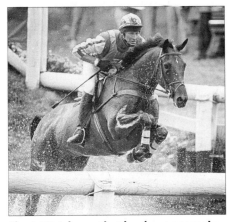

To prevent injury, each workout should include a routine of warm-ups and cooldowns before and after exercise. Muscles, ligaments and tendons should be properly prepared for the demands of athletic exertion. This preparation involves at least 15 – 20 minutes of warm-up to stimulate blood circulation to

Fig. 6.20 A horse that has been properly warmed up before competition performs better and more safely.

the tissues, and to slightly raise body temperature a few degrees. Warmth and circulation improve the flexibility of the musculoskeletal system, improving efficiency of muscle work and reducing the risk of injury to ligaments, tendons and joints.

Warm-Up Exercises
Walking

Walking is a preliminary exercise to gradually increase the respiratory rate and heart rate, flushing the muscles with blood and oxygen. Walking lightly stretches tendons and ligaments to improve their elasticity as the tissues heat up from movement. Joints are also warmed and lubricated.

Walking can be done under saddle, in hand, on a lunge line, or by using a walker. Brisk walking for 5 – 10 minutes sufficiently prepares the musculoskeletal system for more work.

Trotting

After walking, the horse can then be trotted for another 5 – 10 minutes to further warm the muscles and to stretch tendons and ligaments. Urge the horse forwards at a vigorous pace, which further improves the respiratory intake of oxygen and accelerates the heart rate. These physiological changes allow the musculoskeletal system to handle increased stress.

Manual Stretching Exercises

Once the muscles, tendons and ligaments are warm, manual stretching exercises add flexibility. If a muscle is stretched 100% of its functional length before contraction, the strength of the muscle contraction works at maximum efficiency. Most horses are trained at a muscle exertion of only 60% of maximum contraction length, leading to tight, unsupple muscle with a diminished range of motion. Sudden loading of a short, tight and inelastic musculotendinous unit may tear muscle or tendon fibres. To maximize muscle and tendon elasticity, apply stretching exercises in both warm-ups and cooldowns.

During a stretch, maintain each limb in a slightly flexed position to avoid strain to the tendons and ligaments of the lower leg. Grasp the limb above the knee or just below the hock. Each pull should be concentrated above the knee or hock for a greater range of motion in the shoulder or hip joints and their associated muscles.

Hold each stretch for 15 or 20 seconds. It may take several days of practice for a horse to become accustomed to the strange feel of these stretches without resisting. Do not force the stretch. Ask the horse to passively 'let go' in response to a gentle tug.

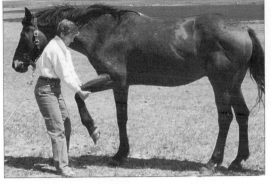

Fig. 6.21 Foreleg stretch.

Forelegs

Pick up each front leg individually and gently pull it forwards to stretch the shoulder and forearm muscles. Then ease the limb forwards and across the body towards the other foreleg. Also pull the leg gently to the outside, and then backwards towards the hind legs.

Hind Legs

Hind leg stretches are similar to foreleg stretches. Each hind leg is first stretched directly behind the horse, then towards the opposite hind leg. The hip and upper leg are then stretched forwards towards the front legs, and finally gently tugged out to the side.

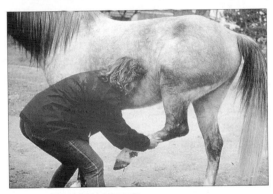

Fig. 6.22 Hind leg stretch.

Suppling Exercises

While mounted, relax the horse's neck and back muscles by bending the head and neck to the side (towards the rider's leg) with a slight jiggle of the rein. This technique softens the poll and jaw as the horse gives to the rein.

A long, downwards stretch of the head and neck can be accomplished by making the horse reach down for a carrot or other treat. This stretch loosens the back and loins, while the horse also relaxes mentally.

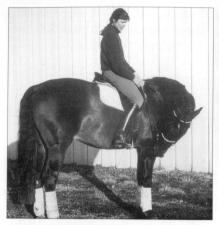

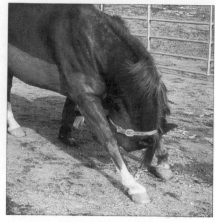

Fig. 6.23 Bending the head to the side softens the poll and jaw.

Fig. 6.24 Bending for a carrot stretches the back and loins.

Moving in circles, figure eight patterns and serpentine patterns asks the horse to step under the body with the inside rear leg, stretching the back and haunches.

Lateral exercises such as leg yields or side-passes supple the poll, neck, shoulders, back and haunches. The horse gradually begins to actively carry itself by using muscle groups in concert.

Long-Term Benefits

Stretching and suppling exercises have more long-term benefits than just the immediate improvement of tissue elasticity. Daily application of stretching exercises both before and after exercise ultimately:

- develops a longer stride as shoulders move with greater freedom
- improves the range of motion in both shoulder and hip muscles to facilitate lateral movements
- improves flexibility in the upper limbs, reducing the risk of injury during stressful demands
- causes less fatigue because muscles and joints are pliable
- improves circulation to all the tissues, requiring less effort during a warm-up and conserving energy for the athletic exertion

Specific Sports Warm-up

The entire warm-up process, exploring all varieties of stretching and suppling exercises, can take as long as 30 minutes. As the warm-up intensifies after the first 20 minutes, a jumping horse might be asked to trot cavallettis or jump several small obstacles (less than 2 feet high). A long distance riding horse could gradually begin a mild incline after 10 or 15 minutes of trotting. A racehorse would be breezed at a slow canter after the initial warm-up to gradually increase cardiac output and blood flow to the muscles.

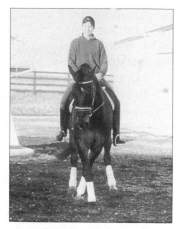

Fig. 6.25 Side-passes supple the poll, neck, shoulders, back, and haunches.

Cool-Down Exercises

Cooling down is as important as warming up. After a horse has finished a workout, devote 15 – 30 minutes to cooling down at a walk or slow trot. It is best to keep a horse moving during a cool-down to dissipate heat generated by working muscles. Dissipating heat will cause muscle and body temperature to slowly decline. Blood that was routed to the muscles is gradually redirected back to internal organs. Oxygen is replenished to muscles that reached an oxygen debt, and accumulated lactic acid is flushed from the muscles. Removal of lactic acid from the muscles is important for alleviating muscle soreness that can occur after exercise.

Post Exercise Stretches

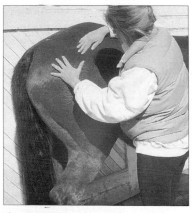

Fig. 6.26 Massaging relaxes tight muscles after exercise.

While walking, a loose rein encourages the horse to stretch its own neck and back, relieving tension on overworked muscles that might begin to tighten. Once dismounted, the same manual stretches that were used during warm-up can also be used in a cool-down. Stretching reduces post exercise muscle soreness.

Muscle Massage

Muscle massage relaxes tight muscles, improving oxygen circulation in the muscles and removing toxic by-products. The large muscles over the hip, neck, back and thighs particularly benefit from 20 – 30 minutes of massage.

With firm pressure, use the heel of the hand or the fingertips to create a circular massaging motion over each muscle group. The horse will relax and most likely will lean into the pressure. As a finishing touch, apply a thick rubber curry comb in a circular motion to stimulate the skin and superficial muscles, while removing sweat and dirt from the coat.

Food and Water

Once the horse's chest is cool to the touch, offer it hay and water. Wait about half an hour after the horse is *fully* cooled down before offering grain. Then blood flow is restored to the intestines, and the horse is less likely to develop colic.

Warm Weather Cool-Downs

During hot and humid weather, a horse may need additional help cooling down. Sponging the head, neck, chest and legs helps remove body heat by improving evaporative cooling. Soak the large blood vessels along the neck and legs for maximum cooling, but stay away from the large muscle groups over the back and hindquarters. Sponging water on overheated, large muscle masses can cause them to spasm, and the horse then ties-up. After a pleasure ride that has stimulated only a light sweat, the horse can be bathed following 15 – 30 minutes of cool-down.

Besides soaking the neck and chest, place the horse in an area shaded from the sun. If the air is particularly still, improve heat dissipation by directing a fan on the horse to push cool air past the skin.

For a horse that exercises during warm weather, it is best to maintain as lean a body weight as possible. Extra body fat delays heat dissipation from the muscles, and dramatically increases the cooling period.

Cool Weather Cool-Downs

It is important to cool down the working muscles adequately after a hard workout any time of the year, but it is essential during the cooler seasons. Working skeletal muscle generates a large amount of heat, and if insufficiently cooled down, or if exposed to cold rain or water directly after a workout, muscle tissue may begin to spasm and cramp.

Insulation Delays Cool-Down

Fat Insulation

Fat is an insulating layer that acts as a 'cushion' against climatic elements. A thin horse has fewer fat reserves against chills than an individual with a healthy covering of flesh.

On the other hand, an overweight horse has the opposite problem from a thin horse. Heat dissipates slowly from an overweight or underconditioned horse. An overweight horse may finish exercising with only a slight dampness around the neck. Then, 2 hours later, it may be soaked in the neck, chest and girth areas because heat loss through the skin continues after exercise.

Hair Coat Insulation

When dry, the horse's hair coat provides insulating protection from chills and damp. A dense winter hair coat protects a horse from the elements, but its length makes it difficult to cool down the horse.

The shortened daylight hours of winter stimulate hairs to grow longer due to the effect of reduced light on the brain's *pineal gland*. A horse with a thick, heavy coat experiences the same phenomenon as a fat horse because the hair layer insulates against cooling. Delayed sweating is a natural occurrence, yet steps must be taken to protect damp horses from drafts and chills.

Horse hairs are evenly distributed on the body, rather than in clusters, as in dogs or cats. The loft in a horse's hair coat insulates it and retains body heat.

Cool-Down Methods

An adequate cool-down permits the circulation to flush away toxic by-products and heat, and prevents tying-up. Consider special cool-down procedures during winter weather such as walking, drying the hair coat, cover-ups, and body clipping.

Walking

Walking for 15 – 30 minutes cools muscles after an exertion, releasing much of the heat that contributes to sweating. Walking is the best way to cool down a horse in cold weather. Either hand walking or mechanical 'walkers' are useful. Walking maintains good circulation to the muscles, which dissipates heat.

Many people mistakenly believe that walking a horse after exercise will dry a damp hair coat. If the sun is shining, it dries a wet coat as the horse walks. However, a dry coat does not mean the horse is fully cool, and a cool horse may also be wet.

As muscles cool down, so do ligaments, joints and tendons. Walking maintains flexibility in these structures, making the limbs less susceptible to injury. Bandages retain warmth and circulatory flow in the lower legs during the walking period. Leave splint boots or leg bandages on during the cool-down period to cool lower limbs slowly.

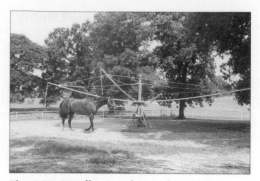

Fig. 6.27 A walker can be used to cool muscles.

Drying the Hair Coat

Sweat scrapers are great for pulling extra moisture from the hair coat to regain loft and insulating capacities quickly. A brisk rubbing with a dry towel or brush also removes moisture from the coat, while exposing more hair surface to the air for faster drying. Towelling also 'polishes' a dull coat. If necessary, an electric hair dryer *(set on low heat)* can be used to speed up drying of a soaked coat.

Body Clipping

To avoid prolonged cool-downs in the wintertime, many horses are body clipped to facilitate heat loss during exercise. Shaving hair away from the chest, abdomen, neck and shoulders exposes a large area for evaporative cooling. Shaving also helps large surface blood vessels in these areas radiate heat away from the horse. However, if a horse has been body-clipped and the insulating hair layer removed, it is very important to cover the horse during resting hours.

Cover-Ups

Rugging serves as a substitute for natural hair on clipped horses, protecting a horse from wind chill or wet weather. Rugs may also give additional protection against the elements for horses with a full hair coat. Many varieties of horse rugs are commercially available, each appropriate for different conditions.

Coolers

'Coolers' wick moisture away from the hair coat while keeping draughts off the horse. A cooler is made of wool, acrylic or a mixture of both. A wool cooler pulls moisture from the coat most effectively, while keeping a horse warm underneath. A cooler is poorly designed for trailer travel. It is too long and wide with no stabilizing straps. A horse can step on a cooler, and pull it off, risking it becoming entangled in the horse's legs.

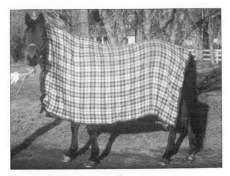

Fig. 6.28 A wool cooler.

Anti-Sweat Sheets

An anti-sweat sheet works well to cool a hot horse. It is form-fitting and made of cotton or polypropylene. Holes or perforations in the sheet allow evaporation of moisture, while providing a protective covering similar to some brands of human thermal underwear.

Once a horse is cooled down fairly well, place another blanket on

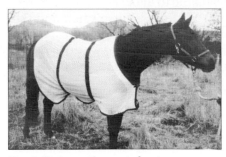

Fig. 6.29 An anti-sweat sheet.

top of an anti-sweat sheet to produce a layering effect. The anti-sweat sheet allows sweat to dry without holding in moisture that could become cold and clammy if kept close to the skin. Heat generated by the horse's muscles collects under the blanket layers, while moisture evaporates away, leaving a dry and warm horse underneath.

Other Cover-Ups

A blanket with a wool liner helps to dry a wet horse while keeping it warm. The outer shell should be a 'breathable' material so moisture can evaporate away from the horse's skin. Check with the manufacturer or tack shop if unsure about the properties of the outer shell.

Common materials used in horse rugs also include Gore-tex® or polypropylene. These materials create a water-resistant barrier, yet a wet horse cloaked in polypropylene or Gore-tex® dries quickly because of the unique 'breathing' properties of these materials. The tight weave of these fabrics also creates a wind breaker effect.

Rugging Wet Horses

Do not rug a wet horse unless it is checked periodically for drying. A rug soaked with sweat provides more surface area for evaporative cooling. More surface area increases the rate of body cooling, creating a 'refrigerator effect', resulting in a chilled and miserable animal. Moisture evaporates from the skin faster than the body is able to warm the skin. Skin temperature decreases, and eventually chills the body as well. Certain fabrics such as cotton and Dacron® enhance evaporative cooling, whereas wool can be wet and still retain some warmth.

Other Options
Enclosed Barn

Access to an enclosed barn provides greater cool-down options in inclement weather. A barn provides a draught-free environment with consistent temperatures. If a barn is well insulated and warm, it is acceptable to wash the horse after a workout. If the hair is matted down by sweat, or caked with mud, vital body heat escapes. Washing sweat and dirt from the hair coat improves the insulating loft once it has dried. It is best to avoid bathing a horse during the winter months unless a warm barn is available to allow complete drying. *Repeated* bathing removes natural oils from a horse's hair and skin and reduces the water repellency of the hair coat. Bathing a horse in cold weather risks accidental chilling, even if using warm water. Use common sense: a dirty horse is better than a sick horse.

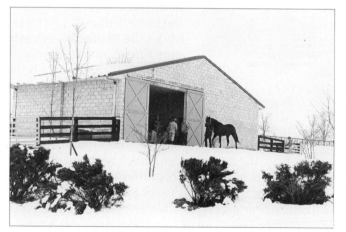

Fig. 6.30 An enclosed, well-insulated, warm barn is the best place to bathe horses in cold weather.

Management

Each horse tolerates climatic changes differently. Consider the horse's body weight, length and distribution of the hair coat, the stabling facilities, and blanketing options available. When cooling down a sweat-soaked horse, an educated approach coupled with instinct and common sense will prevent trouble. Keeping a horse current on respiratory vaccine boosters allows it to fend off chill-related respiratory viruses. Intelligent management can maintain a horse's conditioning programme year-round.

7

NUTRITION FOR PERFORMANCE

With today's technology, hay samples can be submitted to a laboratory for identification of all available nutrients. With this detailed information and the assistance of an equine nutritionist and computer programs, owners and trainers can formulate a tailored diet for each horse. Although such ideal diets are within reach, they are not always practical for the average horse owner, but should be actively considered. Feeding the correct diet is an exact science, and it is frequently better to purchase good quality compounded feed.

Consider each unique situation. A large operation may be able to put up its own hay. However, it is possible for repeated harvest of the same fields to deplete the soil of essential minerals. Hay grown in these fields is then deficient in mineral micronutrients and requires supplementation.

A small farm may only have access to a pasture turnout with ample grass

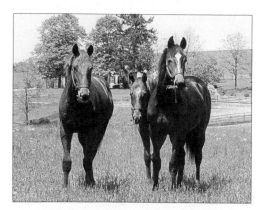

Fig. 7.1 Some farms may have access to good pasture for only a few months each spring.

for a few months each spring. As the pasture is overgrazed, other feeds are required to fulfil basic nutritional requirements. Paddock or stall-confined horses may need hay year-round. Hay is often bought monthly, as budget or storage space allows. It comes from different fields or different harvests, and varies in nutrient content with each truckload.

In implementing a dietary programme for a horse, there are no hard-and-fast rules. Each horse must be fed according to its individual needs. Not all horses need grain in their diet, while others require large amounts. Athletic pursuits and exercise regimens vary between horses, and from day to day for any individual. Genetics and age considerably influence the efficiency of nutrient use.

BASIC REQUIREMENTS

The equine intestinal tract is highly developed to extract nutrients from the digestion of plant matter. Roughage comes in the form of hay or pasture, and serves as the foundation upon which to build a feeding programme. The high fibre content of roughage is essential to normal intestinal function and health. Horses masticate roughage to ensure maximum digestion. The degree of mastication will reduce if teeth are not kept properly rasped.

Energy is one of the basic requirements in a daily diet, yet misconceptions persist about how horses obtain energy. Metabolism of roughage in the large intestine, and fermentation and breakdown of fibre generate large amounts of *volatile fatty acids* (VFA). These along with sugars (glucose) can be used immediately, or are stored as fat. Combining high quality roughage and high-power concentrates (grains and vegetable oil) in a sensible manner allows control of a horse's energy intake, and customizes a ration for each horse's special energy needs.

There are guidelines which can help create a safe diet that best meets a horse's nutritional requirements:

- A horse can only consume 2.5% of its body weight per day in feed. That quantity is simply all the intestines can hold. If the horse weighs 1000 lb, its daily feed limit—grain and roughage combined—is 25 lb.
- At least half of the daily ration, by weight, should consist of roughage in the form of hay or grass, or a combination of the two. A 1000-lb horse with a maximum daily ration of 25 lb should consume at least 12.5 lb of that in roughage. This amount does not provide the entire daily supply of essential nutrients, but it is a starting point on which to build.

- The higher the proportion of roughage, the safer the diet. The more high-power concentrate in a ration, the greater the risk of disease, including founder, colic and various limb deformities that affect growing horses.
- Measure all feed by **weight** and not volume, as the weights of bales of hay or different grain products vary. Weighing the food provides consistency at each feeding.
- Feed at regular intervals, at the same time each day: horses enjoy a regular feeding regime.

Hay

Grass Hay

Alone, quality grass hay provides a nearly adequate diet for a mature, idle horse, meeting its needs for protein, energy and fibre. However, grass hay is relatively low in calcium and high in phosphorus. Therefore, this diet may need calcium supplementation in the form of ground limestone. This supplement satisfies an adult horse's requirement for a calcium-to-phosphorus (Ca:P) ratio of no less than one part calcium to one part phosphorus (1:1).

Cereal Grain Hay

Cereal grain hays, such as oat hay, are similar in nutritive value to grass hays in many respects. However, once the grain heads have fallen from this type of hay, all that remains is straw which is vastly reduced in energy value.

Legume Hay

Legume hays, such as alfalfa or clover, are 20% higher in energy, twice as high in protein, 3 times as high in calcium, and 5 times higher in vitamin A than good quality grass hays. Legume hay therefore gives greater nutrient value than grass hay. However, depending on the amount of legume hay fed, the high calcium content may need to be offset with a phosphorus supplement such as monosodium phosphate.

Nutritional Value

A lot of the nutritional value of hay depends on the stage of harvest and the state of preservation. Most of hay's nutrition (⅔ of the energy and ¾ of the protein value) is within the leaves. Because good quality hay is abundant in leaves, inspect the hay to be sure it is leafy and soft, rather than stemmy and coarse. If hay is stemmy because it was harvested late in the maturation process, or if the leaves have turned to powder and fallen off because it was poorly cured, its nutritional value must be discounted proportionately.

The moisture content should be less than 20% to prevent mould and spoilage. However, excessively dry leaves fall away and the hay loses nutrient value. Shake a flake of hay to see how many leaves fall out, or if they crumble to dust. Check for mould, and break it apart to look for discoloured areas. If the hay is green, smells sweet, holds together well, and is not irritating to handle due to sticks, stems or weeds, then it passes the test for freshness and palatability.

Silage Horse Hage®

Grass is also conserved by ensiling, either in clamps or depends on sealed plastic bags. Success depends on anaerobic conditions being maintained until just before feeding to the horse. Always check for moulds and evidence of a secondary fermentation, which takes place if the product has been exposed to air for more than 1or 2 days. It should look and smell good. Ensiled grass is harvested when the grass is at its highest nutritional value, and is less affected by weather than hay. The nutritional value is such that less concentrate needs to be fed than with grass hay. It is dust-free and therefore of particular use for horses with allergic respiratory disease.

Pasture

The nutritional content of pasture forage varies not only according to plant characteristics, but also by season. Energy and mineral content depend on soil type, but certain rules of thumb help determine how to supplement pasture during different seasons. With rapid spring growth, grasses are high in protein, minerals, and vitamins, but lacking in energy due to the high water content of sprouting plants. A 1000-lb horse has to eat three times as much fresh spring grass as hay to meet its energy requirements. Pasture loses water content as it matures, but it also loses protein and mineral value as its fibre content increases.

Concentrates

Energy is the most critical part of a horse's diet. A primary source of energy is carbohydrates, which are found in the fibre components of hay and grass, and are commonly found in a concentrated form as grain. Grains provide much more energy per pound than hay.

Carbohydrates are easily digested to glucose. Glucose is readily absorbed in the bloodstream and made available to muscles for work, or is stored as fat in adipose tissue or as glycogen in the skeletal muscles and liver.

As an example, the National Research Council stipulates that:

- Light horses at light work require a 25% increase in energy consumption per day.
- Medium work efforts require energy consumption to increase by 50% per day.
- Intense work requires doubling of energy consumption per day.
- Draft horses require a 10% increase in energy consumption for each hour of field work.

When a horse is burning more energy than it is able or willing to eat in forage, grain is the most efficient way to increase energy intake. Grains offer a concentrated source of energy, but are relatively high in phosphorus and low in calcium. Processed grains (rolled, cracked, or crimped) are slightly more digestible than whole grains.

Oats and Maize

Oats and maize are the two most popular feed grains. Oats are higher in fibre content and lower in digestible energy than other grains due to a fibrous hull surrounding each oat kernel. Maize is twice as high in digestible energy as oats. Both oats and maize contain enough protein for mature horses, but oats have up to 12% versus 9% for maize.

Rye and Barley

Rye and barley fall between oats and maize on the energy scale. Barley must be processed to remove its indigestible outer hull. Rye,

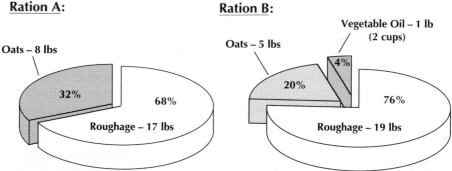

Ration A:

Oats – 8 lbs

32%

68%

Roughage – 17 lbs

Ration B:

Oats – 5 lbs

Vegetable Oil – 1 lb (2 cups)

4%

20%

76%

Roughage – 19 lbs

Fig. 7.2 Ration B, with 3 lb less oats, offers an equal amount of digestible energy as ration A.

when fed alone, is unpalatable. These grains are usually fed in combination with other foodstuffs, in the form of a mixed grain or pelleted feed.

Fat

Fat is an excellent fuel source for working muscles if they are adequately supplied with oxygen during aerobic exercise. (Aerobic exercise generally occurs at speeds of less than 12 m.p.h., or at heart rates of less than 150 beats per minute.) By using fat as fuel and sparing glycogen reserves in the liver and skeletal muscle, a horse on a high-fat diet delays fatigue during aerobic performance. Glycogen remains available as an energy source for anaerobic activity of high speed or sprint efforts.

Fats are up to three times greater in energy density than an equal weight of grain. For example, 1 lb of fat provides the same amount of digestible energy as 3 lb of oats, or 2 lb of sweet feed. However, only a maximum of 12–15% of a ration can be fed in the form of fat. Other feeds such as roughage and grain must complement the use of fat as an energy source.

Vegetable oil as a form of fat is efficiently digested and metabolized. It is not as filling in the digestive tract as grain or hay, and less fat is required to supply a similar amount of calories and energy as found in grain. If the vegetable oil is used, it must be stored properly so it will not spoil or become rancid, It is highly palatable when mixed with grain or bran.

Protein

Because humans have a high demand for dietary protein, they often assume horses have a similar need. Protein is therefore commonly overfed to horses. Horses use it as an energy source only if they lack carbohydrates (hay and grain) or fats. Protein is metabolically inefficient for the horse to process and excrete when fed in excess.

Every horse needs protein, but mature horses require only moderate amounts (8–10% of the ration). Growing horses, pregnant and lactating mares and aged horses need up to 16%. Supplemental protein can be provided with legume hays, or with concentrated grain mixes of higher protein levels.

Maize and oats provide 8–12% protein. Grass hays or pastures are variable in protein content, and for exact values should be analysed at a laboratory. Generally, good quality grass hay contains at least 8% protein. Alfalfa feed products generally provide at least 15% protein, and can be as high as 28%.

As a youngster grows, or as a horse exercises, its appetite normally increases to ingest more energy. With greater feed consumption, the additional protein needs of the growing or exercising horse are usually met.

Calcium/Phosphorous

A quality, well balanced diet probably provides a horse with the vitamins and trace minerals it needs. However, calcium and phosphorus must be present in a horse's diet, not only in sufficient amounts, but also in the correct ratio, and they may require some adjustment. Grains and grasses tend to be high in phosphorus; legume hays provide excess calcium. Therefore, a judicious combination of grain or grass hay with legume hay often achieves an adequate balance of calcium to phosphorus. The ideal ratio of calcium to phosphorus for a mature horse is between 1.2:1 and 2:1. (The maximum Ca:P ratio tolerated by mature, idle horses is 5:1, while a growing horse has a critical need for a ratio of about 1.5:1.)

Feeding bran will alter the Ca:P ratio and must be considered when calculating the diet.

MEETING NUTRIENT REQUIREMENTS
The Pregnant Mare

A pregnant mare has specific dietary demands that affect the health of the growing athlete she carries. Some of the nutrients she receives will be stored by the foal before birth, and used after birth when the mare cannot provide them in her milk. Lack of these nutrients, especially in late gestation, can seriously impair the foal's athletic potential.

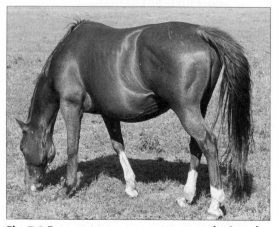

Fig. 7.3 Pregnant mares on pasture need mineral supplements.

For the first two trimesters of a mare's pregnancy, she needs only a normal maintenance diet. Excess vitamin and mineral supplements fed in the beginning months of gestation have negative effects on the foetus, while excess energy causes a mare to become fat.

The Last Trimester

By the ninth month of pregnancy, the foetus starts to grow rapidly; the mare now needs to eat for two. A mare on pasture in her last trimester needs additional supplements to provide adequate nutrition for her growing foetus.

During the last trimester of pregnancy, trace minerals are deposited within foetal liver tissues. Liver reserves of trace mineral micronutrients sustain a foal through a phase of rapid growth during its first 2 – 3 months. If a mare in late stages of pregnancy does not receive enough of specific micronutrients, the potential athlete *in utero* may not store enough reserves in its liver for healthy bone growth. A young athlete's predisposition for developmental orthopaedic disease may begin during late gestation.

Most mares enter this last trimester in late winter or early spring. Rapidly growing spring pasture grass has such a high water content that a mare would have to eat 50 lb daily to consume the 15 lb of dry matter her late pregnancy requires. Not only are her intestines incapable of holding that much forage, but she would have to eat around the clock.

Grain

Mares can be supplemented with maize, oats or sweet feed each day. Be careful when feeding maize: while it is excellent for the hardworking athlete, it is easy to overfeed maize to a broodmare. Weigh the grain rather than feeding it by volume, as oats and maize differ considerably in weight.

Sweet feed typically consists of oats, maize and barley, mixed with 5% molasses to decrease dust and improve flavour. Molasses, with its high calcium content, assists in offsetting the relatively high phosphorus content of the grains. Sweet feed is available with protein levels ranging from 10 to 16%. Choose a feed with a 14 or 16% protein level specifically formulated for broodmares.

Copper and Other Minerals

In addition, pregnant mares experience an increased copper need in their last months of pregnancy because copper is transferred through the placenta and stored by the foal. Ideally, in her last trimester she should receive 30 ppm (parts per million) of copper daily, and it must be balanced with zinc and other minerals. Lack of minerals in the forage can be compensated for only by supplementing pregnant mares with a balanced mineral mix added to grain.

Calcium and Phosphorus

Some grain mixes come already prepared with added minerals. For a mare on grass pasture or hay, buy a specifically formulated mix to ensure she receives an adequate balance of calcium and phosphorus. She will also need a ground limestone supplement to supply ample calcium in her diet if she receives grain without added minerals.

During the last trimester, as the foetus grows and the mare gains weight, gradually increase her grain intake. By the time she foals, she can be eating as much as 6 – 8 lb of grain each day. Another option is to supplement grass hay or pasture with up to 10 lb of good quality alfalfa each day, omitting the grain. Alfalfa provides ample calcium and protein, while pasture furnishes the phosphorus alfalfa lacks. A mare on an alfalfa-rich diet will need phosphorus supplements.

The Lactating Mare

During the first 2 months of lactation, a mare's energy demands increase by 150% over maintenance. Milk *composition* is not influenced by diet, but its *quantity* depends on adequate energy and protein intake. In early lactation, a mare produces as much as 3% of her body weight in milk each day—approximately 30 lb, or 7.5 gallons.

A pasture will mature in summer, losing nutritional value just when a mare needs it most. If her requirements were met with grain, that would be 1.75 lb of grain per 100 lb of her body weight. This would amount to 17 lb of grain a day—a dangerous quantity for any horse. Instead, limit the quantity of grain to 8 lb and provide an equal weight of alfalfa.

Concentrations of trace minerals such as copper, zinc and

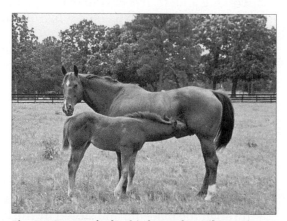

Fig. 7.4 From a foal's third month until weaning the mare's energy demands drop to 50% above maintenance.

manganese in the mare's milk are generally quite low, and cannot give a growing foal its dietary requirements. Despite supplementation of the mare with extra copper, zinc, or manganese, milk concentrations of these micronutrients do *not* increase. A foal depends on liver reservoirs formed in the last trimester of pregnancy, and on dietary supplementation once it begins eating solid food.

From a foal's third month until weaning, it will consume much of its diet as hay and creep feed, reducing its need for milk. Offer 1 lb of grain for each month of age, up to 6 lb a day. As a result, the mare's energy demands drop to only 50% above maintenance. Reduce her ration of grain and alfalfa accordingly, or she is at risk for founder or colic.

The Growing Athlete

The young, growing horse has very specialized dietary demands to build a strong musculoskeletal system for future athletic stress. Normal development of bone, cartilage, joints, ligaments and tendons requires more than just ample amounts of nutrients; the nutrients must also be balanced in respect to each other.

An example of an imbalanced diet would be feeding alfalfa only. Alfalfa has a high protein content (18%), high calcium-to-phosphorus ratio (more than 5:1), and high energy content. It is therefore a valuable feed source, but if fed alone can trigger growth surges that cause *developmental orthopaedic disease* (DOD).

Developmental Orthopaedic Disease

Long Bones

Under normal conditions, the cartilage of growing bone is gradually removed and replaced with bone cells, allowing long bones to elongate while still bearing weight. If this process goes awry, cartilage is retained in some areas where it should have mineralized into bone.

Thickening of cartilage layers in a defective area is accompanied by malnourishment and necrosis (death) of underlying layers of bone *(subchondral bone)*. Weakened bone develops microfractures, with subsequent pain. Or, subchondral bone and defective joint *(articular)* cartilage can separate, forming *osteochondrosis* lesions, which indicates DOD.

Growth Plates

Rapid bone growth due to excessive amounts of protein and energy in the diets of young foals has been implicated in DOD, as has an imbalance of calcium and phosphorus in the diet. An inherited predisposition to rapid growth may also be a component of a DOD syndrome. In a fast-growing foal, nutrients which are essential for healthy bone development are depleted as cartilage matures too rapidly into bone at growth plates and joint surfaces.

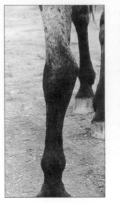 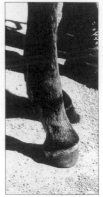

Fig. 7.5 Epiphysitis in knee.

Fig. 7.6 Contracted tendon.

Imperfect maturation of cartilage into bone within growth plates results in *physitis* (commonly known as *epiphysitis*), a form of DOD. *Angular limb deformities* are associated with unequal growth rates along a growth plate, or with malformation or collapse of the multiple bones in the knee or hock joints.

Flexural deformities such as contracted tendons develop as a result of osteochondrosis or epiphysitis, causing pain in joints or growth plates. Upright pasterns, or *club feet,* are another example of a flexural deformity.

Vertebrae

If the vertebrae in the neck develop abnormally, spinal cord compression and 'wobbler' syndrome result.

Abnormally developing cartilage is susceptible to traumatic injury, because even normal activity can damage improperly developing cartilage. Youngsters may show evidence of defective cartilage in joints or growth plates when their maturing body weight excessively loads the malformed joint surfaces.

Preventing DOD

To prevent these crippling syndromes, an intelligent feeding programme is essential for a young horse. Feed a ration combining grass hay, alfalfa hay and grain concentrate. Alfalfa boosts the nutritional value of the grass hay and grain provides phosphorus to balance alfalfa's high calcium content. Grain also provides nutrients without overloading the foal's intestines.

High Quality Diet

Offer the young horse all the hay it will eat, mixing grass with alfalfa in a 2:1 ratio. The alfalfa provides plenty of energy, calcium and protein, including lysine, which is the only amino acid known to be essential for growing horses. Neither grain nor grass hay is a good source of lysine.

A young horse can be supplemented with grain or mixed feed. Care must be taken to give supplementary feed to maintain good growth and body weight. Overfeeding will produce a 'top heavy' foal with increaed loading on bone growth plates and the possibility of epiphysitis. With alfalfa already providing considerable protein, the foal does not need more than a 10% protein sweet feed, or straight corn.

If quality alfalfa is unavailable, replace it with free choice grass hay. Still provide grain as above, but make sure it is 14% protein. Also feed a calcium supplement such as dicalcium phosphate (2 parts calcium to 1 part phosphorus) to replace the calcium alfalfa would have provided.

Trace Minerals

Insufficient dietary intake or a poor quality diet offered to a growing horse reduces the availability of specific micronutrients, such as trace minerals, that are important to healthy bone formation. Trace minerals such as copper are critical for normal musculoskeletal development of the young horse. Copper needs vary from region to region and must be balanced to the amount of available zinc. Trace mineral salt blocks do *not* supply the necessary quantities of minerals. Such blocks are 98% regular salt (sodium chloride) and have very minute amounts of trace minerals. These blocks were developed for *ruminants*, such as cattle, sheep and goats. Free choice consumption by horses does not achieve desired levels of mineral intake each day.

To provide ample concentrations of trace minerals to a growing foal, the minerals must be supplemented in grain. Ask the veterinarian or equine nutritionist for specific recommendations on a trace mineral supplement.

A young horse's skel-

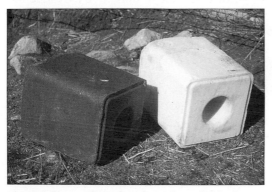

Fig. 7.7 Trace mineral and regular salt block.

etal system continues to form until it is at least 3 years old. During this time, it should remain on a carefully balanced ration. Once near mature size and weight, it can tolerate a greater range of protein and mineral content in the diet without affecting athletic potential.

The Idle and Lightly Worked Horse

An idle, mature horse that is not currently in training needs no special dietary considerations other than maintaining just the right weight. Idle, mature horses fulfil their energy needs effectively with good quality roughage, and need only be supplemented with free choice salt blocks and a balanced mineral mix.

When running the hand along the horse's ribs, only the last two should be felt. Usually the idle horse thrives on a maintenance diet of 1.75 lb quality grass hay per 100 lb. (A 1000-lb horse would receive about 18 lb of hay per day.)

Light Training

When reintroducing a horse to a light training schedule of 3 or 4 days a week of trotting and cantering, feeding demands need only provide 15% more energy than maintenance. To provide the lightly exercised horse with the fuel it needs, feed up to 1.5 lb of sweet feed for each hour of exercise, in addition to quality grass hay. Protein needs do not increase with light exercise, so for an adult horse a 10% protein mix is adequate.

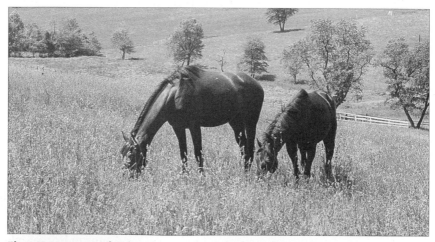

Fig. 7.8 Horses evolved to graze at frequent intervals.

Alternatives to Grain

Hay

Because horses evolved to graze at frequent intervals throughout the day and night, they would much prefer to graze over a long period than to eat only a small portion of grain that disappears quickly. If the horse cleans up its feed and looks for more, offer it extra grass hay while it stands idle in the stall or paddock, or turn it out to pasture.

Beet Pulp

Instead of extra hay, a horse's need for fibre can be satisfied with up to 2 lb (10% of the ration by weight) of beet pulp. Beet pulp is a good roughage substitute because it is relatively low in nutrients and high in fibre (18%). Wet beet pulp swells to many times its original volume. To ensure it will not swell inside the horse and cause colic, soak it in large amounts of water for at least 5 hours before feeding.

Bran

Another low nutritive, but filling, grain product commonly used is wheat bran. Bran is high in fibre, low in energy, and about 15% protein. Not only is it extremely high in phosphorus, but it also binds calcium in a horse's body. This characteristic makes bran useful to balance high calcium diets of legume hays. Half a pound of bran a day is a nice treat and may increase a horse's water consumption, especially if fed as a mash. Although the presence of bran in a horse's diet may increase the volume of its manure, bran is not a laxative. In fact, if bran is overfed, a horse could become constipated.

If a horse is putting on a bit too much weight from an enhanced diet, then exercise it more, or reduce grain. Initially, some adjustments in the diet will be necessary to find just the right amounts of extra feed to keep a horse comfortable and happy while it builds muscle through exercise.

The Hard-Working Athlete

The goal of a feeding and conditioning programme is to improve muscular efficiency and provide fuel reserves for the working muscles. The mental and physical stress of hard exercise on an athletic horse radically increases its energy and trace mineral demands. An equine athlete must be supplied with a quality ration that can be consumed within its intestinal limits (2.5% of its body weight) while providing fuel for locomotion.

Horses involved in sports requiring intense bursts of speed (for instance, racing, polo, hunting and gymkhana) will use aerobic metabolism, but they will also rely on fuel supplied under anaerobic conditions in the muscles. Without ample fuel supplies, a horse will lose its competitive edge as it tires.

Horses in endurance sports (endurance racing, long distance competitive riding and eventing) need large amounts of energy to sustain them through the rigours of prolonged athletic output, in both training and competition. At speeds less than 12 m.p.h. (a fast trot), horses work within aerobic limits, with ample oxygen supplied to working muscles. *(See Chapter 3 for more information.)*

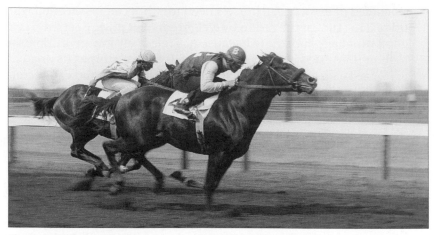

Fig. 7.9 Hard exercise increases an athlete's energy demands.

Replenishing Energy

The diet of an equine athlete must not only fulfil normal metabolic function, but it must replenish energy supplies depleted in strenuous daily workouts. Hay does not offer enough energy to meet the fuel demands of the athletic horse, even if it eats its full intestinal limit of 2.5% body weight every day. The sheer bulk of hay limits a horse's necessary intake.

Although it is difficult to maintain body fat on the hard-working horse, there are ways to maximize a horse's caloric and energy intake without jeopardizing its health or digestive function. To compensate for energy expenditures of rigorous athletics, it is necessary to supplement with concentrates. Up to half the daily intake (by weight) of feed can be supplied in a concentrated form.

Addition of Vegetable Oil

Vegetable oil, mixed into grain, is easily digestible by horses and contributes little to intestinal fill. It provides almost three times as much energy as a similar volume of grain, making it an excellent source of energy. In energy content, 16 oz of vegetable oil is equivalent to 3 lb of oats or 2 lb of sweet feed. For example, feeding 5 lb of maize and 16 oz of vegetable oil a day (divided into 2 – 3 equal feedings) achieves the same nutritional results as 7 lb of maize. The reduced volume of concentrate allows the horse to eat more hay, and the ration is safer. As a bonus, the vegetable oil enhances the lustre of the coat.

A powdered source of fat is available, called Pace®, and it also provides energy for the performance horse. It consists of animal fat and sugars. On a vegetable oil or Pace® supplemented diet, a horse needs to eat 15% less volume to fulfil daily energy needs.

Free-Choice Hay

The active performance horse should always have free choice of good hay so it can eat whenever it has the urge. A horse can consume more dry matter nutrients from hay than it could from pasture, because more than 80% of hay's water content evaporates during the curing process. Use a combination of grass (or oat) hay and alfalfa (up to half), making sure the alfalfa is leafy and of good quality to provide maximum nutrients.

Additionally, roughage in the intestines provides a continuous energy source for an exercising horse, and serves as a reservoir to hold water in the intestines, restoring sweat losses and avoiding dehydration.

Electrolyte Supplements

Although electrolytes are not technically considered 'food', they are essential to a horse's well-being. During training and competition, an athlete may need electrolyte supplements besides the salt block. A good mixture is made with 3 parts Lite® salt (potassium chloride and sodium chloride) to 1 part ground limestone. Another useful mixture combines 2 parts table salt to 1 part Lite® salt to 1 part limestone. Add about 2 oz of either mixture per day to the grain, if necessary. Or, give 2 oz mixed with water orally by syringe every 2 hours during strenuous exercise. Use of electrolytes should be discussed with your veterinary adviser.

Other Supplements

The equine athlete does not need protein supplements. In most cases, an increased intake of food to fulfil energy demands will also supply the added requirement for protein, trace minerals and vitamins without excess supplementation. A particularly heavily stressed horse may benefit from vitamin B and C supplements.

The Aged Horse

As a horse ages, it is often difficult to maintain body weight. Flesh seems to vaporize from the body no matter how much hay is eaten. Harsh winter climates increase the metabolic demands on an old horse's system, making it doubly challenging to keep it in good flesh.

Many geriatric horses are retired campaigners who may live another decade or more when supported by preventative health care (deworming, dental attention) and high quality nutrition. An 'old timer' may not have enough useful teeth to grind hay, or may have problem such as step or wave mouth ; it may be starving in the midst of

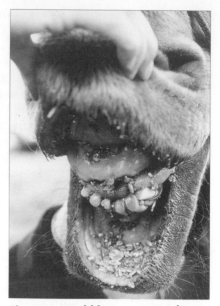

Fig. 7.10 An old horse may not have enough useful teeth to grind its feed.

plenty. To help out, replace hay with a soft gruel of pelleted feed that requires no chewing or grinding for digestion. Alfalfa pellets are an excellent source of fibre, protein and energy. Pellets can be bought 'straight' as compressed alfalfa, or in the form of a 'complete feed' containing up to 25% ground grains in addition to compressed alfalfa. Alfalfa pellets contain at least 27% crude fibre. Ample fibre in the diet is necessary for normal digestive processes for old and young horses alike.

Feed the same amount of pellets *by weight* as hay—do not assume a 1-lb coffee jar holds 1 lb of pellets. If a horse needs 25 lb of hay per day, then give 25 lb of pellets instead, divided into 2 – 4 daily feedings. When soaked in a feed tub for an hour with ample water, pellets swell and soften into a gruel which an old horse can gum and swallow easily.

Advantages of Pellets

Besides supplying highly digestible nutrients, pellets have other advantages. They are easy to transport and store, reduce manure quantity, and because of their compressed size, a horse can eat almost 20% more pellets than hay. Increased intake improves weight gain over the winter months.

Increased Requirements

An 'old timer' reverts to increased dietary needs similar to those of a growing foal. Protein requirements increase to 16%, Ca:P ratios need to be balanced at 1.5:1, and energy needs increase because of reduced intestinal efficiency. The high calcium content of an alfalfa-based diet should be balanced with a phosphorus supplement, such as monosodium phosphate. The geriatric horse may also need vitamin supplements, especially B and C. Age-related changes to the intestines may lead to reduced absorption of nutrients, including vitamins.

Extra Energy

For extra energy, pour 8oz of vegetable oil over the pellet mash twice a day. To satisfy a horse's psychological need to chew, also offer 5 lb of grass hay. The horse may even get some nutrition from it, but the hay must be soft and leafy. Coarse, stemmy hay is irritating to the intestines if not properly ground by the teeth, and can lead to diarrhoea or impaction colic.

Age and Obesity

Some older horses tend to become obese due to hormonal changes associated with age. Usually a diet of excellent quality grass hay avoids obesity and helps to prevent laminitis. These overweight individuals do not need supplementation, but their micronutrient needs must be met with vitamin and mineral additives that balance the ration.

HOT CLIMATE FEEDING

In the summer, many horses are exercised more than during winter months. Exercise burns calories and energy supplies, yet many horses reduce their feed intake by 15–20% during heat spells.

Water requirements vastly increase. Without ample water, a horse may stop eating when it actually needs to replenish its fuel resources.

A horse dissipates heat from actively working muscles through sweating, or evaporative cooling. As a horse sweats, loss of water and electrolytes leads to dehydration and diminished performance unless it can replenish those losses. To compensate for reduced feed intake and loss of electrolytes, it is important to increase digestibility of the diet, and to supply adequate nutrients to an exercising horse. A fit and properly nourished athlete with no excess body fat sweats efficiently. Conservation of body water and electrolytes delays the onset of fatigue or performance failure.

Heat Increment

Diet plays an important role in keeping a horse 'cool' during exercise. Just as working muscle produces internal heat, so does digestion.

The body metabolizes every foodstuff at different levels of efficiency. Digestion and metabolic processes, and the muscular activity involved with eating and digesting each food type, produce a different amount of heat. This amount of heat is a food's *heat increment* (HI). Understanding which foods have low heat increments allows dietary manipulation to improve a horse's cooling ability during hot summer days. The lower the heat increment, the less internal heat digestive processes generate, and the less heat a horse must dissipate in hot weather.

Grains Versus Roughage

Grains are substantially lower in their heat increment than fibrous roughage feeds. Roughage, such as grass hay or pasture, has a heat increment value of 33%, while oats, barley and alfalfa hay have HI values ranging from 15–18%. Maize has an HI of 10–12%. Compare these values with fat at an HI of 3%.

Because it is important to limit heat production in hot climates, and because high environmental temperatures reduce a horse's appetite, the grain portion of a ration may be increased to accommodate special needs. Concen-

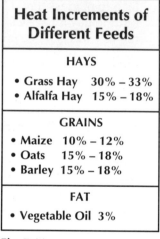

Heat Increments of Different Feeds

HAYS	
• Grass Hay	30% – 33%
• Alfalfa Hay	15% – 18%

GRAINS	
• Maize	10% – 12%
• Oats	15% – 18%
• Barley	15% – 18%

FAT	
• Vegetable Oil	3%

Fig. 7.11

trates are mostly digested and absorbed in the small intestine with little heat generated by metabolism, whereas bacterial fermentation of roughage in the caecum and large intestines generates heat. (This is one reason why extra hay should be fed to horses in wintertime, as large intestinal fermentation generates heat from within.)

Excess Grain

The proportion of grain should **never** exceed 50% of the ration. At least 1% of body weight must be consumed as roughage each day because fibre is essential to healthy equine digestive processes. If grain is fed at greater than 50% of the ration, the high starch content of grain overwhelms the ability of the small intestine to digest it. Excess fermentation of rich carbohydrates can lead to colic, gastrointestinal ulcers, laminitis, or tying-up. Grain concentrates give a horse calories to burn during exercise, but too much grain contributes to deposits of body fat. Insulating fat deposits slow heat dissipation to an extent greater than any value gained by over-feeding grains for their low heat increment.

Maize Versus Oats

Contrary to popular myth, maize is not a 'heating feed.' This mistaken impression may derive from the fact that maize is about two times higher in digestible energy than oats. If maize is substituted for oats at the same *volume* as oats, a horse will receive twice as much energy. The result is a very 'high' or 'hot' horse that may become difficult to handle. An overly energized horse fusses and frets in efforts to vent its fire, and bad behaviour patterns develop. References to such horses have dubbed maize with the misnomer of being a 'hot' food. If maize is substituted for oats, cut the volume in half. However, it is best to *weigh* the feed so there is no question as to how much energy the horse receives.

The HI of maize is actually one-third less than the HI of oats. This difference is due, in part, to the indigestible fibrous hull of oat kernels. As the large intestine breaks down this non-nutritive fibre, internal heat is generated from its metabolism.

Feeding maize instead of oats increases energy supplies. The amount of roughage a horse must eat can then be reduced (within the 50% criterion), and only half the volume of maize needs to be fed as oats. A low HI and compact energy density make maize an excellent carbohydrate to feed in hot summer months.

Fat for Energy

Since the heat increment of fat is only 3%, it contrasts dramatically with other foodstuffs. Feeding 8–16oz of vegetable oil each day provides a valuable source of digestible energy. Because vegetable oil is a fat, adding it to grain has multiple benefits. Vegetable oil is efficiently digested and metabolized, while mini-

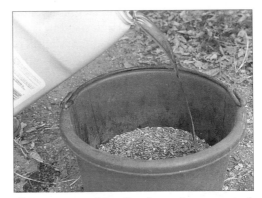

Fig. 7.12 Vegetable oil reduces the amount of concentrate needed and increases the digestible energy.

mizing heat production in the body.

For horses that voluntarily limit feed intake during hot environmental temperatures, adding fat to the diet overcomes the difficulty of supplying ample energy. Fats are up to three times greater in energy density than an equal weight of grain. With fat supplementation it is possible to reduce amounts of other foods and still meet daily energy needs. Feeding 8 oz of vegetable oil twice a day to a 1000-lb horse reduces the amount of grain required to maintain body weight by as much as 25%. There is also a decreased risk of laminitis or tying-up by feeding fat because less grain needs to be fed.

Protein

Role in Sweating

Another mistaken belief of dietary folklore is that exercising horses need extra protein. Protein does *not* serve as a major fuel source during exercise efforts. An insignificant amount of protein is lost in sweat during exercise. Normally, proteins within sweat glands act as 'detergents' to disperse sweat 'water' evenly along the hair shaft, resulting in more effective evaporative cooling. In early stages of training, proteins contribute to the lather of sweat. As a horse is exercised daily in a conditioning programme, proteins are not restored to the sweat glands between exercise periods. Therefore, as fitness improves, the sweat thins and less protein is lost during exercise.

Protein Supplements

Normally, an adult horse thrives on a diet with 8–12% protein. Supplementing protein greater than 15% may be detrimental to an exercising horse. High protein foods also have a high heat increment, making them a poor dietary choice in hot climates. Despite the lower HI value of alfalfa hay (18%) as compared with grass hay (33%), it has a high protein content (as much as 28%). Therefore, feeding alfalfa exclusively has adverse effects.

Protein Requirements

Increased protein in the diet is unnecessary. Any slight increase in protein needs as a response to exercise is usually compensated for by an increase in appetite. During high environmental temperatures, horses that voluntarily limit their food intake need only *minimal* protein supplementation by adding small amounts of alfalfa pellets or alfalfa hay to the ration.

Results of Excess Protein in Hot Climates

Muscle Fatigue

Muscle fatigue during performance is directly related to a build-up of excessive lactic acid. The high protein in an alfalfa diet increases blood and muscle ammonia levels, which results in an increased production of lactic acid in the muscle tissue. Accumulation of lactic acid in the muscle tissue can lead to fatigue and tying-up.

Increased Water Requirements

Nitrogen is a component of ammonia by-products. Excess nitrogen in the body is toxic, and the body eliminates it through the urinary tract. The horse drinks more water to meet the needs of extra urine production. Increased water loss caused by urinary excretion of nitrogen compromises any horse in a hot climate, particularly an exercising athlete.

Respiratory Problems

Besides increased urine production, the nitrogen in urine produces ammonia. Ammonia accumulation in stalls injures the respiratory tract, compromising how well the respiratory system can oxygenate the tissues, and limiting performance. The respiratory tract also helps dissipate heat from the body. While evaporative cooling dissipates most of the heat, respiratory cooling contributes 20% to the cooling process. The healthier the respiratory system, the more a horse benefits in all ways.

Water Requirements

Horses on a hay diet drink almost twice as much water as horses on a grain-supplemented diet. The more hay is provided in the diet, the more water the horse needs for digestion. Ample quantities of cool water must always be available to a horse to ensure efficient digestion and to replenish losses from sweat.

Pellets

Pelleted and extruded feed contains small particles which pull water into the large intestine during digestion. Feeding pellets results in softer manure, but pellets require more water for adequate digestion. Feeding a pelleted ration as a sole feed source may be unwise in a hot climate, because dehydration is a limiting factor of performance.

Roughage

Roughage (hay and pasture) is excellent for retaining water in the intestinal tract. Within reason, water lost in sweat is immediately replenished from a reservoir of water in the digestive tract. During prolonged competition of endurance sports, roughage also supplies energy to a horse long after the meal. It is best to feed 3 – 4 hours before an event, but not too generously, as excess bulk in the intestines limits performance. Balanced proportions of grain, fat and roughage provide maximal energy.

Electrolyte Supplements

Electrolyte losses through sweat are unavoidable and *cannot* be entirely prevented. However, pre-loading long-distance horses with electrolyte supplements within 2 hours of the start of the event will diminish electrolyte and fluid losses within the first 20 miles of exercise. Not only does this supplementation minimize the lag time for electrolyte absorption from the bowels while the horse is exercising, but pre-loading with salts seems to stimulate thirst sooner; horses are then more inclined to drink and maintain their fluid balance. Studies have shown that horses with better electrolyte balances and hydration in the early stages of endurance competition have a greater chance of completing the event successfully. In addition, these horses are able to complete the ride faster than horses that lose more electrolytes and fluids in the early part of competition.

Electrolytes should be supplemented not only before the start of the ride, but also at every rest stop. More benefit may be gained by giving frequent, small doses along the trail every time a horse takes a good drink. Lite® salt in an oral supplement contains potassium, sodium and chloride.

It is unnecessary to supplement light working or idle horses with electrolytes even in hot weather. Such individuals replenish their own needs from a free choice salt block and good quality hay.

Improving Performance

Manipulating meal times and quantities can increase the opportunity for internal heat (generated by digestion and metabolism) to be dissipated throughout the day. Small meals at frequent intervals optimize body cooling mechanisms. During hot weather, feed the largest proportion of roughage at night. While a horse is resting during the cool hours of night, it metabolizes and ferments the fibrous portion of the diet. When there is less fibre in the intestines during exercise on hot days, heat produced from feed is not a limiting factor to performance.

By following some basic principles about which foods are 'cooler' than others, and by discarding obsolete myths about feeding requirements, a horse's diet can be modified to improve mental and physical performance in hot climates.

OBESITY

The subject of a malnourished horse conjures images of an emaciated rack of bones. However, malnourishment has another extreme—obesity. An overweight horse is a statement of dietary imbalance, one that is overabundantly supplied with energy.

Eating Behaviour

A horse accumulates fat for the same reasons people do. Either too many calories for its level of exercise are provided, and/or a bored or greedy horse eats more than it needs. Eating behaviour in horses evolved in an environment where survival of the fittest implied a well nourished and robust individual.

Free Choice Diet

Natural range forage is relatively low in energy, with variable nutritional content depending on season and terrain. In the wild, horses consume moderate amounts of forage at frequent intervals, each meal being about 1 – 3 hours long. Unlike humans, the amount of food consumed is not governed by signals of stomach distension, or 'feeling full', conveyed to the brain, unless the distension approaches pain. A horse with free choice food stops eating before the stomach is fully distended. Therefore, in the wild, stomach distension does not usually occur.

The amount of food a horse eats is governed by the rate of emptying food from the stomach, or the nutritive value of food in the stomach. Cues are sent to the brain from hormonal and nerve receptors that are integrated throughout the gastrointestinal tract and the body. They recognize satisfaction of nutritive needs, and accordingly regulate hunger or fullness by an appetite control centre in the brain.

In a natural state, these integrated signals do not influence the amount or length of a particular meal. Instead, these cues affect the time until the next meal, and the amount then ingested. A horse in this environment eats only enough to maintain good body health.

In an artificial environment where humans dictate when and how much a horse eats, this natural control of eating no longer plays as significant a role. Knowing this fact, we can modify feeding practices to our advantage.

Meal Intervals

Horses with free choice food do not voluntarily fast longer than 2 – 3 hours at a time. A horse that receives only 2 meals a day is psychologically 'starved' by the next meal because of imposed and lengthy fasting between meals. The horse then consumes large amounts rapidly at each feeding, rather than 'grazing' throughout the day. If free choice food cannot be arranged, it is best to feed a *minimum* of three times per day.

Palatable Foods

The actual presence of food induces a horse to eat, but how much it eats is determined by the food's palatability and how easy it is to obtain and eat. A horse's perception of smell, taste and texture decides palatability of the food.

In this modern era, plentiful amounts of tasty and easily consumed feed are available without a horse having to seek it. Many horses eat until all the food is gone. Access to appealing foods may override normal 'regulatory cues' from the gastrointestinal tract and metabolic pathways. A horse continues to eat even though it is physiologically sated in energy and nutrients. Then the extra pounds stack up.

Seasonal Effects

An extensive layer of fat under the skin protects horses from the elements. This insulation diminishes the penetrating effects of wet and cold. Insulating fat deposits maintain a precise body temperature range, and they serve as a readily available source of energy when food is scarce.

Equine feeding behaviour evolved in adaptation to an environment with ample nutrition in the summer and sparse supplies in the winter. During mild months, horses stored sufficient body fat and energy to last through a winter of limited forage. Horses have not yet adapted to the constancy of modern feeding practices that carry them through winter without need of surplus fat deposits.

Competition

Competition within a herd stimulates dominant horses to run others away from the food. Assertive individuals may then have access to

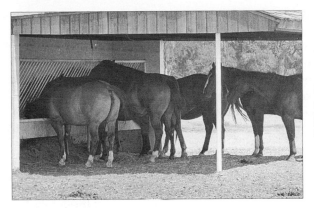

Fig. 7.13 An overly assertive horse often gets more food than it needs.

more food than they need.

If we combine an evolutionary tendency to 'plump' up with easy accessibility to highly palatable and energy dense food, the result is an overweight horse. If exercise is restricted and a horse remains relatively idle, instead of building muscle it continues to put on fat.

The Human Factor

It is much too simple to blame equine obesity on a tendency to overeat; the human factor is important. In some cases, the physiologically ideal body weight a horse carries may not correspond to ideal as viewed through an owner's eyes. Human desires sometimes improperly plump up a horse to 'show' condition.

It is our role to learn what constitutes a healthy body condition so we do not overindulge a greedy individual. It has been proven repeatedly that one of the greatest health hazards for horses is obesity.

Condition Scoring System

One report concluded that racehorses have an optimal racing weight within a range of plus or minus *16 lb*. This range is a fine tuned balance, considering a horse can drink or urinate almost 16 lb in a matter of moments. An average pleasure horse is considered overweight if it carries an excess of 100 – 300 lb of body flesh.

We can fairly evaluate body condition to determine what is the correct weight for an individual, regardless of breed or conformation. Use of a *condition scoring system*, developed by Dr Gary Potter and associates of Texas A&M, accurately estimates stored body fat more effectively than weight, height or heartgirth measurements.

Thickness of fat over the rump and back correlates well with total body fat. Also evaluate rib fat; although it is not as reliable an indicator, it should be considered as part of the whole picture. By feeling the fat cover and visually appraising areas over the back, croup and tailhead, ribs, behind the shoulder, and the neck and withers, a horse is assigned a numerical condition value. This scale is from 1 – 9, or in some cases on a scale of 1–5, from least body fat to most body fat.

Combining a scoring system with conventional methods, such as weighing a horse or measuring heartgirth, achieves fine tuned control of body condition. Gradual weight gains are difficult to appreciate with daily observation. Weight tapes are not very accurate, but are useful to evaluate changes over time. Taking a photograph of the horse at intervals permits an objective, visual comparison of body condition.

Emaciated

An emaciated horse in poor condition has a score of 0 to 1. The spinous processes, ribs, tailhead and hip bones project prominently. The bone structure of the neck, withers and shoulders are pronounced, and no fatty tissue is felt.

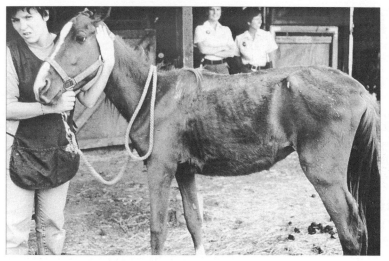

Fig. 7.14 A poor horse—body condition score of 1.

Thin

A thin horse has a score of 3. There is some fat covering the spine— about halfway up the spinous processes, but they are still easily seen. The ribs are visible but have a slight fat covering. The hip bones, tailhead, withers, shoulders and neck are more full, but are discernible. Thin horses do not have enough body reserves to support long

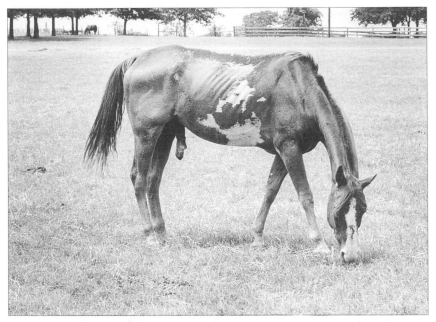

Fig. 7.15 A very thin horse—body condition score of 2.

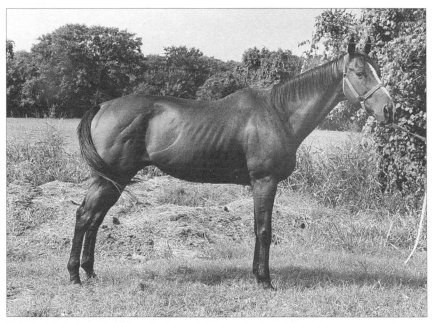

Fig. 7.16 Moderately thin—body condition score of 4.

distance performance. They also chill easily in inclement weather. Many racing Thoroughbreds have a body condition score of 4.

Ideal Condition

A score of 5 corresponds to a 'moderate' condition: the back is level, and the ribs are not visually distinguished but are easily felt when running a hand across them. Fat around the tailhead begins to feel spongy, the withers appear rounded over the spinous processes, with the neck and shoulders blending smoothly into the body. This condition is *ideal*.

Moderately Fleshy

In some cases, it is appropriate for the modern horse to build a 'moderately fleshy' (score 6) body condition. On a horse with a score 6, the fat around the tailhead is soft, the fat over the ribs is spongy, and there is fat deposited along the withers, shoulders and neck.

When a horse is continually exposed to inclement weather in harsh climates, with no access to shelter, a thin layer of fat 'traps' heat within the body. Also, a lactating mare needs plenty of body reserves

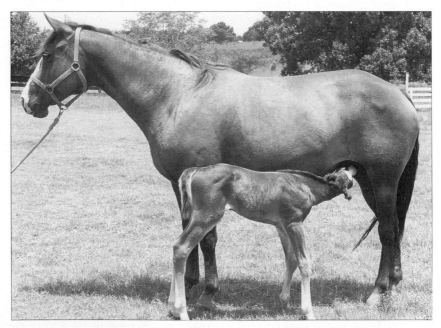

Fig. 7.17 A moderately fleshy broodmare—body condition score of 6.

to manufacture and provide enough milk for her foal, and she should not be maintained too lean.

Overweight

Many overweight horses tend to be fleshy (score 7) or even fat (score 8). Although individual ribs are felt in a fleshy horse, there is noticeable fat between ribs, there is a crease down the back, and the withers, neck and areas behind the shoulders are riddled with fat. It is difficult to feel the ribs at all in a fat (score 8) horse, and the neck is noticeably thickened and 'cresty.' Shoulders, croup and buttocks ripple with fat.

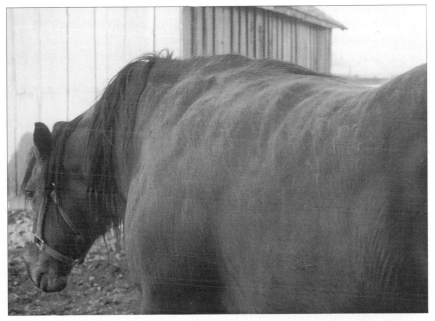

Fig. 7.18 Extremely fat—body condition score of 9.

Extremely Fat

An extremely fat horse tops the scale with a score of 9. Such a horse has a pronounced raingutter-like crease along its back (which in fact will hold water), and patchy fat over the ribs. Fat also bulges around the tailhead, along the withers, behind the shoulders, and along the neck. The flank lacks definition and is filled in with flesh. Ample fat along the inner buttocks causes them to rub together. Serious metabolic problems threaten such a horse if a weight loss programme is not begun immediately.

Obesity-Related Diseases

Obesity is a systemic disease that can lead to serious consequences and metabolic problems in the horse. A list of these problems includes:

- laminitis
- exercise intolerance
- heat exhaustion
- intestinal lipomas
- colic
- tying-up
- musculoskeletal injuries

Obesity and overweight also contribute to developmental orthopaedic diseases such as malformation of joint cartilage (osteochondrosis) or inflammation of the growth plate (epiphysitis) in a growing horse. Pregnant mares may have difficulty foaling due to reduced muscle tone attributable to lack of exercise associated with obesity.

Although they are listed above as a group, each individual syndrome is a separate debilitating condition, potentially resulting in permanent lameness or death. At the very least, an overweight horse cannot perform to potential.

Musculoskeletal Injuries

Another problem arises when a 'weekend warrior' is over-fed daily to compensate for its athletic output which only occurs on Saturday and Sunday. Instead of removing supplemental energy sources from the diet on weekdays when the horse stands idle, an owner continues to provide appetizing food, full of calories. The rider wonders where the horse's exuberance has gone, and why it is now so sluggish and dull. 'Maybe it needs more grain' is a common response to the malady. Insult is heaped on to injury. Feet, tendons, ligaments, joints and bone must withstand excessive concussion and strain. Musculoskeletal injuries develop as the legs are loaded with excessive weight.

Laminitis

Perhaps one day an owner notices the horse is tender on its front feet. The liver can no longer detoxify the continual carbohydrate overload of grain, rich alfalfa, or lush pasture. The resulting systemic metabolic crisis causes severe problems with the blood supply in the feet. The diagnosis: laminitis.

Lipomas

What is seen as deposits of bulging fat on the outside of a horse is a reflection of what is being deposited internally around organs and within the *mesentery*, which is the fan shaped tissue encircling the small intestine.

A horse develops intense abdominal pain, a sudden onset colic crisis that is not responsive to medical therapy. On the operating table, it is discovered that fat stores have been generously deposited within the mesentery. Fat globules have formed a fatty tumour *(lipoma)*. The lipoma hangs from a long stalk that has wrapped around a part of intestine, strangulating it.

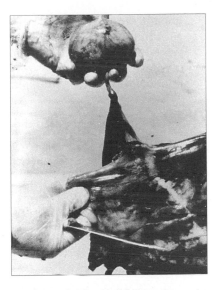

Fig. 7.19 Lipoma in the intestine.

Obesity and the Growing Horse

Excessive body fat in a young, growing horse can overload an immature, undeveloped skeleton, contributing to bone and joint abnormalities. Obesity also amplifies concussive forces on maturing cartilage, resulting in orthopaedic disease.

Cartilage was removed from the knees of growing Thoroughbreds and analysed after 3 months of a high energy, push-fed diet where the horses were encouraged to eat too much too often. Abnormal cellular development of cartilage was evident. After 9 months on a push-fed diet, clinical signs were obvious. Lameness, limb deformities, growth plate abnormalities (epiphysitis), and retarded formation of the cartilage (osteochondrosis) developed from the unbalanced diet.

Hormonal and Mineral Imbalance

Hormones influence cellular processes of maturation, differentiation, and synthesis of cartilage and growth plates. The amount of carbohydrate energy a foal ingests regulates the growth of bone and cartilage by affecting hormonal control. Overnutrition interferes with normal circulating levels of hormones such as *somatomedin* (a growth regulator), *insulin, thyroxine* and *cortisol.* With accelerated growth rates, mineral demands for adequate bone development also increase. Relative excesses or deficiencies of specific minerals result in developmental orthopaedic disease.

Musculoskeletal Failure

An increase in energy and protein consumption of up to 30% greater than the values recommended by the National Research Council does not enhance the biomechanical strength of growing bones of yearlings. Additional body fat loads bones with additional body weight without a proportional increase in structural stability. Under these circumstances, failure of bone, ligament, tendon, or joint structures is inevitable. These syndromes are commonly seen, particularly in overweight individuals.

Preventing Obesity

These medical maladies are easily preventable. Reduce high energy diets of rich alfalfa hay, lush pasture, or supplements of grain or pellets. Substitute instead a diet including grass hay—providing it free choice if possible. Some individuals, however, thrive on a limited amount of grass hay fed daily, so free choice feeding may not be practical.

Within 2 – 3 days of a free choice grass hay diet, appetites usually stabilize. A horse consumes only what is physiologically necessary to maintain a healthy weight. Grass hay is palatable, but not overly appealing as are alfalfa or concentrates. Neurohormonal cues from the gut can once again naturally regulate hunger and satiety.

A common dilemma is in following feeding guidelines. They are just that—guidelines. Each horse has a unique metabolic constitution that dictates how easy or difficult it is to maintain its weight. How much energy a horse burns on a daily basis is determined by:

- age
- temperament
- rider's weight and expertise
- environmental temperature and humidity
- intensity and duration of work
- terrain
- level of conditioning

Losing Weight

It is dangerous to 'starve' an obese horse for rapid weight loss, as starvation leads to high levels of circulating fatty acids *(hyperlipaemia)*. These fatty acids are deposited in the liver, resulting in liver damage. Weight loss should be gradual. Ample roughage will ensure healthy gastrointestinal function, and mental peace of mind. Feeding at least 1 lb of hay per 100 lb of body weight each day maintains intestinal movement and health.

Place an obese horse on a strict diet by restricting high energy foods, or substituting with less energy-rich foodstuffs. Switch from alfalfa hay to grass hay, pull the horse off rich pasture or limit its access to only a few hours a day, and eliminate grain and vegetable oil.

A weight-loss diet for a horse is no different from a human attempt to defeat an overweight problem. Reduce the amount and the quality of food ingested, and provide regular exercise. Not only will a horse look better, but it will feel better, and be able to perform to potential.

Training the Overweight Horse

Along with a sensible diet, exercise is the best way to reduce fat deposits. Walking is an excellent way to slowly increase heart rates and warm muscles. Start the first week with 15 – 20 minutes, every other day or three days that week. Work two-thirds of the time at a walk, and one-third at the trot. The second week, work for 30 minutes, 3 – 4 days. Slowly increase distance in the third week, but keep the speed the same until the horse is working for 30 – 60 minutes. Finally, add longer trot intervals and 1 – 2 minute canter intervals (changing leads) in the fourth week. At the end of one month, the horse should be fit enough to further increase mileage, and then speed.

Fig. 7.20 An over-weight horse benefits from exercise and a lower energy ration.

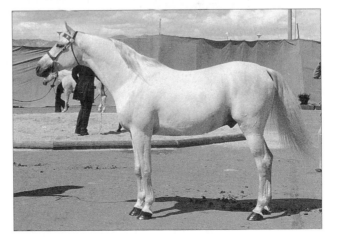

Inability to Control Heat

Working muscles expend energy at 20 – 50 times the resting metabolic rate, and one natural by-product is heat. As internal body temperatures initially rise, most of the blood from cardiac output is diverted to the skin, away from the working muscles. Blood vessels of the skin dilate, transferring excess heat from the muscles to the body surface. This increased blood flow elevates skin temperature, and activates sweat glands to begin evaporative cooling.

As environmental temperatures rise, or as humidity increases, evaporative cooling becomes less efficient. For heat loss to result, the outside air must be cooler than the inside of the horse. Also, sweat must evaporate to transfer heat from the skin to the air. High humidity limits complete evaporation, and therefore reduces the effects of evaporative cooling.

An athletic horse should have enough fat reserves to burn going into the training season, but there can be too much of a good thing. For the athletic horse, fat can dramatically hamper performance.

An obese horse is in extreme danger of being unable to regulate its own temperature even under the best conditions. Extremes in environmental temperature and humidity increase this danger. In the summer, follow a careful exercise approach for the overweight horse.

Reduced Heat Dissipation

A fat horse carries an added insulating layer under the skin. A fat and unconditioned horse must work harder at a given effort, generating more body heat than a fit horse. It is difficult for a fat horse to dissipate heat away from working muscles because fat slows the conduction of heat to the skin periphery. The same fatty tissue that conserves body heat in cold weather interferes with evaporative cooling on hot days.

Because they cannot efficiently conduct or sweat the heat away from the body, fat horses are prone to exercise intolerance, fatigue, and heat stress. As a horse sweats in large quantities, it loses vital body fluids and salts, contributing to dehydration and electrolyte imbalance. At first, performance may suffer, but with continued fatigue there is a rapid decline toward heat exhaustion and metabolic failure.

Tying-Up

Once surface evaporation can no longer keep up with the heat build-up, internal temperature continues to rise. This heat impairs muscle contraction, adding to fatigue and exhaustion. Loss of electrolytes through the sweat, and an increased muscle temperature spark a chain of abnormal biochemical events in the muscles, resulting in the paralysing cramps of tying-up.

Inversion

If a horse cannot rid itself of enough heat, it may start panting to remove heat through the respiratory tract. This problem is seen as an *inverted* pulse rate to respiratory rate ratio, with the breathing rate above the heart rate.

Slow Cardiac Recovery

Cardiac recovery is difficult as the body struggles to eliminate internal heat. The circulatory system cannot keep up with the competing demands of the working muscles, the increased metabolic rate, or the need to increase blood flow to the skin.

Elevated Temperature

Continued inadequate dissipation of heat leads to rising and persistently elevated body temperature. Rectal temperature over 105.8° F results in heat-induced injury of nerves, with irreversible systemic collapse, shock and death.

These events may also occur in a horse that is not overweight but is underconditioned for the work effort, or in any horse exercised in excessively hot and humid climates.

Increased Energy Needs

Body condition has a more pronounced effect on performance than environmental temperature. Not only does additional body fat impair performance, but the effort required to move additional body mass also increases a horse's energy expenditures. After exercise, faster pulse and respiration recoveries are noted in moderate body condition (score 5) horses than in fleshy (score 7) individuals. Unconditioned horses do not metabolize fat as efficiently as fit horses because their enzyme systems have not been 'trained' to effectively use fat as fuel.

Heat dissipation requires additional calories. A fat horse tends to consume more energy-dense feed after a work effort than does a fit, sleek horse. A fleshy horse requires an increase in total energy intake for both maintenance and performance simply to remain in an overweight condition. The average obese horse consumes about 5 lb more feed per day than a moderately conditioned horse. Such an appetite compounds the problems of obesity.

8

FITNESS EVALUATION

The goal of the rider or trainer in any equine sport is for the horse to compete in top form with minimal stress. At the end of the performance, the horse should have enough zest to continue if asked. This is the ultimate test of stamina, strength, speed and *heart*.

Each horse is a unique individual. The best way to keep a horse out of metabolic danger is to know the horse. Know its normalcies, abilities, and most of all its limits. Metabolic problems often begin subtly. The rider or trainer should be able to recognize warning signs of impending fatigue, or metabolic disaster. An aware and sensitive rider can stop the spiral leading to exhaustion and crisis before it begins.

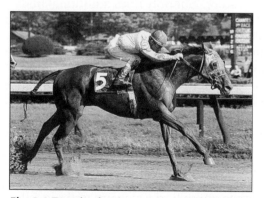

Fig. 8.1 Terrain, footing, and weather must be considered when evaluating a horse's fitness for an event.

FITNESS INDICATORS

Competition places critical physiological demands on a horse at every moment. A horse's level of fitness is not the only influence on its ability to perform well. Also consider the horse's metabolic condition and body weight, the age, the weight of the rider relative to the horse's size, the terrain or footing, and the weather.

Specific criteria determine how a horse is holding up under stress, and its ability to continue a performance. One general fitness indicator is the horse's attitude. The look in the eyes, the degree of alertness, the impulsion of stride, and the way the horse holds the body and ears indicate its overall well-being.

Heart Rate Recovery

One objective criterion is the horse's *heart rate recovery* after a performance. During exercise, the heart rate can increase to eight times the resting rate, increasing blood flow and oxygen to working muscles. For example, if a horse's resting rate is 30 bpm, its heart rate at maximal exertion could be 240. In a normal recovery the heart rate falls rapidly in the first minute after exercise, then decreases more slowly over the next several minutes.

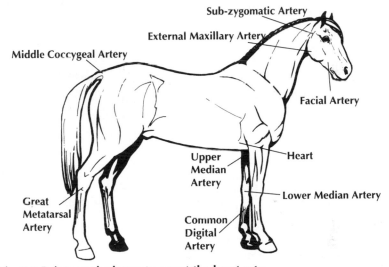

Fig. 8.2 Points on the horse to count the heart rate.

The recovery rate depends on fitness, environmental temperature, and the type of athletic exertion. For an endurance horse, the heart rate should drop below 60 – 70 beats per minute (bpm) within 10 minutes after exercise has stopped. For a sprint horse, the heart rate should drop to 150 – 180 bpm after 30 seconds, and 100 – 140 bpm after 1 minute. Within 30 minutes, the heart rate should be below 60 bpm after any kind of exertion.

Cardiac Recovery Index

Once the horse's heart rate is less than 60 – 70 bpm, a *cardiac recovery index* (CRI) is enormously helpful in uncovering subtle problems before they become serious. Determine the resting level by counting the heart rate for 15 seconds. Trot the horse out 125 feet and back the same 125 feet. This distance usually takes about 25 seconds to complete. Start the stopwatch as the horse begins the trot, and stop it at 1 minute *(about 35 seconds after the horse returns)*. At this point, count the heart rate for 15 seconds. The heart rate of a normal horse that is not suffering from metabolic or musculoskeletal problems returns to the resting rate, plus or minus a beat, at the minute check.

A CRI heart rate that is two or more beats above the resting rate may indicate exhaustion or pain. An example of its use is in endurance events. The CRI is one of the parameters used to determine if a horse should be held at the check for a longer rest period, or should be taken out of the competition.

Capillary Refill Time

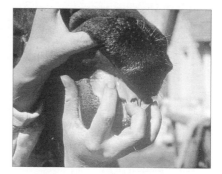

Fig. 8.3 Press the gums with a fingertip to check capillary refill time.

Gums should be a healthy pink colour, and if blanched (pressed) with a fingertip they should become pink again in approximately 2 seconds. This method shows that the circulatory system is in good shape, pumping blood to all parts of the body. The time required for this response is called the *capillary refill time*. Capillary refill time should only be considered with other parameters as it is not a reliable indicator on its own.

Jugular Refill

Another method of evaluating circulatory efficiency and hydration is achieved by pressing a finger into the jugular furrow (groove) and watching how long the jugular vein takes to fill with blood. Every horse's exact jugular refill time will be different; however, the jugular vein should fill to the size of a pencil within 2 seconds. Checking the jugular refill time at the beginning of the event helps the rider monitor dehydration during the event. If the refill time is longer than it was at the beginning of the event, then the horse is dehydrated because the circulating blood volume is lower, or there may be a cardiovascular problem. When the head is held in normal head carriage, there should only be the slightest pulse visible in the jugular vein.

Gut Sounds and Intestinal Activity

Intestinal activity and the associated gut sounds heard on both sides of the flank are important indicators of normal physiological function. An exercising horse may have fewer gut sounds because a large percentage of blood goes to the muscles. Less blood reaching the intestines slows intestinal activity. However, the intestinal tract should not be silent. Also, a horse's appetite should be active, preferably greedy, at rest stops or after a performance.

If a horse is operating anaerobically, it can be watered and fed hay after it is cool to the touch on the chest—after about 20 – 30 minutes. After 30 minutes to 1 hour, the horse can safely be fed grain.

If a horse is operating aerobically, and it continues to exercise after a rest period (1 hour maximum), it is safe, indeed necessary, to allow the horse to drink water and eat hay or grass. If desired, a small amount of grain may be given to a horse that is still operating aerobically. After exercise, cool the horse out as above before watering or feeding, to allow time for the blood to flow back to the intestines.

Veterinary Evaluation

When available at equine sports events, a veterinarian can play a crucial role in achieving safe and successful competitions. Rely on this resource. Communicate with the veterinarian, and ask questions. Point out inconsistencies in the horse's performance.

In addition to evaluating a horse's metabolic condition at rest stops during endurance events, veterinarians also recognize swelling in the limbs, or an obvious lameness that might prevent a horse from competing. They may also point out nicks, scrapes, minor injuries and sores from improperly fitted tack that the rider may overlook.

STRESS INDICATORS
Persistent Heart Rate Elevation

Persistent elevation of heart rate may indicate an impending metabolic collapse. The heart rate remains high if a horse is near exhaustion. Pain also elevates the heart rate. If other metabolic signs such as attitude, gut sounds, level of fatigue, level of dehydration, and body temperature seem normal, seek out a source of pain, particularly in the limbs or muscles.

Respiratory Rate

The respiratory rate should decrease with the heart rate recovery. Preferably, the respiratory rate will drop below the heart rate after about 10 minutes. However, environmental conditions, hair coat, obesity, and level of fitness influence this drop. For example, in hot and humid climates, horses may pant in rapid, shallow respirations. A high respiratory rate is also associated with high body temperatures.

Inversion

Whenever the respiratory rate remains faster than the heart rate, it is called an *inversion*. Even an inexperienced eye will observe that an 'inverted' horse appears to pant. Respiration is shallow and rapid, and the horse's flank moves in and out with each breath.

If the heart rate recovers within 10 minutes but the respiratory rate remains high, the horse is not necessarily in trouble. It may need help in ridding its body of the extra heat. After extended exercise, spend a few minutes walking the horse so the circulation continues to flush heat and lactic acid from the muscles. Soak the head and neck with water to speed cooling.

Dehydration

There are many levels of dehydration, and there are variable indications of it. A rough estimate of dehydration is made by pinching a fold of skin on the point of the shoulder or the eyelid, and noting how quickly it snaps back into position. If a horse is not dehydrated, blood flow to the skin is normal so the skin snaps back immediately. Pinched skin that remains 'tented' and does not return to normal indicates a dangerous level of dehydration.

A horse with mild dehydration of 2–3% may have a prolonged capillary refill time, a dry mouth, or dry mucous membranes. Other signs of dehydration include depressed intestinal activity, and slow heart rate recovery. However, even low levels of dehydration can adversely affect the performance horse. At about 5% dehydration:

- the eye sockets appear sunken
- skin elasticity is markedly reduced
- the horse is weak, and appears dull

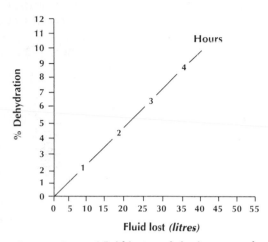

Fig. 8.4 Litres of fluid lost, and the increase of dehydration during a long distance activity on a hot day.

Mild dehydration with a slight decrease in circulating blood causes the sodium, chloride and potassium (electrolytes, or body salts) in the bloodstream to stimulate thirst. With progressive dehydration and an excessive loss of sodium, chloride and potassium, the stimulus to trigger thirst is eliminated. By not drinking, a horse worsens the dehydration problem. **Just because a horse will not drink does not mean it does not need fluids.** It may be on the edge of a serious electrolyte imbalance, and in need of immediate intravenous fluid and electrolyte therapy.

On a hot day, it is possible for a 1000-lb long distance horse to lose 2 – 3 gallons (7.6 – 11.4 litres) of fluid each hour of exercise, or 6 – 12 gallons (22.7 – 45.5 litres) during the entire activity. This amount of fluid loss can lead to **severe** dehydration of 7% – 10% and circulatory collapse.

A racehorse can lose up to a half gallon (0.4 litres) of fluids during a mile race. On a hot, humid day, even mild dehydration can affect race performance.

If an overheated horse abruptly stops work, blood pools in the muscles. This accumulation reduces the amount of circulating blood, contributing to the horse's relative dehydration. If an exhausted horse refuses to move, massaging the major muscle groups in rhythm with the heartbeat can help circulate blood through the muscles.

Preventing Dehydration

Conditioning helps prevent dehydration. The more fit a horse is, the less demand exercise places on the body, and the less heat is produced by exercise. Therefore, conditioning reduces fluid loss from sweat. By sweating less, the body conserves vital electrolytes and body fluid.

Allow the horse to drink at every opportunity. A hot horse can be allowed to drink as long as it continues to move afterwards. Otherwise, cool out slowly and offer small amounts of water at frequent intervals.

It may be appropriate to consider the use of electrolyte solutions for drinks during and/or at the end of endurance events.

Doctoring Drinking Water

Some horses simply do not like the taste of strange water and will refuse to drink. If a horse is finicky about water, begin to 'doctor' the drinking water at home with a small amount of cider vinegar or sugar about a month before competitions. The vinegar or sugar disguises the strange water source and encourages a horse to drink. As an alternative, carry water from home to a competition.

Body Temperature

Working muscles expend at least 20 times the energy of their resting metabolic rate, with the natural by-product being heat. A *thermoregulatory centre* in the horse's brain sets the normal temperature and maintains it within a very narrow range. To control body temperature within this limit, the body needs to dissipate the heat produced by working muscles. A high body temperature often corresponds to a high respiratory rate, and both these factors are monitors for thermoregulatory control within the horse.

The rectal temperature is a good indicator of internal temperature. It is normally 98–101° F. After prolonged exercise, it is normal for the rectal temperature to reach 103–104° F, but the temperature should return to normal within 15 – 30 minutes after exercise.

A rectal temperature persisting above 105° F reveals metabolic problems, and may result in weakness and incoordination. Loss of muscle control and strength can lead to serious accidents. An exhausted horse may stumble and fall, or it may not safely clear an obstacle—placing both horse and rider in jeopardy.

Natural Cooling Methods

The body dissipates a vast amount of heat produced by muscle metabolism through evaporation. A smaller amount of heat is lost through respiration.

Evaporative Cooling

To remove most of this heat, a horse sweats. As body temperature initially rises, most of the blood is diverted to the skin for heat dissipation, and away from the working muscles. Water vapour on the skin, produced from the sweat glands, pulls heat from the blood vessels, and the outside air evaporates the warm water. This process is called *evaporative cooling.* Along with heat loss, evaporative cooling also releases large quantities of fluid and electrolytes.

Respiratory Cooling

As body temperature rises, another far less effective mechanism helps dissipate heat. Just as a panting dog moves air across its hanging tongue, a horse breathes rapidly to cool the body. Warm blood, flowing from heated muscles, circulates to the lungs. Warm air in the lungs is exhaled. With each incoming breath, cool air (including oxygen) is exchanged for warm air. Respiratory cooling does not release fluids or electrolytes, but it contributes only a small amount to the cooling process.

Other Cooling Methods

Cool Water Application

Soaking the neck, chest and legs with water creates the same effect as sweating. Cool water applied over the large, superficial blood vessels of

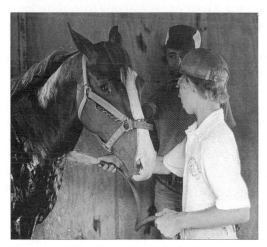

the head, jugular region of the neck, armpit and forelegs dissipates internal heat. The water temperature is not critical provided the large blood vessels in these areas are repeatedly soaked. A single bathing is not enough. Continuously apply water until the respiratory rate lowers, or drape wet towels over the head and neck while the horse walks.

Fig. 8.5 Soaking the neck cools the horse.

Cooling down a horse too rapidly leads to chilling and shock. The body temperature of a severely overheated horse should lower 1° F every 15 – 30 minutes when bathing the head and neck with water.

Never apply water to the large muscles in the back or hindquarters of an overheated horse! Walking and natural cooling best dissipate heat from these muscles. If these muscles cool too rapidly, muscle reflexes will cause the blood vessels to constrict away from the skin. Less blood flow to the skin surface allows heat to persist within the muscles.

Also, the muscle tissues still retain lactic acid that needs to be carried away by the bloodstream. Muscle cramping associated with vessel constriction also reduces oxygen to the muscles. After a hard workout, it may take a couple of hours until it is safe to give the horse a full body bath. After a pleasure ride that stimulates only a light sweat, the horse may be bathed after 20 – 30 minutes of cool-out.

Dangers of Cold Water

Applying cold water to the heavy muscles of the back and hindquarters can cause myositis or rhabdomyelitis (tying-up). (*See Chapter 3 for more information.*) A tied-up horse has these symptoms:

- refuses to move or appears very stiff if it tries to move
- exhibits signs of 'colic' due to pain from muscle cramping
- sweats, paws, or attempts to roll
- heart and respiratory rates climb in response to pain

A trainer or veterinarian can evaluate muscle suppleness, as well as tenderness to hand pressure along the large muscle groups of the back or hindquarters. A normal horse has a fluid stride in contrast to one that is beginning to tie up. Tight or excessively firm muscles or obviously cramping muscles indicate fatigue and electrolyte abnormalities.

As muscle fibres spasm and contract, more heat is produced in already overheated muscles. Retention of body heat increases both heart and respiratory rates to cool the body. The result is a very slow recovery time, and metabolic problems. Avoid such a scenario by resisting the urge to fully sponge down a horse until it completely cools out.

Heat Stress

Heat stress occurs when the body temperature climbs above 105° F and the body cannot efficiently cool itself. Internal temperature continues to rise. Usually, heat stress develops from overexertion leading to overheating, rather than external heating by the sun's rays. However, exhaustion or heat stress can develop if weather conditions have overtaxed a horse's ability to dissipate heat, or have interfered with proper fluid and electrolyte levels of the body.

Hot Weather

Hot weather limits a horse's ability to shed heat from the body. The horse sweats, but sweating is not always enough to stay ahead of the heat build-up. As either environmental temperature or humidity increase, the evaporative cooling of sweating becomes less efficient. In a horse experiencing heat stress, internal heat continues to rise once evaporation from the skin can no longer keep up to rid the body of heat.

Level of Conditioning

Hot weather is not the only factor contributing to heat stress. A horse that is ridden *too fast for its level of condition* produces excess body heat. A horse with many fat layers under the skin cannot dissipate heat effectively. Not only does excess fat impair normal cooling processes, but it directly relates to a horse's level of fitness.

Preventing Heat Stress

Conditioning builds muscle in place of fat. Conditioning also develops capillary beds, improving the circulation of oxygen in the tissues and flushing heat to the skin surface.

Training during hot and humid weather, especially interval training or multiple workouts, can cause heat stress. The horse should be monitored closely for signs of heat stress on hot, humid days. Workouts should be less intense or shorter to prevent heat build-up in the working muscles. Also, wetting the neck, chest and forelegs of the horse before and during exercise can delay heat build-up on a hot day.

Determining the Danger of Heat Stress

A simple formula adds the environmental temperature to the per-

Levels of Heat Stress (Temperature + Humidity)
If the sum of temperature and humidity is less than 120, normal cooling mechanisms are sufficient unless a horse is obese or has a long hair coat.
If the sum is greater than 140, a horse relies mostly on sweating to dissipate body heat.
If the sum is greater than 150, and especially if humidity is more than 50% evaporative cooling is severely compromised.
If the sum is greater than 180, there are no natural means for the body to cool itself; internal temperature will continue to rise, resulting in heat stress.

Fig. 8.6

cent humidity, determining the danger of heat stress on any given day. If, for example, the temperature is 90° F and the humidity is 75%, the sum is 165. At this level, evaporative cooling may not be enough to cool the horse.

As the horse loses vital fluids through sweating, it will steadily dehydrate if they are not replenished. Dehydration reduces blood flow to the skin. The body responds by limiting sweating to conserve body fluids. Heat continues to build within the horse with no outlet, stimulating a decline towards exhaustion.

Anhydrosis

In hot, humid climates, a horse may experience a syndrome called *anhydrosis.* This syndrome is a loss of the ability to sweat. A horse that does not sweat cannot cool itself. Body temperature rises, the horse pants, and performance suffers. A horse that has ceased to sweat needs medical attention and should be kept still and quiet.

Tissue Hypoxia

At higher temperatures, muscles (and all body tissue) have a greater demand for oxygen. If these metabolic demands cannot be met, muscle contraction is impaired, contributing to fatigue. If a horse's body temperature exceeds 106° F, the body demands more oxygen than can be supplied by the respiratory system. Tissue *hypoxia* (lack of oxygen) results, leading to kidney, liver and brain damage. At temperatures greater than 107° F, a horse may go into convulsions or a coma, and die.

Warning Signs of Fatigue

The body has developed obvious alarm systems to alert the astute observer to beginning failure, preventing serious metabolic problems such as dehydration, exhaustion and heat stress. A knowledgeable rider or trainer will notice many of these signs of fatigue:

- slow heart rate recovery
- elevated heart rate for over an hour
- high respiratory rate, often shallow and inefficient
- deep, gulping breaths that persist for over 1 minute
- high rectal temperature for longer than 30 minutes
- dehydration with dry or pale mucous membranes, prolonged capillary refill time, jugular refill time, lack of intestinal sounds, and/or lack of skin elasticity
- depression
- lack of interest in surroundings

- lack of appetite or thirst
- muscle tremors or twitching
- muscle cramping
- thumps *(synchronous diaphragmatic flutter)*

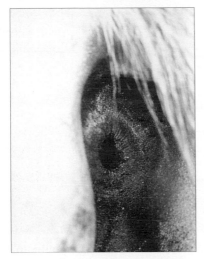

Fig. 8.7 Flaccid anal tone indicates exhaustion.

An exhausted horse with these symptoms is in need of medical attention. Without therapy, it can progressively decline and go into shock.

Other Stress Indicators

Diarrhoea is an indicator of stress, and contributes to loss of fluid and electrolytes through the faeces. Dry and scant faeces warn of marked dehydration. Anal sphincter tone should be strong; a flaccid anus is a sign of exhaustion.

ELECTROLYTES

For racing and other short-term events, a primary problem is heat dissipation from working muscles. For horses in longer events, the problem of *electrolyte* loss also must be addressed. Electrolytes are the body salts that contribute to all biochemical functions. A delicate balance in the amounts of these salts is essential for normal bio-chemical functions, such as muscle contraction, and normal intesti-nal function. Not only does extreme and prolonged sweating lead to dehydration, but horse sweat consists of more than just water. Sweat releases important electrolytes and minerals, including:

- sodium
- calcium
- chloride
- potassium
- magnesium

Lack of Electrolytes

Loss of abundant electrolytes contributes to a foamy, white and thick consistency of the sweat when they are released from the skin. The better conditioned a horse is, the 'thinner' the sweat becomes.

After a performance, small amounts of electrolytes are replenished by making a salt block available to the horse or by adding them to the feed. If losses are extreme, a veterinarian can give fluids and electrolytes by stomach tube or intravenously.

If essential amounts of electrolytes are lost in a horse's sweat and not replenished, a cascade of events contributes to a horse's decline. Correct balances of sodium, potassium, calcium, and magnesium control *neuromuscular irritability*, which is the ability of a muscle to respond to nerve impulses.

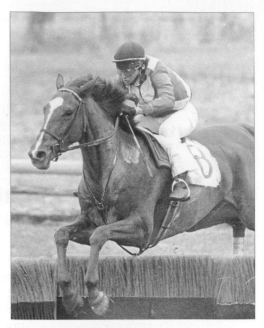

Fig. 8.8 Loss of electrolytes contributes to white, foamy sweat.

Neuromuscular Depression

A lack of certain electrolytes leads to neuromuscular depression, which means that the muscles respond slowly or not at all to nerve signals. Sodium, chloride, and potassium, three of these electrolytes, are major components of sweat. Working muscle releases these electrolytes through the sweat.

Loss of Sodium

A loss of sodium in the bloodstream depresses neuromuscular activity, impairing muscle contraction. A horse with a sodium deficiency is prone to fatigue and performance falters. Not only is sodium crucial to neuromuscular function, but it also helps retain body fluids so a horse does not become dehydrated. Sodium is not available to the horse in feed, so it must be offered as a supplement on the grain or by syringe.

Loss of Chloride

With exercise of a short duration, chloride loss is not usually a concern, but extended endurance exercise stimulates the kidneys to compensate for a loss of chloride by retaining bicarbonate (similar to the bicarbonate of baking soda) from the blood. Bicarbonate retention by the kidneys results in a mild *alkalosis,* or high pH of the bloodstream.

The competitive endurance horse operates aerobically until it fatigues or must sprint or climb. During these difficult efforts, working muscles generate lactic acid by anaerobic metabolism. Yet, not enough lactic acid is produced to lower the pH level of the blood and counteract the bicarbonate. A long distance horse is therefore more likely to have a metabolic alkalosis than a racehorse, for example. In view of this alkalosis, it is **dangerous** to feed sodium bicarbonate or inject a sodium bicarbonate solution into an endurance athlete.

Loss of Potassium

Potassium is an important electrolyte controlling the force of contraction in the muscles, both skeletal and heart. It is also responsible for dilating small arteries to improve oxygen supply to the tissue. If oxygen and blood supply to the muscles are compromised with potassium depletion, tying-up develops. Potassium loss also results in fatigue.

Hay is rich in potassium so this mineral is normally replenished when a horse stops working and eats. If exhaustion or metabolic problems depress the appetite, potassium must be replenished by supplements.

Neuromuscular Hyperirritability

Neuromuscular *hyperirritability* means that the muscles respond too much, or cannot stop contracting. Calcium relates to hyperirritability in two ways. First, too much calcium in the muscle cell and a lack of energy molecules contributes to hyperirritability. Second, if a horse loses excess calcium or magnesium in sweat, the neuromuscular system can becomes hyperirritable, as shown by muscle twitching and nervousness. If there is a profound lack of calcium, there is inability of the muscles to contract.

Hard work increases the demand of calcium and magnesium for muscle contraction, and therefore accelerates their depletion. A horse with excessive losses of calcium and magnesium from the bloodstream may develop multiple syndromes, including:

- intestinal shutdown
- colic
- heart arrhythmias
- tying-up
- thumps (synchronous diaphragmatic flutter)

Electrolyte supplements may be necessary during a long distance event to prevent the occurrence of these syndromes.

Excess Calcium in Muscle Cells

Normal contraction of muscle fibres depends on a calcium balance in the muscle cells. Each muscle fibre has a 'pump', fuelled by energy molecules, that removes calcium from the cell. Without energy the pump cannot remove calcium from the cells. Excess calcium in muscle cells creates persistent contraction, or spasms of muscle fibres.

Lactic acid accumulated in muscles changes the pH to an acid environment, which also interferes with the activity of the calcium pump and energy use. Imbalances of sodium, chloride, potassium and magnesium also impair muscle function and pump activity. Fatigue and tying-up result. *(See Chapter 3 for more information on tying-up.)*

Lack of Calcium in the Bloodstream

Calcium or magnesium loss from the bloodstream through the sweat can lead to *stress tetany*, which is a visible form of hyperirritability. Muscles and nerves become hyperirritable; a horse becomes nervous and jumpy, the muscles twitch or spasm, or the limbs stiffen.

Thumps

Thumps, or synchronous diaphragmatic flutter, is not a disease in itself, but it is a distress flag indicating electrolyte imbalances. The *phrenic nerve* passes directly across the heart muscle as it runs to the diaphragm, and provides nerve impulses for contraction of the diaphragm muscle. Excess loss of calcium and magnesium through the sweat, and rising levels of lactic acid in the body sensitize the phrenic nerve. It begins to respond to the electrical discharges of the heartbeat. Then the diaphragm contracts at the same time as the heartbeat. This contraction is seen as a twitching in the flank, or felt as a thumping if the hand is placed against the flank. The twitching is not related to respiratory movements.

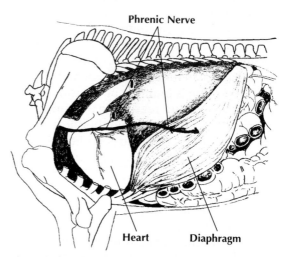

Phrenic Nerve

Heart **Diaphragm**

Fig. 8.9 The phrenic nerve and the interaction with chest anatomy.

Dietary Cause of Thumps

Hard work and hot, humid weather promote loss of calcium and magnesium through sweat. As a horse sweats, hormones from the parathyroid gland must remove calcium from the bones to the bloodstream, and the kidneys must retain the calcium to prevent its loss through urine. This system maintains calcium levels in the bloodstream.

Alfalfa hay is rich in calcium. A horse that is fed a diet primarily of alfalfa hay is predisposed to thumps and tying-up. A consistently high dietary intake of calcium 'turns off' the parathyroid gland. It is unable to mobilize calcium from bone stores during periods of excess calcium loss in the sweat. A horse can be fed alfalfa hay during and after a competitive event to replenish these losses, but should not be fed excess alfalfa between events.

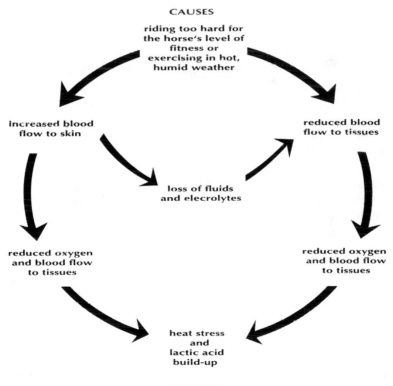

CAUSES

riding too hard for the horse's level of fitness or exercising in hot, humid weather

increased blood flow to skin

reduced blood flow to tissues

loss of fluids and elecrolytes

reduced oxygen and blood flow to tissues

reduced oxygen and blood flow to tissues

heat stress and lactic acid build-up

EFFECTS

Fig. 8.10 Dehydration cycle leading to heat stress and lactic acid build-up.

Electrolyte Imbalance: A Dehydration Cycle

Once changes in the electrolyte balance begin, deterioration proceeds in a domino-like cascade, preventing a return to normal. Continuing dehydration diverts the blood away from the muscle, liver and kidney tissues, to the skin for heat dissipation through sweating. Additional electrolytes are lost through the urine and sweat, and dehydration continues.

Sweating may not be enough to cool the horse, and initially the body sweats more profusely, losing more fluids in an attempt to dissipate heat. As the horse's internal temperature rises, it succumbs to heat stress.

With less body fluid, blood volume lowers, and blood circulation to all tissues diminishes further, which reduces oxygen availability. Then lactic acid collects in oxygen-starved tissues, biochemical reactions falter, and cell death occurs. Ultimately all body parts fail together. Without medical intervention, the result of this process is shock and death. The key to a horse's safety and performance stamina is to prevent it from nearing a state of heat stress or exhaustion.

PREVENTING METABOLIC PROBLEMS

Good nutrition, during both training and performance, can diminish stress and fatigue. Feed is the substance on which a horse refuels.

To prevent metabolic problems, condition the horse properly before any event or race, and ride logically without overstressing it.

Properly warm up a horse for 15 minutes before a competition so that muscles, tendons and ligaments receive adequate blood flow and flexibility before speed begins. An adequate cool-down is important after a stressful exertion to remove toxic by-products from muscle, and to dissipate heat from the horse's internal core.

Acclimatization

With training, a horse becomes accustomed to environmental influences. However, the athletic horse often performs away from home in a different environment. Ideally, if a horse is going to perform in a location that has dramatically different environmental conditions than it is used to, it should be moved to the location about 3 – 4 weeks beforehand. This will help to acclimatize it to the different stresses. If the horse is not moved soon enough, performance may suffer.

High Altitude

Below 7000 feet, the atmosphere usually supplies adequate oxygen to fuel the body. At 10000 feet, a horse consumes 10% more oxygen for the same task performed at sea level. Working muscles operate less efficiently if oxygen supplies are not sustained. Rapid fatigue and excess body heat result.

The enormous storage capacity of oxygen-carrying red blood cells in the spleen allows a horse to respond immediately to a higher elevation. As a survival response to a lack of oxygen, the spleen dumps extra red blood cells into the circulation, providing more oxygen to the demanding tissues.

Low oxygen in the blood turns on a special hormone *(erythropoietin)* that stimulates the bone marrow to make haemoglobin, and more red blood cells to hold the haemoglobin. The blood thickens, but unlike the thickening associated with dehydration, the new red cells are more laden with haemoglobin and oxygen. This adaptive process takes several weeks. After this time, the body is supplied with ample oxygen. Within a month, a horse should be well-acclimatized to the added demands of a high altitude environment.

Another temporary, but immediate, response to altitude within the first week or two is an increased heart rate and cardiac output, pushing more blood and oxygen to the tissues. The horse breathes deeper, and the respiratory rate rises, gathering more oxygen to be absorbed into the bloodstream. The competitor that has not been properly acclimatized may have slower heart rate recovery times than usual.

Initially after relocating to a higher altitude, a horse will urinate more frequently. Increased urination is a normal response to lower oxygen levels. However, it can lead to greater body fluid loss and relative dehydration. In addition, the reduced efficiency of working muscles produces more internal body heat. Then the horse sweats to rid the body of heat, losing body fluids and electrolytes. If the horse does not drink enough to compensate for fluid losses in the urine and sweat, the body slowly dehydrates.

Some individuals may also go off their feed in the first week after relocation. Then the horse will lose weight, and will not get valuable nutrients—energy, protein and electrolytes.

Immune System

A horse that is moved to a new environment is exposed to strange bacteria and viruses. The psychological stress of transport and new surroundings depresses a horse's immune system, making it more vulnerable to viral and bacterial attack. The immune system can respond to these foreign bodies by making antibodies against them. At least 2 weeks is required to activate the immune system to provide disease protection. This protection is particularly important to prevent respiratory disease that can severely impair performance.

Observation

For endurance and other long distance events, allow the horse access to water and food to restore fluids and energy. Provide electrolyte supplements to restore those losses from sweat. Cool the horse down at rest stops by sponging the head, neck and legs.

It is essential to take careful note of the horse throughout a performance. The horse cannot speak; its only defence against trouble is to communicate by body posture, or lack of interest or energy. Pay complete attention to the horse, and 'listen' to it. In this way, an owner or trainer ensures the horse's durability and excellence in its competitive athletic endeavours.

9

LEG SWELLING: CAUSES AND CURES

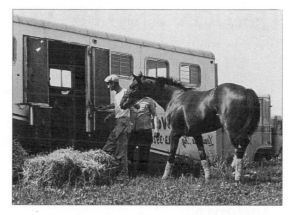

Fig. 9.1 Careful attention to a horse's safety is important in avoiding leg injuries.

DETERMINING THE CAUSE

After discovering a mysterious leg swelling on a horse, begin a systematic analysis of the situation. Leg swelling can result from a traumatic injury, or from a systemic illness that affects the entire body. Tissues of the leg do not have a great ability to expand. Limb swelling causes discomfort as the skin stretches to accommodate the enlarged size. The first step is to gather information.

Determine if the horse is lame on the affected limb. Observe it at the walk, and then, if it appears to be moving well, observe it at the trot. Then examine the limb to identify the exact source of the problem, whether it be skin or soft tissue swelling, tendon swelling, or joint swelling. Look closely for nicks, scrapes or puncture wounds. If

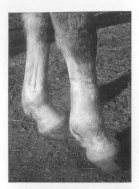

Fig. 9.2 Swelling in the right front cannon bone area.

the pastern area is swollen, pick up the foot and look carefully for a nail or other sharp object. Take the horse's rectal temperature, which is normally less than 101° F. Check to see if more than one leg is swollen.

Reconstruct the workouts from the last few days. Was the footing good? Could the horse have slipped? Was it ridden on hard ground too long or too fast? Was it turned out to pasture—alone or with others?

These questions may provide data to identify the cause of the swelling. An inflammatory response can be controlled in many different ways, and it is wise to consult the advice of a veterinarian before beginning any therapy.

TENDON AND LIGAMENT INJURIES

Any trauma, stress or strain to tendons or ligaments in the leg may begin as a slight filling along the back of the cannon or in the pastern area. In any inflammatory condition, proteins *(polypeptides)* are released into surrounding tissues. They summon white blood cells (WBCs) to 'clean up' the problem. Cellular 'water' enters with them, and the limb swells more. As the WBCs finish their job and die, they release enzymes that are toxic to surrounding cells. More WBCs, and water, invade the area. The inflammatory cycle continues, and the swelling remains.

Oedema

Normally, fluid that diffuses from the capillaries into tissues brings WBCs, nutrients and oxygen to the cells. The function of the *lymphatic system* is to retrieve this fluid and return it to the circulatory system. With an inflammation the lymph system cannot remove the fluid, and then the cells and intercellular spaces swell with the excess fluid. This swelling results in *oedema*. If one pushes on the swollen tissues, the fluid may be displaced, especially in regions

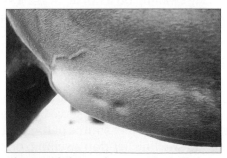

Fig. 9.3 Pitting oedema on the belly.

where the skin is able to stretch more, leaving an indented impression of the fingertip. This characteristic is aptly termed *pitting oedema*.

Oedema of the limb is self-perpetuating. When the tissue expands, it increases the distance over which nutrients must cross to reach the cells. Swollen tissue compresses blood vessels and further limits fluid movement out of the cells.

JOINT INJURIES

Joint swelling can be serious, and should receive veterinary attention. Trauma to a joint, such as a fall or a kick, or bone fracture respond well to immediate application of ice until the veterinarian arrives.

Windgalls

Windgalls, or inflammation, of the fetlock joint, occur as a result of heavy work, nutritional deficiencies, or trauma. Windgalls may also occur when a horse that has been heavily worked suddenly stops work for a few days. In this situation, the windgalls may abate with exercise.

In most cases, there is no pain, heat, or lameness associated with windgalls. Once a windgall has begun, it may remain for life. A long-standing windgall may also harden. However, unless lameness develops, treatment other than light exercise or improvement in the diet is usually unnecessary.

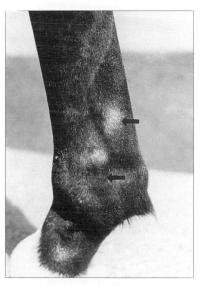

Fig. 9.4 Two windgalls.

Dislocations or Punctures

Dislocations or punctures within a joint show pronounced swelling and lameness. Successful management of these injuries with return to soundness is dependent on rapid and aggressive professional treatment. Treatment of puncture wounds of tendon sheaths and joints within 1 to 2 hours of the injury, and certainly within 6 hours maximum, significantly increases the possibility of a successful outcome.

Joint Inflammation in Foals

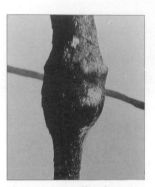

Fig. 9.5 A swollen knee on a foal.

A foal with one or more swollen joints may be suffering from *navel ill*, an infection within the joints that entered at the umbilicus and spread through the bloodstream. In the very young foal, rupture of the *common digital extensor tendon* at the front of the cannon bone results in a full swelling on the outside of the knee or hock.

A weanling or yearling may suffer from *epiphysitis* (inflammation of the growth plate) that appears as an hourglass-shaped fetlock, an overly knobby, swollen of the and painful knee or swelling of the bones either side of the fetlock.

THERAPY FOR LEG SWELLING
Cold Therapy

By understanding the physiology of swelling, certain principles can be applied to control it. Examples of injuries that benefit from cold therapy are:

- strained tendons or ligaments
- splints
- muscle injury
- joint injury
- kick injury
- interference trauma (striking one leg with another)

Ideally, apply cold for the first 48 – 72 hours after an injury occurs, beginning immediately. Water immersion (in buckets, boots, or a running stream) or ice massages are the best forms of cold therapy. Wrap ice in towels to prevent freezing the superficial skin layers.

Effects of Cold Therapy
Decreasing Inflammation

Cold therapy stops the inflammatory process by decreasing blood flow to the area as capillaries constrict from the cold. By slowing microscopic bleeding and haematoma formation, fluid leakage into the injury site is controlled. Haemorrhage and oedema disrupt tendon or ligament fibres. With healing, excessive fibrous scar tissue forms and thickens the tendon. This scarring is minimized with the initial use of cold treatment and a compression bandage.

Pain Relief

Cold also provides pain relief *(analgesia)* because nerve signals are limited at temperatures of 50–59° F. Analgesia lessens the muscle and tendon spasms which occur because of pain.

By 'cooling' a tendon, pain and lameness subside and give a false impression

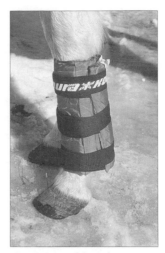

Fig. 9.6 A cold pack.

of a 'cure'. But cold therapy also increases the stiffness of the collagen in tendon or ligament fibres, reducing the elasticity of these structures. Although the horse may not be visibly lame, premature or strenuous exercise is extremely detrimental to the limb and may result in additional injury. **Rest** is the time-honoured therapy for treatment of most tendon strains.

Length of Application

Muscle tissues require cold application for about 25 minutes to achieve the desired effect. Initially, muscle temperature rises due to a reflex which increases the circulation. Then the temperature begins to decline in the deeper muscle layers, and continues to drop up to 10 minutes after cold application has been discontinued. If no activity follows therapy, the muscle tissue will not warm up to normal temperature for 4 hours. Therefore, confining the horse ensures prolonged cold therapy effects. Deep muscle massage will also loosen spasms in the fibres.

Joints cool more slowly than muscle, and remain 'cooled' for up to 2 hours. If a joint can be safely moved, intermittent flexion during cold therapy hastens the cooling process.

In deeper structures such as muscles and joints, cold deters swelling, but at temperatures less than 59° F, subcutaneous oedema (beneath the skin) is increased. A light pressure bandage controls the swelling caused by cold therapy. However, the benefit derived from the cold therapy far outweighs this mild superficial oedema.

Bandaging

After cooling down a strained tendon, a splint, or an injured muscle or joint, carefully bandage the limb when possible. The benefits of bandaging include:

- reducing swelling
- encouraging the tissues to heal with limited scar tissue
- supporting damaged structures
- preventing the spread of swelling to other areas of the leg

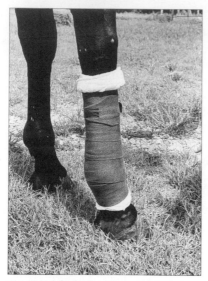

Fig. 9.7 A light bandage controls swelling and discourages scar tissue from forming.

If a horse 'does a tendon' at exercise, a support bandage should be fitted before it is travelled home or for treatment. A modified Robert-Jones bandage is appropriate. This can be achieved in the field by applying a couple of layers of Gamgee® or cotton wool to the leg, from the hoof to the knee, with firmly applied stable bandages over. The stable bandages should overlap one-half width on the way down and come back up in the same manner (forming a crossover pattern). With two or three layers of padding it is not possible to over-tighten the bandages.

Gravity encourages swelling of the structures below the injury site. Therefore, if the injury is above the fetlock it is best to bandage from knee to hoof, or hock to hoof. Also, a bandage is less likely to slip into a position where it hinders blood flow if the entire lower limb is bandaged.

If swelling appears above the bandage, or if a horse chews at the bandage or stamps its foot, check for excess tightness of the bandage. Cotton padding prevents inadvertent tightening of the bandage materials that could hinder circulation or compress tendons. Apply bandages uniformly, with no bumps or wrinkles.

Heat Therapy

Begin heat therapy **after** 2 – 3 days of cold therapy. Heat therapy works by warming the tissues around an injury site. This warming actually stimulates the body to 'cool' the area by dilating vessels and increasing blood flow. The oxygen supply is improved, and blood components such as WBCs, antibodies and nutrients are delivered to the tissues. The lymphatic vessels can once again remove waste products and excess oedema fluid. Pain decreases, and wound healing is enhanced. Increased circulation to the area leads to mild oedema in the subcutaneous tissues. Therefore, light bandaging after heat therapy is advantageous.

Hair and the thick layer of horse hide serve as an insulating barrier to heat, and more time is required to warm deeper structures than surface structures. Applying heat to a limb for 20 minutes is usually adequate. Problems that benefit from heat therapy include:

- contusions (bruising)
- mild sprains
- strains
- muscle or nerve inflammation
- joint arthritis

Water immersion or hot water bottles are more effective than dry heat, such as an electric heating pad. Place a towel between the skin and the hot pack to prevent burning and to insulate the pack. Never apply anything too hot to a horse's skin. A temperature of about 125° F is sufficient.

If circulation and tissue metabolism were increased by erroneously applying heat immediately after the injury, further damage and swelling would occur. But now, 3 days later, microscopic bleeding has ceased, and the healing process has begun. At this time, heat therapy decreases spasms in the area to provide pain relief, and promotes clean up of the injury.

Sweating

'Sweating' is another one-step method of heat therapy. An effective leg sweat is prepared by combining DMSO (dimethyl sulphoxide) and a nitrofurazone preparation. 'Sweat' bandages work by increasing heat and circulation to an area to remove swelling. A plastic wrap placed under a standing wrap traps sweat produced by the leg, creating a fluid barrier and retaining heat by preventing evaporative cooling. To prevent skin rash, do not leave a sweat bandage on for more than 48 hours.

Epsom Salts

Adding Epsom salts (magnesium sulphate) to wet heat therapy helps draw swelling from the tissue. Dissolve 16 oz Epsom salts per gallon of warm water, and soak the injured site for 20 minutes.

Poultices

A commercial poultice preparation 'pulls' swelling from an inflamed area in the same way Epsom salts do. Apply a poultice compound under a layer of absorbent material, such as roll cotton. A poultice pulls swelling away from the tissues, and creates a warm, moist, environment. Place a light pressure wrap over the cotton to hold the preparation in place, and to support soft tissue. Zinc oxide-impregnated bandages, and Animalintex® pads serve as excellent, ready-made poulticing materials, and need only be covered with an elastic, adhesive bandage.

Liniments and Balms

Many old-time horse liniments and leg balms also create heat and increase circulation by chemical action and by mild irritation of the skin. Human and equine athletes use these balms to advantage, but most should not be applied under a bandage as there is a real possibility of 'burning' the skin. Always read the labels and follow the instructions of the manufacturer.

Other Beneficial Therapies

DMSO

When applied in the same manner as a poultice, dimethyl sulphoxide (DMSO) is a very effective anti-inflammatory agent. It occasionally irritates the skin, and may result in mild hair loss. Do not apply it to any raw or deep wound surfaces. Wear protective gloves when applying DMSO as it easily penetrates human skin.

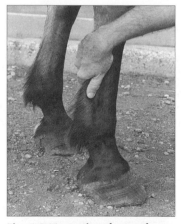

Fig. 9.8 Massaging the tendon.

Massage and Hydrotherapy

Deep massage is beneficial to an injured muscle or tendon along with cold and heat therapy. It increases circulation and breaks down adhesions formed by scar tissue. Massage by hand manipulation, or by hosing the limb with a forceful spray of water (hydrotherapy). Whirlpool boots are also commercially available. A whirlpool can be made by reversing a vacuum cleaner to convert the sucking air into blowing air. The hose inserted in the water achieves a turbulator effect, but exercise extreme caution and only use equipment designed for use with water and fitted with a circuit breaker fitted at the plug.

Exercise

Hand walking, or self-exercise in turnout, also enhances circulation to a limb, and reduces the build-up of fibrous scar tissue adhesions in tendon or ligament injuries. Light exercise can begin after the acute inflammatory stage has subsided, which may be from 2 days to 2 weeks after the injury. *'Stocking up'* from confinement, or swelling created by pregnancy responds quickly to light exercise.

Drug Therapy

Drug therapy is used in conjunction with hydrotherapy and rest of an injured leg. Commonly used drugs are the non-steroidal anti-inflammatory drugs (NSAIDs), such as phenylbutazone, or Finadyne®. NSAIDs limit the inflammatory process before it begins, and limit oedema, swelling and pain. However, NSAIDs can mask a severe problem. They may hide an injury that requires professional attention. They also enable a horse to inflict further injury by lessening a protective pain response.

SYSTEMIC ILLNESS

During the analysis of the injury, note if more than one limb is swollen. If so, it is advisable to contact a veterinarian immediately.

Do not overlook the obvious — simple stocking up from sluggish circulation caused by standing in a stall or small pen. Advanced pregnancy often slows circulation in the tissues, resulting in swollen, stocked up legs. However, complete swelling of more than one leg may signal a systemic problem which affects

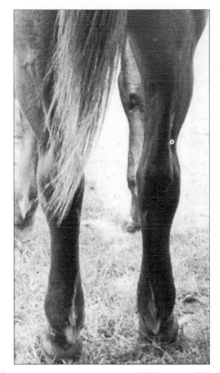

Fig. 9.9 'Stocking up' caused by poor circulation.

the entire body. These diseases include:

- heart disease
- a tumour or abscess that blocks the lymph system
- a dietary protein deficiency
- protein loss due to intestinal parasitism, or liver, kidney or intestinal disease
- viral infections, such as equine influenza or *equine viral arteritis*
- vaccination reactions
- an allergic form of strangles *(Streptococcus equi)* called *purpura haemorrhagica* which causes blood vessels to leak *(vasculitis)*

Horse owners have treated sore legs with cold and then hot packs for centuries. Modern science has only explained the treatment in medical terms, and defined the limits of this method of therapy. Done properly, the system still works.

10

TENDON INJURIES: PREVENTING AND MANAGING

As the horse evolved to flee predators, the bones in the lower legs telescoped in length. Longer bone provides a lever arm which increases the contraction of the muscles to propel a horse across the ground. When the strap-like tendons that connect muscle to bone cross over a joint surface, the bending motion of the joint amplifies muscle contraction. Elastic energy transmitted within a ten-

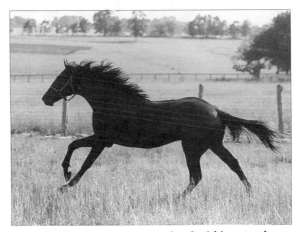

Fig. 10.1 Elastic energy transmitted within a tendon produces locomotion.

don produces locomotion. The athletic horse is at risk of tendon injury because every step stresses these elastic structures.

Tendinitis is an inflammation which involves only the tendon, while *tenosynovitis* is inflammation of the tendon and its sheath. An owner or trainer may see a tendon injury as a *bowed tendon*. This results from an inflammatory condition in the tendon that causes it to thicken with scar tissue.

There are several kinds of bowed tendons, each classified according to their position on the limb. A low bow is in the lower cannon area near the fetlock joint. A middle bow is in the middle of the cannon area. A high bow is in the upper cannon area. A full bow involves all three areas. If a horse suffers from tendinitis or a bowed tendon, its athletic career is not necessarily over. Proper management and healing of the original injury greatly influence how well a tendon regains function and resists repeated trauma.

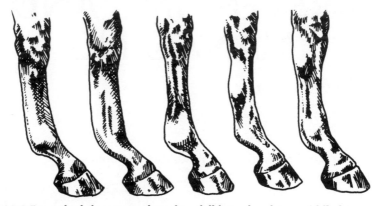

Fig. 10.2 From the left, a normal tendon, full bow, low bow, middle bow and high bow.

A study by Dr Roy Pool (University of California at Davis) found that 25% of clinically 'normal', symptomless horses have some microscopic abnormality in the tendon, suggesting a degenerating area of tendon. If this unhealthy spot increases and a tendon is continually or abruptly overstretched, clinical tendinitis results.

STRESS HANDLING OF TENDONS
Tendon Structure

Tendons are made of bundles of longitudinally oriented collagen fibres. Most tendons are surrounded by sheaths. The tendon sheath allows the tendon to glide smoothly over the structures of a limb. As the limb bears weight, a tendon normally extends within a narrow range of elasticity. When reasonably stretched (as with weight-bearing), the collagen fibres maintain their linear and parallel order. Once the load is removed they snap back to the original position.

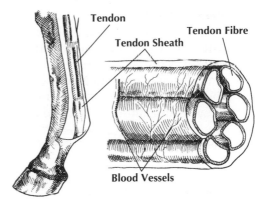

Fig. 10.3 Tendon structure and sheath.

Tendon Injury
Tendon and Muscle Interaction

One of the normal functions of the flexor tendons along the back of the cannon bone is to stabilize the fetlock. These tendons prevent the fetlock from collapsing on to the ground when the limb is supporting weight. Normally, the muscle decreases the stress on the tendon, which attaches the muscle to the bone. When the muscle fatigues, vibration in the muscle and tendon *(musculotendinous unit)* increases strain on the collagen fibres of the tendon. As groups of muscles fatigue, the limb sinks into unnatural configurations. An example is *dorsiflexion* of the fetlock, when the fetlock sinks towards the ground, overstretching the flexor tendons.

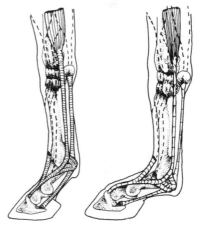

Overloading Tendons

Initially, a tendon adapts to the stretch, but increased loading of a limb may extend a tendon beyond its elastic limit. If a

Fig. 10.4 On the left, a normal fetlock. On the right, dorsiflexion of the fetlock.

tendon is stretched beyond 5–6% of its length, the fibres stiffen, and irreversible structural damage results. Like a rubber band that has been overstretched, once the excessive weight-bearing strain is removed an overstretched tendon does not regain its original pattern. If a tendon is stretched beyond 8% of its length, it can rupture.

Conditioning Tendons

Overstretching a tendon through overloading results from excessive athletic demands for which the horse is not conditioned. Conditioning is one way to prevent and manage tendinitis, or a bowed tendon. Light and repeated loading of tendons through conditioning and training stimulates the tendons to respond to mechanical strain. They become more elastic and resist being overstretched.

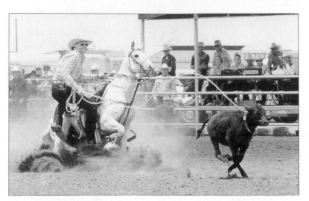

Fig. 10.5 Sports involving sudden twists and turns can cause tendon injury.

If a horse is fatigued, or if a training programme incorporates too much speed, jumping, uneven terrain, or sudden twists and turns, tendons lose stability when the corresponding muscles become exhausted or are overloaded. It is therefore important to properly condition a horse for the intended sport. Other mechanical factors, such as poor footing, unbalanced feet, poor conformation, and high risk activities also contribute to tendon injury and should be avoided.

Mechanical Factors Leading to Tendon Injury

Poor Footing

If a foot is not picked up quickly enough as the body advances across the ground, the *superficial digital flexor tendon* is overstretched. The *superficial flexor muscle* contracts as a horse propels forward. The complementary tendon should be shortening, but if the pastern is not picked up and moved forward quickly enough, the fetlock sinks to the ground (dorsiflexes) while the body continues forward. The tendon will then overstretch.

Situations that can cause poor footing and tendon injury include:

- Slippery ground that encourages a hoof to slide backwards, simulating a situation where the leg is too far under the body

where it cannot advance or be lifted quickly
- Deep footing, such as mud, sand or snow, which causes a foot to sink—it may not elevate in time to avoid tendon injury
- Shoe caulks, trailers, or studs on the shoes which make the foot 'stick', delaying lift and advancement of the foot as the body moves forward.
- Uneven footing which excessively loads the tendons beyond normal stress limits

Unbalanced Feet

Unbalanced feet simulate uneven footing, causing a leg to twist unnaturally because it is unevenly loaded. Once it was thought that raising the heels on a tendon-injured horse would decrease the stress on the tendon. This idea is incorrect: raising the heel lengthens the distance the tendon drops with weight-bearing and increases tension on an already-injured tendon. A serious bow may benefit from slightly lowering the heels, but it is best to trim the feet at a proper and reasonable angle.

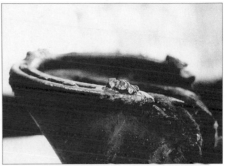

Fig. 10.6 Shoe caulks can make a foot stick, thereby delaying lift and advancement of the foot.

A broken hoof–pastern axis angle also interferes with a smooth breakover of the limb. For example, a long-toe – low-heel (LTLH) configuration slows lift and delays advancement of the foot as it travels.

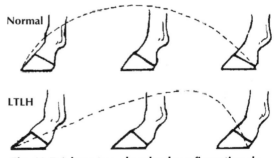

Fig. 10.7 A long-toe – low-heel configuration delays lift and advancement.

Poor Conformation

A calf knee conformation functionally mimics LTLH hoof, delaying breakover and stressing the flexor tendons. A long, upright pastern conformation predisposes to tendon injury by increasing the fetlock drop experienced with weight-bearing.

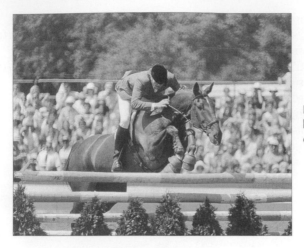

Fig. 10.8 Jumping is a high risk activity which can injure a tendon.

High Risk Activities

Certain activities contribute to dorsiflexion of the fetlock, increasing the risk of overstretching a tendon. Jumping not only abnormally loads the forelegs upon landing, but often involves sudden and tight turns, or uneven terrain. Polo is another example of an activity that abruptly loads the forelegs as a horse is turning or moving at speed. Long distance riding, negotiating downhill terrain, and the speed work of racing place excessive demands on the entire musculotendinous unit.

In some cases, it is necessary to change the athletic pursuit of an injured horse to ensure a successful career. For example, a jumping horse can be converted to a pleasure or equitation candidate. A racehorse can become a hunter/jumper, dressage or driving horse.

INJURY-PRONE AREAS
Cannon-Bone Area

There are several areas on equine legs where injuries most often occur. The *superficial digital flexor tendon* along the back of the cannon bone

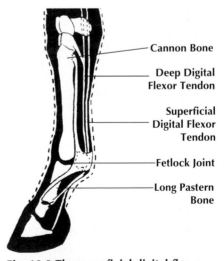

Cannon Bone

Deep Digital Flexor Tendon

Superficial Digital Flexor Tendon

Fetlock Joint

Long Pastern Bone

Fig. 10.9 The superficial digital flexor tendon is especially prone to injury.

is predisposed to injury because it is under the greatest amount of tension. It is also furthest from the centre of rotation of the fetlock joint. Many injuries occur at the point where the superficial digital flexor has the smallest cross-sectional area, which is in the middle of the cannon bone area. As the tendon's cross-sectional area decreases, it becomes stiffer and less elastic. In addition, there is an increased force per unit area on this narrower segment of the tendon.

Fetlock Area

Another area highly susceptible to injury is the fetlock area. If the *deep digital flexor tendon* is injured, a low bow results. Tendon injuries in the fetlock area or below have a poorer prognosis than injuries higher on the limb. Because of the digital sheath over the tendon in this area, more connective tissue develops beneath the skin (subcutaneous) in the healing process. This tissue restricts gliding of the tendon through the sheath.

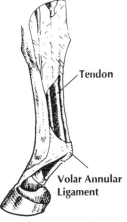

Fig. 10.10 The volar annular ligament will bind down an inflamed tendon.

The *volar annular ligament*, a non-elastic band of dense connective tissue, runs horizontally across the back of the fetlock, and may be involved in a low bow. The volar annular ligament does not stretch as the deep digital flexor tendon swells, therefore the ligament binds down the inflamed tendon. This unrelenting pressure reduces blood flow to the tendon over time. Fibre death, reduction in gliding motion, and development of adhesions which bind the two structures together result from a reduced blood flow. The ligament constricts, resulting in a visible depression over the back of the fetlock, with a pronounced bulge above and/or below, near the digital tendon sheath.

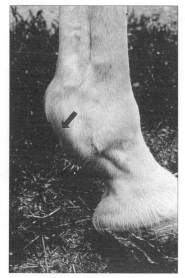

Fig. 10.11 The 'dent' in the swelling is due to volar annular ligament constriction.

251

With immediate surgical intervention to release the constricting ligament, there is a more favourable prognosis for a horse to return to function. If adhesions are allowed to progress too long before surgery, they 'glue' the structures together, permanently restricting the tendon and causing pain.

TENDON REPAIR

What begin as small microscopic tears in the orderly tendon fibres may expand to a large tear. Accompanying inflammation produces clinical symptoms of pain, heat, or swelling. Capillary bleeding within the tendon triggers an inflammatory response. Oedema and bleeding interrupt the normal tendon fibres' pattern of tight, longitudinally oriented and parallel bundles. The tendon is weakest at 5 – 7 days after injury, with the acute inflammatory stage lasting up to 14 days.

Tendons are excellent at repairing themselves if given the time and help they need. To better understand how to aid healing and speed a return to function, it is helpful to study the healing process within an injured tendon.

Fibrin and Granulation Tissue Repair Process

Fibrin is a blood component which binds together torn tendon collagen. In the first 3 weeks after injury, this fibrin forms a *fibrovascular callus* around the injured tendon. The fibrovascular callus connects the wounded structures, in effect hardening the fibrin cells into a scaffold in preparation for repair. Then, like a skin wound, the body repairs the tendon injury with *granulation tissue* and more fibrous connective tissue.

The blood supply within the tendon only nourishes about 25% of the tendon volume. But because inflammation limits internal blood flow, healing compo-

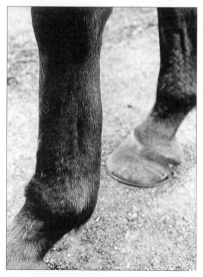

Fig. 10.12 A bowed tendon is thickened with scar tissue.

nents must come from the tissue around the tendon (peritendinous). The more the peritendinous cells contribute to healing, the greater the development of adhesions and scar tissue. Adhesions restrict the normal gliding ability of the tendon through the sheath, and scar tissue limits its elasticity.

During this repair period, granulation tissue forms and then organizes into fibrous tissue. The inflammatory process permanently thickens a tendon with scar tissue, giving the visual impression of a bow where there had been a straight structure.

During the next few months, a tendon repair 'matures'. Collagen fibres redevelop to a normal, longitudinal orientation. Usually, by 6 weeks after injury, collagen formation exceeds collagen breakdown within the tendon. By 3 months, collagen fibres begin to form discrete bundles. The bundles are similar to normal tendon by 4 months.

Exercises That Promote Healing

During the repair process, controlled passive motion exercises realign collagen fibres longitudinally by placing mild tension on the tendon. These slow, range-of-motion exercises include manual flexion and extension of the limb for 10 – 15 minutes, two or three times a day. After the acute inflammatory stage, begin light hand walking. Progressively increase these exercises over the months. It is not known how much passive physical therapy is appropriate, therefore it is wise not to overdo this practice.

Aggressive physical activity interferes with repair, and re-injury can occur. Attempts to forcibly break down adhesions are counterproductive, whereas gentle lengthening and stretching of scar tissue give better results.

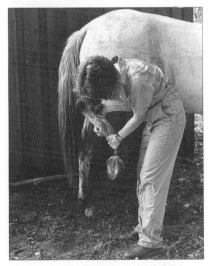

Fig. 10.13 Manual flexion of the injured limb realigns collagen fibrils.

Healing Time

The time required for healing varies, depending on the extent of the injury. A minimum recovery period for slight tendon tearing may require only a month. More severe injuries require *at least 10 months* for a tendon fibre to heal completely. It may be necessary for a horse to recover for 1 – 1½ years to achieve optimal repair. It is essential that veterinary recommendations be followed, so that a performance horse is given a long enough recuperative period to prevent a relapse.

Indications of 'healing' can be misleading. Many horses at 10 weeks after injury may not respond to finger pressure over the tendon. They may also have no heat or swelling in the area. However, there are still areas of tendon damage that are in the earlier healing stages and require a longer rest period than other areas of the same tendon.

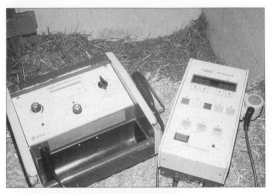

Fig. 10.14 Two types of ultrasound machines.

Ultrasound Evaluation of Injuries

Ultrasound is a useful tool to evaluate tendon injuries and to monitor healing. Before the introduction of ultrasound, only certain clinical signs could be used to evaluate tendon healing. A study by

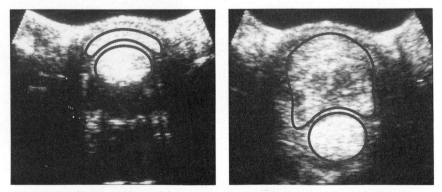

Fig. 10.15 Ultrasound is used by veterinarians to diagnose and monitor an injury. For example, on the left is a normal deep digital flexor tendon and superficial digital flexor tendon. On the right, the deep digital flexor is still intact, but the superficial digital flexor tendon is disrupted and severely injured.

Dr Virginia Reef (University of Pennsylvania) revealed that specific, outward, clinical appearances have little relationship to the severity of a tendon injury as evidenced by ultrasound.

In her study, heat was felt in only 17% of injured tendons. Heat diminishes long before healing is completed, therefore it is not a reliable indicator of readiness to return to work. Similarly, only 19% of the horses in the study were sensitive to finger pressure over the afflicted tendon. Only 40% had an associated lameness, while swelling or filling of the leg was apparent in 85% of the horses. These numbers illustrate that the degree of lameness or swelling is *not* a reliable indicator of the severity of an injury. Accurate assessments of the extent of tendon damage and the progress of healing require the use of diagnostic ultrasound technology.

How it Works

With diagnostic ultrasound, high frequency sound waves are transmitted to a tendon. The denser the tissue, the more resistant it is to sound waves, and the sound waves bounce back off the tissue surface as an 'echo'. The denser the tissue, the greyer the projection seen on the screen *(echogenicity)*. If the sound waves pass freely through blood, fluid or oedema, the image appears black on the screen because the sound waves do not produce an echo.

In this way, a tendon is 'imaged' to measure the extent of an injury in both width and length. The monitor shows areas of fibre disruption, or swelling of a tendon.

For example, a common tendon injury is a *central core lesion* associated with severe fibre disruption and haemorrhage. On the screen, the lesion appears as a black hole in the centre of the tendon. The size of the hole determines the severity of the injury and prognosis for return to athletic soundness.

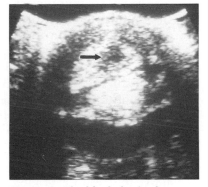

Fig. 10.16 The black dot in the middle is a central core lesion.

Both mild and severe injuries initially give similar outward appearances of pain, swelling and heat. However, the prognosis for healing is radically different between a severe central core lesion and a tendon that is merely swollen. Ultrasound discerns these differences at the onset.

Monitoring Healing

Ultrasound is useful to monitor the healing process over time. The increasing greyness on the screen reflects the stage of healing. This information helps to plan a strategy for returning a horse to performance. After an appropriate lay-up period, and as the echogenicity of the lesion increases, longer and faster workouts can be used to restore tendon strength. Exercise reorients the fibres along the plane of tension. Ultrasound diagnostics are repeated at 2–3 month intervals to monitor progress for as long as 1–3 years after an injury has occurred.

RECURRENCE OF TENDON INJURY

A recurrence of a tendon injury is possible if the tendon is prematurely stressed while an injury is visible on ultrasound as a 'discrete healing lesion'. Also, not all fully healed tendon injuries are immune to further damage. A prior tendinitis does not result in loss of strength in the tendon, but it does result in reduced elasticity. A previously injured tendon, bowed or not, may be unable to withstand normal stresses placed on it by exercise.

Transition Zone

Subsequent tendon damage does not necessarily occur at the site of the original injury. It often occurs just above or below the point where tendon structure least resembles normal structure. These areas are called *transition zones* because they are between the normal areas and previously injured areas of the tendon. Adhesions in the transition zones may prevent the fibres from orienting longitudinally as they heal. Instead, they orient abnormally and may prematurely tear before they reorganize in a longitudinal pattern. Fibres with a loosely structured and random pattern are a weak link in the collagen chain.

Adhesions are unyielding, causing the inelastic tendon tissue above or below the original injury to 'super stretch'. Continued microtrauma in this area enlarges the traumatized area, and causes lameness due to chronic inflammation.

TENDON THERAPY

There are many approaches to therapy for tendinitis or a bowed tendon. The ultimate goal is to restore elasticity and gliding function to the tendon. As indicated, lameness, heat, sensitivity, and filling of the tendons are unreliable indicators of actual injury in the area, yet these may be the only indicators if ultrasound is not available. Once these symptoms appear, take emergency measures to minimize damage.

Controlling Swelling

Local swelling and haemorrhage further damage tendon fibres. Therefore, controlling swelling is essential if the tendon is to heal well and with limited adhesions. If a horse shows lameness in a previously bowed limb, or if it is sensitive to pressure over an affected tendon, ice the leg immediately or hose it with cold water to limit swelling. A light pressure bandage controls swelling beneath the skin, which is associated with cold therapy, until a veterinarian arrives. Non-steroidal anti-inflammatory drugs control swelling. DMSO applied to the tendon area under a light bandage also exerts strong anti-inflammatory effects. After acute inflammation has stopped, warm soaks improve circulation and elasticity of the tendon and assist the healing process. Depending on the extent of the injury, the acute inflammatory stage may last from 2 days to 2 weeks.

Surgery

For superficial digital flexor injuries, Dr Larry Bramlage (Rood and Riddle Equine Hospital, Lexington, Kentucky) has suggested cutting the superior check ligament just above the knee to release tension on the scarred tendon. Performing this surgery during the initial repair stage significantly reduces scarring in the tendon. The superior check ligament becomes longer as it heals, reducing tension on the injured tendon. Its transitional zone is not subjected to much stress because both the muscle and tendon above the knee actively assume some of the load of weight-bearing.

Bandaging

After a layoff for a tendon injury, support wraps are useful during reintroduction to work by delaying the onset of fatigue in an injured leg. It is speculated that a bandage also limits dorsiflexion of the fetlock when the limb is fatigued. A leg bandaged with the Equisport® (3-M) bandage or equivalent can absorb up to 39% more energy, for example on dorsiflexion of the fetlock, than an unbandaged leg. With its elastic properties, the bandage assumes the elastic function of the tendons as the fetlock sinks with weight-bearing, reducing strain on the tendons.

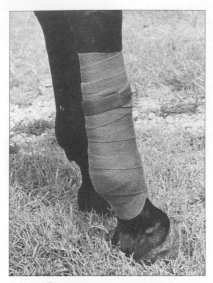

Fig. 10.17 Bandages support injured tendons and are sometimes used to protect sound legs from interference injury.

The supportive capabilities of a bandage depend on the tension with which it is applied, and the bandage configuration. The tighter the bandage is applied, the greater is its energy-absorption capacity. Be sure not to apply the bandage so tightly as to cut off the circulation. If in doubt, consult a veterinarian.

The most versatile method of applying such bandages is at half-stretch tension in a low figure eight, starting just below the knee and spiralling down with a two- to three-layer figure eight over the fetlock, and the bandage spiralled up again to the knee. Applied in this manner the bandage does not inhibit fetlock mobility, and at half-stretch tension it should not impair local circulation or constrict the tendons.

Materials that absorb the most energy also tend to wear out fastest. Bandage support of a limb declines rapidly with an increasing number of fetlock dorsiflexions. Studies with the Equisport® bandage focus mainly on racetrack application where the bandage only needs to aid limb support for about 2 – 5 minutes. This limitation must be considered when bandaging a long distance riding horse or a dressage or jumping horse. Bandages may be more of a hindrance than a help if they are too tight and impair local circulation, or if they partially restrict the range of motion of the fetlock joint.

MANAGEMENT

After a tendon injury the horse should be stalled for at least 2 – 3 weeks to restrict movement of the limb. This enforced rest prevents further damage to the tendon.

To promote proper realignment of the fibres by passive motion therapy, the ankle can be alternately flexed and extended for short periods several times daily after the acute inflammatory stage has subsided.

Ultrasound documents the initial injury and monitors its progress to recovery. Follow a conservative approach based on recommendations by a veterinarian and ultrasound information before returning a horse to active work.

There is no substitute for appropriate conditioning or proper choice of athletic function. In managing an old injury, the importance of a warm-up and cool-down for a horse (and tendons) cannot be overstated. Good circulation in the limbs improves the elasticity of the musculotendinous unit and helps to avoid tendon injury.

11

HIGH-TECH THERAPY
FOR INJURIES

For any athlete, pain can be the difference between a poor performance and one that is brilliant. Equine athletes may only be able to communicate subtle pain by a decline in their athletic output. High-tech therapies, used along with conventional medicine, can relieve pain and heal injuries.

HIGH-TECH THERAPY APPLICATIONS
Diagnosis

An honest evaluation of a technique's effectiveness requires accurate diagnosis of the injury. Adding technological advances, such as heart rate monitors, to a training programme lends insight into the level of discomfort a horse experiences while at work. Previously 'inexplicable' impairments in performance can now be documented. A sustained, higher than normal heart rate at a given work level reflects pain induced by exercise stress.

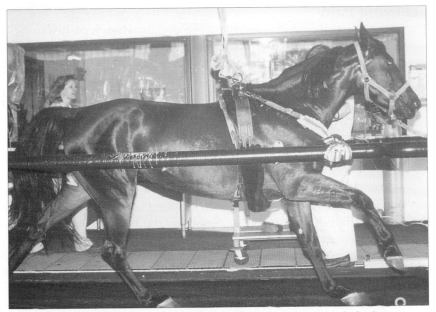

Fig. 11.1 Gait analysis using a treadmill and video cameras can help detect subtle problems before they become serious.

A gait analysis monitor is an imaging device that shows how well a limb is moving on a treadmill. In addition, video cameras can record and exactly measure the length and cadence of strides to detect subtle problems before they become serious. Infrared thermography is a diagnostic tool which images heat gradients. It detects inflammatory conditions, particularly of the lower limbs, spine, face and superficial muscles. Such devices often foretell impending failure.

Injury Management

Not only is sophisticated technology used to define a problem, but these tools are also applied to manage a healing process and to facilitate the horse's rapid return to soundness. Recently, researchers have dedicated their efforts to evaluating high-tech therapies—such as lasers and ultrasound—for injury management. In many cases conventional medicine is insufficient to 'cure' a lameness. Therefore it is understandable that a frustrated owner or trainer may seek high-tech alternatives to alleviate a chronic problem that has not responded to standard treatment.

Relieving Pain

No single approach is infallible, especially when it comes to the healing process. The medical profession can only assist nature and manipulate biological processes to proceed along a desired course. Many high-tech options such as *Transcutaneous Electrical Nerve Stimulation* (TENS) provide pain relief without actually 'curing' the injury.

When an injury occurs, the body's guarding response increases muscle tension with a subsequent decrease in blood flow. This decrease causes waste products to accumulate in the injured area. In addition, the body's natural inflammatory response to the injury includes continued production of prostaglandins and other chemicals that reinforce inflammation, heat, swelling and pain. Pain relief limits the inflammatory response, enabling the body to heal quickly. Although the problem remains, it does not interfere with performance to the same degree. TENS, electroanalgesia, lasers and ultrasound provide pain relief. Laser radiation and ultrasound, however, also promote healing.

Promoting Healing

Using scientific evidence about biological factors that promote healing, high-tech options such as lasers and ultrasound attempt to stimulate circulation to the tissues. Electrical Muscle Stimulation (EMS) also promotes healing. Healing requires adequate circulation of oxygen and nutrients to the tissues, and removal of waste products from the tissues. Lasers, ultrasound and EMS accomplish these goals similar to how conventional procedures use pharmacological drugs, hot and cold therapy, or poultices.

When a horse is in obvious need of conventional surgical or medical treatment, alternative therapies do little to repair the injury. However, the use of high-tech alternatives along with conventional surgery, pharmacological drugs, and physical therapy enhances the probability for successful treatment.

ANCIENT ARTS, NEW TECHNOLOGY

Several new technologies capitalize on 'modern' knowledge of the healing process, while instituting the ancient principles of the arts of *acupuncture* and *acupressure* to manage an injury. These high-tech therapies are a blending of Eastern and Western medical philosophies.

Acupressure and acupuncture operate by stimulating specific nerve tracts and meridians that directly interact with the injured body part. These 'points' can now be stimulated by high-tech tools in a variety of ways.

Acupuncture

The ancient art of acupuncture stimulates specific nerve fibres with needle penetration. There are many good books on the market today regarding the pure forms of acupuncture and acupressure. This chapter deals only with the modern applications of those arts, using high-tech equipment. High-tech ways of stimulating acupuncture points are:

- heat application to the points
- acu-injection of drugs or saline at the points to prolong stimulation of the nerve
- electrical stimulation of the points

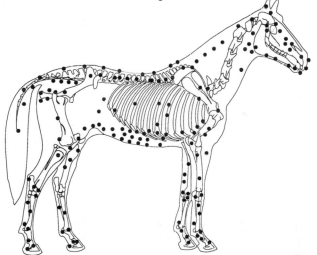

Fig. 11.2 An overview of the numerous acupuncture points of the horse.

Acupressure

Acupressure is an off-shoot of acupuncture. It seeks to stimulate the same points as acupuncture, but without penetrating the skin. Because it requires no technical knowledge, there are many ways to use acupressure. One way to use acupressure on the horse is massage therapy. Another common acupressure tool is the twitch.

The Twitch and Endorphin Release

A nose twitch 'sedates' and relaxes the horse while a mildly painful procedure is performed. Heart rates decrease up to 8% while using a twitch, just the opposite response expected from a painful or frightening experience.

It is hypothesized that the twitch stimulates specialized sensory fibres in the skin, resulting in a release of chemicals from the central nervous system. These chemicals, similar to morphine, are called *endorphins* and *enkephalins*.

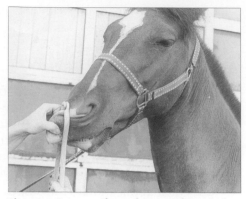

Fig. 11.3 Pressure from the use of a twitch releases endorphins and enkephalins.

They reduce and suppress perception of pain. Scientists at the University of Utrecht in The Netherlands analysed levels of these substances in the blood and discovered that endorphin levels increased by 81% during twitching and returned to normal within 30 minutes after the twitch was removed.

ELECTRICAL THERAPIES
Transcutaneous Electrical Nerve Stimulation
Relieving Pain

One method of electrically stimulating acupuncture points is Transcutaneous Electrical Nerve Stimulation, known as TENS. This point stimulation provides relief from pain symptoms.

Conventional TENS therapy provides a voltage of electrical pulses high enough to stimulate the acupuncture points, but low enough to avoid sustained muscle contractions. Impulses are passed to the nervous system us-

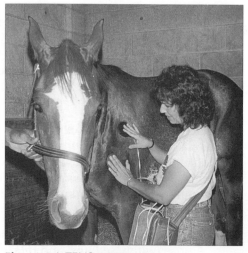

Fig. 11.4 A TENS set-up.

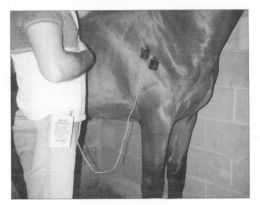

Fig. 11.5 Another TENS set-up.

ing a padded electrode placed over the skin. The electrodes send impulses to nerve receptors in the skin and in the superficial tissues. Sensory information is relayed to the central nervous system by specific pain receptors *(nociceptors).*

These nociceptors are located in areas of motor and trigger acupuncture points. A motor point excites muscle tissue and causes it to contract. Trigger points define hypersensitive areas afflicted with inflammation and tenderness.

Many acupuncture points are located in the superficial skin layers, where nerves and nociceptors transmit impulses from both the internal and external environments to the central nervous system. Stimulation of these nerve fibres and pain receptors by TENS results in the production and release of endorphins and enkephalins from the brain. Whereas the half-life of enkephalins is as brief as 1 minute, endorphins have a half-life of 2 – 3 hours, providing opiate-like pain relief.

The Gate Theory

TENS provides pain relief by a 'gate theory'. Repeated, *nonpainful* stimulation of the sensory nerve fibres causes the nerve endings to fatigue. Then they are unable to transmit pain sensation to the brain. This overload of stimulation also causes a release of *serotonin*, a chemical which blocks pain impulses and reception by the brain, and, in effect, 'closes a gate'. Then the brain 'ignores' the less intense stimulus of the injury.

Diagnosis

TENS is also a valuable diagnostic tool, particularly if used in conjunction with infrared thermography. Infrared thermography shows heat gradients, detecting inflammatory conditions. An inflamed area is already stimulated by pain reflexes because it hurts. Therefore, less voltage is required from TENS to 'fire' a trigger point nerve. TENS finds the more sensitive nerve tracts, which are in an inflamed area. This method confirms an infrared thermograph which shows acute inflammatory heat patterns. Conversely, in structurally sound areas with no inflammation, infrared thermography shows 'cold' patterns. Appropriate therapy can then be directed at the specific injury site.

Electroanalgesia

Another type of electrical stimulation, electroanalgesia, is very similar to TENS therapy, but uses different frequencies than TENS. Unlike conventional TENS, electroanalgesia mildly amplifies electrical output to produce visible muscle twitches.

Low-Frequency Electroanalgesia

Low-frequency electroanalgesia (LFEA) may provide pain relief for 1 – 3 days. LFEA is especially helpful for the chronic pain of degenerative joint disease because it stimulates large nerve fibres in the joint to elicit a central pain-suppressing effect.

High-Frequency Electroanalgesia

At a higher frequency than used for TENS, electroanalgesia also provides pain relief by the gate theory (ignoring the less intense stimulus of the injury), and by releasing endorphins. *High-frequency electroanalgesia* (HFEA) relieves pain more quickly than LFEA, but pain relief is sustained for shorter periods than LFEA.

Electrical Muscle Stimulation

High voltage *Electrical Muscle Stimulation* (EMS) has been reported to exercise atrophied muscles by passively producing muscle contractions. Muscles are strengthened through this process because it 'retrains' the biochemical and enzymatic reactions vital to adequate muscle contraction. A limb that needs rest for bone, joint, ligament or tendon repair can be 'exercised' without weight-bearing and is not unduly stressed while healing. Also, the pumping action of these electrically produced muscle contractions indirectly improves circulation to the area. Therefore, improved blood flow enhances the healing process while removing waste products, and oedema formed by a stagnant circulation is reduced. EMS may also improve cases of laminitis by improving circulation to the foot.

Pulsing Electromagnetic Fields

Still another high-tech method allegedly improves oxygen supply and increases temperature within the tissues (particularly

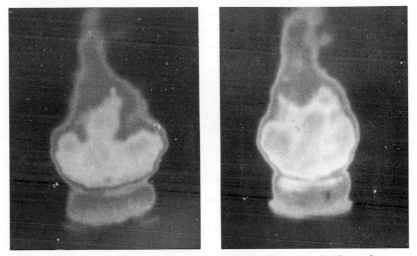

Fig. 11.6 Thermograph showing increased blood flow into the foot after EMS. On the left, before treatment. On the right, after treatment the light area, signifying blood flow, is lighter and larger than before.

bone) by improving dilation of blood vessels and circulation. This in turn promotes healing. This technique uses *Pulsing Electromagnetic Fields* (PEMF). It is sometimes used for bone injuries, especially long bones, such as bucked shins or splints.

Usually two electromagnetic coils are placed on opposite sides of the injured area, with each coil 'capturing' the electromagnetic field of the other to align it into a uniform field. This uniform field supposedly produces a uniform electric current within the tissues.

Normally, bone has an electrical polarity. The pulsing field generated on the coils mimics the long bone's normal electrical potentials, stimulating faster healing.

Theoretically, varying wave patterns and pulse rates determine the biological response. There is still no evidence as to which specific pulses and waves affect what or how. It is speculated that magnetic fields increase oxygen levels in tissue and improve energy production to fuel healing processes. Improving circulation and oxygen to the tissues may also limit the pain created by lack of oxygen.

A similar principle attempts to use biomagnetic, flexible, rubber or plastic pads surrounding a foil. The foil contains a magnetized iron compound, producing alternating magnetic fields. Foil pads are bandaged in place to increase circulation when applied over blood vessels.

The principle of PEMF is good in theory, but controlled research projects comparing different electromagnetic devices show no improvement in the healing rates of bone or tendon.

LASERS

A recent method of wound healing and pain relief is using *laser* radiation as a 'light-needle' to stimulate acupuncture points. The word 'laser' is an acronym for *Light Amplification by Stimulated Emission of Radiation.*

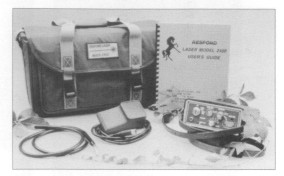

Fig. 11.7 Portable laser unit and components.

Laser radiation is generated by electromagnetic waves of the same wavelength that are aligned in both time and space, and travel in nearly parallel directions. These characteristics allow the waves to be focused as a thin beam onto a very small spot. The intensity of this beam can be magnified to cut directly through living flesh. Laser radiation is used as a surgical tool for intricate procedures such as eye or urogenital surgery. A less intense beam can coagulate tissues to control bleeding during surgery.

The most common commercial laser uses 85% helium and 15% neon to produce a beam of radiation at the far end of the visible light spectrum. Because a red beam is visible to the human eye, it can be accurately applied.

Benefits of Soft Laser Treatment

The intensity of the laser is lowered by deliberately broadening or de-focusing the beam to be used on a larger area of the horse. The result is called 'cold' heat, or soft laser treatment (SLT). SLT may stimulate wound healing reportedly by modifying biochemical responses,

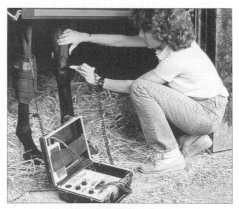

Fig. 11.8 Laser application therapy.

particularly collagen (connective tissue) repair, and increasing energy production. It may also alleviate pain by releasing endorphins.

A threshold of laser energy must be delivered to affect the tissues, but not enough energy to be destructive. In some situations, a pulsing wave is more beneficial than a continuous beam. With a continuous beam, damage to the tissues due to overheating is possible. As yet, the threshold level has not been exactly defined, and depends on the type of tissue, whether bone, muscle, tendon or ligament.

More important, the tissues must receive the laser energy at a wavelength that can be absorbed and not reflected. Commercially available lasers differ in the amount of energy they deliver to the tissue, and these products are not standardized.

Relieving Pain

The most profound effect of laser therapy may be pain suppression by stimulating acupuncture points. Cells absorb laser energy readily due to the laser's interaction with normal cell processes. For example, lasers favourably affect the sodium potassium pump that is the essence of intracellular communication and biochemical reactions, which causes cellular functions to speed up.

Because absorption is so great, laser energy usually penetrates 3.6 – 15 millimetres, which although only skin deep may activate acupuncture points to release endorphins. Endorphin and enkephalin levels increase in the blood and in the cerebrospinal fluid to provide pain relief. SLT also suppresses pain transmission by nerves, reducing nerve tissue excitability.

Promoting Healing

At present, researchers are still speculating about how SLT accelerates healing. The laser energy itself may affect the tissues as a whole by 'vibrating' the cells at a specific wavelength. Or, a particular frequency of applied energy may effect specific cellular functions of the 'lasered' tissue.

Biochemical functions may be stimulated to respond rapidly to an injury. The 'cold' heat generated by soft laser energy excites protein synthesis, cell replication, and communication between the cells. The biochemical signals tell the injured body part to heal faster, which intensifies the immune response.

Developing blood vessels within the tissue improves circulation, reducing swelling and oedema. Fibroblasts, the precursors of connective tissue, are stimulated to produce collagen faster and correctly.

Wounds

Because it excites the natural immune response, soft laser therapy can be used to heal open wounds. The wound is stimulated to heal more quickly than with conventional medicine alone.

Day 1   Day 15   Day 35

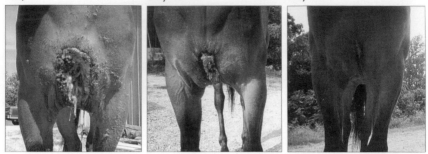

Fig. 11.9 The accelerated healing process of a wound treated with soft laser therapy and penicillin.

Laser is particularly applicable to horses with retarded healing processes such as old wounds with necrotic (dead and dying) tissue. Collagen deposit is enhanced in such cases, reawakening and accelerating healing without risking excessive scar formation.

Internal Injuries

Use of cold laser is not limited to open wounds. It helps heal bowed tendons, curtails ligament injuries, and curbs sore throats from an overreacting lymph system. Used correctly, it is a safe tool for non-invasive therapy, where cellular membranes remain intact and no detectable changes occur in the cells.

This non-invasive characteristic is the magic of laser therapy. Initially, therapy is applied once or twice a day. Then the intervals between applications are progressively lengthened.

The arts of acupuncture and acupressure have been used successfully for thousands of years by Eastern approaches to medicine. Through our unfailing worship of high technology, the West may have inadvertently stumbled on to the healing applications of these ancient arts.

ULTRASOUND

Ultrasound has been a major benefit to medical diagnostics. It identifies illness or injury of internal body organs or musculoskeletal structures. *(See Chapter 10 for more information.)*

Ultrasound is also a therapeutic tool because it 'heats' musculoskeletal components that may be too deep, too large, or too dense to benefit from hot soaking. We are all familiar with the healing effects of deep heat. For human athletes, heating pads, hot whirlpool baths, hot tubs and saunas relax aching muscles and improve circulation in the body. Since it is impractical to immerse a horse in a steaming water bath for 20–30 minutes, we must resort to other measures.

The penetrating warmth of ultrasound therapy reduces spasms in muscles or tendons, particularly in the large muscles over the back, buttocks and shoulders. It is especially difficult to use conventional heat therapy in these areas because only superficial warming would result. (Ultrasound should **not** be used over open and contaminated wounds, because it can drive bacteria further into the tissues, spreading infection.)

Mechanics of Ultrasound

Ultrasound's therapeutic advantage comes from its mechanical effects. As sound waves enter the tissues, the tissue molecules 'vibrate'. Energy created by the friction of sound waves entering the tissue generates heat. Ultrasound energy is barely absorbed by skin, but is well absorbed in tissues with a high protein and low fluid content, such as muscles tendons and ligaments. Muscle absorbs 2½ times as much of this energy as fat, and bone absorbs 10 times as much energy as muscle.

Types of Ultrasound

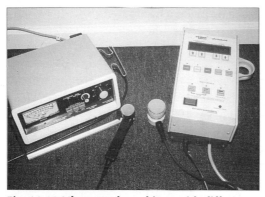

Fig. 11.10 Ultrasound machines with different sized heads for different areas of the horse.

Continuous Waves

Ultrasound is used as either a continuous wave, or as a pulse at regular intervals. Continuous wave ultrasound provides deep heat, improving elasticity and pliability of tight, thickened and scarred tissues. Horses involved in sports that require collection, pushing from behind or stretching the back can form scar tissue in their backs. These sports include endurance racing, eventing, jumping and dressage. Or, scar tissue can form as *fibrotic myopathy* within the thigh muscles. The deep heat of ultrasound therapy benefits these injuries.

Problems With Continuous Wave

If ultrasonic waves are generated continuously, excessive heat builds in

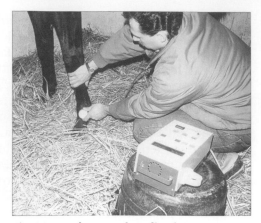

Fig. 11.11 Ultrasound application.

the shallow tissues. Ultrasound can raise tissue temperature by 7 – 8° F at 2 inches below the skin surface if applied continuously over one spot or for too long. This method is counterproductive because too much heat injures the tissues, resulting in permanent damage to bone and surrounding tissue. The appropriate amount of time depends on the type of tissue and the injury involved, and as yet has not been defined.

Bones are very dense, and the sound waves cannot pass all the way through them. The energy reflects back to the source, overheating

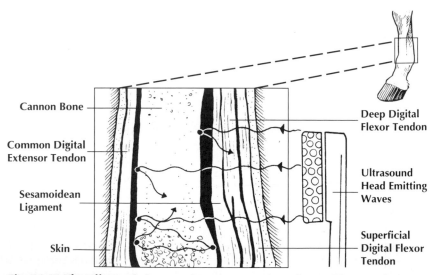

Fig. 11.12 The effects of ultrasound waves on various tissues. The sound waves bounce off and inside the bone, causing heating.

the bone and surrounding tissue. Ultrasound should not be applied directly to bone since this would be painful to the horse.

Ultrasound treatment of fractured inflamed or growing bone results in excessive blood circulation to the bone, with resultant demineralization and thinning of the affected area. Excessively heating bone and surrounding tissues destroys the blood supply, causing part of the bone to die and separate from the healthy bone.

Pulsing Waves

Pulsated waves can be compared to waves crashing on a beach. Unlike the ocean, however, medical pulsing waves can be adjusted to penetrate the exact distance desired into the tissues, limiting overheating. For example, a greater intensity of ultrasonic waves increases the tissue absorption of the waves. Not only can the ultrasonic waves be adjusted to limit penetration, but the interval between pulses allows heat dissipation from the tissues.

Applications of Ultrasound
Reducing Swelling

Ultrasound therapy is useful for tendon, ligament or joint injuries to the limbs. A useful application of ultrasound is to combine it with cold therapy. Apply an ice pack or cold water for 20 minutes, then pulse at 25% frequency (every fourth wave) for 20 minutes. A massaging effect known as 'micro-streaming' or 'acoustical streaming' encourages moving molecules to go from areas of high concentration to areas of low concentration. Applying ultrasound in this way improves circulation, limits the onset of oedema and pulses the swelling out of the limb.

Place a 'sweat' bandage on the limb for 24 hours after using a combination of cold and ultrasound therapy. The second day, use ultrasound over topical medication *(phonophoresis)*. Ultrasound encourages small, molecular-weight molecules, such as topical corticosteroids, to penetrate up to 2 inches. For this reason, ultrasound is **not** used over open and contaminated wounds, because it can drive bacteria deep into the tissues, spreading infection.

Relieving Pain and Promoting Healing

The deep heating of ultrasound relieves pain by changing the rate at which the nerves react and by limiting tissue spasms. Warmth restores the pliability of collagen fibres and relieves joint stiffness. Deep heat enhances circulation and production of energy which accelerates the healing process.

Ultrasound and Physical Therapy

When combined with range-of-motion exercises, optimal results are achieved from ultrasound. These exercises include physical therapy in the form of flexing and extending the limb immediately after ultrasound treatment.

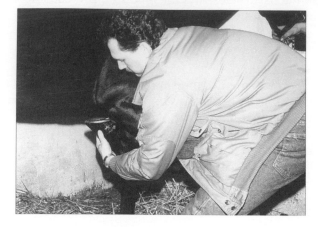

Fig. 11.13 Ultrasound therapy should be followed by physical therapy.

Many injuries can be avoided with adequate conditioning and training. However, chronic injuries such as arthritis or constrictive scar tissue deposits benefit from the enhanced range-of-motion and pliability afforded by ultrasound.

BENEFITS OF HIGH-TECH THERAPY

To return an equine athlete to soundness, the owner or trainer must achieve specific goals. It is paramount to reduce pain, to regain full use and movement of an injured area, and to restore or enhance strength to the injured area.

High-tech alternatives can provide pain relief, and, in cases of reparable injuries, may help speed the healing process. Physical therapy by flexing and extending the limb, along with controlled exercise and balanced shoeing, can also help return a horse to performance.

Ours is a highly technological society, and some people have invested an enduring faith in promoting the 'magic' of such wonders. To date, few specific *scientific* studies have been conducted that support the results of any of the high-tech equipment in use. Currently, most results are based on trial-and-error experimentation, along with individual, anecdotal testimonials to the success of these devices. Many products claim successful results where other, conventional modes of treatment, including prolonged rest, have failed.

Expectations must remain realistic—these devices will not cure the incurable. Instead, a horse may regain enough strength, elasticity, and pain relief to be serviceable in instances where pharmacological alternatives provide little comfort.

12

MANAGING CHRONIC LAMENESS

For the performance horse, one occupational risk is the development of a lasting lameness. Not all chronic pain can be corrected or cured, but some solutions offer the horse relief from continual discomfort. A complete list of potential debilitating lameness conditions would be very long. The most common situations include:

- chronically bruised feet
- navicular syndrome
- chronic back pain
- conditions of *degenerative joint disease* (DJD)

Bruised feet result from improper trimming or shoeing. For example, a flat-footed horse is prone to sole bruises. Bruises may also be caused by riding on rough terrain.

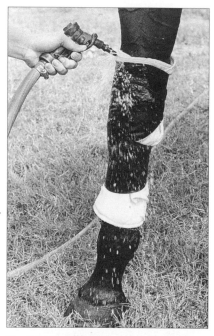

Fig. 12.1 Good management can give a horse relief from chronic lameness.

Improper shoeing may also be a cause of navicular disease, especially in horses that engage in rigorous, concussive activities such as jumping, racing, or polo. Inflammation of the feet causes damage to the deep digital flexor tendon and its associated navicular bone, resulting in chronic lameness.

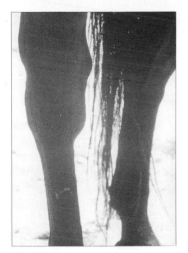

Fig. 12.2 Bone spavin.

Chronic back pain may develop as a consequence of pain in one or both hind legs, or from a poorly fitted saddle or poor riding technique.

Examples of degenerative joint diseases include:

• bone spavin (arthritis of the hock)
• high ringbone (arthritis of the pastern joint)
• low ringbone (arthritis of the coffin joint)
• stifle arthritis
• arthritis in any other joint

A veterinary lameness workup will identify the cause, allowing the problem to be appropriately addressed.

CAREER OPTIONS
Changing Disciplines

Every horse has a different pain tolerance. Some sports are too demanding for a horse with chronic pain, and a solution is to change disciplines. Jumping, hard stops, speed work, and collection aggravate many chronic pain conditions. A horse that cannot perform to a minimum standard in a sport should be converted to another career. Changing disciplines is better than causing excessive pain while trying to achieve the impossible. Suitable alternatives include using the horse as a school horse for beginner riders, or as equitation horse for light pleasure riding.

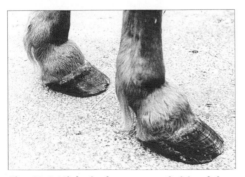

Fig. 12.3 High ringbone, or arthritis of the pastern joint.

Lowering Expectations

A horse that can withstand a rigorous athletic task to some degree may be able to continue competing in that sport, yet the owner should lower his or her expectations of the horse. Accept a lower level of performance in the chosen discipline. Entering fewer events each season, and spacing them apart can also help the chronically lame horse. Also, be prepared to scratch from a competition at the last moment if the horse is moving poorly that day.

If the horse cannot perform to a level of expectation, retire it, or put it in an environment with lower athletic demands. Lowering our expectations is more humane than asking a horse to suffer pain.

TRAINING AND FITNESS LEVELS

The greatest problem with managing the chronically sore athlete is maintaining a competent level of training and fitness. The work required to keep such a horse fit may make it impossible to participate in demanding sports like racing, polo or jumping.

The better the horse is trained when a chronic lameness problem surfaces, the less effort is required to retain its level of training. Moving a novice horse with chronic pain to higher levels demands far more effort than maintaining a lame but highly skilled horse at current levels. A novice horse may be unable to progress through the transition phases of training. Set realistic expectations and goals, and modify both as the horse's condition allows.

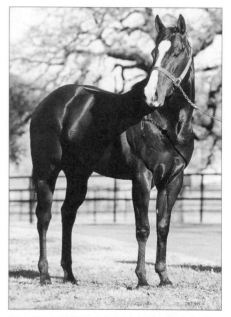

Fig. 12.4 Maintaining good body condition minimizes stress on the musculoskeletal system.

Not only is the horse's level of training important, but conditioning the whole body is critical to success. Maintaining the horse in as good a condition as possible for its intended athletics helps the body compensate for the lameness. Strengthening muscles, ligaments, and tendons compensates for the load on a sore joint, muscle or tendon. A tired horse is likely to take a misstep or overtax the musculoskeletal system. Fitness minimizes the development of fatigue.

Another example of maintaining condition is body weight. It is important to maintain the horse's body weight at a reasonable level. Obesity compounds the stresses on joints and support structures in the limbs. A horse that carries excess weight, either its own or too heavy a rider, overloads the injured area.

Record Keeping

A log of the horse's performance can track its responses to athletic demands, without guessing about what is and is not working. Including these items in the log helps avoid guesswork:

- training schedule
- productive output
- mental and physical attitude
- types and frequency of medication and therapy
- daily performance results

Rushing Training

Do not rush a horse to compete by a predetermined date. Allow the horse to progress at its own pace of learning and conditioning. Rushing the training overtaxes both its physical and mental states, and inevitably leads to a debilitating lameness.

BALANCED SHOEING

One of the most critical steps in managing the chronically lame horse is a regular schedule of balanced shoeing. A balanced foot is better able to dissipate concussion stresses evenly up a limb. Unlike in foals, conformational defects are not correctable in a mature horse. Stresses and strains continue on twisted joints and

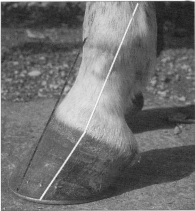

Fig. 12.5 A broken hoof-pastern axis angle, shown by white line. The black line shows the proper angle.

279

ligaments despite the best shoeing techniques. Yet, without the stable foundation of a balanced foot, conformational defects are magnified to seriously crippling levels.

Of utmost importance is correcting a broken hoof–pastern axis angle to reduce stress on the navicular bone, deep digital flexor tendon, and support structures of the coffin joint. *(See Chapter 4 for more information.)* For example, eliminating a long-toe–low-heel foot configuration reduces stress on these structures, improving navicular disease, low ringbone (coffin joint arthritis), and high ringbone (pastern joint arthritis). In addition, each foot should be balanced so that it impacts the ground equally on both sides.

Special Shoes and Pads

Horses with lower limb problems such as hoof cracks, high ringbone, low ringbone, or navicular disease benefit from an *egg-bar shoe*. Egg-bar shoes enlarge the foot's base of support for loading forces down the limb. Bone spavin (arthritis of the hock) also benefits from egg-bar shoes because the shoe limits the twist on the painful joint, and provides stability and support throughout the limb.

Conditions such as bruised feet or inflammation of the coffin bone (pedal osteitis) improve with protection from stout hoof pads. A wedge pad is often used to treat navicular disease by raising the heel to decrease the pull on the deep digital flexor tendon as it passes behind the navicular bone and bursa.

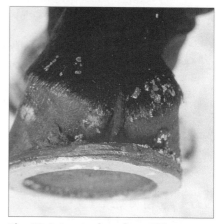

Fig. 12.6 An egg-bar shoe with a wedge pad.

TREATMENTS
Medications

Many horses with a chronic lameness condition can continue to train and perform if appropriate medications are given. However, different associations and racing commissions have different rules concerning anti-inflammatory drugs. Always check with the show steward or racetrack officials about the types and amounts of anti-inflammatory drugs legal for competition. Find out what forms must be filed and when. If a drug must be withdrawn before competition, find out how long is required for withdrawal. If a veterinary certificate is required, contact the veterinarian soon enough to obtain the necessary document.

NSAIDs

Anti-inflammatory medications are an essential part of chronic pain management. The most common pain relievers are the non-steroidal anti-inflammatory drugs (NSAIDs) such as, Finadyne® Ketofen®, phenylbutazone and naproxen. It is sometimes helpful to use low doses of NSAIDs the day before, the day of, and the day after a demanding exercise period. However, maintaining the horse on daily doses could create intestinal or gastric ulcers.

For endurance or competitive riding, NSAIDs must be withdrawn 3 - 4 days before the event. *(For more information on NSAIDs, see Chapter 18.)*

Adequan® Therapy

For joint pain, additional options are available. Intramuscular injections with Adequan® provide horses in both the acute and chronic stages of DJD with considerable relief. Adequan® improves the lubricating properties of joint fluid and exerts some anti-prostaglandin effects, reducing the destruction of joint cartilage by inflammatory enzymes.

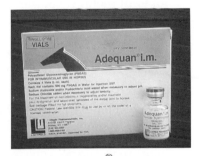

Fig. 12.7 Adequan® therapy.

An oral supplement containing mussel shells allegedly increases the chondroitin sulphate component of joint fluid to achieve similar effects to the Adequan® therapy. There is no current scientific proof of these compounds' true value, despite anecdotal reports of favourable results, particularly if the horse starts these oral supplements after Adequan® therapy.

Hyaluronic Acid Injection

Multiple injections of *hyaluronic acid* (HA) at 2 – 3 week intervals into a singly affected joint is an effective deterrent to the progression of arthritis. HA improves joint lubrication and has anti-inflammatory effects, but its usefulness is limited to inflammatory conditions in joints that have not yet developed cartilage damage.

Corticosteroids

Injecting a corticosteroid, a potent anti-inflammatory drug, gives immediate but short-term relief. Long-term use can lead to irreversible cartilage degeneration, therefore corticosteroid injections should be restricted to joints that are not responding to other methods of therapy. Moreover, the potent anti-inflammatory effects of a corticosteroid injection may mask enough pain that the horse will overuse the joint and further damage the cartilage. Usually a couple of weeks' rest following a steroid injection minimizes the potential of overuse damage of the joint.

Topical Anti-inflammatory Medications

DMSO (dimethyl sulphoxide) is a powerful anti-inflammatory agent that will reduce inflammation in the soft tissues around a joint, and is particularly beneficial for ligament or tendon injuries. However, topical anti-inflammatory medications cannot penetrate to joint depth when applied to the skin, and are not considered useful for joint therapy. For this reason, topical liniments or blistering agents also have limited value for joint pain.

Surgery
Joint Fusion

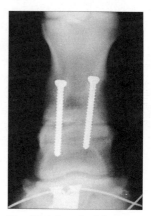

Some lameness conditions respond favourably to surgery. It is possible to surgically fuse *(arthrodese)* specific low-range joints in the horse, such as the lower joints of the hock or the pastern joints. Rehabilitation takes up to a year to return a horse to athletics. Success rates range from 60 to 80% depending on the original problem. Conditions that also involve soft tissue injury, such as a rupture of the collateral ligament, may not heal as quickly or as successfully as those with strictly joint problems.

Fig. 12.8 Surgical fusion of the pastern joint.

Neurectomy

A common surgical option to treat navicular disease is neurectomy, which is a complete cutting of the nerve supply to the back third of the foot. This surgery can keep a horse working comfortably for a year or more. A neurectomy provides pain relief for up to 3 years for about 60% of navicular horses. This procedure is not a cure; it simply

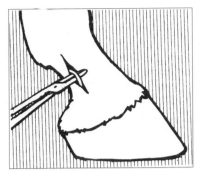

Fig. 12.9 The digital nerve is cut in a neurectomy.

buys time. *(See Chapter 4 for more information on navicular disease.)*

WORKOUTS FOR THE LAME HORSE

Daily physical therapy encourages limberness in a chronically sore horse. These horses are often tense and rigid in many parts of their bodies from attempting to guard against anticipated pain. Relaxed muscles are less prone to injury.

Warm-Up

The chronically lame horse needs to be especially coddled in warm-up and cool-down periods. Warm it up with slow, low-stress work, incorporating stretching exercises into the routine. Start with at least 10 minutes of brisk walking followed by 10 minutes of light trotting before asking for more demanding work. A proper warm-up increases circulation to the muscles and improves suppleness while gently stretching tendons and ligaments before applying extreme stress to the limbs. Walking is an excellent way to limber a horse and improve blood circulation throughout the body with a minimum of stress impact.

Massaging and Stretching

Massaging the heavy muscle groups of the hips, thighs and back improves relaxation. Also, manually stretching each leg several times before exercise helps the suppling process.

Mounted stretching exercises are particularly valuable for

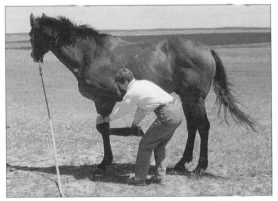

Fig. 12.10 Manual stretching relaxes and limbers up tense muscles.

treating a horse with back pain. Encouraging a horse to work in a long and low frame stretches the topline and relaxes back muscles. The reins should be loose so the rider's hands create no restriction to a full stretch. *(See Chapter 6 for more information.)*

Strengthening Muscles

Strengthening the support structures of muscles, ligaments and tendons allows them to assume some of the load, placing less stress on the stifle joint. Resting a horse with stifle lameness can be counterproductive. A horse with stifle arthritis particularly benefits from conditioning and development of the muscles in the hind legs. Easy long distance riding can benefit a horse with hock problems by strengthening the gluteal and quadriceps muscles. Circle work, however, places increased torque (twisting) stresses on the limbs. Therefore, minimize its use as a training technique for the chronically lame horse.

Each day of exercise, allow the horse to dictate how much it can tolerate in the workout. Be sensitive to behavioural clues that signal increasing soreness. A horse in pain develops bad habits, and its attention is distracted from the training and the task at hand. If the horse hurts, it is better to stop for the day than to persist at the athlete's expense.

Soft Footing

A horse with navicular problems works best on soft footing. For the footsore horse, minimize downhill riding to reduce the concussion impact on the horse's feet. Jumping, uneven terrain and hard stops are activities that worsen foot soreness, and they should be avoided.

At a competition, remember that the footing in the barn or training area may be better than the footing at a competition or in the warm-up arena. Seek another area for a warm-up if the footing is unsatisfactory.

Cool-Down

Walking after exercise relaxes the chronically lame horse. A 15-minute walking cool-down removes toxic by-products and heat from the tissues, and safely restores stretch to muscles and tendons.

Hydrotherapy

Hydrotherapy is an ideal means of managing arthritic joints or sensitive tendons. Hosing a limb with cold water or icing a limb immediately after a workout session minimizes the inflammatory response to exercise. Joints may need 30 – 60 minutes under an ice wrap to cool down enough to elicit an anti-inflammatory response. After icing, apply a standing bandage to limit rebound swelling.

13

AVOIDING DIGESTIVE DISORDERS

For the performance horse to reach maximum potential, it must be in the best of health. Good feeding management and good health care maintenance play key roles in maintaining a strong metabolic constitution and avoiding digestive disorders.

THE DIGESTIVE PROCESS
Eating Habits

The horse evolved as a grazing animal, serenely munching on sweet grasses of the plains, moving with the herd in search of available forage. The intestinal system was accustomed to small and frequent meals. The horse ate plants moist with dew and containing natural water. It cropped grasses as they grew, slowly adapting the microflora in the intestinal tract to changes in the nutrient value of plants as they responded to season and climate. As available food sources dwindled, the horse moved on, not stopping long enough to contaminate its feed with droppings that might reinfest it with parasite eggs. In this idyllic state, the horse moved about, maintaining muscle tone and good circulation.

Today, horses live quite differently. Urban development and time constraints compel us to confine horses for convenience. Horses in a natural state graze continually. By providing meals designed by humans we drastically alter how the intestinal tract handles food. People are now faced with management of an animal not naturally equipped to deal with imposed diets, feed schedules and exercise routines.

The Teeth

Once food is in a horse's mouth, the teeth begin the digestive process by grinding the food, making it easier to digest. Horses chew their food in a rotary grinding motion, and the teeth of the upper jaw are wider than those in the lower jaw. These factors cause an uneven wear pattern. The outer edges of the upper teeth and the inner edges of the lower teeth develop sharp points, reducing the amount of chewing and grinding and possibly creating ulcers and sores in the cheek or tongue.

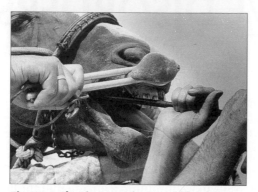

Fig. 13.1 Floating (rasping) smooths sharp points.

The teeth should be checked annually by a veterinarian so the sharp edges can be smoothed by rasping them down with a file, a process also known as *floating*. If the upper teeth are ahead of the lower teeth, hooks often develop on the front premolars and the rearmost molars. These hooks can pose problems for chewing and bridling.

Wolf Teeth

Examine a young horse for *wolf teeth*, which are vestigial premolars located at the front of the molars in the upper jaw. A wolf tooth should not be confused with canine teeth. Most male horses grow canine teeth which sit in front of the bit, about halfway between the incisors and the molars. Some mares also grow canines, but not as commonly as males.

A wolf tooth is very small, but its location coincides with the place a bit rests in the horse's mouth. It has been suggested that, to avoid bad habits, wolf teeth should be removed before training begins. Horses with tooth problems from either large hooks or wolf teeth resist the bridle, and many throw their heads to avoid the painful bumping of the bit on the offending tooth.

Wave Mouth

Older horses often lose teeth, which causes no immediately apparent problems. But the absence of a tooth allows the corresponding tooth on the opposite jaw to overgrow. The horse's teeth eventually develop a *step* or a *wave mouth*. Then the teeth cannot efficiently grind the food for digestion. These horses can be prone to diarrhoea, impactions, colic or choke.

The Digestive System

Changes in a daily routine can result in digestive disorders. A detailed look at the equine digestive system shows how sensitive it can be to management situations.

The Stomach

The stomach of a 1000-lb horse is equivalent in size to the stomach of a large man. The relatively small equine stomach capacity is approximately 4 gallons.

Eating stimulates regular stomach contractions to move feed into the small intestine. Normally, the stomach empties its contents, called *ingesta*, into the small intestine within 2 – 3 hours. When the stomach contracts, the intestines contract as well. Progressive propulsion of ingesta towards the large intestine is essential for digestion, nutrient absorption and gas elimination. Roughage moves out of the stomach rapidly, while grain concentrates remain longer.

A horse is unable to vomit due to muscular limitations of the oesophagus, even if the stomach overdistends with fluids or gas. Excess fermentation and overfilling of the stomach can cause pain, and can lead to rupture and death.

The Small Intestine

The small intestine regulates passage of the ingesta into the caecum and prevents backflow of gas from the caecum. Feed moves rapidly (compared with the rest of the digestive process) through 70 feet of small intestine taking only 3 – 4 hours to be admitted into the caecum's fermentation chamber.

The Large Intestine
Fermentation

A horse's intestinal tract is like a fermentation vat, capable of processing fibre and cellulose due to the bacteria and protozoans within it. In the horse, fermentation occurs after the small intestine in the caecum and large colon. Here, proteins, carbohydrates and cellulose are broken down by bacteria into nutrients, which are absorbed along with fluids. This process is improved by the grinding of the fibre and by breaking the shiny outer covering with the teeth. Cellulose breakdown by bacteria produces large volumes of gas that have no escape through the oesophagus, and must travel hundreds of feet through the intestinal loops to the rectum.

Within the large intestine near the *pelvic flexure* is a regulator that coordinates muscle movement of the intestines and the progression of ingesta through the various loops of bowel. Large particles may be delayed for up to 72 hours to allow bacterial digestion to degrade fibre into fuels. At the same time, more easily digested foodstuffs and gases are propelled towards the rectum for elimination.

The Large and Small Colon

The large colon has five segments. At several junction points where the segments anatomically blend into one another, the diameter of the bowel abruptly decreases. It is at these points of stricture that ingesta or foreign bodies can cause an obstruction, and prevent normal outflow of gas and materials. The small colon has a similar function as the large colon, but it is smaller. The ingesta therefore become smaller as the faeces are prepared to be passed from the body.

All segments of the intestine are interrelated by allowing normal function of the other parts to continue. Consistent waves of contractions *(peristalsis)* and a healthy blood supply to and from the

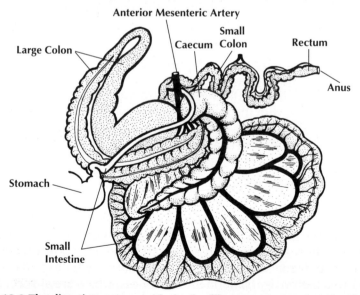

Fig. 13.2 The digestive system, with the fan-like mesentery supporting the small intestines.

intestines are vital to a horse's overall well-being. Interruptions in either of these features can set off a series of events that result in digestive disorders.

DIGESTIVE DISORDERS IN FOALS

Manage the foaling environment appropriately. A newborn foal is susceptible to *meconium impaction* if the first faecal balls are not passed soon after birth. Meconium is dark, pelleted faeces which consist of accumulated cellular debris and waste materials during foetal development. Failure to pass the meconium within 24 hours of birth requires immediate attention, possibly by your veterinary surgeon.

Foals are notoriously bad about tasting and eating everything in sight. Foreign body obstructions often cause colic in young horses. Fibres from rubber tyre feeders, baling twine, wood pieces, and rubber balls have all been incriminating items. Twigs, rubber tyres, and plastic have been implicated in some oesophageal obstruc-

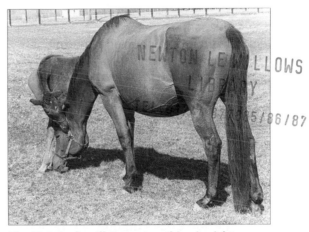

Fig. 13.3 Foals will taste everything in sight.

tions. Foals are also susceptible to sand colic as early as the first few months of life.

Foals will often consume their mother's manure *(coprophagy)*. This is thought to 'seed' the gut with bacteria for digestive purposes, but it may continue as a 'bad habit', making them subject to heavy parasitism, which can also cause impaction colic. Their environment should be routinely cleaned and the mare and foal dewormed every 6 – 8 weeks.

Foals have a markedly smaller diameter and volume digestive tract than an adult horse, which hastens the onset of signs. A very young foal may show signs of a colic by rolling on to its back with legs in the air, neck outstretched in obvious pain.

Up to a year of age, foals are prone to *gastric ulcers* if medicated with non-steroidal anti-inflammatory drugs. *(See Chapter 18 for more information on NSAIDs.)*

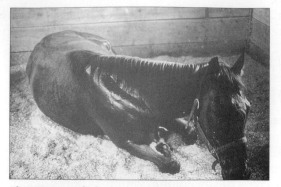

Fig. 13.4 A colicky horse may sweat and lie uncomfortably.

COLIC

Colic is not a disease in itself, but rather it is the word used to describe abdominal pain. Most commonly it is a symptom indicating a digestive disorder but the abdominal pain may be from other causes, such as urinary problems. Colic is a word that conjures up visions of a horse in distress—nostrils flared, pawing at the ground, kicking or biting at the belly, rolling on the ground, and sweating. It may be a form of 'butterflies in the tummy' which passes off without any action needed. The horse may stretch out as if to urinate, but it is too uncomfortable to apply an abdominal press to empty the bladder. It may stand depressed and dull, not wanting to eat. It may lie down, then get up, only to lie down again to relieve the discomfort coming from within the belly.

Colic must be differentiated from other problems not directly related to the gastrointestinal tract. Examples are pain from:

• ovulation	• foaling	• founder	• tying-up
• bladder stones		• laminitis	• fever

The horse has a unique intestinal system. The distinctive anatomy of the intestines predisposes to a variety of syndromes that cause pain. Pain of colic is a result of excess tension or stretching of the bowel lining or of the mesentery, that serves as a supportive sling of the intestines within the abdomen. Spasms of the bowel lining, due to irritation or a decrease in blood supply, also result in pain.

Horses require up to 2.5% of their body weight in feed intake per day, equivalent to 25 lb for a 1000-lb horse. At least 50% of that feed should be in the form of roughage. This fibre component stimulates intestinal movement. Also, a horse that is fed complete pelleted rations, condensed hay cubes, or limited quantities of hay suffers from boredom. Its natural urge to chew finds it devouring fence boards, eating dirt and sand off the ground, or consuming its own manure.

Spasmodic Colic

Spasmodic colic is due to a gut that moves too much. Nervousness and excitability, sometimes induced by sudden weather or barometric pressure changes, may result in this colic. Stress from transport or athletic competition can upset normal nerve impulses to the intestine and change intestinal movement. Certain drugs and organophosphate dewormers also overstimulate intestinal movement.

Intussusception

Severe changes in intestinal movement may cause a segment of bowel to telescope into an adjacent segment. This *intussusception* effectively acts as an obstruction, yet the condition of the horse rapidly deteriorates as gangrene and bowel death *(necrosis)* develop. It is an exceedingly painful and potentially lethal syndrome, requiring rapid surgical intervention.

Impaction Colic

Impaction is one of the most common causes of colic. An obstruction, or *impaction* in the large colon takes many hours to days to fully form and cause outward signs of pain or discomfort. Once an impaction becomes extensive enough, it places pressure on the bowel, or alters normal movement of the intestines. Abnormal intestinal contractions or gas distension cause pain. This mild or intermittent pain may be accompanied by depression and lack of appetite.

Intestinal tumours or abscesses can mimic an impaction. The tumour or abscess pushes on the bowel lining, causing discomfort, or it reduces blood flow and alters normal movement. Although the horse did not have an impaction before, changes in the normal intestinal function can cause an impaction, called a *secondary impaction.*

Causes of Impaction Colic

Obstructions of the bowel are commonly caused by decreased muscular movements of the gastrointestinal tract. As foodstuffs accumulate and sit in the bowel, water is removed. Once an impaction begins, the smooth muscle of the intestinal walls contracts in an attempt to move it along. This contraction may not only generate pain, but it also squeezes out more fluid, worsening the problem. Now the ingesta are no longer pliable and movable, and form an obstruction. Impaction colic can be caused by:

- limited exercise
- coarse food
- enteroliths
- consumption of foreign materials
- decreased water intake
- consumption of bedding
- heavy parasite load

Limited Exercise

Limited exercise reduces blood circulation to all muscles, including the intestinal muscle. A sluggish circulation changes normal intestinal movement, which may cause an impaction. During cold or wet weather, horses used to being outdoors may be brought into a stall. Then even low-level exercise is restricted.

Decreased Water Intake

Digestion of the great amounts of fibre a horse eats each day requires large volumes of water to fuel normal metabolic processes and maintain body fluid levels. A horse consumes 5 – 15 gallons of water each day in cool weather. Excessively hot weather, sweating and dehydration may remove water from the gut and dry out the ingesta. Obstructions also occur due to limited access to clean or ice-free water. Frozen water or even excessively cold water discourage drinking.

As horse owners, we have been told that feeding extra hay during cold weather generates internal heat as a by-product of fibre breakdown in the large colon. So, obediently, we add hay to the pile, which under normal circumstances is the correct thing to do. However, if a horse is not drinking enough, this practice compounds the problem by increasing intestinal bulk without adequate water to process it. Moreover, coarse feed materials or concentrated food require more water to properly digest.

Coarse Feed

Excessively dry or coarse feed can create an obstruction within the bowel. In addition, any dental problems can add to the problem by decreasing the ability to adequately grind coarse feed or fibre.

Consumption of Bedding

Shavings or straw bedding may seem unnaturally palatable to a bored horse. A horse may overconsume bedding to satisfy a fibre deficiency. These materials commonly form an impaction. Or, a pregnant mare may eat her bedding when suddenly confined in a new environment for observation and foaling.

Enteroliths

In certain areas, water and soil conditions contribute to an *enterolith* obstruction. Enteroliths are mineralized salts surrounding a pebble or small object. Over long periods, progressive layers of mineral deposits build around the central core. Once an enterolith enlarges enough to obstruct flow of ingested materials or gas, a symptomatic colic results.

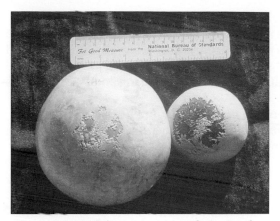

Fig. 13.5 Enteroliths can vary greatly in size depending on their age.

Warning Signs of Impaction Colic

Advance warning signals include mild depression, decreased appetite, lying down frequently, and scanty, hard and dry faecal balls, if any. The normal number of bowel movements per day averages 8 – 12. Faecal passage may diminish over a period of days before a problem is evident.

The earlier an impaction is recognized, the better the prognosis for successful medical treatment using oral laxatives, restorative intravenous fluids, and pain control. Occasionally, surgery is necessary to remove the obstruction. Excess pressure on the bowel or stagnant blood flow causes gangrene in a loop of intestine. Surgical removal prevents septic shock and death.

Preventing Impaction Colic

Prevention seems simple: ample water, high quality feed, and exercise. A special effort should be made to ride in the winter, or to find a large turnout area. Induced exercise by lungeing, or playtime in a herd is preferable. Vary the daily routine so confined or exercise-restricted horses do not become bored and eat bedding or foreign objects.

Fresh, ice-free water should always be readily accessible. Tank heaters keep water at an acceptable temperature in the harshest winters. Make sure the heater does not short out and shock the

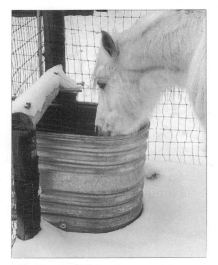

Fig. 13.6 A tank heater prevents water from freezing.

horse every time it tries to drink. If a dominant herd member hogs the trough, add another water tank to ensure equal opportunity.

Feed good quality hay that is neither excessively coarse nor fine. A bran mash does not act as a laxative due to the unique structure of the equine intestines, but a mash will encourage water consumption. Adding 1 – 2 tablespoons of salt to the mash further encourages drinking, but do not give extra salt to a horse that is drinking poorly, as salt worsens dehydration.

Careful observation of the number and quality of bowel movements each day, the amount of water consumed, and the horse's general attitude help prevent serious impaction colic.

Gaseous Colic

Any change in normal movement patterns in the intestines can cause problems. When bowel movements cease altogether, it is called an *ileus*. Fermentation continues, but gas does not move towards the rectum. As gas builds within the intestines, the overdistension results in pain. Bacterial overgrowth occurs in the stagnant gut, and bacteria begin to die. The death of certain types of bacteria release endotoxins that can result in shock, laminitis or death.

Building gas in a stagnant gut compromises the blood supply by exerting excess pressure and tension on the blood vessels. Portions of the bowel may be displaced as the segments balloon with gas and attempt to fully occupy the abdominal cavity. The left side of the large intestine normally floats freely in the abdomen with no supporting attachments to the body wall or other organs. The large intestine is therefore prone to great movement within the abdomen.

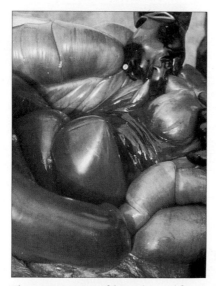

Fig. 13.7 A rotated intestine, with gas distention and gangrene where the blood supply was cut off.

Intestinal Torsion

Abnormal contractions, aided by gravity, may cause an actual rotation of the intestine, and result in an intestinal twist *(intestinal torsion)*. The free suspension of the left large colon, coupled with gas distension, abnormal peristaltic waves, or an ileus (ceased bowel movements) can result in a torsion or a portion of the gut may become displaced.

It is largely myth that a horse rolling around in pain will cause twisting of the intestines. Twisting can happen, but intestines can twist even if a horse is standing. Allow a colicky horse to lie quietly if it will, but prevent the horse from rolling so it does not hurt itself or the handlers. Forcing the horse to walk or trot may be beneficial for 10 – 15 minutes, or may keep a restless horse moving until veterinary help can arrive. However, hours of forced movement only exhausts a horse and handler. Prolonged, forced walking depletes valuable energy and calories needed to combat the illness.

Diet

Many colics are caused by inappropriate dietary management. An overabundance of excessively rich feeds (grain, alfalfa hay, lush pasture) stimulate excess gas production within the stomach or large intestines.

Sudden changes in feed are detrimental to the bacterial microflora in the gut and predispose to overproduction of gas or endotoxins. Mouldy food, or rapid introduction of large amounts of grain or legume hay will upset the system.

Feeding After Exercise

Feeding immediately after vigorous exercise can be dangerous. At this time, blood is still circulating in the muscle tissue, and is shunted away from the stomach. This lack of blood flow delays emptying of food from the stomach, promoting excess fermentation. After the horse is cool, the blood supply is diverted back to the intestines and then it is safe to feed. The time required to cool down the horse depends on its condition, the environmental temperature and humidity, and the demands of the workout.

Cold Water After Exercise

Drinking excessively cold water after exercise may set off spasms at the *pyloric sphincter* located between the stomach and the small intestine. Pyloric spasms delay movement of ingesta out of the stomach. Overdistension of the stomach with gas is quite painful, causing a sudden and violent colic.

Cribbing

Cribbing is a behavioural vice that is a liability for a performance horse. Cribbers do so out of boredom, then out of habit. A horse that cribs grabs onto a firm object like a fence rail or post, a water tank, or a stall door. It then pulls back on the object and sucks air into the

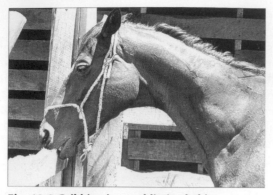

Fig. 13.8 Cribbing is an addictive habit.

stomach with each pulling exertion. Not only does a cribbing horse turn away from eating and drinking to nurture its addictive habit, but it is at risk of developing gaseous colic. It is hard to keep weight on a 'cribber,' and performance suffers. This vice also causes management problems because the horse's teeth wear down fencing, stall doors, etc.

It is easy to identify a cribbing horse by examining the incisors for abnormal wear. The incisors will be excessively worn and rounded. A cribbing collar limits the behaviour by causing pain as the horse pulls back and flexes its throat and upper neck. The collar bites into its flesh, making cribbing physically uncomfortable.

A surgical option is available, but it has limited success of less than 60%. It involves cutting the nerve supply to the muscles under the neck that enable a horse to crib.

Colic From Lipomas

An overweight horse is predisposed to *lipomas,* which are tumours of fatty tissue. As fat accumulates in the body, it builds into lumps within the mesentery. Gravity may pull these lumps of fat into one large mass with a stalk attaching it to the mesentery. It is possible for a loop of small intestine to become entrapped around this stalk, and strangulate (see Fig. 7.19).

Colic From Parasites

Internal parasites create areas of inflammation and irritation as they migrate through the intestinal lining or the blood vessels supplying the intestines. Bloodworms interfere with blood supply and intestinal movement, while roundworms form obstructions within the cavity of the bowel *(lumen).* Interrupting blood flow diminishes oxygen to bowel loops, and interferes with nerve input to the intestines. Waves of contractions then become disorganized, or may cease altogether. Other internal parasites damage and erode the bowel lin-

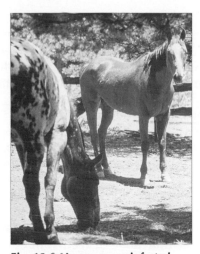

Fig. 13.9 Horses are reinfested with parasites by eating manure.

ing, causing leakage of faecal contents into the abdomen. The resulting infection and inflammation are called *peritonitis*. This condition is painful and potentially lethal.

The role of parasites in colic cannot be overstated. Adequate cleaning of paddocks and stalls, along with an aggressive parasite control programme at least every 2 months, markedly reduces this cause of serious colics. *(See Chapter 14 for more information.)*

Sand Colic

Over time, horses can consume a large amount of dirt or sand, which can weigh heavily in the gut and severely abrade the intestinal lining. Due to the insidious nature of this sanding syndrome, a long period may be required before it progresses to the point of overt abdominal pain.

Sand colic is not solely a problem in areas, that are very sandy, for example sand dunes. Anywhere there is sand, decomposed granite, or just plain old dirt, sand colic can arise. Many people cover paddocks or arenas with sand or road base to improve footing, so even if these soils are not naturally found in the environment, they can be delivered to it.

Mechanics of Sand Colic

The design of the equine large colon, with its narrowing segments, encourages deposition and trapping of sand in constrictive areas. If excessive sand accumulates in the large colon, it obstructs passage of food materials. This unmovable impaction causes gas to build up behind it, with associated pain as segments of bowel distend and swell. Pain reflexes and spasms around an impaction may shut down movement. Abnormal peristaltic contractions in the gut can lead to a displaced or twisted intestine.

At the site of the impaction, the heavy and abrasive material can erode through the intestinal lining. Pressure necrosis on that portion of bowel causes the intestinal contents to leak into the abdominal cavity. Inflammation and infection of the abdomen *(peritonitis)*, *en-dotoxic* and/or *septic shock*, and death can result. A similar situation occurs if a swollen or weakened bowel ruptures.

Symptoms of Sand Colic

Several symptoms are tip-offs to a problem from excess sand ingestion. Often a persistent diarrhoea develops (in about 35% of afflicted horses) before the onset of painful symptoms. Because it abrades the lining of the intestinal tract, sand impairs absorption of nutrients and fluids. As intestinal movement slows, diarrhoea intensifies.

In some individuals the only signs may be depressed appetite and weight loss. Performance may suffer because of chronic discomfort or reduced nutrient efficiency. Other horses experience low grade, mildly painful bouts of colic that appear as intermittent but recurrent episodes. Sometimes a colic crisis starts during or after riding, possibly because the sandpaper-like abrasion stimulates painful spasms of the intestine. Imagine a sausage of concrete lining the gut, as it is subjected to extreme physical exertion.

Any horse that experiences chronic diarrhoea or recurrent episodes of mild colic should be examined by a veterinarian. The key is to diagnose the problem early, before it becomes too advanced to rectify.

To give a mental picture of how serious sand accumulation can be, consider results of necropsies on horses that died due to sand colic. Up to two-thirds of the intestinal space was full of sand, wall to wall. In some places this material could be crumbled between fingers; in others it was so tightly packed that it could not be manually broken up.

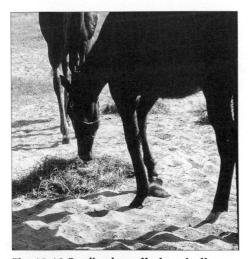

Fig. 13.10 Feeding hay off of sand offers a high potential for causing sand colic.

Managing Sand Colic

Feeding Systems

Feeding off the ground may simulate natural grazing, but consider what happens when hay is thrown on the ground. The horse spreads it around to pick out the tastier morsels. It may step in it, grinding it into the dirt. When it finally gets down to the leftovers, a still-hungry horse consumes the rest, sand included. If alfalfa is fed, the leaves drop out, and the horse snuffles around in the dirt to get every last tasty leaf. Tipped-over feed buckets spill grain on to the ground and, with attempts to pick up each piece, dirt is also ingested. Horses foraging on overgrazed pastures will eat cropped grasses and roots, with soil attached.

Horses on a pellet diet quickly finish their feed. Either lack of fibre or boredom may cause them to eat manure (with dirt), board fences, or dirt. Also, a fibre deficiency limits normal stimulation of the large colon, resulting in sluggish intestinal movement that allows sand to separate out into the intestine.

If the only available water source is a shallow, muddy or sandy pool, soil in the water will separate out inside the horse.

Diagnosing Sand Colic
Gut Sounds

Occasionally, a veterinarian can listen to the abdomen in front of the naveal with a stethoscope and hear sounds similar to what one hears in a conch shell, that is, surf on sand. These sounds may also resemble the sound made by slowly rotating a paper bag partially filled with sand. Not hearing these sounds does not mean that sand is not present. For 'sand sounds' to be heard, the bowel must be heavy enough to be lying next to the abdominal wall, and the bowel must be moving.

Sand in the Faeces

Any sand or grit in the faecal material is significant. Lack of sand does not guarantee that it is not present in the gut. A simple test can be performed to monitor sand build-up. Take six faecal balls from the centre of a fresh pile of manure where it has not contacted the ground. Mix the faeces in a quart of water. Once the solid material separates out, measure the amount of sand in the bottom of the vessel. More than one teaspoon per six faecal balls is abnormal.

Rectal Examination

Rectal examination of the intestinal tract does not always reveal definitive information. If a large amount of sand is present in the gut, it may pull the intestines downwards to the bottom of the abdomen and out of reach.

Belly Tap

A belly tap *(abdominocentesis)* involves inserting a needle into the abdomen to determine fluid character and volume. This technique is not generally used to diagnose sanding, but if such information is accidentally obtained this way it clarifies a tentative colic diagnosis. Sand may be obtained through such a tap because the weight of the sand pushes the intestines along the belly wall, and the needle may inadvertently penetrate the intestine.

X-Ray Films

X-ray films of the abdomen can positively diagnose sand in the intestines. This procedure requires powerful X-ray equipment, often available only at a university veterinary teaching hospital.

Treating Sand Colic

Water

Medical therapy of a 'sanded' horse must ensure adequate hydration, by oral and intravenous fluids, of the intestinal contents to help the horse pass the sand. Ample water moves material through the gut and prevents dehydration and a resultant impaction.

Laxatives

Laxatives are administered by stomach tube. The best medication is *psyllium hydrophilia mucilloid*, commonly known as Metamucil®. Psyllium was once thought to move sandy material out of the gut by lubricating it in a gelatinous material. Now it is thought to stimulate movement of the bowel, and to pull fluids into the intestine.

A study at Colorado State University radiographically illustrated that only 2 days of psyllium therapy resolved chronic diarrhoeas caused by sand. However, because sand builds up over a long time, it may require a lengthy period to pass it out. Treating seriously 'sanded' horses includes stomach tubing with psyllium for 2 – 5 days, followed by feeding ½ lb twice a day to adult horses, or ¼ lb twice a day to foals. This regimen is carried out for 4 – 5 weeks. Sand is inconsistently found in the faeces during psyllium therapy, so treatment should not be prematurely discontinued.

Pain Relievers

Pain relievers, such as non-steroidal anti-inflammatory drugs, help resolve a sand impaction. They reduce spasms around the impaction, and allow gas to escape so water can enter and soften the obstruction. By relieving pain from abrasion, water and food intake improve.

Hay

If a sanded horse has only mild pain and is still having bowel movements, high quality hay promotes movement of sand out of the intestinal tract.

Surgery

Surgery for sand colic may be necessary if:

- there is a limited response to medical treatment within 48 – 72 hours
- vital parameters such as heart rate, capillary refill time, and mucous membrane colour deteriorate
- pain persists and worsens

Surgery may be the only alternative — to physically remove the sand from the gut. How aggressively the horse is treated affects its chances survival. A University of Minnesota study determined that horses undergoing surgery of sand colic experience a 50% survival rate. A study at the University of Florida revealed that those cases treated surgically had a survival rate of 92%, because of the aggressive treatment before the bowel became gangrenous and necrotic.

Bran

Contrary to popular myth, bran is neither therapeutic nor preventive. Due to peculiar equine intestinal anatomy, by the time the relatively small amount of bran reaches the large intestine of the horse it can hardly exert any laxative effect. The equine gastrointestinal system is radically different from a human's. Bran encourages water consumption, which indirectly improves intestinal movement and passage of material through the bowel. If peristaltic contractions move feed along normally, then faecal contents will not stay in the bowel long enough for sandy material to separate out.

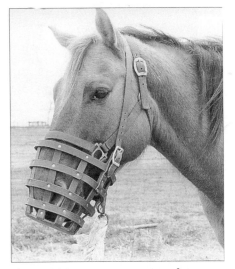

Fig. 13.11 In a rare case a muzzle may be needed to prevent a horse from eating dirt.

Preventing Sand Colic

Monitor each horse for differences in eating habits, especially those that eat anything, or that search the ground all day. To prevent sand colic in these horses, feed more roughage, or feed more often, and provide more exercise to curtail boredom. A rare individual may need a muzzle to prevent it from eating dirt.

Changing Feeding Practices

By recognizing an evolutionary need for horses to frequently eat small amounts of good quality fibre, feeding practices can be modified not only to prevent sand colic, but also to improve the health of the digestive system and the horse's mental happiness. A horse performs better if the natural urge to constantly nibble is satisfied. This urge is satisfied by free choice grass hay, and supplementing only hard-working individuals or difficult keepers with alfalfa and grain. Feeding enough hay, or feeding at frequent intervals can also eliminate behaviour such as licking the ground or eating dirt. By not overstocking pastures, ample forage is available so horses do not consume dirt. A diet of free choice grass hay, salt, and adequate water limits sand and dirt ingestion.

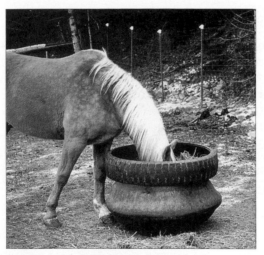

Fig. 13.12 Tyre feeders limit sand intake.

Using Feeders

Removing the hay from the ground is essential for prevention. Using racks, hay nets, or tyre feeders minimizes spillage. Feeding on rubber mats or concrete pads may be an alternative in special cases. Overhead feeding arrangements present another problem. A horse with an overhead feeder is prone to respiratory problems. It cannot clear foreign material and mould spores from the respiratory tract, because the head is held up in an unnatural position. Also, hay is pulled out of overhead feeders and scattered on the ground. Rubber tyre feeders better ensure that the feed material stays put. They allow head-down feeding, and are relatively safe.

Be aware that young foals can get trapped inside such feeders and be injured. Youngsters (and some adults) also like to chew on the rubber feeders, eating white walls or rubber material, and may develop a severe impaction colic.

Providing Clean Water

Check water tanks to see if sand is in the bottom of the tank. Sand in the water tank is a signal that the horses' mouths are full of sand. Clean, fresh water encourages drinking which promotes intestinal health and normal peristaltic movement.

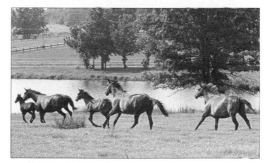

Fig. 13.13 Clean, fresh water promotes intestinal health.

Preventative Medications

Along with changes in feeding practices, preventative medication with psyllium products can prevent sand colic. Feed 8 oz a day of psyllium for 5 consecutive days each month. Lengthy treatment is unnecessary because the laxative effects slightly disturb normal electrolyte and fluid balances. For stubborn cases, or horses attended by a veterinarian, long-term psyllium treatment may be necessary.

Choke

Horses can choke on their food, but rather than an obstruction blocking the airway as in people, food is lodged somewhere along the oesophagus, making it impossible to swallow.

The first impression as a horse suddenly turns away from its food and stops eating is that it is colicking. Initially, a horse appears distressed and agitated, exhibiting colicky type behaviour. It stretches the neck to relieve the pressure, or paws, sweats, or rolls on the ground. Saliva foams from the mouth, and there can be greenish froth coming from the nostrils, often accompanied by gagging and coughing.

Problems Associated With Choke

Aspiration Pneumonia

Choke is a true emergency, requiring immediate veterinary attention. Food, mucus and saliva that are regurgitated from the mouth and nostrils can be inhaled into the lungs as a horse struggles to relieve the oesophageal obstruction. Material inhaled into the lungs and airways rapidly leads to an *aspiration pneumonia*.

The horse may panic and may be difficult to handle and possibly dangerous

Electrolyte and Fluid Loss

A choked horse suffers serious electrolyte imbalances, as well as dehydration. Not only does an oesophageal obstruction prevent drinking, but the horse loses saliva as it drools from the mouth. Saliva contains large quantities of sodium and chloride, and is essential for recycling these salts through the intestinal tract where they are reabsorbed by the body. A horse experiencing a prolonged episode of choke is unable to swallow the saliva, and needs intravenous fluids and electrolytes.

Treating Choke

With immediate veterinary attention, the majority of chokes are easily resolved without complications. While awaiting a veterinarian, it is helpful to place the horse on an incline with the head facing downhill. Such a small change in position helps drain regurgitated material out of the mouth and nose and minimizes the chances of its being inhaled into the airways. Remain calm and talk soothingly to help control the horse's anxiety. If the ball of food is visible on the left side of the neck as a bulge, *very* gentle massage may help break it down.

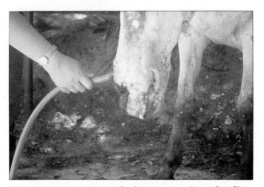

Fig. 13.14 During a choke, green tinged saliva froths from the nostrils.

Sedatives administered by a veterinarian position the head and neck downwards, and relax the muscles spasming around the food mass. A stomach tube is passed into the esophagus to the level of the obstruction, and a gentle stream of water breaks it up. Non-steroidal anti-inflammatory drugs minimize scar tissue formation once the obstruction is dissolved. Broad spectrum antibiotics prevent infection of the oesophageal lining.

Feeding After a Choke Crisis

Follow-up care after a choke crisis is critical. Withhold food from a sedated horse until it is fully recovered, because both the cough reflex and swallowing apparatus are depressed under the influence of sedatives. In some cases, it is necessary to entirely withhold food for the first 24 – 48 hours. For a horse to safely swallow food, it must be adequately chewed and softened liberally with saliva. Pre-soaking pellets in ample water for 20 – 30 minutes breaks them apart and softens them. This gruel slips easily down an irritated oesophagus, allowing it to heal, and inflammation to subside. When it is safe for the horse to eat again, feed the gruel in small amounts, several times daily for up to 2 weeks after the episode. During this time, a horse is highly susceptible to a recurrent episode of choke, so care must be taken to remove all coarse or dry feed from the diet.

Preventing Choke

Implementing certain management procedures prevents choke, or prevents a reoccurrence in a previously choked horse. Most chokes are caused by large pelleted concentrate, or by coarse hay. These feeds are easily eliminated from the diet. If pellets are fed, they should be the small variety. Grass pasture and hay cubes rarely cause a choke; however, competition with herd-mates may make a horse bolt its feed. Such a horse should be separated at feeding time to encourage it to eat slowly. If a greedy horse seems to 'inhale' grain or pellets, place smooth rocks (2 inches minimum size) in the feed tub with the concentrate. The rocks slow intake because the horse must rummage around them.

Inadequate water intake can result in a choke. Drinking plenty of fresh water ensures ample saliva, and adequate water for intestinal digestion. During transport it is important for a horse to drink enough to limit dehydration. Some horses stressed by trailering may snatch and gobble hay or grain. It is best to withhold feed from anxious horses.

Dental problems may cause a horse to swallow food before it is chewed properly. Teeth should be checked and floated regularly.

Introduction of new or palatable bedding materials, such as straw or wood shavings, should be monitored carefully to ensure a horse does not eat them.

Some instances of choke are unpreventable if caused by tumours, space-occupying abscesses, or scar tissue from an old injury. These problems functionally decrease the diameter of the oesophagus. If there is suspicion of such a malady, a veterinarian can diagnose it with an endoscope or by contrast radiography. With contrast radiography, a radio-opaque material is injected into the oesophagus and X-ray films are taken of the area.

Diarrhoea

Inflammatory conditions of the large intestine can lead to diarrhoea. The performance of an equine athlete suffers as a result of diarrhoea because it loses valuable electrolytes and fluids in the faeces. Persistent diarrhoea also leads to weight loss or colic. With careful management practices, many cases of diarrhoea in the mature horse can be quickly resolved.

Causes of Diarrhoea

Poor Dental Care

Poor tooth care is a common case of diarrhoea, especially in the aged horse. If feed is not properly ground, it irritates and inflames the intestine. Coarse food or chronic sand ingestion creates a similar irritation leading to diarrhoea. Regular tooth care, premium hay quality, and not feeding on sandy soil are easy ways to eliminate these sources of diarrhoea.

Overfermentation in Bowel

A horse that is fed an abnormally high grain ration or mouldy food may develop diarrhoea due to overfermentation of bacteria in the bowel. Bacterial endotoxin or fungi inflame the bowel. An inflamed bowel cannot absorb nutrients, water and electrolytes, so they are lost through the faeces. Feeding at least half of the ration as roughage ensures normal intestinal function. Discard all spoiled feed.

Nervousness

A nervous horse or a horse verging on exhaustion may have temporary diarrhoea due to changes in intestinal activity. These horses may benefit from electrolyte supplements during transport or competition. It is equally important that they have frequent access to fresh water to restore fluid losses.

Parasites

Infectious organisms also contribute to diarrhoea in horses. Parasite infestation of the intestines creates inflammation in the intestinal lining, the intestinal blood vessels, and the abdominal cavity. A heavily parasitized horse often has loose stools along with an unthrifty appearance and a loss of performance.

Other Causes

Intestinal bacterial and viral organisms infrequently infect adult horses and lead to diarrhoea. A veterinarian should evaluate such ailments so effective treatment can be instituted. Liver disease, intestinal cancer, heart failure, and poisoning by medications, plants or heavy metals are rare causes of diarrhoea.

14

INTERNAL PARASITE CONTROL

A key feature of equine health management is effective control of internal parasites. Horses continually reinfest themselves with parasites while eating on ground contaminated with manure. Given the opportunity, most horses will defecate in an area separate from their feed supply. Heavily populated pastures do not provide horses enough space to separate a pasture into roughs (ungrazed grass around fences) and lawns (grazing areas). Studies in England and Ohio have shown that twice weekly removal of faeces from pastures or paddocks is an even more effective method of parasite control than dewormer treatment at 4 – 8 week intervals. Combining manure removal and dewormer medication promotes a healthy and minimally parasitized horse. If left unchecked, the impact of intestinal worms on the horse's health is dramatic.

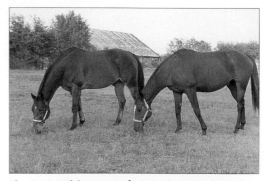

Fig. 14.1 Without good pasture management, grazing horses can easily be reinfested with parasites.

TYPES OF INTERNAL PARASITE

An understanding of the various species of worms and their life cycles helps eliminate infection within an individual and a herd. In general, horses obtain infective larvae through contaminated feed or water, manure eating *(coprophagy)*, or contaminated pastures. Adult worms are rarely seen in the faeces unless a horse is severely parasitized. The various egg stages of the worms can only be viewed through the microscope.

Large Strongyles
Bloodworms

One common internal parasite is the large strongyle. The three most common species of large strongyles affecting the horse are *Strongylus vulgaris, Strongylus equinus* and *Strongylus edentatus*. These bloodworms are examples of the complex life cycle of intestinal worms.

Life Cycle

An infected horse passes eggs in its faeces, where the eggs hatch. A hatched egg develops into a first stage then a second stage larva and finally the infective third stage larva. If a horse ingests the third stage larva of *S. vulgaris*, the larva penetrates the wall of the large intestine. For about 7 days it remains there, developing into a fourth stage larva. Then the fourth stage larva wanders through the bloodstream for about 8 more days.

By 2 weeks after infection, the worms are in the cranial mesenteric artery and adjacent vessels. These vessels provide the main blood supply to the intestinal tract. The larvae remain there for 3 months. As they develop to fifth stage larvae, damage to these blood vessels reduces blood flow to the intestines and surrounding tissues.

Once developed to the fifth stage, the larvae return to the large intestine and mature to egg-laying adults, and the cycle repeats. The period from ingestion of infective larvae to egg-producing adults is called the *prepatent period*. For *Strongylus vulgaris* this period requires 180 – 200 days. Whatever strongyle larvae a horse acquires today will not complete its cycle or associated damage until 6 – 7 months later. Since strongyle larvae require 4 – 7 days to reach the infective stage, cleaning up manure deposits twice weekly reduces the risk of a horse consuming them.

Prepatent periods for *Strongylus equinus* and *Strongylus edentatus* are 9 months and 10 – 11 months, respectively. These large strongyles migrate through the abdominal cavity, liver and pancreas, causing damage to these internal organs.

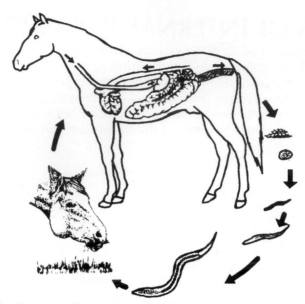

Fig. 14.2 The life cycle of large strongyle takes 6 – 7 months to complete.

Symptoms

Clinical signs of strongyle infestation are:

- diarrhoea
- colic
- weight loss
- poor hair coat
- unthriftiness, depression, poor appetite or dullness
- anaemia, resulting in reduced athletic performance or growth
- changes in intestinal movement resulting in impactions, intestinal twists or death
- obstructions of the blood vessels, leading to death

Small Strongyles

Another group of parasites that has recently received much attention is the small strongyles. Their life cycle and biology are similar to those of the large strongyle except the fourth stage larvae do not invade the blood vessels of the intestinal tract. Instead, they move to the lining of the large intestine, causing diarrhoea and/or constipation, and ill-thrift.

Normally, the prepatent period for small strongyles is 2 – 4 months; however, a larva may remain as a *cyst* in the tissues for up to 2½ years. Frequent deworming is essential to control these parasites.

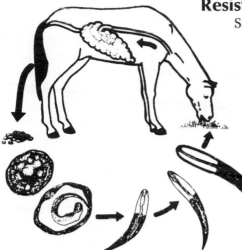

Resistance to Dewormer

Small strongyles have developed resistance to a common group of drugs, the benzimidazoles. Adult small strongyles genetically pass the resistance on to future generations. Routine faecal exams check for this parasite and determine its potential resistance to dewormer products.

The product used should be varied to avoid resistance developing.

Fig. 14.3 The life cycle of the small strongyle.

Ascarids

The most important parasite infecting the small intestine is the ascarid (roundworm). Ascarid eggs are extremely resistant to environmental conditions and persist in the environment for years. Usually, they require 2 weeks to hatch to infective second stage larvae.

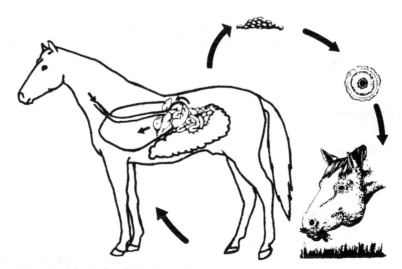

Fig. 14.4 The life cycle of the Ascarids.

Life Cycle

After ingestion of infective larvae, the journey through the body begins in the small intestine and continues through the circulatory system reaching the liver, heart and the lungs. As ascarid larvae mature, they travel up the airways of the lungs and trachea into the mouth. There they are swallowed, and again pass into the small intestine where the larvae mature into the adult egg-laying stage. The prepatent period (time between ingestion of infective larvae to egg-producing adults) for the ascarid is 10 – 12 weeks.

Symptoms

Clinical signs of ascarid infestation include an unthrifty, poor-doing horse with a rough hair coat. Diarrhoea and gas, alternating with constipation, are fairly common. Many Ascarid-infested youngsters have a potbelly and fail to gain weight.

Not only do the migrating larvae damage the lungs, but viruses and bacteria can invade the damaged respiratory lining. Respiratory infections induced by migratory, immature forms often occur, particularly if the horse is 1 – 2 months old.

If many adult worms ball up in the small intestine, the obstruction leads to colic, peritonitis (inflammation or infection of the abdominal cavity), or death.

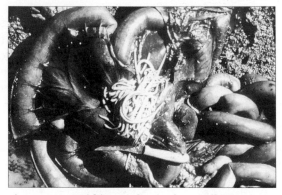

Fig. 14.5 Ascarid impaction in the small intestine.

Roundworms in Young Horses

The age of a horse greatly affects ascarid infection. Horses develop an acquired immunity with age until about 15 years old. Ascariasis is a problem in young horses less than 2 years old, and in older horses over 15 years old.

Not only are foals extremely susceptible to ascarids, but foals tend to consume the mare's manure (coprophagy). If the manure is loaded with ascarid eggs, a foal becomes heavily infected. Both mare and foal should be dewormed often, and the environment cleaned of faeces. Mature horses are rarely heavily infected unless the immune system is compromised by disease or stress.

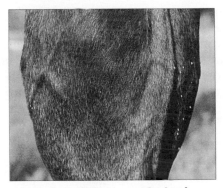

Fig. 14.6 Bot fly eggs attached to leg.

Bots

Bot 'worms' are not actually worms at all, but are the larvae of the bot fly, *Gastrophilus sp.* (all species of the genus *Gastrophilus)*.

The bot fly lays its eggs on the leg and chest hairs. When the horse licks or rubs the hairs, the eggs are transferred to the horse's mouth. Unhatched bot eggs can survive for up to 6 months on the hairs.

Life Cycle

Once in the mouth, hatched larvae burrow into the tongue and tissues of the mouth and oesophagus. While in the mouth tissues, the bot larvae may cause pain with chewing, or may impede swallowing because of throat swelling. After about 3 weeks, the larvae travel to the stomach.

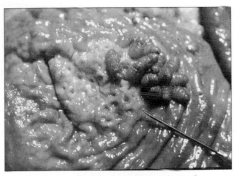

Fig. 14.7 Bot fly larva on the stomach.

The larvae attach to the stomach lining, and can cause ulcers, food impaction, colic or peritonitis (inflammation of the abdominal wall). Although rare, the stomach may rupture and cause death. Bot larvae require about 10 months to develop once they enter the mouth. Certain species of bot larvae attach to the rectum as they pass to the anus. Their presence causes irritation and tail rubbing, and is often mistaken for pinworm infestation.

Use of ivermectin (Eqvalan®) in the autumn will remove the bots from the stomach. Frequent grooming to remove the eggs from the coat will reduce the bots in the stomach.

Stomach Worms

Life Cycle of *Habronema*

Stomach worms, *Habronema sp.*, pass their eggs through the faeces, and then fly larvae ingest the eggs. The horse either ingests

313

the fly larvae and stomach worm egg, or infected adult flies deposit their larvae around the mouth and lips of the horse. From there they pass directly into the stomach and develop to the egg-laying stage, repeating the cycle. Larvae in the stomach may stimulate an immune response, forming large, tumorous masses. Although these disappear once the larvae are gone, areas of glandular stomach tissue are replaced with scar tissue.

Summer Sores

The most significant damage caused by *Habronema.* is summer sores. If a horse's skin is broken from a wound or abrasion, flies feeding on the injury may infect it with larvae. The larvae do not grow or develop here, but they cause a pronounced tissue response. A non-healing sore persists that is easily invaded

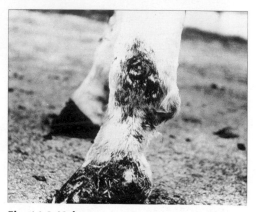

Fig. 14.8 *Habronema* causes summer sores.

by bacteria. Deworming a horse kills the larvae, reducing its chances of contracting this parasite.

Life Cycle of *Trichostrongylus axei*

Another stomach worm is *Trichostrongylus axei*, a common parasite of cattle and other ruminants. Infective larvae develop similarly to large strongyles, but only require 3 days to become infective. Horses infected by this worm exhibit a loss of condition, with diarrhoea and/or constipation, protein loss and anaemia. A chronic inflammatory response develops in the stomach.

Other Worms

There are a variety of less important parasites to consider that may affect the health and well-being of a horse.

Pinworms

Pinworms, or *Oxyuris equi*, ingested from feed contaminated with manure, develop in the caecum (part of the large intestine). Then, a fertilized adult female enters the rectum, passes through

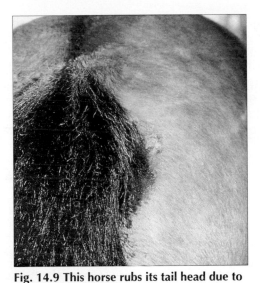

Fig. 14.9 This horse rubs its tail head due to pinworms.

the anus, and deposits her eggs around the anus and/or vulva. These eggs drop on to the ground or on to food that has been placed on the ground. The entire prepatent period is a rapid 52 days. An affected horse itches and rubs the tailhead leading to an associated loss of hair.

Intestinal Threadworms

Intestinal threadworms, *Strongyloides westeri*, are primarily a problem in foals and have been implicated in foal diarrhoea and scours. The infective stage of the larvae is passed through the mare's milk, or penetrates the skin. As with ascarids, immunity to infection increases with age; by 4 – 5 months of age, foals are resistant to infection. Because of the association of foal scours with the life cycle of this parasite, deworming of scouring foals is recommended.

Lungworms

Although their natural host is the donkey, lungworms can infect horses. Usually donkeys do not show clinical problems, but will pass larvae in their faeces. Horses pastured with donkeys are at high risk of infection, but it is possible for horse-to-horse transmission to occur. Associated problems due to lungworms include a chronic cough, pneumonia and pleuritis.

Tapeworms

Tapeworms are becoming more common in the horse population. Their life cycle depends on a mite which the horse ingests while eating pasture or hay. Development in the mite requires 2 – 4 months, while in the horse the adult tapeworm takes another 6 – 10 weeks to develop. Heavy infestations lead to intestinal perforations, peritonitis, colic or intestinal inflammation *(enteritis)*.

MANAGING INTERNAL PARASITES

A century ago, during the rise of the industrial age, crowding of horse populations within increasingly urban areas resulted in enormous worm infestations and ill health in horses. An excerpt from Miles' *Modern Practical Farriery* (1896) comments: 'Whoever will take the trouble to visit a knacker's, and to turn over the dunghill in its yard, will find it to be composed quite as much of worms as of excrement.'

Parasite control methods diminish the number of infective larvae available to a horse. Twice weekly removal of manure from pasture and paddocks is a very effective method. Deworming medications are the other ingredient to a comprehensive parasite management programme.

Less than two decades ago, veterinary medicine only offered an arsenal of fairly potent chemicals to kill adult worms. These chemicals were not without hazard. Many of them were toxic to the horse, in some cases lethal, and they needed to be given in large quantities to be effective. The best way to administer the medication rapidly was to give it by stomach tube. Before safe paste formulas, and with extreme risk of drug toxicity reactions, stomach tube deworming was the only way to go.

Horses living on the uncrowded, open range may have only needed a drench once or twice a year. However, in these days of concentrated housing where horses are at continual risk of reinfesting themselves, they should be dewormed at least every 6 – 8 weeks. Deworming at this interval interrupts the damaging life cycle of internal parasites.

Ideally, aggressive deworming programmes of monthly treatments between April and October will kill most internal parasites. During the winter, due to dormancy and reduced maturation of worms in the body, deworming every 2 months is usually enough.

Deworming Products

The pressures of urban living have promoted intensive research over the last decade into newer, more efficient and safer dewormers in the form of pastes and powders.

Everyone says: rotate, rotate, rotate. Many conflicting ideas on what rotate exactly means further confuse the issue. Every time a deworming product is given, the horse is being administered a drug. It is important to know what the chemical is, and what its purpose is. Learn about the nature of the chemicals in these compounds, taking note of the active ingredient listed under the brand name.

Dewormer Classification

There are so many anti-parasite products available on the market today for a horse that, it is no wonder that confusion exists. By simplifying the list of dewormers, a strategy can be devised to limit the parasite burden of a horse by reducing the number of infective larvae. Our chemical arsenal revolves around six different classes of dewormers.

Fig. 14.10 Various brands of dewormers.

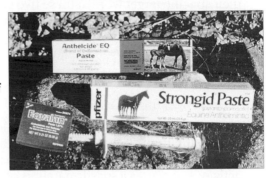

Benzimidazoles

The benzimidazoles, include products with chemical names of oxibendazole, oxfendazole, mebendazole, fenbendazole, thiabendazole, cambendazole, to name a few.

Febantel

A second drug class, called the pro-benzimidazoles, includes only one drug, febantel. Febantel has effects similar to those of the benzimidazoles. For the sake of convenience these two drug classes are considered as one, the benzimidazoles.

Pyrantel

A third drug class called the tetrahydropyrimidines is commonly known as pyrantel (Strongid®). Pyrantel comes in pellets and pastes.

Ivermectin

A fourth class called avermectins describes the drug ivermectin (Eqvalan®), produced by bacterial fermentation.

Organophosphates

Organophosphates are a fifth drug class, and their active ingredient is either dichlorvos or trichlorfon. This drug class is specifically targeted at bot fly larvae in the stomach.

Piperazine

Piperazine belongs to the sixth class, and is effective against ascarids.

Although the organophosphates and piperazine are effective against their specific target worms, these two classes are obsolete due to the development of safer, broad spectrum products found in the other drug classes which are effective against all parasites.

From six classes, we have simplified to three:

- Benzimidazoles
- Pyrantel
- Ivermectin

Each drug kills intestinal worms by a different mechanism e.g. ivermectin interferes with neuromuscular coordination of the worm, causing a flaccid paralysis. Pyrantel also interferes with neuromuscular activity, but causes a spastic paralysis of the worm. Benzimidazoles interfere with energy metabolism, and the worms die of starvation.

Preventing Resistance

Specific strategies can be used to maximize the effect of dewormers. Currently, it is feared that by exposing parasites to a rapid rotation of different drug classes every few months, we may inadvertently select parasites that develop resistance to many of these chemicals. Resistance allows the worm to tolerate dewormer doses that previously killed them.

Based on current research, an optimal strategy is one of slow rotation of dewormers at 1-year intervals. More frequent rotation may result in multiple drug resistance to several different classes at once. Ideally, one product should be used during the season of maximum egg transmission. In this way, a single generation of parasites (of 1 year) is not exposed to different and multiple drug classes. By slowly rotating at yearly intervals, each generation is only subjected to one mechanism of action by a drug, and is subsequently less likely to develop drug resistance. The next year another drug class is used, the third year a third drug class, the fourth year returns to the first year's product, and so on.

Resistance to Benzimidazoles

To date, many of the 40 species of small strongyles have developed resistance to the benzimidazoles. Not only are adult worms able to develop resistance, but they genetically pass resistance genes along to future generations. Of the benzimidazoles, the only drug currently available that the small strongyles cannot resist is oxibendazole.

Ivermectin

As yet, no parasite resistance has developed to either pyrantel or ivermectin. Using ivermectin twice a year at 6-month intervals in addition to pyrantel should eliminate damaging migratory forms of the parasites. Ivermectin can also be incorporated into a system of slow rotation, but should not be used exclusively so resistance does not develop.

Recommended Deworming Schedules

Different climatic conditions dictate how a management programme should be approached. For instance, in warm and moist environmental conditions peak strongyle egg counts occur in the spring and summer with release of larvae from the intestinal walls. There is vast contamination of pastures and paddocks at this time of year. Moisture and warm temperatures speed larval development into an infective stage.

The infective larvae are at their peak between April and October when temperatures range between 30 and 85° F. They can survive freezing temperatures, emerging in the spring with warmth and moisture.

Deworming	
YEAR	**TYPE AND FREQUENCY OF DEWORMER USE**
Year 1:	Ivermectin every 2 months.
Year 2:	Benzimidazole, but use ivermectin in June and December to kill bots. Deworm every 2 months.
Year 3:	Pyrantel, but use ivermectin in June and December to kill bots. Deworm every 2 months.
Year 4:	Back to ivermectin every 2 months.

Fig. 14.11

In southern climates, warm and moist environmental conditions encourage persistent development of infective larvae year-round. Overcrowding or excessively unsanitary conditions may also require the deworming schedule to be increased. Each horse's immune response is different. A sick or unthrifty horse may have trouble ridding its body of parasites even with the aid of dewormers, especially if it is continuously re-exposed to infective larvae in mounds of uncollected manure.

Deworming

If a horse is not at high risk from environmental factors, an example of an effective deworming programme is as shown in Fig. 14.11.

This programme is an example of a deworming strategy that will achieve effective and safe parasite control, but should **not** be construed as the only possible approach.

Administering Dewormers

The individual horse, management and hygiene practices, and expertise at handling and restraining a horse determine how consistently the deworming task is performed. The method by which a dewormer is given is not nearly as important as the frequency, the drug used, and the assurance that the **entire dose** is received. If uncertain, discuss with the veterinarian about what would be best for the horse. Deworming with a medication spray 'gun' ensures that a liquid drug is given at the appropriate dose and that all of it reaches its destination, the stomach. Yet, pastes or powders can be used with equal effectiveness.

Effective Deworming Technique

Dosages

Effective deworming depends on knowledge of body weight. Read package inserts about the toxic levels particular to a drug. Adjust upwards of suspected weight, but **keep out of the toxic range**. A wide therapeutic index indicates the safety margin that protects a horse from toxic levels but is a strong enough dose to kill the parasite. As examples of safety margins, oxibendazole can be given up to 60 times the recommended dose before toxic effects are seen. Pyrantel has a safety factor of 20 times, while ivermectin has a safety margin of 6 times the recommended dose.

There is **no reason** to administer such a walloping amount. Usually, overestimating an adult horse's weight by 200 – 300 lb when determining the correct dose will not produce any adverse effects, **except** if using organophosphates. *(Even the recommended dose for organophosphates can be toxic to a horse.)*

Be sure to check specific products for safety claims regarding use in pregnant mares or foals. If in doubt, consult a veterinarian about what amount and which product to use.

Paste Dewormers

If a paste dewormer is correctly administered, it is absorbed in the stomach and alters biochemical pathways necessary for parasite survival but not to the host horse. There is no reason to deworm on an empty stomach as was done in the old days. In fact, feeding enhances absorption of a drug from the stomach.

However, when paste is given, be sure all food is out of the mouth, then place the syringe on the back of the tongue. Gently hold the horse's head up while depressing the plunger. Stimulate the tongue to move back and forth so the horse swallows the paste.

To avoid mistakes it is helpful for a veterinarian to give instructions in paste administration. Paste deworming should be executed with confidence, and with certainty that the drug has been received by the horse. If a horse is particularly fractious, a veterinarian can perform the necessary task every 6 – 8 weeks.

Powder Dewormers

If dewormers are given in powder form on feed, the total dose must be consumed within 8 hours to be effective. Powder is an uncertain method of delivery. It is ineffective if feed spills from a bucket, food is spat or dribbled on to the ground, or if the powder is filtered out by the horse and pushed to the side. Mixing powdered medication with molasses or corn syrup into a small amount of grain or bran improves chances of consumption of the entire dose. Watch the horse eat to be confident of success, or aware of failure.

Ineffective Deworming Technique

Deworming failure occurs if an inappropriate dose is given, or if a horse does not actually receive all, or any, of the medication. With paste dewormers, a common error occurs when a horse suddenly moves as the plunger is depressed and part of the medication shoots out of the side of the mouth. Another way a horse will not receive an appropriate dose is if it has food in its mouth at the time of paste administration. As the dewormer syringe is removed, the horse might spit out the food and paste. A drink at the water trough immediately after deworming causes loss of a considerable amount of medication.

Although an owner may deworm every 2 months with an approved product, a horse may still show obvious signs of parasitism: poor hair coat, potbelly and unthriftiness. In some instances, a horse may fail to gain weight, or performance may suffer. These problems disappear within weeks of a *proper* deworming: an adequate dose is given and received by the horse. Such horses respond magically; they bloom and flourish.

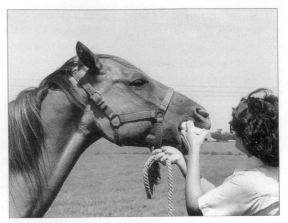

Fig. 14.12 Proper administration of a paste dewormer.

Underdosing Causes Drug Resistance

Consistent underdosing can lead to larger problems than not deworming at all. Constant exposure to doses not large enough to kill but large enough to stress the worm promotes the worm's drug resistance. When finally exposed to adequate levels of a drug, resistance capabilities prevent the worm from dying. Moreover, it genetically passes on such resistance to its offspring. Despite the deworming, a horse retains an overwhelming parasite load.

Egg Count

If a horse does not respond to a regular parasite control programme, a faecal exam analysed 2 weeks or more after deworming determines the number of parasite eggs, or egg count, per gram of faeces. Parasites such as the ascarids may produce 100 000 eggs per day, while large strongyles may only produce 5000 eggs per day. Pinworm eggs are not normally seen in the faeces, but are obtained by pressing cellophane tape against the anus.

Large numbers may mean the worms are resistant to a dewormer product. Faecal analysis by a veterinarian allows close monitoring of a parasite load within a horse, and observations of hair coat, body condition, weight gain, attitude and performance provide other clues. A veterinary exam may reveal other metabolic, nutritional or dental problems contributing to a horse's unthrifty health. Not all illness can be blamed entirely on worms.

Efficacy of Dewormers

Another important characteristic of dewormers is described as efficacy, which is the effectiveness in achieving the desired result (greater than 85% kill of a particular parasite). Oxibendazole has 95 –100% efficacy against both large and small strongyles, 90–100% against ascarids, and zero effect against bots. Pyrantel has 92–100% efficacy against *Strongylus vulgaris*, 86–100% for mature ascarids, 100% for immature Ascarids, but is only 50–70% efficacious against pinworms, 65–75% against *Strongylus edentatus*, and zero for bots. Ivermectin possesses 95–100% efficacy against large and small strongyles, pinworms, ascarids and bots.

Efficacy of Dewormers		
OXIBENDAZOLE	Large Strongyles	95% – 100%
	Small Strongyles	95% – 100%
	Ascarids	90% – 100%
	Bots	0%
PYRANTEL	Large Strongyles:	
	S. vulgaris	92% – 100%
	S. edentatus	65% – 75%
	Ascarids:	
	Mature	86% – 100%
	Immature	100%
	Pinworms	50% – 70%
	Bots	0%
IVERMECTIN	Large Strongyles	95% – 100%
	Small Strongyles	95% – 100%
	Ascarids	95% – 100%
	Pinworms	95% – 100%
	Bots	95% – 100%

Fig. 14.13

Immunity to Parasites

Normally over time, a healthy horse develops some degree of immunity to certain parasites and can fend off massive infestation. The body's immune system recognizes the parasite's proteins (antigens) as foreign and launches an immune attack by forming antibodies. The more antigens are in the horse's body, the more anti-bodies are formed.

Dewormer efficacy of 100% may not be advantageous, because it eliminates the source of the antigens. Then, a horse's uneducated im-mune system cannot defend against future parasite infec-tion.

Foals and young horses under 2 years old that have not yet developed immunity may suc-cumb to overwhelming parasite loads by ascarids or large strongyles if not regularly de-wormed.

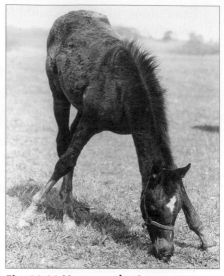

Fig. 14.14 Horses under 2 years can have an overwhelming parasite load.

Allergic Reaction

When a horse with an overwhelming infection is dewormed for the first time, the destruction and breakdown of the worm expose the horse to foreign proteins. This exposure can result in an aller-gic reaction, or severe inflammation in the intestine where the parasite attaches, causing oedema and thickening of the intestine. These reactions decrease absorption of nutrients and fluids, and may be accompanied by temporary diarrhoea. An overwhelming infection produces a similar response, resulting in chronic diar-rhoea or colic, common signs of intestinal parasitism.

It is far better to have a consistent deworming programme than to subject a horse to continual internal damage, or to side effects associated with deworming an older horse for the first time. The objective is to allow a horse's normal immune system to deal with a very small load of parasites.

Preventive Management

By minimizing an internal parasite burden in the horse, health and performance flourish and gastrointestinal disturbances are averted.

Controlling internal parasites with dewormers is an essential part of management, but should be combined with intelligent husbandry.

Introducing New Animals to a Herd

New individuals should not be introduced to the herd immediately, but should be isolated. Before allowing them to join the herd, deworm new arrivals two or three times, at 3 – 4 week intervals. This practice protects from reinfection those horses that have received excellent deworming management.

Concurrent Deworming Schedules

All members of a herd, including foals, should be dewormed at the same time. It serves little purpose to deworm only a small percentage of a herd, because untreated horses continue to excrete eggs in their faeces, recontaminating not only themselves but the treated horses as well.

Maintaining Pasture

Contaminated forage results in reinfection with worm larvae. Careful pasture management prevents overgrazing that would otherwise encourage manure deposits to outstrip available forage. Removing manure manually by shovel or pitchfork twice weekly will control parasite populations. Chain dragging a pasture spreads the manure and prevents overgrazing of certain areas, while also breaking parasite life cycles. If economically feasible, mechanical removal of faeces by pasture vacuums provides excellent parasite control. Harrowing spreads the larvae throughout the grazing area and damages the forage, therefore it is not advised.

Collected manure should be composted before spreading it on a pasture. Heat within the compost pile kills infective larvae and prevents pasture contamination. Rotating pastures with other species, e.g. cattle or sheep, will help to keep the parasite burdern down and the grass in better condition.

Maintaining Pens and Paddocks

Manual cleaning of manure from pens and paddocks twice a week removes parasite larvae before they become infective. By cleaning pens, the frequency of treatments between April through October is reduced to every 2 months instead of the recommended monthly administration. The more often a dewormer is given, the greater the possibility for drug resistance to develop.

Monitoring With Faecal Analyses

To monitor the parasite control programme's effectiveness, faecal analyses can be performed, comparing a faecal sample before deworming treatment with one obtained exactly 2 weeks after treatment.

Most dewormers result in decreased egg shedding of strongyles for 4 – 6 weeks after treatment, while ivermectin depresses egg shedding for up to 8 weeks. Because large and small strongyles create such havoc and danger within a horse, a primary goal in any deworming programme is to concentrate efforts on removal of these particular parasites.

15

SKIN AILMENTS: AVOIDING AND CURING

The condition of a horse's coat is a reliable reflector of internal body health. External parasites, fungal infections, scratches, skin growths or saddle sores can mar any coat and create performance problems.

EXTERNAL PARASITES

Flies and Midges

Horse Flies

Flies cause troublesome skin irritations. One such culprit is the horse fly, *Tabanus*. Its bite is painful and causes nodules on the skin. The most commonly affected areas are along the neck, withers, back and legs.

Stable Flies

The stable fly, similar to the common house fly, also pierces the skin with its mouthparts, irritating the horse and leaving behind nodular swellings. Stable flies are poorly named because they really prefer light and sunny areas, only going inside during rainy weather. They lay eggs in decaying urine-soaked straw and manure. Adequate manure removal and stall cleaning, along with the use of insecticides, control the stable fly population to a manageable level.

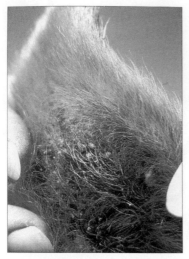

Fig. 15.1 Blackflies feed in the ears.

Blackflies

Blackflies (Simulium), commonly known as ear gnats, feed on blood drawn from the flat surface inside the ear *(the pinna)*. They can also cause irritation around the eyes. Blackflies are found particularly near running water, which is a breeding ground for the pest. Adults travel great distances, up to 100 miles, therefore control is nearly impossible.

Blackflies are tiny insects that reach a maximum length of 5 millimetres, about the size of an apple seed.

As the blackflies feed on the delicate lining of the ears, toxins secreted in their saliva increase permeability of capillary beds, improving access to blood meals. Oozing and blood-encrusted scabs form where blackflies have fed. The discomfort from an intense inflammatory response causes the horse to become head-shy. What begins as an instinctive response to avoid pain and discomfort can develop into a habit of head-shyness even after the ears are healed.

Allergic Reaction

Some horses respond to blackfly bites with a severe allergic reaction. Horny growths, or *plaques*, develop inside the ear. These cauliflower-like plaques peel away easily by rubbing with a thumbnail or a piece of gauze (if the horse allows them to be touched). Their easy removal distinguishes them from more tenacious sarcoid tumours often found in the ears.

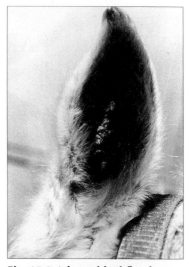

Fig. 15.2 A large blackfly plaque resembles a cauliflower.

Once blackfly plaques are removed, applying a topical corticosteroid ointment reduces the severity of the allergic response. A horse can be encouraged to accept daily topical medication inside the ears by quickly applying ointment while it is distracted with a bucket of grain. Prevention is better than treatment to avoid the horse's becoming head-shy when handled close to the ears.

Effects on the Ears
Pigmentation Loss

A persistent inflammatory response to blackflies causes a horse to permanently lose skin colour inside the ears. This white patch is of only cosmetic significance, and does not interfere with the skin's return to function or health.

Treatment

Immediate recognition of a problem helps to correct it before poor behaviour or white patches develop. Normally, hair in the ear protects the deeper ear canal from collecting dirt or debris and keeps insects or ticks from crawling into the ear canal.

Hair Removal

If a horse has blackflies, trimming or shaving away all fine hairs lining the ear pinnae helps restore health to the ear. Wads of cotton should be inserted into each ear before clipping to prevent particles of hair or debris from falling into the deep ear canal where they can stimulate an infection. It may be necessary to have a veterinarian tranquillize or sedate a head-shy horse. A sedative also encourages the horse's head to droop, and allows more thorough cleansing of afflicted skin in the ears. After shaving, be sure to remove the cotton wads.

Removal of hair inside the ears allows thorough inspection of scabs or sores. Without hair for scabs and oozing serum to cling to, the tender skin inside the ears heals quickly. Without the presence of blood to attract blackflies to a 'banquet', it is easier to provide relief for the horse. Anti-inflammatory corticosteroid creams or topical roll-on insect repellants are easily applied to hairless skin. Spray insecticides into the ears with caution, taking care not to accidentally spray an irritating substance into an eye.

Once ear hair is removed, smearing the inside of the ears with a light layer of a petroleum-based salve also deters blackflies from reaching the skin for feeding. Only products intended for use in the ear should be used, or a veterinarian should be consulted. Body heat causes salves to melt into the deep ear canal.

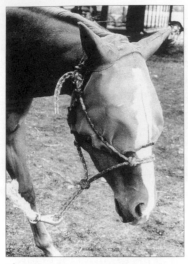

Fig. 15.3 An ear net protects from insects.

Prevention
Ear Nets

To prevent blackfly irritation, ear nets can be purchased as part of a netted face mask. Mosquito net material forming the mask covers the face and eyes, and extends over the poll and ears to keep insects off all structures of the head.

Blackflies feed mainly during the day, so in areas of high blackfly populations an allergic horse can be stalled indoors during those hours. However, other insects, such as *Culicoides* midges, emerge at dusk.

Culicoides Midges

The bite of the Culicoides midge may cause an allergic reaction, called *Culicoides hypersensitivity*, Queensland's itch, sweet itch, or summer eczema. The midges feed along the topline of the horse, and the horse self-mutilates to appease an intense itching *(pruritus)*. It starts by rubbing the mane and tail down to raw and bleeding skin. As the syndrome worsens, all body areas itch and the horse traumatizes its neck, chest and belly. In a delirium of itching, it pauses over bushes to rub its belly, and abuses fence posts, stall doors and sides of barns.

Not only does a horse destroy its hair coat and skin with this behaviour, producing a scruffy appearance, but the horse becomes

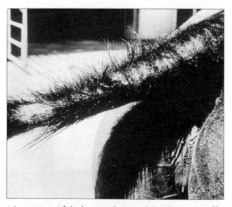

Fig. 15.4 This horse has rubbed away all its tail hair due to itching.

depressed and irritable. It may become belligerent to handlers. Even if it is ridable (depending on the degree of skin damage), its performance suffers.

There is a hereditary predisposition to Culicoides hypersensitivity. Usually it surfaces in horses over 2 – 3 years old, and the allergic response worsens with age.

This ailment is seasonal, showing up from late spring through late autumn as it coincides with warmth and the fly season. Culicoides midges prefers areas of high humidity such as damp pastures, edges of ponds, or areas around wet, decaying plants. The midges are evening feeders, particularly around dusk, so management control of this syndrome is best aimed at stabling the horse from dusk to dawn.

Mosquito netting or screening over the stalls keeps Culicoides out, and a protective 'fly sheet' minimizes bites. Frequent and repeated applications of insect repellants are advantageous, and automatically timed mist sprayers in the barn help kill the midges and flies.

Unless a horse is relocated to a different environment that is not a favourable breeding ground for the midges, it is almost impossible to entirely protect an allergic horse from bites. Corticosteroid medications, at a dose recommended by a veterinarian, have been used to reduce the allergic response to a manageable level throughout the fly season. Prevention with insert repellants and barrier creams is preferable.

Ailments Similar to Culicoides Hypersensitivity

It is important to differentiate pinworms and bot fly larvae from the more dramatic Culicoides hypersensitivity reaction. These parasites cause similar symptoms.

Pinworms

Initially, Culicoides hypersensitivity is confused with pinworms due to the horse's tendency to rub away the hair on the tailhead. However, Culicoides hypersensitivity progresses along the topline of the horse, whereas pinworms or a normal oestrus cycle cause a horse to concentrate on rubbing the rear end only.

By applying adhesive tape to the skin around the anus, and then pulling it off again and sticking it on to a microscope slide, a veterinarian can microscopically examine the sample for pinworm eggs.

Bot Flies

As bot fly larvae mature and travel from the stomach of the horse to the rectum and anus, they spend a short time attached to the lining of the rectum. These parasites also can cause itching of the tailhead.

If there is any doubt about the possibility of infection with either bots or pinworms, it is simple to administer an appropriate deworming paste and see if the itching disappears in about a week.

Horn Flies

To make matters even more confusing, another fly bite hypersensitivity reaction—which is easily confused with Culicoides hypersensitivity—is called *focal ventral midline dermatitis*. As the name of this problem suggests, it is found only under the belly. The skin around

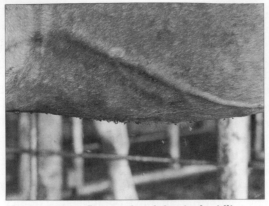

Fig. 15.5 Horn flies on the abdominal midline.

the navel is scaly, crusty and ulcerated, and lacks hair *(alcopecia)* and colour. This reaction is due to the horn fly, *Haematobia*, which prefers to obtain a blood meal along a narrow strip on the abdominal midline. The horn fly can be recognized by its peculiar feeding position with the head pointing towards the ground. Use of fly repellants and corticosteroid–antibiotic combination creams minimize inflammation and any secondary bacterial infection.

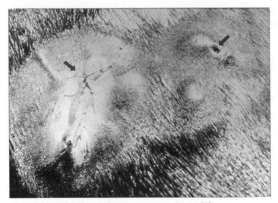

Fig. 15.6 The breathing pores of warbles.

Warbles

If a large single nodule on the horse's back has an opening, it is most likely the breathing pore of a warble called *Hypoderma*. The warble, also called a heel fly, lays eggs on a horse's hairs. Once these eggs hatch, the *Hypoderma* larvae migrate through the skin, arriving at the back about 4 – 5 months later during the antumn and winter months. On rare occasions, the warble could migrate to the brain instead of the back, resulting in severe neurological problems. Warbles are common to cattle, so horses pastured with or near cattle are at risk. Always consult your veterinarian before using insecticidal or anthelmintic preparations as a nasty abscess may form where the larva is killed.

Other Causes of Nodules

If there is no breathing pore, the nodule may instead be a nodular *necrobiosis*, which is the result of cell death and scar tissue build-up. This nodule is caused by reaction around a particle of synthetic material from a saddle pad, or from a mini-infection from a recent fly bite. These firm lumps are easily seen and felt in areas along the withers, back, thorax or belly. They are not usually painful and there is no skin ulceration or reddening over the lumps.

Applying a topical corticosteroid cream may cause the knot to disappear. The nodule normally regresses within about 3 weeks. During the healing period, it is important that no tack pressure be placed over the lesion. If the nodule persists, or if it is constantly aggravated by tack, it may be necessary to surgically remove it. The nodule does not grow back, but healing takes longer than treatment with corticosteroids. In most cases the nodules cause no problem and may have been present for some time before being noticed by the rider.

Fly and Midge Bites and Their Symptoms	
Horse Flies	Nodules on the neck, withers, back and legs.
Stable Flies	Nodules on the entire body.
Blackflies	Oozing, blood-encrusted scabs, inflammation, perhaps loss of skin colour or cauliflower-like plaques inside the ear canal. Erosion of skin at corner eyes.
Culicoides Midge	Itching starts at the tail and mane, then spreads to the withers and to the entire body.
Horn Flies	Scaly, crusty, ulcerated lesions, lacking hair and colour around the navel.
Warbles	Large nodules with a breathing pore on the back.

Fig. 15.7

Mites

Mites can be identified on examination, by your veterinary surgeon with a microscope, of skin scrape microscope, of skin scrape samples. There are seven main types, which will now be considered in turn.

Mange Mites

Many other parasites cause intense itching in the horse. *Mange mites* stimulate severe itching around the head and neck and can progress over the entire body. There are many species of mange mites, most of which are difficult to see. Mites are usually transferred by direct contact of horse to horse, or via contaminated grooming tools, blankets and tack. Treatment with ivermectin twice at a 2-week interval usually controls these parasites.

Mites and Their Symptoms	
Mange Mites	Itching starts at the head and neck, then spreads to the entire body.
Scabies	Itchy, thickened skin in skin folds, throat and ears.
Sarcoptic Mites	Itching starts around the head, neck and shoulders.
Demodectic Mites	Nodular lesions on the head, neck and withers.
Chorioptic Mites	Cracked, greasy lesions on the abdomen and lower limbs, especially the hind legs. Stamping feet.
Straw Itch Mites	Small, crusty, non-itchy weals.
Harvest Mites	Crusty, scaly, scabby, colourless papules on the neck, thorax and legs.

Fig. 15.8

Scabies

Scabies or *psoroptic* mites prefer areas of skin folds, the throat, and even the ears. Intense itching may cause the skin to thicken and the horse to self-mutilate affected areas.

Sarcoptic Mites

Sarcoptic mites can be a moderately serious skin ailment in the horse, beginning around the head, neck and shoulders, accompanied by intense itching. This type of mange mite is contagious to humans.

Demodectic Mites

Demodectic mites are extremely rare, producing nodular lesions of the head, neck and withers. They burrow deeply into the skin to the base of the hair follicles. Consequently, a very deep skin scraping is necessary for microscopic identification. Demodectic mites may inhabit the skin of up to 50% of normal horses, but usually elicit no disease symptoms unless a horse suffers from immune suppression or deficiency.

Chorioptic Mites

Chorioptic mites are a problem in winter, involving the abdomen or the lower limbs, especially the hind legs. The horse tends to stamp its feet and break the hairs on the leg from rubbing. Due to the cracked, greasy appearance of the skin of the lower leg, a case of chorioptic mites may be confused with 'scratches' or 'grease heel'. Normally, scratches are *dermatitis* caused by a skin irritant, or a bacterial and/or fungal infection around the back of the pastern. Dermatitis is inflammation of the skin. Its symptoms include painful, itchy, weeping red and inflamed skin. Some or all of these symptoms may be present, depending on the cause. If a case of dermatitis does not respond to conventional treatment with anti-fungals, antibiotics and anti-inflammatory topical ointments, chorioptic mites may be the cause.

Straw Itch Mites

The *straw itch mite* causes small raised areas of oedema *(weals)* on a horse's skin. They are non-itchy, crusty eruptions. The straw itch mite normally parasitizes grain insect larvae and is commonly found in alfalfa hay or straw. Humans are also affected by this mite, with intense itching. The problem usually recedes within 3 days without special treatment.

Harvest Mites

Infestation with harvest mites is called *trombiculiasis*. It can be a problem in late summer and autumn. Horses pastured in fields and woods may develop crusty *papules* (elevated areas with a defined border) on the face, neck, thorax and legs. Commonly, the lips and face are involved, with scaly, scabby areas lacking colour, which may or may not itch. It is easy to mistake affected lesions around the muzzle as areas of *photosensitization*. (Photosensitization, discussed later in this chapter, is an abnormal reaction of the skin to sunlight, causing sunburn and dermatitis.)

OTHER EXTERNAL PARASITES
Onchocerca Worm

External parasites come in all shapes and sizes, and inflict damage in a variety of ways. Some parasites may be transmitted to a horse by a biting insect. The microscopic *Onchocerca* worm lives along the crest of the neck in the nuchal ligament. Adult *Onchocerca* produce larvae *(microfilariae)* that migrate just under the skin to the abdominal midline, to the head and face, or into the deep tissues of the eye.

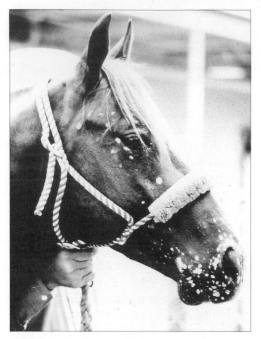

Fig. 15.9 *Onchocerca* **lesions are scaly, crusty, and lack colour.**

The Culicoides biting midge serves as a vehicle for spread of the *Onchocerca* among horses. A horse with an *Onchocerca* infection often has scaling, crusty lesions around the face and eyes, under the belly, along the neck, and over the topline. The lesions are hairless and usually lack colour.

A mild allergic reaction causes the involved areas to become itchy. As a horse rubs the itch, the areas inflame further. This skin problem is common during warm weather due to transmission by Culicoides midges, and a more active microfilaria production by the *Onchocerca* adults, as they are stimulated by longer daylight hours.

Diagnosis of *onchocerciasis* is made by microscopic examination of affected tissue obtained by surgical biopsy, or skin scraping. Seeing microfilaria through the microscope positively identifies the skin ailment.

Moonblindness

If the microfilariae migrate through the eye, *periodic ophthalmia*,

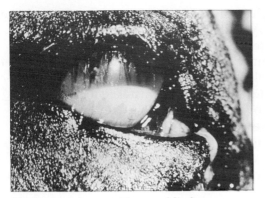

Fig. 15.10 A horse with moonblindness.

or 'moonblindness', can result. Moonblindness is accompanied by chronic attacks of *anterior uveitis*, which is an inflammation of structures surrounding the pupil. Uveitis is painful, and symptoms include tearing, squinting, and sensitivity to bright light *(photophobia)*. Corneal ulcers develop subsequent to swelling of the eye's internal structures.

Fortunately, the incidence of onchocerciasis has dramatically diminished due to the drug ivermectin which effectively kills the parasite. Ivermectin has reduced the reservoir of the *Onchocerca* worms, and today it is rare to see well maintained horses with this skin problem. However, there may be horses with eye damage from previous exposure to migrating microfilariae.

Pelodera strongyloides

The symptoms of a microscopic parasite that affects the skin of the thighs and belly, called *Pelodera strongyloides*, may be mistaken for urine or manure scald. This parasite causes *rhabditic dermatitis* which is itchy and painful. Usually, sanitation of the environment controls this problem. Diagnosis is often only accomplished by a skin biopsy.

Lice

Onchocerca and *Pelodera strongyloides* are invisible to the naked eye. But carefully brushing the hairs the wrong way may lead to the discovery of more obvious skin predators, such as *lice*.

Infestation with lice is called *pediculosis*. Typi-

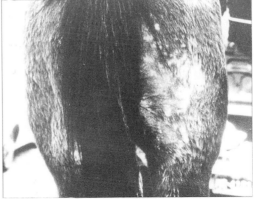

Fig. 15.11 The hair coat of a horse infested with lice appears moth-eaten.

cally, this parasite is a problem in winter, because the eggs *(nits)* thrive in the deep layers of a fuzzy winter hair coat. Lice are host specific, meaning that a horse louse will not infest a person, dog or cat.

The louse spends its entire life cycle on the host. They can be seen along the topline and look like 'walking dandruff'. The nits are cemented to the hairs, and should not be mistaken for bot fly eggs. Nits are white and more oval than the yellow bot fly eggs normally found on the legs. Using a magnifying glass aids identification.

Lice cause intense itching, and a horse self-mutilates to satisfy the itching. The hair coat may appear moth-eaten in places, and large areas of hair will be rubbed out, especially over the buttocks, thighs, neck and head.

Poor sanitation, overcrowding and undernutrition cause lice infestation. They are transmitted directly from horse to horse, or by brushes, blankets and tack. Specific louse shampoos are necessary to treat the horse, while tack and equipment should be soaked in a sterilizing solution.

Ticks

Spinous Ear Tick

The spinous ear tick, *Otobious*, inhabits the ear canal. These ticks remain attached for up to 7 months, feeding off lymph secretions and causing irritation and head-shaking. Sometimes a horse may droop a particularly affected ear, or rub incessantly on a post. The intense inflammation caused by these ticks makes their attachment sites susceptible to bacterial infection. It is often necessary to sedate the horse to properly examine the ear canals and remove the ticks.

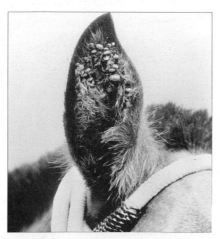

Fig. 15.12 An ear infested with ticks.

Hard Ticks

The bites of hard ticks are quite painful. These ticks are also found along the mane and tail, withers, and flank. Ticks irritate soft-skinned areas around the groin, under the tail, around the anus and vulva, and under the throat and belly, so look carefully in these areas.

Ticks burrow their heads into the superficial skin layers. Secondary bacterial infections around these bites can occur, and occasionally oedema and soft tissue swelling result even after the tick has dropped off.

It is important to remove the head by grasping the tick and slowly easing it out of the skin. Burning it with a match while still on the horse, or applying alcohol or turpentine are not advised methods for tick removal. These techniques do not induce the tick to release itself, and may irritate or chemically burn tender skin.

Ticks can transmit serious infections, such as Lyme Disease and protozoal diseases. Providing they do not carry a disease, ticks generally cause little harm to the horse, although a heavy infestation may signal a suppressed immune system. A horse could easily develop anaemia from blood loss if a heavy enough tick load occurs.

Summer Sores

A syndrome caused by abnormal larval migration of the stomach worm, *Habronema*, is called *summer sores* or *cutaneous habronemiasis*. During the warm months when house or stable flies are active, larvae from the stomach worm are passed in the faeces and ingested by larvae of these host flies. Once the fly larvae hatch and begin feeding on the horse, they are deposited at feeding sites. If worm larvae are deposited in areas other than around the mouth, such as the mucous membranes of the eyes and prepuce, or on wounds or traumatized skin, they migrate underneath the skin, causing a severe allergic hypersensitivity reaction.

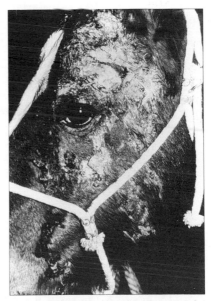

Fig. 15.13 Summer sores are caused by *Habronema* larvae.

The lesions that develop appear ulcerated, raw and bleeding, and are very painful and itchy. A horse may bite at and traumatize the lesions. Although they may regress during winter, the lesions reoccur the next year at the same time and in the same place.

Summer sores resemble proud flesh, *fibroblastic sarcoids*, or a *squamous cell carcinoma* tumour. Biopsies must be performed to differentiate from these other problems. Surgically cutting away dead and dying tissue, along with non-steroidal anti-inflammatory drugs and antibiotics, help control tissue proliferation. Ivermectin is effective in killing the worm larvae.

Other External Parasites and Their Symptoms	
ONCHOCERCA WORM	Scaly, crusty, hairless, colourless lesions on the face and around the eyes, under the belly, on the neck and topline. If the microfilariae migrate through the eye, moonblindness can result.
PELODERA STRONGYLOIDES	Painful, itchy dermatitis on the thighs and belly.
LICE	Intense itching, 'walking dandruff' especially around the mane and tail.
TICKS Spinous Ear Tick	Irritation, head shaking, drooping, or rubbing of ears; found inside ear canal.
Hard Tick	Feed inside ears, around mane, tail, withers, flank, groin, under throat and belly.
SUMMER SORES	Ulcerated, raw, bleeding, painful, itchy lesions in old wounds or on mucous membranes of the eye, mouth, and prepuce.

Fig. 15.14

FUNGAL INFECTIONS

A fungus is a living organism invading the hair coat. Small, firm, pea-sized bumps in the skin, skin flaking, or hairlessness signal the beginning stages of fungal infection. A fungus cannot grow in living tissue, but produces toxins to create an environment in which it can thrive.

These toxins cause an inflammatory reaction in the skin, with resultant oedema, necrosis (tissue death), or an allergic hypersensitivity reaction. Because the fungus weakens the hair shaft, the hair easily breaks off.

Ringworm

Fungal infections called *ringworm* or *girth itch*, often result in circular patches of hair loss, with scabby or flaking skin beneath, and broken hairs visible in the lesions. In horses under 2 years old, the immune system is less developed, and the entire body may be overwhelmed by the disease.

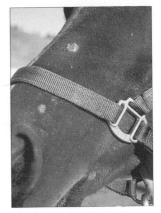

Fig. 15.15 The beginning signs of a fungal infection.

The fungus can persist in the environment for up to a year, and it is transferred by brushes, blankets, clothing, rake handles, etc. Ringworm is extremely contagious from horse to horse, and to small children. Wash hands thoroughly with povidone-iodine after handling an infected horse, and soak all tack and equipment in a diluted sterilizing solution straight povidone-iodine, or a 3% Captan solution (approximately 33 parts water to 1 part Captan 50% Powder). (Captan 50% Powder can be found at nurseries as an orchard spray.)

Ringworm spores are known to be extremely difficult to clear from rugs and girths. The use of 5% lime sulphur or placing the kit in a black polythene bag with a formalin 'bomb' has been suggested as being the most effective treatment.

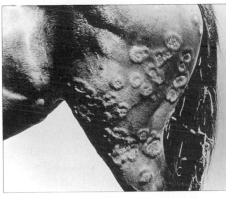

Fig. 15.16 An unusually severe reaction to ringworm.

Sunshine helps to rid the environment of fungus, which is why many dark, damp barns provide a perfect environment for fungal growth. Fungal infections are common in autumn and winter when sun rays diminish, dampness prevails, and horses are housed inside.

Diagnosis and Treatment

A veterinarian can diagnose a fungal skin infection by obtaining a scraping of an affected area, and examining it with a microscope. It may on occasions be necessary to grow it on dermatophyte test medium, which is a gel-like nutrient medium especially for fungus. Results usually require 4 – 14 days to confirm the presence of a

Fungal Infections and Their Symptoms	
General Fungal Infection	Small, firm, pea-sized bumps, skin thickening and roughening, scaling and crusty skin, hair loss.
Ringworm	Circular patches of hair loss, scabby or flaking skin, broken hairs.

Fig. 15.17

disease-causing fungus by culture methods

Normally, fungal infections resolve by themselves within 1 – 3 months, unless a horse has an immune deficiency, another debilitating disease, malnutrition, or stress from overcrowding or poor sanitation. Such horses are unable to rid their bodies of the fungal infection, or may be persistently reinfected.

Treatment requires shampoos using povidone-iodine, followed by a rinse with Captan 50% Powder, mixed at 2 ounces per gallon of water. On localized spots, specific anti-fungal ointments may be used. If the entire body is involved, or if a case does not respond to topical treatment, then griseofulvin powder may be prescribed by a veterinarian. (Do not use griseofulvin on a pregnant mare.)

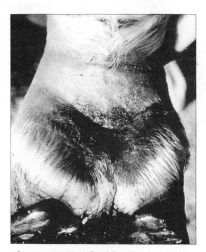

Fig. 15.18 Cracked heels occur at the back of the pastern.

CRACKED HEELS (SCRATCHES)

White markings on a horse's legs add flash to its overall appearance. Beneath the white fur lies pink skin, which under most circumstances poses few problems as the hair coat protects pink skin from sunburn.

However, legs marked with white socks or stockings are prone to irritation. Irritation creates a skin inflammation (dermatitis) of vulnerable tissues at the back of the pastern. The syndrome has many names, each a description of either the cause or symptoms of the problem. Commonly called *cracked heels,* other descriptive terms include *grease heel, mud fever, scratches, white pastern disease* and *dew poisoning.*

Under the right conditions, any horse can develop cracked heels. Like chapped hands, the skin is painful and is often accompanied by localized swelling and lameness. Initially, there is no visible evidence of an inflammatory crisis, but in a short time hair loss occurs along with weeping, red skin at the back of the pasterns. Constant motion of the pastern causes the skin to crack and form fissures. Ulcerated and raw sores persist beneath the scabs.

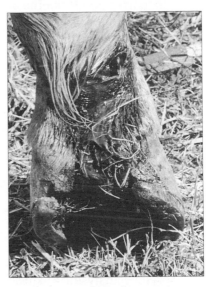

A cracked skin surface that is caked with dried and moist serum appears greasy, hence the name grease heel. Over time, inflamed skin overreacts by growing thickened, horn-like proliferations called 'grapes'. These growths must be removed surgically to treat the underlying skin.

Typically cracked heels are confined to a small area with swelling beginning directly around the lesions, but some cases may be aggravated by sun exposure and are called *photoaggravated vasculitis.* (Vasculitis is inflammation of blood vessels.) Ultraviolet radia-

Fig. 15.19 Grease heel.

tion may trigger cases during the long days of summer.

Usually only white-marked limbs are affected, and swelling and lameness are out of proportion to the mildness of the skin lesions. As a case of cracked heels progresses, swelling may encompass the entire lower limb. Lesions weep and ooze serum. Sores develop not just on the back of pasterns, but also on the sides and fronts of pasterns and fetlock. If pink skin ascends the leg, the dermatitis may spread to the cannon area.

Causes of Cracked Heels

Rough stubble in a field, sand, soil and grit of training surfaces, and muddy pastures irritate the skin on the lower legs. Unsanitary conditions of urine-soaked and dirty bedding lead to caking on the feet and pasterns of stalled horses, creating chemical and bacterial irritation to skin.

In horses with particularly long hairs down the back of the legs, such as the feathering common to certain draft breeds, cracked heels occur even under the best conditions. Long hair traps moisture and debris, which are prime conditions for dermatitis.

Other Related Problems

Skin irritation is not the only cause of cracked heels. Infectious organisms, mites or *photosensitization* can cause dermatitis or can complicate an existing case.

Fungal Infection

Fungus proliferates in dense hairs and the unsanitary skin environment common to the lower limbs and may be mistaken for cracked heels. However, a fungal infection may also occur on a darkly marked limb or on other parts of the body. Skin scrapings grown by a veterinarian on a special nutrient medium can identify a fungus.

Chorioptic Mange Mite

Another organism that invades long hairs around the pastern is a *chorioptic mange mite.* Draft horse breeds are particularly susceptible. This mite causes an intense itching in the invaded area, causing horses to stomp or bite at their legs in agitation. This mite is diagnosed by analysing a skin scraping under a microscope.

Rain Scald Mud Fever

In moist areas or during warm and rainy spring months in any region, a common problem is infection with the *Dermatophilus* bacteria. Spores are continually present in the environment and are activated by moisture. Commonly seen along the back, loins and croup, *Dermatophilus* infection is called *rain scald.* Activated spores infiltrate skin traumatized by flies. Lower limbs are affected in areas of moist terrain, earning it the name mud fever. *Dermatophilus* dermatitis which is limited to pastern areas is often mistaken for cracked heels (scratches). Daily antiseptic cleansing of afflicted skin assists a normal immune system to defeat infection by *Dermatophilus.*

White Pastern Disease

Bacterial organisms can cause or complicate a case of white pastern disease. Specifically, a *staphylococcal* bacteria infection is the most common cause. A veterinarian can diagnose and treat these infections. Unlike cracked heels, only one limb may be affected.

Treating Cracked Heels

Various home remedies are concocted to treat cracked heels, including sauerkraut poultices. People struggle for months using home remedies trying to rid a horse of cracked heels, to no avail. There is no substitute for cleaning affected legs and shaving away the hair so that topical salves and bandages can be applied.

The first step in treating cracked heels is to soften and remove matted hair and crusts. Gently soap the area with warm water and an antiseptic scrub, such as tamed iodine (Betadine®) or chlorhexidine (Hibitane®). An antiseptic scrub also treats any superficial bacterial infection.

Once all of the crusts and mats are loosened and the hair is towelled dry, clip all hair away with electric clippers. Residual particulates, crusts and contaminants are removed along with clinging hair. Many horses resist scrubbing and clipping. Veterinary help and sedatives may be necessary for treating objecting horses.

If crusting tissue adheres tightly to underlying, ulcerated skin, removing the scabs forcefully causes more harm than good. Instead, coat matted areas with a salve and bandage them for a day or two. Then, crusts, mats and scabs easily peel away from the skin without further trauma.

Once the crusts and hair are removed, apply a topical antibiotic–corticosteroid combination cream or ointment. Not only is this preparation soothing, but it restores pliability to cracked tissue. A light bandage over the wounds keeps them clean and protects pink skin from ultraviolet rays. Also, a bandage supports damaged tissues and promotes healing.

If a case of cracked heels has developed beyond a local irritation to a grease heel, apply zinc sulphate (contained in white lotion) or calamine lotion to suppress serum production and weeping. After a day or two, apply an antibiotic–corticosteroid cream and bandage as above. The tissues should never be dried out with astringent products such as copper sulphate or lime, because they worsen the dermatitis and substantially slow healing.

NSAIDs

Inflammation and tissue swelling impair circulation to the area, and must be controlled for healing to advance. This goal is accomplished with non-steroidal anti-inflammatory drugs, such as flunixin meglumine (Finadyne®) or phenylbutazone ('bute'). In photoaggravated vasculitis cases, corticosteroid medications may be necessary.

Preventing Cracked Heels

It is of little benefit to address the symptoms of the problem without also addressing the cause. Unsanitary housing conditions should be improved. A horse pastured in irrigated fields, moist grass or mud should be removed from this environment until the legs are healed, or until the environment dries up. If sunshine aggravates the condition, the legs should be covered with bandages, or the horse should be housed indoors during the daytime.

For light or Warmblood breeds, shaving the back of the fetlocks maintains cleanliness. If feathering down the legs is desired for draft breeds, diligent attention to hygiene is essential. Careful daily inspection of all limbs identifies a beginning problem before it gets out of hand.

Cracked Heels and Similar Ailments	
Symptoms of Cracked Heels	Dermatitis, consisting of painful, inflamed, cracked, weeping, red lesions at the back of the pastern. Also, hair loss and 'grapes'.
Problems Similar to Cracked Heels	Fungal Infection Chorioptic Mange Mite Rain Scald/Mud Fever White Pastern Disease Photosensitization

Fig. 15.20

PHOTOSENSITIZATION

Photosensitization occurs when the skin overreacts to sunlight, causing sunburn and/or dermatitis. It is difficult to distinguish from cracked heels, especially the more severe photoaggravated vasculitis. Photosensitization is caused by a breakdown product called *phylloerythrin*, which is released from plant chlorophyll.

Certain plants, such as ragwort, cause liver disease. Liver disease prevents normal body excretion of phylloerythrin, and the chemical accumulates in the skin. A horse with either plant-induced or metabolic liver disease can develop photosensitization.

Phylloerythrin accumulates in skin tissues where it absorbs ultraviolet light. Sunburn results, leading to tissue oedema, inflammation, and cracked, peeling skin that weeps serum. The matted, crusty appearance of the skin and hair closely resembles the symptoms of cracked heels. As scabs peel away, ulcerated, raw areas are revealed underneath.

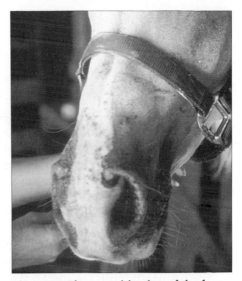

Fig. 15.21 Photosensitization of the face and muzzle.

Other plants, such as St. John's Wort, contain excess amounts of a chemical which accumulates in the skin. The chemical causes the skin to absorb UV rays of the sun, and photosensitization results.

Because sunburn only affects pink skin, photosensitized horses react on areas of the legs with white markings. Distribution is similar to that of cracked heels, but photosensitization reactions may also include other white areas, including the face and muzzle. One way to distinguish cracked heels from liver disease is that with liver disease the mucous membranes of the gums and eyes are jaundiced.

Differentiating between a dermatitis that involves all four limbs and possibly the muzzle, and a photosensitization reaction to a plant (with or without liver disease) can be difficult. Dermatitis can be caused by parasites, bacteria or fungus. Photosensitization can be caused by certain plants or liver disease. Biochemical analysis of liver enzymes in the bloodstream can diagnose liver disease.

ALLERGIES
The Role of the Immune System

The world teems with invisible organisms. Under the right conditions, these microbes colonize the body, afflicting an animal with disease symptoms. Normally, the immune system keeps the organisms at bay.

These disease-producing organisms are made partly of proteins. Inflammatory cells recognize these proteins, called *antigens*, as foreign, and wage invisible battles when they attempt to invade the body. Antigens then stimulate the body to launch an immune response.

The immune system responds by manufacturing other proteins, called *antibodies*, which are weapons against a specific antigenic target. Pre-programmed antibodies set off a cascade of biochemical events. Localized inflammation starts within minutes.

Normally the immune system works in harmony with other biochemical responses to keep a horse disease free, healthy and vital. Occasionally however, the body rebels and an immune response is blown out of proportion. This hypersensitivity response is called an *allergy*. It can range from a serious, life-threatening reaction within the respiratory tract to mild but disagreeable skin reactions, called *hives* or *urticaria*.

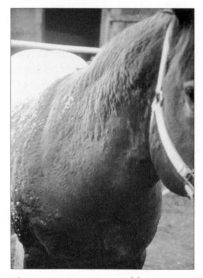

Fig. 15.22 Large, round bumps are characteristic of hives.

Hives/Urticaria

Hives are areas of oedema (swelling of cells with fluid) that begin as small lumps. Then they grow together into large, elevated, round, flat-topped bumps with steep sides, about the size of a fingernail. Pressing one leaves an impression of a fingertip; is called *pitting oedema*.

They initially form on the neck and shoulders and along the thorax. If the symptoms are not stopped early, the entire body may become involved, especially the upper hind limbs. An affected horse appears droopy and depressed as the immune system wages a silent war.

Hives usually appear 12 – 24 hours after exposure to the foreign protein, and resolve as quickly. Because hypersensitivity reactions take months or years to develop, a sudden onset of hives is *not always* a result of a very recent change, making it difficult to locate the source of the problem.

Causes of Hives

Most hives are caused by an allergic response to a plant, food or drug, although the specific cause is isolated less than half of the time. Blood transfusions, ingestion of certain plants, or feed additives can be responsible for hives. Liver disease is sometimes associated with recurrent hives; in those cases once the liver heals, hive episodes abate.

Drug Allergies

Medications such as non-steroidal anti-inflammatory drugs like flunixin meglumine (Finadyne®) or phenylbutazone, and procaine in procaine penicillin may cause allergic reactions. Hives can also occur after administration of equine influenza vaccine or tetanus antitoxin.

Food Allergies

Certain food substances, particularly those with high protein contents, cause hives in some horses. This allergic reaction is accompanied by small, raised areas, or weals, that itch intensely and cause the horse to rub its tail.

Pollen and Moulds

Inhaled allergens, such as pollen or moulds, are common sources for hives. Antigens inhaled into the lungs stimulate swelling in the respiratory tract, similar to asthma in people.

Topical Applications

Not all incidents of hives are caused by intake of a foreign substance. Localized, topical application of tamed iodine scrub, liniments, insecticides or contact with bedding may also spark an allergic reaction.

Insect Bites

Insect bites often stimulate an outbreak of hives. Isolated groups of bumps that appear rapidly, especially in thin-skinned areas, may be allergic reactions to mosquito bites, Culicoides midge bites or *Onchocerca* parasites. Most insect bite reactions resolve with no treatment within 12 – 72 hours. These weals are mildly tender and flat. Insect bites rarely cause hives on the entire body unless it is overwhelmed by the bite toxin. Usually the weals are confined to one area.

Other Forms of Hives

Ehrlichia equi

An odd form of hives develops secondary to some bacterial or viral infections, and specifically to *Ehrlichia equi*. Infection causes fever, depression, weakness and poor motor coordination.

E. equi forms unique 'target' lesions, called *erythema multiforme*, that remain for weeks or months in a fairly symmetrical distribution. These hive-like lesions have an area of central clearing, and look like doughnuts or bull's eye targets.

Purpura Haemorrhagica (See also Chapter 5)

An unusual allergic response to *Streptococcus* species of bacteria including the one responsible for strangles *(Streptococcus equi)* can cause *purpura haemorrhagica*. A month or two after a bout of strangles, a Streptococcal respiratory infection, or influenza, the horse appears stiff from muscle soreness. It is unwilling to walk or move its sore neck. The limbs are stocked up, and oedema extends into the belly and prepuce. Urgent veterinary attention is required.

Hives can appear on the entire body in a case of purpura, due to a breakdown in blood vessel walls. The breakdown occurs because of an immune response to the *Streptolysin O* toxin remaining from the *Strep equi* infection. Small blood spots are visible on the mucous membranes of the gums, eyes and inside the vulva. As the syndrome progresses, swelling increases in the legs, and the skin begins to ooze serum.

To combat an allergic response to the Strep toxin, massive quantities of penicillin and potent anti-inflammatory agents (corticosteroids) are administered for weeks until the symptoms abate.

Angioedema

Profound hypersensitivity allergies occasionally result in a syndrome called *angioedema*. This reaction is more severe than simple hives. The head and respiratory tract swell, and respiratory swelling moves downwards. The weals are infiltrated with cellular components, turning soft, pitting oedema lesions into firm bumps.

Anaphylaxis

Angioedema is a life-threatening condition: it can rapidly progress to *anaphylaxis* and death. Anaphylaxis begins with muscle tremors and patchy sweating. The horse appears anxious or colicky. Respiratory distress quickly follows, due to pooling of blood and fluid in the lungs. The horse collapses and may go into convulsions before death.

Anaphylaxis can occur rapidly and progress to an irreversible condition within a few minutes. Hives is a precursor to angioedema which is a precursor to anaphylaxis, so it is important to summon a veterinarian if a horse has hives. There is not always the luxury of seeing an allergic response before it becomes a death warrant to a horse. If a horse's specific drug allergy is not known, accidental administration of an offending medication can cause immediate disaster.

Preventing Hives

When buying a horse, question the seller about previous allergic responses the horse may have experienced. Inform the veterinarian, trainer and stable manager about these allergies. A big sign written in red should be placed outside the horse's stall describing known allergies.

Determining the Cause of Hives

If a horse erupts in hives, discontinue new medications or food supplements immediately. To determine if the hives is a result of a food allergy, change the grain and hay ration for at least 2 weeks. Slow 'introduction' of an original feed may stimulate reappearance of the hives, which will determine the food that sparks an

Allergies and Their Symptoms	
HIVES	Small, elevated, flat-topped lumps that grow together into large lumps. Appear first on the neck, shoulders and thorax, eventually spreading to the entire body, especially the upper hind legs.
Ehrlichia equi	'Target' lesions, with fever, depression, weakness, poor motor coordination.
Purpura Haemorrhagica	Stiffness, stocking up, then oedema extends to the belly and prepuce, until the skin oozes fluid. Hives on the entire body, with blood spots on mucous membranes.
Angioedema	Hives are firm, the head and respiratory tract swell and breathing is difficult.

Fig. 15.23

allergic response.

If hives occur as an isolated incident, the cause may never be discovered. However, if hives is a recurrent problem, tracking down the source includes intradermal skin testing for pollen (plants, bushes and trees), moulds, grasses, weeds, dust and farm plants such as maize, oats, wheat and mustard.

Most horses affected with a case of hives usually recover uneventfully with little cause for concern. Pay attention to recent changes in diet, environment, medications, vaccinations, or stress factors that may cause the immune system to overreact.

SKIN GROWTHS

Skin growths are a form of cancer, and may be either *benign* or *malignant*. Benign means the growth is of only cosmetic significance and it does not spread to other organs. Rarely, skin growths become malignant, which means the cancer spreads to internal organs. Cancers of the skin are rarely life-threatening in horses as they are in dogs or people, but skin growths do detract from a horse's appearance. However, any skin growth that appears suddenly or enlarges rapidly should be examined by a veterinarian.

Sarcoids

One of the common skin growths found on horses is the *sarcoid*. It is a benign tumour unique to equine skin. The term 'tumous' is misleading since a sarcoid growth is usually localized to a small area and does not invade underlying tissues or lymphatic vessels. Unlike malignant and life-threatening growths, sarcoids do not spread to internal organs. They remain an external, cosmetic blemish, but may occasionally interfere with tack or skin mobility and if traumatized a sarcoid can become ulcerated or infected. Over 50% of horses with a single sarcoid ultimately develop multiple sarcoids.

Sarcoids are thought to develop from an infective virus that enters a break in the skin, or as a transformation of cell components in an abnormal response to trauma. Areas of skin subjected to trauma are predisposed to sarcoids. These tumours can be transmitted from one part of a horse to another by biting, rubbing or contaminated tack.

Almost half of all sarcoids are found on a horse's limbs, while 32% are located on the head and neck, especially the ears, eyelids and mouth. Other locations for sarcoids include the chest and trunk, the abdomen and flank and the prepuce.

Verrucous Sarcoids

Verrucous sarcoids are wart-like, dry, horny masses, resembling a cauliflower. They are usually less than $2\frac{1}{2}$ inches in diameter. Verrucous sarcoids can appear spontaneously without any prior trauma or wound of the skin. They are difficult to distinguish from warts except that verrucous sarcoids tend to lack hair, partially or totally, while warts have hair growing up to the edges and often regress spontaneously. Verrucous sarcoids do not regress as do warts.

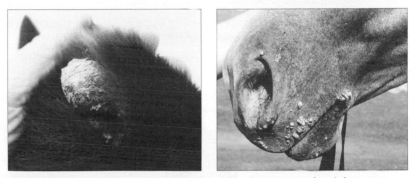

Fig. 15.24 On the left, a verrucous sarcoid in the ear. On the right, warts.

Warts

Warts are usually seen in young horses under 2 years old, particularly around the muzzle, but they can also appear on the legs, prepuce, ears or abdomen.

Fibroblastic Sarcoids

If a verrucous sarcoid is traumatized, it can develop into a *fibroblastic sarcoid*. Fibroblastic sarcoids often develop subsequent to a wound, and are difficult to distinguish from normal granulation tissue. These masses are like proud flesh, and may enlarge and expand to greater than 10 inches in diameter. A fibroblastic sarcoid may remain as a small lesion for years, and then suddenly erupt into a nasty-looking sore. Or, it can start as a rapidly and aggressively growing tumour. A wound that refuses to heal and is repeatedly ulcerated and infected may actually be a fibroblastic tumour.

Mixed Sarcoid

Both the verrucous or fibroblastic types are further classified as broad-based (sessile), or with a stalk (pedunculated). A mixture of verrucous and fibroblastic forms represents the third type, a *mixed sarcoid.*

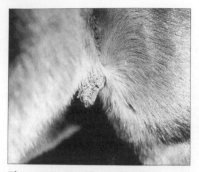

Fig. 15.25 A pedunculated sarcoid on the flank.

Occult Sarcoid

Flat tumours represent the fourth type, the *occult sarcoids*. They are usually flat or very slightly raised, the skin is thickened, and the surface roughened. They may even resemble ringworm, or skin crusting from a bacterial infection or poor skin health. Occult sarcoids typically appear around the head, especially the ears and eyelids. If aggravated by a surgical biopsy, they may revert to the fibroblastic form. Rubbing or traumatizing an occult sarcoid can also stimulate conversion to a fibroblastic sarcoid.

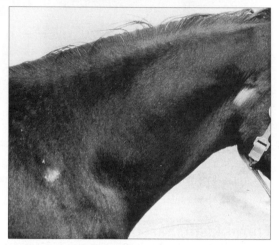

Fig. 15.26 Occult sarcoids are often found on the neck.

Recognizing Sarcoids

It is virtually impossible to determine the exact nature of a growth based on appearance. Fibrosarcomas, neurofibromas, neurofibrosarcomas, and squamous cell carcinomas are all malignant tumour types easily confused with a sarcoid. Fibromas, although mistaken for sarcoids, easily shell out and are well defined, while a sarcoid infiltrates around its margins, without a neat border. Summer sores caused by *Habronema* fly larvae also develop ulcerated masses not readily distinguishable from sarcoids. Keloids are made of collagenous, connective tissue that may resemble a sarcoid.

Often, it is difficult to identify the exact nature of a growth without a complete or partial biopsy of the enlargement. The biopsy will show any abnormal cells. However, a biopsy or surgery may stimulate an occult sarcoid to revert to the fibroblastic form, therefore occult sarcoids should be left alone.

Treating Sarcoids

Unless a sarcoid obstructs performance or tack or is an ugly and ulcerated mass, or its location causes a horse to become head-shy, it is best to leave it alone. Carefully monitor the sarcoid for any growth or change.

If treatment is necessary, various techniques are available for different types and locations of sarcoid tumour. The most difficult sarcoids to remove are those on the limbs. If multiple sarcoids are present, a complete cure is less likely.

Along with a treatment, most of a growth must be surgically removed. With surgery alone, 50% recur within 3 years, often within 6 months. By combining surgery with another treatment, such as cryosurgery, immunotherapy or hyperthermia, greater success may be achieved.

Cryosurgery

The most successful therapy to use along with surgical removal is *cryosurgery*. It is up to 80% effective if performed correctly. The lesion is frozen rapidly to –20° C and then allowed to thaw slowly to room temperature, whereupon it is refrozen, followed by a slow thaw. It may even be frozen a third time.

Before a cryosurgical site has healed, it normally develops a noticeable inflammatory reaction with swelling, oedema and discharge. This reaction may last for a week. Complete healing may take up to 2 months for the body to reject all the dead tumour tissue.

Drawbacks

Although cryosurgery is a preferred treatment, it does have some drawbacks. It is not useful in locations around the head and ears, the eyelids, thin-skinned areas directly over a protuberant bone such as the hip, or points on the lower limbs over joints. In these locations, there is risk of injuring tissue beneath the sarcoid with freezing.

Usually, scarring is minimal. The area loses hair colour due to hair follicle and pigment-producing cell *(melanocyte)* destruction by freezing.

Immunotherapy

An alternative treatment is *immunotherapy*. The success of immunotherapy demonstrates that the health of the immune system plays a large role in the development and regression of the sarcoid tumour. Two different methods of immunotherapy have been used, BCG injection and sarcoid tissue insertion.

BCG Injections

The first and most successful treatment involves a tuberculosis vaccine called Bacillus Calmette-Guerin, or BCG. BCG is made from the cell wall of the organism which causes tuberculosis, the *Mycobacterium*. Success depends on the horse's ability to develop a delayed hypersensitivity response to activate the cellular immune system.

BCG mobilizes specialized white blood cells that 'reject' a sarcoid, much as bacteria and viruses are rejected from the body. It is injected directly into a tumour. The normal immune response removes this foreign protein while at the same time recognizing the tumour cells as foreign. Tumour cells are then destroyed.

Following injection of BCG, a local inflammatory reaction and swelling occur within the first 24 – 48 hours. Sites of BCG injection usually worsen before they improve. To achieve adequate regression of a tumour, three to six injections of BCG are required at 2 – 3 week intervals. BCG injection of a head or ear sarcoid may also stimulate regression of other sarcoids on the legs or flank.

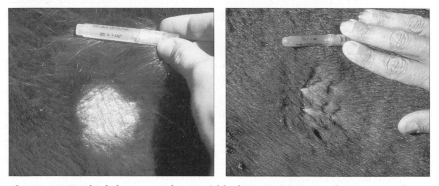

Fig. 15.27 On the left, an occult sarcoid before BCG immunotherapy. On the right, the same sarcoid after four BCG injections.

BCG is best applied to tumours less than 2½ inches in diameter. With multiple or excessively large lesions, injecting excessive amounts of BCG vaccine may be necessary to achieve the desired results. These excessive amounts can cause adverse systemic reactions, such as hives or anaphylaxis. Current products of BCG on the market are highly purified protein derivatives of tuberculosis bacteria. Purification decreases the risk of adverse systemic reactions.

Success rates of 50–80% are achieved with BCG application combined with surgical removal. Over 90% of flat sarcoids on the head or neck regress with BCG therapy.

Sarcoid Tissue Insertion

Another way to stimulate an immunotherapeutic response is to implant match-size slivers of sarcoid tissue just under the skin of the neck. These slivers should be frozen before implantation to prevent new sarcoid formation at an implant site. This method typically takes 6 months to achieve sarcoid regression.

Hyperthermia

A less common therapy for sarcoids is *hyperthermia,* which uses a radio-frequency current to heat the tissue to 50° C for about 30 seconds. This technique may be repeated up to four times at 1 – 2 week intervals, depending on the size of the tumour. A cosmetic advantage of hyperthermia is that the hair follicles remain functional after treatment, and a natural hair colour grows back.

In general, sarcoids do not pose a major health hazard to a horse. Because it is a common ailment of the equine skin, monitor any skin growths so benign tumours can be differentiated from dangerous ones.

Melanomas

As horses tend to live outside under all sorts of conditions, skin pigmentation is advantageous to their survival. Melanin is a substance produced by pigment-secreting skin glands; it protects against 'sunburn' of the skin from ultraviolet radiation. Horses with black hides are rarely bothered by the sunlight. However, black skin can harbour a tumour of abnormal pigment-producing cells *(melanoblasts).* The tumour, called a *melanoma,* forms when melanoblasts increase their metabolism and reproduce in localized areas of the skin. The black skin of a grey horse with excessive skin pigment can develop melanomas.

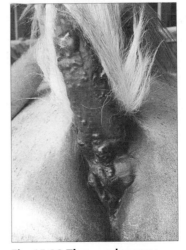

Of grey horses over 15 years old, 80% ultimately develop some form of melanoma. Most melanomas begin as slow-growing, encapsulated, and relatively benign growths. The tumours develop just under or above the skin with hair

Fig. 15.28 These melanomas may or may not be malignant.

at first obscuring them until they become large enough to be visible. It can take years (as long as 10 – 20) for a melanoma to become hyperactive to the point of concern. Once a melanoma displays an accelerated growth rate, the malignant cells rapidly invade surrounding tissue.

Tissue around the tumour cannot keep pace with the consumptive tumuor cells so tissue dies and ulcerates. Then the horse has bleeding or infected skin sores that fail to heal. Surrounding normal tissue may be displaced or replaced with the invasive melanoma.

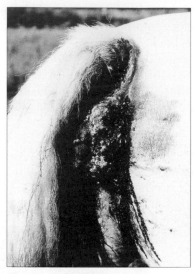

Fig. 15.29 A melanoma can grow to severe proportions.

Location of Growth

Melanomas develop around the anus, tailhead, vulva or prepuce, and occasionally are found around the parotid salivary gland, head and neck. However, they can be found anywhere on the body, with a rare report of location within a hoof.

Normally, melanomas take a long time to spread to internal body organs, such as the spleen and lungs. It usually takes years to wreak detrimental changes on the body and metabolism. It is not usually life-threatening, but when a tumour rapidly invades tissue around the anus or urinary tract it may interfere with a horse's quality of life. In these cases, the humane option is to euthanaze the horse to end pain and discomfort caused by ulcerated skin masses or obstructed bowels.

Treating Melanoma

If the tumours are isolated and single, it is advisable to leave them alone. Treatment by surgical removal tends to 'anger' the skin. Not only do many of the tumours regrow, but they become more aggressive than before. Multiple melanomas spread over much of the body are not only a cosmetic problem. These melanomas are difficult to manage if they interfere with saddling or with the ability of a mare to breed or foal without discomfort.

Cimetidine

A new form of chemotherapy offers an exciting possibility for treatment of melanomas. The oral drug cimetidine (Tagamet®), commonly used for treating stomach ulcers, has successfully stimulated remission of melanomas in horses. The medication can be used by itself or along with surgical removal to halt progression or recurrence of melanomas.

Method of Action

It is thought that cimetidine modifies the immune system to control the cancer. Under normal circumstances, white blood cells called *suppressor T-cells* stop the attack of other white blood cells once an infection or 'foreign' protein is defeated. This cellular check-and-balance system prevents an immune response from raging out of control. Cancer patients have an excessive number of suppressor T-cells that suppress the anti-tumour defence mechanism.

Squamous Cell Carcinomas

Horses with too little pigment in their skin can also develop skin cancer. *Squamous cell carcinomas* are cauliflower-like growths that tend to be ulcerated and bleed easily. They occasionally spread to other organs, like the lymph nodes. Pink-skinned horses, such as Appaloosas and Paints, are predisposed to squamous cell carcinoma around mucous membranes where there are no hair and no melanocytes to protect the skin from ultraviolet rays.

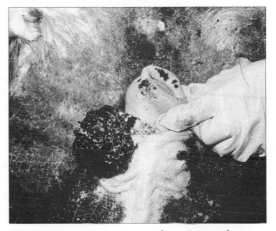

Fig. 15.30 Squames commonly occur on the prepuce.

'Squames' mostly occur around the anus, vulva, prepuce or eyes of pink-skinned horses. Ultraviolet radiation may cause normal cells to change into tumorous cells, but squamous cell carcinoma also develops in areas never exposed to the sun.

The only cure is surgical removal, or cryotherapy (freezing the tissue). Horses with pink skin around the eyes may benefit from fly face

Skin Growths and Their Symptoms	
WARTS (papillomatosis)	Highly infectious viral skin disease of horses up to 3–4 years of age. Most slough in 3–4 weeks of reaching maturity but treatment may be necessary if fly-strike and secondary infection.
SARCOIDS	Non-malignant. Appear on the limbs, head, ears, eyelids, mouth, neck, chest, trunk, abdomen, flank, and prepuce.
Verrucous	Dry, horny, wart-like, hairless, cauliflower growths.
Fibroblastic	Lesions resembling proud flesh, growing to greater than 10 inches in diameter.
Mixed	Mixture of verrucous and fibroblastic sarcoids.
Occult	Flat or slightly raised, thick, rough lesions.
MELANOMAS	Benign or malignant, slow-growing, encapsulated just under or above the skin surface. Appear around the anus, vulva or prepuce, parotid salivary gland, head and neck.
SQUAMOUS CELL CARCINOMAS	Cauliflower-like growth on pink skin, appearing around the anus, vulva or prepuce and eyes.

Fig. 15.31

masks to reduce the penetration of ultraviolet radiation. These mosquito-netted masks can reduce ultraviolet rays by 70%. Zinc oxide or sun-blocking agents can be applied to the face, reducing sunburn that may ultimately create tumours on the lips or muzzle.

DIAGNOSING SKIN DISEASES

In the field of veterinary dermatology sometimes the disease cannot be positively identified, but rarely are skin diseases life-threatening. When a blemish is discovered, it is best to get veterinary advice for rapid treatment. Diagnosis of any skin disease requires more investigation than a simple glance. Try to identify the type of lesion found.

- How many are there, and how big are they?
- On which parts of the body are they found?
- Is the skin scaly or scabby or crusty?
- Are the hairs broken, or do they pull out readily?
- Do the hairs mat together?

- Is there hair at all?
- Is there a firm nodule, or a soft swelling?
- Is there any redness?
- Is there a lack of colour?
- Is the affected area moist or dry?
- Is the skin of normal texture, or thickness?
- Is there granular material? What colour is it?
- Does the horse itch and scratch?
- Are the areas sensitive when touched or pressed?

Consider also whether the horse is pastured or stalled, what sort of diet or medication it may have received, and its age and breed. By examining the horse carefully, and noting these particulars on the checklist, an owner or trainer can help portray a clinical picture to a veterinarian about the progression of a skin problem.

A careful veterinary examination combined with further diagnostic aids facilitates a rapid diagnosis of the skin problem. To track down the source of a skin malady the veterinarian may take skin scrapings for microscopic examination to identify mites and ticks, cultures and antibiotic sensitivities to define bacterial infections and specific treatment, fungal cultures to identify ringworm, and skin biopsies to identify *Onchocerca*, summer sores, or allergic reactions.

See that manure and soiled bedding are removed to reduce breeding grounds for flies. Deworm regularly to reduce internal parasites, such as pinworms, bots and stomach worms that could infect a horse's skin.

Keep brushes and tack separate for each horse so a communicable disease will not reach epidemic proportions if transferred from horse to horse. In summer, bathing with insecticide shampoos not only deters bites and skin irritation, but removes dirt and sweat from the skin, allowing the coat to bloom and shine. Massage from currying, brushing, and shampoos enhances the lustre of the coat.

SADDLE SORES

Sometimes it is hard to detect problems that occur with saddle fit until an obvious soreness or wound develops. Not all horses provide clues that tack is ill-fitting. If a horse shows progressively poor behaviour such as tail wringing, back humping, crankiness, or sluggishness when asked to move forward, look for saddle problems. Some self-preserving individuals have less subtle behaviour changes. They stop in their tracks, refusing to move until an offending article is removed.

Even with a custom-fit saddle, problems can arise. Uphills and downhills in steep terrain cause a saddle or girth to shift, creating friction points. Changes in physique accompany changing seasons. A summer fat or winter lean frame changes saddle fit.

A tired horse may subtly alter its gait. Then, imperfectly fitting tack chafes in unlikely places.

Different breeds of horses are prone to saddle sores. Thoroughbreds are known for their thin, tender skin. Thin-skinned Arabians are also at greater risk of saddle sores.

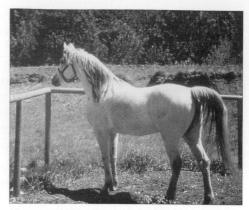

Fig. 15.32 Thin-skinned Arabians are prone to saddle sores.

Signs of Saddle Sores

There is no substitute for well-fitted equipment and diligent monitoring for problem spots. Signs of impending saddle sores include subtle behavioural changes, and raised swollen areas of the skin. Swelling is caused by a serum leak beneath the skin, along with oedema due to poor circulation beneath a pressure or friction point. These spots are often tender to finger pressure, and are red, inflamed or ulcerated.

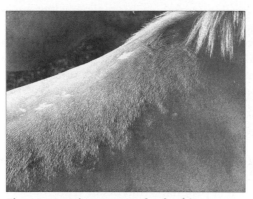

Fig. 15.33 Hair may grow back white on a coloured horse and black on a grey horse.

Other warning signs are isolated spots of missing hair with a pinkish tinge to the skin, indicating mild abrasion at a friction point. Note isolated dry areas under the saddle after a workout. Dry heat builds under pressure points where the skin cannot sweat and breathe.

Hair follicles and pigment-producing cells (melanocytes) may succumb to localized heat production, resulting in growth of black hairs on a grey horse, or white hairs on any other coloured horse. This destruction of melanocytes results not only from heat injury to the skin, but from any form of physical trauma.

If sweat and caked-on mud remain on a horse after a workout, they irritate the skin, creating conditions that favour bacteria. Commonly, staphylococcal organisms that normally live on the skin invade irritated tissues. Initially, a small nodule is felt. The nodule develops into a painful pustule that ruptures.

Leaking pus and serous material form small crusts and scabs, further matting down the hair. Low grade bacterial infections are easily avoided by rinsing hair and skin after a workout to remove accumulated sweat and debris.

Preventing Saddle Sores

To prevent saddle sores, many factors should be considered, including selecting the right saddle and accessories, and grooming and stretching the horse. Also, rider expertise is important. When a horse carries an unbalanced rider, the tack should be checked frequently. A rider sitting off centre may grip more with one side of the body than another, or may dig in with calves or heels. Sores may be found under the leg skirts or stirrup leathers.

Selecting the Proper Saddle

The type of athletics pursued is critical when selecting a saddle. Using a dressage saddle on a long distance horse invites problems with sore backs, for both horse and rider. When a horse is working hard for many hours, a heavy saddle also contributes to heat build-up.

Grooming

Before saddling, carefully curry and brush the horse so grit does not embed in the skin. Dirt particles abrade protective hair from the skin, contributing to skin chafe. Saddle pads should be cleaned of matted hair and sweat-caked dirt before the next use, so no friction points develop under the saddle.

Saddle Pads

Moisture and salts from sweat need to be removed from the skin by an absorbent saddle pad that can breathe and release accumulated moisture. Wool has always been a favoured material for this purpose.

Saddle pads should be uniformly thick and smoothed out so there is no material bunching up. When saddling, put the saddle pad on the horse's neck, and slide it backwards into position in the same direction that the hairs lie. This method flattens the hairs beneath the pad. Saddle pads should not be used to compensate for a poor saddle fit.

Sacks

A simple trick prevents saddle sores from developing. Jute sacks serve as girth sleeves, saddle pads or as padding over hobbles. The sack material is absorbent and soft and breathes, making it an excellent way to prevent a mild chafe from worsening.

Stretching the Legs

Some horses develop fat rolls or loose skin around the girth area. Once the saddle is on and the girth tightened, pick up each forelimb and stretch it forwards to relieve pinching of loose skin rolls.

Girth Sleeves

Fleece-like girth sleeves can be fitted over an English or Western girth to absorb moisture and prevent pinching of the skin between the elbows and the girth. Cord girths configure more exactly to skin contours as a horse moves, and an English figure-eight girth also conforms better than a straight piece of leather.

Rubberized, elastic pieces at the top of an English girth connect to the billets to allow greater flexibility in the girth. Flexibility is helpful for a horse that negotiates trails and hilly terrain. Elasticized rubber gives as the abdomen and thorax expand when a horse travels uphill. The horse breathes better, and saddle sores are avoided.

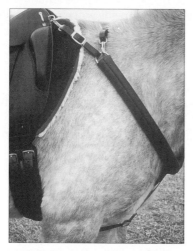

Fig. 15.34 Neoprene breast plate and girth.

Neoprene Equipment

Recently, tack has been made of rubber neoprene to prevent chafing in areas commonly rubbed by conventional equipment. Neoprene breastplates and girth covers are used for horses worked under saddle for many hours. The skin beneath the neoprene does not overheat from contact with the equipment. Neoprene tack slides over sweaty skin and fur with ease. Cleaning neoprene tack is a horse owner's dream — it is hosed off after each use to remove sweat and mud, and hung up to dry.

Healing Saddle Sores

Most superficial skin abrasions heal rapidly within 10 – 21 days provided reinjury does not occur. If a girth or saddle sore is discovered and treated immediately, it remains only in the outermost tissue layers, capable of healing in 1 – 2 weeks. If deeper tissues are injured, the wound may not fully heal for up to 3 – 6 weeks.

Cleansing the wound with a dilute tamed iodine/salt water solution removes superficial bacteria. The wound should be softened with an antiseptic ointment, and the scab removed daily, or bacteria trapped beneath the scab will reproduce in a moist, warm environment. Use of a low pH cream, such as Dermisol®, is also effective.

The main objective in encouraging healing is to prevent further trauma to the area. The saddle should be locked in the tack room, and not brought out again until the wound is healed. In a mild case, a doughnut shape can be cut out of a thick foam or felt pad to prevent saddle contact. Any pressure around a sore limits the circulation necessary for wound healing.

16

WOUND MANAGEMENT

Of all the medical incidents with which a horse owner or trainer is confronted, the most common are skin wounds. In most instances, a veterinarian is not present at the time of injury, and hours may pass before a veterinarian is summoned and can arrive.

INITIAL TREATMENT

Initial treatment greatly influences the outcome and duration of wound healing. Many people assume that applying a topical salve is sufficient while waiting for the veterinarian, but this erroneous notion can do more harm than good.

When the protective skin layer is broken open, environmental and skin contaminants are introduced into the wound along with dirt, gravel, and foreign materials such as wood, paint or hay. Certain soils, clay, and organic matter inhibit the immune action of white blood cells, antibodies, and antibiotics, and also interfere with the normal antibacterial activity of serum. A wound should be cleansed of all foreign material as rapidly as possible to prevent bacteria from gaining a foothold and deeply invading the tissue. Normal immune mechanisms at a local tissue level effectively deal with up to 1 million bacteria per gram of tissue. More than 1 million per gram will overwhelm the immune system, creating infection. Antiseptic ointments, creams or sprays cannot reach deep into a wound if devitalized tissue and foreign debris obscure it. It is better to wash the wound with warm salt water, if available. If the wound is clean and likely to become soiled on the way home, apply a dressing before moving the horse.

Debridement

Once the skin surface is broken and the underlying tissues have lost their protective barrier to bacterial invasion, wound margins are colonized with bacteria within 2 – 4 hours after injury.

A wound that has been present for more than 1 – 3 hours is probably already so contaminated that a topical antibiotic does little to fend off infection. Extensive cleansing and *debridement* (cutting away devitalized tissue with scissors or a scalpel) of the wound is necessary for successful treatment.

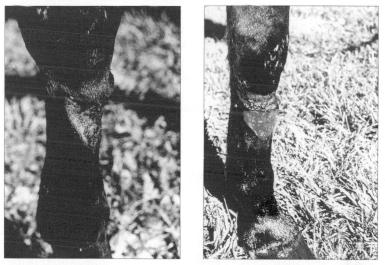

Fig. 16.1 On the left, a non-healing wound. On the right, the same wound after debridement, which will allow the wound to heal.

Hose the wound for 5 or 10 minutes while waiting for the veterinarian to arrive. Gentle water pressure mechanically loosens debris and grit that has adhered to the area. This action substantially reduces the numbers of contaminating bacteria at the wound site.

Shaving

If possible, hair should be removed from the edges of a wound to prevent it from acting like a foreign body or harbouring bacteria or dirt. Hair obscures drainage, and prevents thorough examination of the extent of the wound. Before shaving, cover the wound with a water-soluble, sterile K-Y® lubricating jelly or moist gauze sponges to prevent shaved hairs from falling into the wound.

Cleaning Compounds

While certain compounds are beneficial to healing, others are useless as antiseptics. Some may even slow healing by irritating the wound or causing cell death.

It is best to use a mild salt solution when scrubbing equine tissue. Plain tap water is better than distilled water, but both of these salt-free solutions have a lower electrolyte content than the wound tissues. Consequently, the tissue will 'drink up' the salt-free water. The cells swell, contributing to localized oedema and cell death.

If physiological sterile saline or Lactated Ringer's solution is unavailable, a home-made salt solution can be made to wash the wound. To approximate the physiological salt content of a horse's tissues, dissolve ½ tablespoon of table salt into 1 litre of water. Add an antiseptic to the solution, such as povidone-iodine (Betadine®) or chlorhexidine (Hibitane®).

Correct dilution is essential to avoid furthur damage to wound edges.

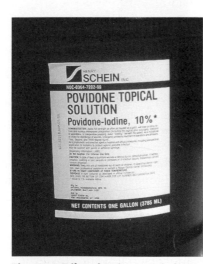

Fig. 16.2 Diluted PI is a good cleaning compound.

Povidone-Iodine

To commercially make povidone-iodine of a 0.5% preparation, tincture of iodine (7%) is combined with a polyvinyl substance to decrease staining, stabilize the iodine, and reduce its irritability to tissues. Tincture of iodine is an excellent antibacterial agent, but it is **too strong** for wound cleansing.

To make a scrub for wound cleansing, povidone-iodine (PI) solution is added to the salt water to a concentration that visually approximates weak tea. To achieve this concentration, add 10 millilitres (ml) or less of the PI solution to 1 litre of salt solution. For the horse, the best antibacterial and least tissue-toxic effect of PI occurs at concentrations of less than 1%. At a low concentration of less than 0.03%, white blood cells of the immune response are stimulated to migrate to the wound to perform their clean-up function. Conversely, at concentrations of 5–10%, iodine dramatically hinders the immune function of white blood cells, increasing a wound's susceptibility to infection.

The antibacterial activity of PI lasts for only 4 – 6 hours in the wound without any residual effect. Because a horse is so large, absorption of iodine into the body is insignificant. However, humans, who must frequently apply this solution should wear rubber gloves to avoid absorbing iodine in toxic amounts.

Chlorhexidine

Chlorhexidine (Hibitane®) is an excellent cleaning solution, effective against bacteria, viruses and fungi. An ideal concentration of 0.05% for wound cleansing is prepared by mixing 25 ml with 1 litre of salt water, or 1:40 dilution. Not only does chlorhexidine work against a broad spectrum (many kinds) of bacteria, but its effects persist in the tissues because it binds to skin proteins. Therefore, its antibacterial effects outlast those of PI.

Both PI and chlorhexidine are available as antiseptic scrubs, and should be diluted with a salt water mixture when scrubbing the wound. Adequate rinsing removes sudsy cleanser from the wound once it has been thoroughly cleaned and investigated.

Ideally, anything that is put into a wound should be so mild that if it were instilled into the eye it would not irritate mucous membranes or the eye itself. Following this principle avoids trouble.

Compounds That Slow Healing

Using other types of soaps in a wound slows healing and increases the susceptibility of a wound to infection. Detergents and soaps are toxic to the cells, causing them to swell and break which adds to devitalized tissue. Only wound-specific, soapy antiseptics should be applied to equine tissue, such as chlorhexidine scrub or PI scrub. If these are unavailable, Phisohex® soap (containing chlorhexidine) can be used with ample rinsing.

Tincture of Iodine

Tincture of iodine (7%) is a strong antibacterial agent. However, it is so destructive to tissue that the only safe application is to the soles and frogs, to control thrush or toughen the feet. It should not be applied to intact skin because it will irritate, causing a rash or skin inflammation. Healing tissues are also negatively affected by tincture of iodine.

Hydrogen Peroxide

People commonly pour 3% hydrogen peroxide into a wound. Peroxide is useful on human skin for wounds with *anaerobic* (oxygen-free) bacterial growth, because the foaming action increases the oxygen tension in a wound, which destroys anaerobic bacteria. However, hydrogen peroxide is toxic to equine cells, especially to migrating fibroblasts that produce collagen to repair a wound. Peroxide also causes blood clots in microvessels, interfering with oxygen supply to the tissues. Reduced oxygen results in more devitalized tissue, and delayed healing. Hydrogen peroxide should be reserved only for cleaning off blood that has splattered the hair *below* a wound.

Alcohol

Alcohol (isopropyl or rubbing) should never be applied to open wounds because it destroys protein in the open tissues. It can be used to wipe *around* a wound perimeter to loosen debris, but should not contact open skin.

Evaluation

While scrubbing, evaluate the wound and determine its depth and seriousness. It is possible for soft tissue planes to separate, leading into a tunnel much like a puncture wound. Sometimes these 'punctures' pass unnoticed at the time of the injury unless veterinary care is obtained.

Exudate

Initial examination of a wound identifies its smell, if any, and the amount and character of the discharge *(exudate)*. The exudate may be nothing more than shedding dead and dying tissue, and white blood cells. It does not necessarily include bacteria. However, an odd or foul odour or a large amount of exudate is highly suspect of infection and requires immediate veterinary care.

A veterinarian should be summoned for such wounds, or if a wound is deeper than a superficial laceration. Foreign bodies in the wound need to be extracted, and skin flaps removed or sutured by the veterinarian to maintain adequate blood supply.

Once a wound has been scrubbed and debrided to healthy-looking tissue, the next step is to maintain it in a moist and clean environment. Appropriate antiseptic ointments and bandages promote tissue healing.

PROMOTING WOUND HEALING

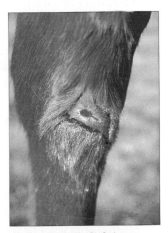

Healing begins with fibrous connective tissue collagen, or fibrin strands, which are made of proteins. *Fibroblasts*, which manufacture the fibrin, migrate into the wound by the third day. Budding blood vessels appear after the fibroblasts.

As *granulation tissue* (made of capillaries and fibroblasts) fills in the wound, it provides a surface along which *epithelial cells* (new skin cells) will migrate. Regrowth of skin between the wound margins is called *epithelialization*. Not only does bacteria slow healing, but it produces potent enzymes that destroy fragile and newly formed skin cells.

Fig. 16.3 Epithelial tissue surrounds the granulation tissue in the middle.

Contraction

Wound size reduces through a process known as *contraction*. Adjacent, full-thickness skin at the wound margins is pulled in towards the centre of a wound by the action of *myofibroblast cells* (specialized cells that convert from fibroblasts to act like muscle cells).

In a chronic wound, granulation tissue consists more of fibrous connective tissue, and is relatively sparse in myofibroblasts. Debulking with a scalpel removes a stagnant granulation bed, or proud flesh. Fresh tissue replaces it, including myofibroblasts capable of reducing wound size over time.

Factors Affecting Contraction Rate

Contraction rates of 0.2 millimetres per day during the first few months can only reduce a scar to half the original size. Continued remodelling of a scar over the next 6 – 12 months further reduces its size.

Skin Tension

The size of a wound does not affect contraction rate, but skin tension does. Lower leg wounds tend to have taut skin edges and contract slowly. Also, dry wounds are tighter and therefore contract slower than moist wounds.

Any excess tension, oedema, or movement of a wound interferes with function of the myofibroblasts. Then, contraction is limited, and may cease prematurely before the wound edges meet. A water-soluble dressing with a pressure bandage (such as a modified Robert–Jones bandage) should be applied while waiting for veterinary attention. This will help to control any bleeding, reduce swelling and keep the wound edges together.

Hydration and Warmth

Because the mammalian body is made of almost 70% water, skin dehydrates if a wound is left open to the air. Dehydrated tissue eventually becomes devitalized tissue and compromises healing.

The skin on the lower limbs of a horse inherently lacks blood supply and warmth as compared with the skin of humans or many other animal species. For the processes of skin repair and wound closure to advance, a wound needs to be maintained in a warm, moist environment, especially during the early stages of tissue repair.

The length of time from when the injury occurred to when it receives professional attention affects the extent of tissue dehydration and onset of infection. While awaiting professional medical evaluation, apply a water-soluble dressing and a light bandage to the cleaned wound to limit tissue dehydration. A bandage maintains a moist environment and retains a moderate amount of body heat at the wound site; both features enhance the early stages of healing.

Sutures

Since initial evaluation of a wound does not always determine if it can be surgically repaired and sutured, assume that it will be sutured, and proceed accordingly. If a wound is to be sutured, no ointments, sprays or creams should be applied. Medications that are not water-soluble stick to the tissue, preventing the edges from touching when they are stitched together. Insoluble substances are also difficult to remove from the deeper tissues of a wound, which interferes with how well a suture will hold. The decision to stitch a wound depends on:

- location of the wound
- skin tension at that site
- configuration of the wound
- degree of tissue damage
- tissue contamination

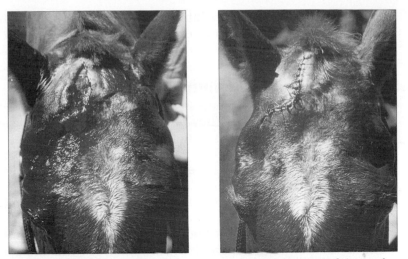

Fig. 16.4 On the left, a clean, shaven head wound before suturing. On the right, the wound after suturing.

Facial wounds or wounds on the torso respond well to suturing efforts even if discovered days after an injury. However, a limb wound may not be amenable to sutures even if evaluated within a few hours of injury.

Topical Ointments

No matter what is applied to an equine skin wound, little can be done to accelerate healing. However, the natural healing process can be delayed by infection or tissue dehydration.

Blunt trauma, such as a blow from a kick, fall or collision with a solid object, damages the surrounding tissues considerably, making the wound edges jagged. Such wounds are at significantly greater risk of infection due to compression of blood vessels, an increased area of devitalized tissue, swelling and oedema. They also do not suture well. All these factors contribute to an environment right for bacteria.

If a wound is so traumatic that suturing will not work, or so mild that veterinary care is not needed, topical ointments prevent a wound from drying out. Each veterinarian has his or her special recipe or topical medication for treating wounds.

Water-Soluble Ointments

Only water-soluble ointments should be applied to a wound that is to be sutured, or on open, contaminated wounds until the wound has filled in completely with granulation tissue.

373

The list of commercially available wound preparations is exhaustive and it is best to consult a veterinarian before applying them to a wound.

USP-Petrolatum-Based Ointments

Petrolatum-based ointments are used on the normal skin around a weeping wound. They protect the skin from skin scald, caused by the protein-rich serum that drains from a productive injury.

A variety of these products are available, yet when applied directly to a wound, certain topical ointments interfere with healing if their pH or ingredients are inappropriate. Their *antimicrobial* agent has little actual effect on wound healing, and the carrier base compound dramatically **slows** healing. Any product that contains a USP-petrolatum ingredient slows skin growth, and delays wound healing. It is best to use tissue-soluble compounds that are not lethal to the cells. Consider the chemical compositions of antibacterial ointments that are purchased at feed and tack stores. Those products with a USP-petrolatum ingredient irritate the tissue and slow healing.

Amount of Ointment

Only a very thin layer of antiseptic ointment is necessary to achieve the desired effect. Too much ointment has adverse effects, including:

- encouraging excessive exudate and wound debris by impairing normal drainage
- reducing air circulation to the tissues
- attracting dirt and soil to a wound, which negates all positive effects achieved by a previous scrubbing

Antiseptic powders or sprays also obstruct natural drainage, leading to accumulation of exudate. These substances dry out the skin margins, inhibiting normal skin cell growth.

Antibiotic Absorption

The penetration of antibiotics in a wound is influenced by different factors. Inflammation causes an increased blood supply. Increased circulation enhances antibiotic (both injected and topical) penetration to a wound site.

Dead and dying tissue and white blood cells cause an acidic pH in the wound site. The presence of pus and serum, along with an acidic pH inhibits the antimicrobial action of many antibiotics, such as the sulpha drugs. After healing begins, fibrin or blood clots in the wound further block antibiotic penetration.

Ointment Contamination

When using large jars of ointments, be careful not to contaminate them with dirt, hair and debris so bacteria are not placed into a wound. Use tongue depressors, clean rubber gloves, or gauze to remove medication from a jar, keeping the ointment clean for future use. Pay attention to the expiry dates on products containing antibiotics, and discard outdated ointments because time renders them ineffective.

Bandaging

A study done at the Kansas State College of Veterinary Medicine compared four types of treatment regimens on equine skin wounds.

- Group 1 received daily irrigation with physiological saline for the first 11 days, and then a 5-minute tap water lavage from day 12 on. No medication or bandage was applied to these horses.
- Group 2 received daily application of a nitrofurazone ointment only.
- Group 3 received nitrofurazone ointment plus a bandage.
- Group 4 received a bandage and the wound was lavaged with tap water every third day.

The results showed marked differences between treatment regimens. Wounds from Groups 1 and 2 formed hard, thick scabs that were persistently contaminated with dirt and bedding, resulting in increased inflammation of the wounds. In contrast, the bandaged wounds had less inflammation, less dehydration, and less contamination than the unbandaged wounds.

Healthy granulation tissue formed faster under a bandage, with those wounds healing faster (63 days) than the wounds left open to the air (96 days). Faster healing may have been caused by reduced contamination or inflammation in the earlier healing phases.

Yet, once the bandage was removed, the wounds from Groups 3 and 4 seemed prone to trauma and loosening of the fragile new skin. In the unbandaged wounds, the collagen organized faster than under a bandage, possibly due to tension forces in surrounding skin that resulted from mild dehydration by air exposure. Though the unbandaged wounds healed slower, they were not as prone to reinjury.

Despite these results, many bandaged wounds often progress faster and more successfully than wounds that are left open to the air. In many cases, healing progresses slowly without the protection and moisture-retention achieved from a bandage. Although more granulation tissue formed under bandages than on unbandaged legs, bandaged wounds had less scar tissue and an improved scar contraction.

Bandaging Recommendation

These results indicate a wound should be kept bandaged until an intact, healthy granulation bed is present. Once a layer of granulation tissue has filled in a wound, a bandage may do more harm than good by reducing oxygen to the wound, and by trapping an accumulation of inflammatory cells (pus). A lack of oxygen causes tissue to die. The dead tissue and an accumulation of pus leads to an acidic pH.

To counteract these conditions, a wound produces more capillary buds to compensate for an oxygen deficit, while fibroblasts are stimulated by the acid environment to produce more collagen. The result is production of proud flesh.

Benefits of Bandaging

Retaining Moisture

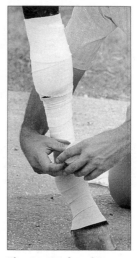

Covering a wound with a bandage reduces evaporative fluid loss from the surrounding and involved tissues. If a wound surface is moist and oxygen-rich, new skin growth proceeds at up to 0.2 mm per day on the lower limbs. On the torso, progress may be as rapid as 2 mm per day. If a wound dehydrates, the decreased circulation deprives the wound of the internal oxygen source. Then cellular migration proceeds at less than 0.1 mm per day in any area.

Bandaging does reduce the wound's uptake of atmospheric oxygen. But keeping the wound moist, and therefore allowing the circulation to flow freely, compensates for a relatively minor deprivation of atmospheric oxygen. Bandaging also helps a wound to absorb atmospheric oxygen.

Fig. 16.5 A bandage keeps a wound warm and moist.

Protection From Distortion

A bandage also provides a stable support for migration of new skin cells across a wound. Distortion of a wound surface due to excessive movement, oedema, or trauma disrupts myofibroblasts and epithelial cells that are moving across to bridge the gap. Collagen fibres and capillary buds are also broken by such distortions. A bandage protects a wound from further trauma and excessive movement and reduces oedema swelling. The slight pressure exerted by a bandage reduces the development of proud flesh, provided the bandage is not wrapped so tightly as to interfere with limb circulation.

Retaining Body Temperature

Temperatures of approximately 86° F promote wound healing, while temperatures less than 68° F result in a 20% reduction in tensile strength. Possibly, cooler temperature at a wound site constricts superficial vessels to the skin, resulting in reduced blood and oxygen supply to the wound and its healing connective tissue components. Applying an insulating bandage over a wound retains body temperature to provide the healing benefits of warmth.

Removing a Bandage

The appropriate time to stop bandaging is determined by examining the colour of the skin cells. While the newly formed skin is still a thin layer, there is an apparent colour difference between the thicker, outer margin and the thin skin layer covering the granulation bed. Once the skin has uniformly thickened, it is the same colour, indicating that it may be appropriate to remove the bandage.

Slow Healing

If a horse persists in traumatizing a wound, or a wound remains subject to irritation from manure, mud or flies, the protective wrap which allows healing to continue to completion, is repeatedly disturbed. This slows the healing process and allows the formation of granulation tissue which extends above the wound edges and is known as proud flesh. Healing ceases at this point, and the layer of proud flesh grows without restraint. In such cases, a light pressure bandage may temporarily stop the build-up of proud flesh. It may be helpful to use a padded pressure bandage to reduce the possibility of proud flesh. Use of a neck cradle may be necessary to stop a horse chewing bandages or even chewing wound edges.

Controlling Proud Flesh

Steroids

Corticosteroid added to a salve aids healing by controlling proud flesh. Steroids stabilize the release of enzymes from local white blood cells that begin an inflammatory response, therefore granulation tissue formation is slower. Also, corticosteroids inhibit new capillary growth, so by decreasing surface blood vessels granulation tissue production is reduced.

However, steroids inhibit skin cell growth and stop a healing process if applied for too long. Steroids should never be placed in a deep wound before the granulation bed has formed, because they depress normal function of the immune system and can promote infection.

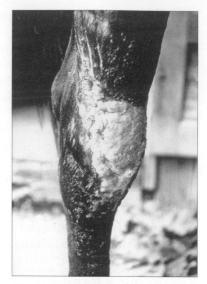

Fig. 16.6 Proud flesh formation.

Nitrofurazones

Certain compounds contribute to the formation of granulation tissue. Nitrofurazones, used on deep wounds, delay new skin growth by 30%. A thick scab forms over the wound surface, preventing healing from the 'inside out'. However, on superficial skin abrasions, nitrofurazones keep the skin moist and supple so hair quickly grows back.

Damaging Chemicals

Other substances have been used to stop development of proud flesh, such as copper sulphate, bleach, lye, and similar caustic chemicals. By chemically cauterizing proud flesh, they also damage the migrating skin cells, and ultimately slow healing if used to excess.

An old-time, but destructive 'remedy' applies a mixture of lye and bacon grease to wound surfaces. In principle, the salty bacon grease may 'pull' swelling from a wound, as would a poultice. Lye is destructive to bacteria, and grease keeps a wound soft and pliable. However,

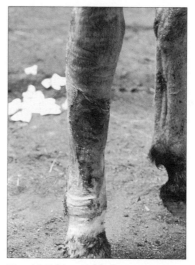

Fig. 16.7 Lye and bacon grease damage a wound.

lye is also toxic to fragile skin cells and deeper tissues. Too much salt dehydrates the tissues. Grease attracts dirt and grit to the wound surface. The result is a non-healing, open wound which develops profuse amounts of proud flesh.

Surgical Removal

It is better to surgically remove proud flesh than to resort to chemical irritants. Caustic substances cause tissue death, with redevelopment of proud flesh that persists as a non-healing, grotesque wound.

For a non-complicated wound that is clean and uninfected, healing proceeds in spite of our ministrations. In many cases, time and cleanliness are the best remedies.

Remodelling of the Tissue

The ultimate tensile strength of a wound allows tissue to sustain normal mechanical stress so it does not tear or break open. Complete remodelling and contraction of a scar from a skin injury occur rapidly for 3 – 6 months, the tissue reaching maximum tensile strength up to 1 year after injury. Collagen, rapidly manufactured by fibroblasts during the first 2 – 4 weeks, is responsible for tensile strength of a wound as it organizes. By 40 – 120 days, skin regains 50–70% of its original strength. Collagen continues to remodel for 1 – 2 years. Epithelial cells and fibroblasts produce enzymes to break down existing collagen. Newly deposited collagen fibrils more tightly interweave, with a corresponding increase in tensile strength and flattening of the scar.

Despite a horse's apparent tendency to self-destruct, regeneration and repair of skin wounds can return an injury to not quite, but almost, as good as new. Usually, wounds that do not penetrate all the way through the skin form tissue identical to the original skin, without scar formation. In actuality, however, large connective tissue and collagen components may not regrow to their original pattern. Although 'healed' epithelial tissue appears identical to original skin, the new connective tissue is functionally less efficient. Even under ideal conditions, the scar tissue ultimately remains 20% weaker than the original tissue.

Managing a skin wound with rapid and aggressive veterinary treatment significantly reduces the time required for healing. Risk of infection is diminished, and a wounded area heals with an acceptable cosmetic appearance and return to function.

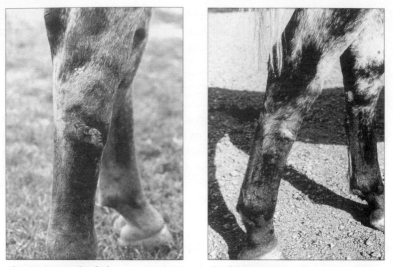

Fig. 16.8 On the left, a puncture wound which remained untreated for 10 days. On the right, the scar would be smaller if treatment had been sought immediately.

PUNCTURE WOUNDS

In the most carefully managed stabling operation, horses are often surrounded by man-made objects such as fences that splinter or crack, nails, gates, latches, stable tools and farm equipment. A horse can accidentally snag itself on any of these objects.

A superficial-appearing abrasion can disguise a deeper, penetrating hole through the skin. Long hairs, mud, and dirt can mask the extent of an injury.

Anaerobic Bacteria

If left unattended, puncture wounds have serious consequences, despite a mild appearance. Of the many kinds of bacteria introduced into a wound, the potentially life-threatening organisms include those that live in an environment lacking oxygen (anaerobic).

When the skin is punctured, germs are introduced beneath the flesh. The small portal of entry through the skin often seals over, providing an oxygen-depleted environment ideal for growth of anaerobic spores. As a wound festers, devitalized and dead tissue in the wound encourage the anaerobic bacteria to prosper.

Clostridium is one genus of anaerobic bacteria. With only 20 minutes, exposure to oxygen, these bacteria can be inactivated.

Clostridial bacteria are common inhabitants of the digestive tract. They are passed as spores into manure, soil and decomposing organic matter. The spores can survive in the soil for years, so any wound is at risk of contamination.

Tetanus

One of the most common anaerobic bacteria associated with equine pureture wounds is *Clostridium tetani*, the organism responsible for *tetanus*. In the decades before vaccines were available, tetanus infected an alarming number of horses, causing a prolonged and painful death.

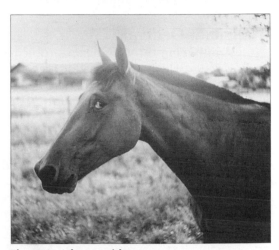

Fig. 16.9 A horse with tetanus.

As the tetanus bacterium dies, an *exotoxin* is released. The exotoxin reaches the brain through the bloodstream, or migrates up peripheral nerves to the central nervous system. It slows normal nerve transmission by preventing release of a chemical neuro-transmitter, *acetylcholine*, and by preventing release of an inhibitory transmitter, *glycine*, at the neuron. Rapid paralysis descends from head to toe.

Symptoms begin in the head and forequarters, as spastic contraction of skeletal muscle results in 'lockjaw'. Facial muscles become rigid. The horse cannot acquire, chew or swallow food. Nostrils flare, the third eyelid descends over the eye, and the ears remain rigid and upright due to persistent spasms of the facial muscles.

As exotoxin progressively paralyses the body, the horse assumes a stiff 'saw-horse' stance with legs extended. If the horse goes down, it is unable to rise due to the rigidity of legs and neck.

Afflicted animals arc hyper-responsive to external stimuli, especially noise, convulsing as muscles spasm and contract incessantly. Eventually, paralysis of the diaphragm or complications of aspiration pneumonia cause a horse to suffocate. Or, it may succumb to dehydration or malnutrition.

Today, such an unfortunate demise from a wound is rare. If a horse is injured and has not been on a regular immunization programme that includes a yearly booster of tetanus toxoid, it should receive prophylactic or preventative tetanus therapy. This tetanus antitoxin neutralizes exotoxin circulating outside the nervous system. If the horse has not received a tetanus toxoid booster in the past 8 – 12 months, boosting it stimulates sufficient immunity in the face of an increased risk.

Malignant Oedema

Another life-threatening anaerobic bacterium is *Clostridium septicum*, which is responsible for a syndrome known as *malignant oedema*. This organism produces a large amount of gas in muscles, creating a crackling feel *(crepitation)* beneath the skin over the wounded area. The wound site is hot and painful, and swollen with oedema and gas. An accompanying fever may spike to 106° F. Toxins released from the bacteria rapidly spread through the body, and are capable of killing a horse in less than 2 days.

Although infection with tetanus or malignant oedema is uncommon, such possibilities cannot be ignored. Penicillin injections kill anaerobic bacteria, and anti-tetanus prophylaxis protects the horse.

Treating Puncture Wounds

Initially, hair is clipped or shaved away from the wound edges so it will not interfere with healing. The puncture opening is then vigorously scrubbed with antiseptic to prepare for examination. Thorough wound cleansing prevents infection from contaminating organisms, removes devitalized tissue, and flushes away exudate that interferes with healing.

Puncture wounds are irrigated with antiseptic electrolyte solutions under mild pressure to loosen hair and dead tissue. It is important to cleanse wounds of soil particles, because certain soil types inhibit the immune response. Immediate veterinary attention is also essential for any puncture wound.

Evaluating the Wound

If it is difficult to see if the skin has been punctured, prepare the wound for further evaluation by scrubbing thoroughly around the injury so no contaminants will be carried into a deep wound. Gently insert an antiseptic-soaked cotton swab into the wound to see if a hole or pocket is present. Do not attempt to completely probe the hole with the cotton swab; cotton fibres or broken swabs discourage healing.

This procedure evaluates if a wound is more than a superficial abrasion. A veterinarian should be summoned if any swelling, pain or heat accompanies a wound. Because a hole is often too small to scrub deeper tissue, a small, seemingly superficial wound may require professional care.

A puncture into a joint, tendon sheath or bone requires immediate professional expertise to prevent crippling consequences. The extent of tissue damage can be assessed by a veterinarian. The wound is probed for foreign bodies such as wood, plastic, glass or metal fragments, and it is determined if tendon sheaths or joint capsules have been penetrated, or if a wound tract leads down to muscle or bone.

Drainage

If a pocket has formed below a puncture, it is often necessary to establish a drainage hole at the low point of the wound so serum does not accumulate. A serum pocket slows healing because it prevents tissue connection and harbours bacteria. Accumulated serum flows from the pocket once there is an opening at the lowest point of the wound.

The original puncture may also need to be enlarged so a wound can heal from the inside out, without obstruction to drainage. Similarly, any scab that forms over the top of the wound should be removed. If a wound seals too quickly, trapped bacteria rapidly infect it.

Local antibiotics are infused into a wound; these liquid antibiotics do not obstruct drainage from the puncture. Covering the hole with thick ointments or creams obstructs drainage and attracts dirt and manure to the wound.

If a wound is left unbandaged, a petrolatum-based ointment can be applied to normal skin *below* the wound to prevent scalding of skin and hair loss from irritating serum that drains from the opening.

Bandaging

A puncture wound on the lower limb is usually bandaged to protect it from contaminants and further trauma. The bandage should not be applied too tightly or it will impair drainage. Some puncture wounds develop localized or gravitational swelling that is relieved by a light pressure bandage. As oedema decreases, drainage improves so healing can proceed faster.

Poultice

Application of a poultice or 'sweat' to a puncture site draws away the swelling or pulls the infection out for further cleansing of the wound. Warm Epsom salt soaks, 2 – 3 times daily, serve a similar purpose.

Wound dressings should be absorbent and should not block drainage. Change bandages frequently to assess healing and to remove encrusted material. Initially, bandages are changed every 2 – 3 days, or more frequently depending on the seriousness of an injury.

Identification of Bacteria

Most puncture wounds heal uneventfully within 1 – 2 weeks after treatment is begun. If a wound remains undiscovered for even a day or two, it may be valuable to obtain a bacterial culture and antibiotic sensitivity. Before cleaning a wound, a sterile swab placed into the wound soaks up secretions, and then it is replaced into its sterile sleeve. The swab is sent to the lab for cellular examination and bacterial growth.

Accurate identification of bacteria defines appropriate antibiotic treatment. For the next 2 – 3 days, while the lab is growing the culture, the horse receives broad spectrum antibiotic injections, which are selected by a veterinarian according to the greatest likelihood of success.

Kick Wounds

Kick wounds are similar to puncture wounds because blunt impact from a hoof causes a small break in the skin. Deeper connective tissue separates from the blow, leaving a tunnel along which bacteria can travel. If the blow is over a muscle, the wound heals with few complications when appropriately treated. If the kick is over ill-protected bone, a crack can form in the bone, a piece can be chipped off, or inflammation of the bone may interfere with its blood circulation.

If a kick wound is deep or traumatic enough to affect underlying bone, a *sequestrum* may develop. A sequestrum is a fragment of bone that has broken off with the initial impact of trauma, or has become devitalized due to reduced blood supply from infection. This dead bone fragment acts like a foreign body. The wound may initially heal, only to break open again. A chronic, draining tract persists until a sequestrum is surgically removed.

Tendon or Joint Punctures

If a puncture endangers a tendon sheath or joint space, special X-ray films can show the extent of injury. Injection of a sterile, radio-opaque dye into a wound is immediately followed with radiographs to outline the entire depth of the puncture tract with the dye. Such films are called *fistulograms*. Dye also passes around foreign bodies such as wood, plastic or glass that do not show on regular survey films because of their similar density to soft tissue.

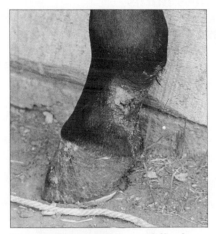

Fig. 16.10 Rope burns are difficult wounds to manage.

ROPE BURNS

A horse's hide is a tough but resilient structure, providing a thin, protective armour against perils in the environment. A common hazard to horses is a rope. As a rope entwines around a horse's leg, it often causes the horse to panic. The horse fights to get free of the entrapment, and as it kicks and struggles—without regard to any injury it inflicts upon itself—living hide disappears, revealing muscle and sinew beneath.

Characteristics of Rope Burns

Rope burns exhibit some unique characteristics. They are initially difficult wounds to manage, and require prolonged healing time. The friction can generate enough heat to burn or thermally injure the tissues.

Although rope burns are similar to lacerations, they are considered burns due to the heat created by rope sliding across skin. If tissue is heated to more than 140° F, thermal injury results.

A large amount of heat is necessary to raise tissue temperature high enough to damage tissue proteins. However, considerable time is required for heat to dissipate from the burned tissue. Because of this time lag to restore an area to normal temperature, injury continues despite removal of the rope from the leg.

Classes of Burns

Instead of classifying rope burns as first, second or third degree, it is more informative to assess thermal injury in terms of depth of skin and tissue damage. Rope burns are classified as:

- superficial
- partial-thickness
- full-thickness

Superficial and Partial-Thickness Burns

A *superficial* (minor) burn reveals reddened, thickened skin only. A *partial-thickness* burn is accompanied by oedema beneath the skin, intense inflammation, and pain. Damage to lymphatic vessels, along with increased leaking of capillaries, causes seepage of protein-rich fluids into the subcutaneous tissues. This material provides the structural basis for fibrin clots to stop bleeding, repair a wound, and provide a scaffold for healing. However, a high protein concentration in damaged tissue also serves as a nutrient medium for bacteria, with the potential for infection.

Full-Thickness Burn

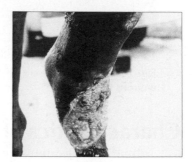

A *full-thickness* (major) burn results in profound limb swelling, and tissue appears 'tanned' and leathery. Because pain fibres are disrupted in a deep wound, the area is numb.

Although many rope burns are relatively minor and do not often progress beyond a partial thickness depth, any minor rope burn can become a full-thickness wound if inappropriate topical medications are applied, or if a bacterial infection overwhelms the healing process.

Fig. 16.11 A full-thickness rope burn.

Treating a Rope Burn

Wounds that appear minor may disguise extensive tissue damage caused by crushing and thermal injury when the horse struggled against the rope. The deeper the 'burn', the longer the healing time, and the greater the likelihood of tendon or ligament involvement. From the onset, rope burns should receive aggressive medical treatment to aid healing and limit scarring.

Immediate application of ice (wrapped in a towel) to the injury arrests persistent heat damage. Even a seemingly mild rope burn should be treated in this manner. What appears as a relatively superficial friction burn early presents a serious appearance days later,

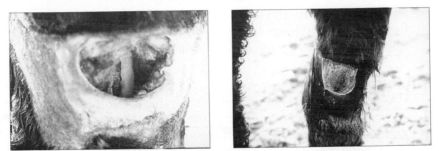

Fig. 16.12 This open wound was not sutured (left), but was bandaged. Bandaging allowed granulation tissue to form (right).

accompanied by swelling and lameness.

Because most rope burns tend to worsen dramatically before they improve, it is impractical to suture them. Instead, they are allowed to heal by *second intention,* that is, as an open wound that will fill in with granulation tissue. The same principles applied to any open wound also apply to second intention healing of rope burns.

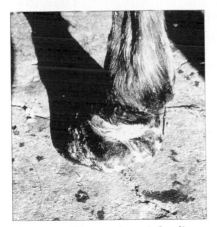

Fig. 16.13 This rope burn is healing well, but should stay bandaged.

Cleaning the Wound

Soil, manure and hair ground into the wound encourage rapid bacterial colonization of dead and dying tissue. To keep injured tissue as healthy as possible, immediate and thorough cleansing of a rope burn is important. Vigorous scrubbing with moist gauze sponges and an antiseptic electrolyte solution removes devitalized tissue, blood clots, large particles of debris, and skin contaminants.

High pressure irrigation (flushing) with antiseptic solutions cleans the wound of deeper bacteria and debris. It may be necessary to debride discoloured areas, because devitalized tissue contributes to the inflammatory response and provides nutrients for bacteria. A dark red or purple tissue colour represents congestion and stagnant blood caused by bruising and crushing.

Heat damage interferes with a normal immune response within a wound, making it susceptible to infection. Use of a cream containing silver, with or without aloe vera, protects tissue from drying. Silver ions in this preparation prevent the antibiotic from being inactivated by debris and discharge from the wound. The wound must be frequently cleaned, dressed, and bandaged to prevent infection.

Inflammation

An intense inflammatory response to thermal injury changes the way cells flow into the wound. White blood cells stick to vessel walls, and red blood cells mass together *(agglutinate)*. Toxins are released from dying cells, resulting in progressive tissue death. As blood vessels are blocked and constrict in response to injury, oxygen supply is reduced to the damaged area, leading to more cell injury and death—a vicious circle.

Corticosteroids and NSAIDs

Initially, a wound is isolated by the immune system and cleaned up by inflammatory cells. However, with excessive inflammation, oedema and oxygen deficiency result. Corticosteroid or non-steroidal anti-inflammatory medications encourage dilation of the blood vessels, reduce cell adhesiveness, and enhance blood circulation, minimizing this process.

Aloe Vera

Aloe vera is useful in managing burns because it stabilizes blood vessels in damaged tissue, reducing leakage. Other reports find that aloe vera has an antibacterial effect as well. *(Use only straight aloe vera extract, as mixtures containing aloe vera may be combined with potentially harmful chemicals.)*

Once a healthy granulation bed has developed over a rope burn, healing proceeds as it would for any other skin wound. With the presence of granulation tissue, the wound is as resistant to infection as is intact skin.

Eschar Formation

A coagulated crust of skin debris forms over the top of a rope burn. This crust is called an *eschar*. Not only does an eschar encourage harmful bacteria by providing nutrients, but it delays penetration of antibiotics to deeper tissues. An eschar that is brown–black in colour is probably invaded by bacteria.

Oxygen is important to cellular metabolism, particularly the processes involving wound healing. Further, oxygen enhances the activity of white blood cells responsible for cleaning up dead tissue and bacteria. An eschar prevents atmospheric oxygen from reaching the underlying wound. As a wound heals, fragile, newly formed skin cells compete with collagen-producing fibroblasts for oxygen.

An eschar should be removed from a wound as often as possible, to allow healing from the inside out. Its removal maintains a moist environment which aids the process of skin repair. Any remaining eschar usually separates from a wound as a granulation bed forms over a 2 – 4 week period.

Keloid Formation

A *keloid* may develop as a skin-like covering over proud flesh. This exaggerated scar protrudes above skin level. The wound surface resembles skin, but it remains fragile, dry, and crusty and lacks elasticity and strength derived from an underlying skin layer. Such wounds may require skin grafts to replenish a skin layer, or they are subject to chronic cracking and bleeding.

17

INJECTABLE MEDICATIONS

Many pharmacological and biological products available for the horse come only in injectable form. As the number of available equine medicines increases with improved vaccines, antibiotics and anti-inflammatory medications, more people are giving their horses injections.

When a veterinarian prescribes a course of therapy, the following factors are considered before any medication is given:

- Of primary consideration is the therapeutic goal: what specific disease process are we trying to alter, and what medication will do that?
- Is there an oral alternative that effectively side-steps the need for injections, or is more cost effective?
- What dosage is appropriate for the individual, and how often must the drug be given to maintain effective blood levels?
- How long must the therapy continue for therapeutic success?
- How can one evaluate a response to treatment?
- Will one drug interact adversely with another which is given at the same time?
- Does the horse suffer from a liver or kidney problem that might

prevent normal excretion of the drug from the body?
- Is the horse pregnant or lactating, thereby precluding use of certain drugs?
- What adverse or allergic reactions might be anticipated from the medication?
- Can the horse be monitored for adverse reactions, and can rapid control of any allergic response be initiated?
- Are there competition rules that refer to the drug?

Consideration of these factors for an entire course of therapy should be left to a veterinarian's expertise. However, for the confident horse owner, administration of injectable products can save both time and money provided safe principles are followed under veterinary advice.

Any time a substance is injected into a horse, be well-advised and educated about what the product is, what it will do, why it is necessary and how to administer it. Good common sense about both purchase and storage of drugs can build a complete and safe equine emergency first aid kit.

Medicating with any drug should not be a haphazard 'shot in the dark'. Advice from a veterinarian can direct an owner or trainer to safe and effective formulations for an emergency. It is important to examine selection and storage of these drugs and to have plan of action.

THE LABEL
Generic and Name Brands

Many products are available as both a generic or a proprietary name brand. In many instances, a generic product is pharmacologically identical to the more expensive name brand. However, in other instances, the carrier vehicle, preservative, or suspension material of a generic form results in delayed or reduced absorption of the drug as compared with the name brand. Unless cost is prohibitive, it is better to purchase the proprietary name brand drug to ensure appropriate absorption and distribution of the active ingredient in the product.

Active Ingredient

It is equally important to carefully note the active ingredient of the drug or drugs. As an example of a confusing label, suppose the aim is to treat a horse with penicillin. For many years the familiar bottle of Pen-Strep® was thought to serve this purpose. However, careful note of the label reveals that penicillin (at 200 000 units per ml) is combined with *dihydrostreptomycin*, another antibiotic which is a treatment of infections in cattle. Because of the way this combination antibiotic is formulated, a recommended dose of Pen-Strep® provides plenty of dihydrostreptomycin for a horse, but *underdoses* the penicillin. If the injection's volume is increased to supply adequate penicillin, then dihydrostreptomycin is *overdosed* with possible side effects, including toxicity to the kidneys. Very few bacterial organisms contracted by a horse are susceptible to dihydrostreptomycin. It is therefore best to buy straight, uncomplicated procaine penicillin G (at 300 000 units per ml).

Refrigerated Medications

If products needing refrigeration, such as penicillin or vaccines, are shipped, they should arrive in an insulated container with cold packs that are still chilled. Many products, especially vitamins and vaccines, become unstable when exposed to heat, and are rendered inactive if they become warm for even a short period. Only deal with reputable sources such as your local veterinary clinic.

Expiry Date

When purchasing injectable products, check the expiry date. Make sure there will be enough time for all the product to be used before that date. The date indicates that if a drug is stored in the recommended manner, and if given at the recommended dose, the product will be effective until that date. Throw away a drug that is past its expiry date, especially antibiotics and if they are known, or suspected, to be contaminated.

Outdated drugs do not often cause harmful reactions, but their reduced effectiveness can result in serious consequences, particularly with antibiotics for bacterial infections. Just as consistent underdosing of dewormers leads to resistant parasite strains, reduced effectiveness of antibiotics leads to antibiotic-resistant strains of bacteria, and consequently to severe infections. Therefore, outdated products do little to improve the success of therapy.

Type of Drug

Intravenous drugs should not be injected into muscle, because they may cause irritating muscle reactions. As an example, there is currently no intramuscular preparation of phenylbutazone. Injection of the intravenous preparation into a muscle results in massive skin sloughing and pain. Then secondary bacterial infections of the skin develop. Myoglobin released from massive muscle breakdown travels to the kidneys and may obstruct their filtering systems, resulting in renal failure.

Moreover, injecting intramuscular medications, such as vaccines or penicillin, into a vein can cause an anaphylactic (severe allergic) reaction and death. Be sure to read all labels, and consult a veterinarian if there is any question about drug type.

SAFE STORAGE

Injectable drugs come in many forms:

- single-dose vials
- multiple-dose vials or bottles
- glass ampoules
- prepackaged, single-dose, plastic syringes

Many drugs come in liquid form, already mixed with a saline solution. However, some drugs and vaccines are unstable in solution and are therefore freeze-dried (lyophilized). Then they are mixed with a saline solution or sterile water immediately before injection so the active ingredient is not degraded by storage.

If bottles of vaccine or other drugs sit for long periods, sediments may form in the bottom. Sediment particles may be important molecules of active ingredient that are no longer equally mixed in the solution. These substances should not be injected into muscle as sediments can create a noxious reaction at the injection site. If a drug has sedimented out, shake it. If it returns to normal and is not past its expiry date, it is still acceptable. If it does not mix together with shaking, or is past the expiry date, throw it away.

With lengthy storage, the tops of the vials may get dusty. It is best to clean the top of a bottle by swabbing it with alcohol before inserting a needle or withdrawing any medication. A dust-free cabinet or storage box reduces settling of grime and dust on the rubber stopper.

Storing injectable drugs in syringes for a lengthy time can result in injection of an inadequate dose, as some compounds are absorbed into the plastic walls of the syringe. When this happens, the horse does not receive the entire dose.

Any medication, whether in a bottle, vial or syringe, should be carefully stored *out of reach of children or pets*, preferably in a locked cabinet or box. Needles accidentally discovered by children are a hazard to their safety. Accidental ingestion of many drugs can be poisonous to children or pets.

Environmental Stresses

Chemical incompatibilities within some drug preparations may result in premature precipitation of sediments, colour changes, gas formation, or gelatinization (residue clinging to the sides of the bottle). Or, the drug may be inactivated without any visible change. These changes may occur due to interaction with preservatives or solvents in the drug, particularly if caused by pH changes, heat or cold.

Injectable vitamin preparations are some of the products especially sensitive to environmental stresses. Most vitamin preparations are stable at acidic pH, from pH 2.0 to 6.5. The higher the pH, the less stable the preparation. In the presence of ultraviolet rays of sunlight, many vitamin preparations are inactivated. Heat greater than 75° F, or aeration by shaking, also contributes to vitamin instability. Contact with certain metals, especially in the presence of light, heat, or aeration, promotes rapid oxidation of vitamins. Trace elements of iron, copper or cobalt will destroy the B-complex vitamins in a vitamin–mineral mix, therefore it is useless past the expiry date. Likewise, storing the mix in a metal container can also cause vitamins to become inactivated.

Vitamin Injection Storage

To effectively maintain the recommended shelf-life of vitamin injections, store them in a dark, cool place, free from any shaking. If the preparation is outdated, throw it away as it is probably ineffective.

Vaccine Storage

Heat stress is also dangerous to vaccines. They should be kept under refrigeration, and not stored on the dashboard or seat of a truck for even a short time. When transporting vaccines, it is best to pack them in a small ice chest to keep them cool. A small amount of heat can make the product inactive. It is then better to throw a questionable product away, and purchase a fresh batch.

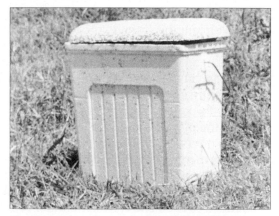

Fig. 17.1 Some drugs require refrigeration.

Contaminated Medications

Most injectable products have been heat sterilized, or filtered through Millipore® filter systems to reduce the risk of contaminating bacteria or foreign proteins. To limit the number of adverse reactions to injections, the products are ideally free of insoluble foreign particles or pyrogens, which are fever-producing substances.

If multiple-dose vials are used, as with flunixin meglumine (Finadyne®), corticosteroids, certain hormones, tranquillizers or sedatives, or vaccines, beware of contamination of these bottles with dirt or used needles that can transfer blood or particles into the bottle. Any bottle suspected of such contamination should be discarded.

PRE-INJECTION PROCEDURES
Reading the Label

Before giving an injection, read the label several times to be certain it is the correct item. A wise practice is to read the label while picking up the bottle, read it again while withdrawing the medication, and once again while putting the bottle down prior to injection. Be sure the solution is well mixed.

Using Clean Needles and Syringes

Whenever an injection is given to a horse, a brand new sterile syringe and needle should be used. Needles should *never* be transferred from horse to horse because of risk of transfer of serious infections, such as equine infectious anaemia or protozoan blood parasites such as *Piroplasma*. Needles are inexpensive; there is no reason to save or salvage them.

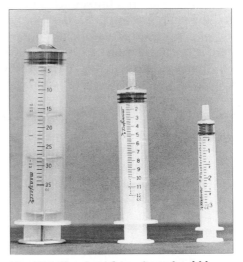

Fig. 17.2 The size of a syringe should be appropriate for the dosage to be given.

Vials, syringes and needles should be disposed of promptly so children or pets have no access to them. Burning these items after use is the preferred method of disposal, especially for biological products such as vaccines. Advice should be given by your veterinary surgeon.

Cleaning the Site
Alcohol

Proper technique is essential to ensure a safe and clean injection. Choose a clean, unsoiled dry area. Many people still squirt alcohol (70% ethanol or isopropyl) on the area before needle insertion. However, studies have shown that even shaved or hairless skin must remain moistened in alcohol for *at least* 2 minutes before any antiseptic action is achieved. Moreover, not all microorganisms are susceptible to alcohol. A quick squirt of alcohol on top of fur and skin may remove some debris and dirt, but it accomplishes little more.

Effective Antiseptic Solutions

Combining 1.5% tamed iodine (Betadine®) or 0.5% chlorhexidine (Hibitane®) with 70% alcohol greatly enhances its antiseptic action, although the solution still must contact every microscopic particle of hair and skin for 2 minutes.

Surgical scrubbing with tamed iodine solutions before injection is impractical but certainly provides a less contaminated injection site. Remember that horses are quick to learn about painful procedures—the next time surgical soap is applied, the horse will be planning an exit from the situation, and the target will be a lot less stationary. Horses have long memories for painful experiences. It is no wonder that a horse responds to the sight of a syringe and needle in hand, or to the smell of alcohol applied to the skin just before the needle is inserted.

Handling the Horse

Always untie a horse before giving an injection, and have a restrainer hold the head. The restrainer should stand on the same side as the person with the needle. The horse's head is pulled towards both people, and if it decides to kick, it automatically spins the hind end away.

If a horse is tied and violently reacts to needle insertion, it may lunge and throw itself against the rope. The horse's fright increases when it is unable to get free, and it can injure itself or a person in the struggle.

INTRAMUSCULAR INJECTIONS

Most of the time a horse suffers no ill consequences from an intramuscular (IM) injection given by a knowledgeable person. However, there are risks and adverse side effects that should be considered. It is important to understand how to give intramuscular injections and what adverse reactions to watch for.

For a less experienced horse owner, some rules-of-thumb should be followed. The objective is to perform the procedure as quickly and painlessly as possible.

Injection Targets

Define the target for the injection ahead of time to avoid blind stabbing. The anatomy of the horse provides many major muscle groups which are safe for IM injection. Intramuscular injections can be given in the neck, rump and thigh, and occasionally the pectoral muscles of the chest. Certain landmarks guide injection in each location.

Neck Injection

To avoid being kicked and hurt by a resentful horse, the neck and rump are the safest targets.

If the neck is used, note the triangular-shaped area of muscle bordered above by the nuchal ligament, below by the cervical spine, and behind by the

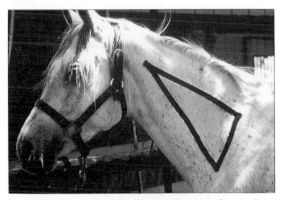

Fig. 17.3 The triangle indicates the area for IM injections in the neck.

shoulder blade. If an injection is deposited within the ligament, it will not be appropriately absorbed. Be sure to stay away from the spine or the bony shoulder blade. Close to the spine is the *jugular furrow (groove)* which contains major blood vessels such as the carotid artery or jugular vein.

If vaccine or medication that is not intended for intravenous (IV) use is deposited in these vessels, serious and potentially fatal reactions can occur. Also, drugs injected around major nerve branches running along the jugular furrow may be harmful.

Rump Injection

The rump muscle is a large 'muscle mass located far from any vital structures. (At this location, it is also possible to avoid a kick that states an objection to the shot.)

On the large rump muscles (gluteals), the target site for injection is defined by drawing a line from the top of the croup to the point of the buttocks, and another line from the point of the hip to the dock. The intersection of these two lines is a safe muscle injection site.

There is a disadvantage in using the gluteal muscles, in that an abscess may form at the injection site. Because these

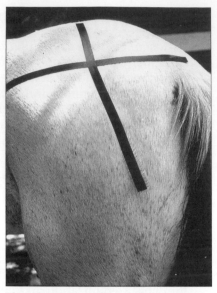

Fig. 17.4 Intersection of the two lines is the IM injection site on the rump.

muscle bundles are encased in a large, continuous sheet of connective tissue *(fascia)*, an abscess can form under the tissue layers and spread up the loin and back. This spreading potentially leads to massive skin destruction and sloughing. Moreover, because the hip is located in an uppermost position, it is difficult to drain an infected injection site.

Thigh Injection

To avoid abscesses, inject into one of two large muscles that make up the thigh, along the back of the leg. These muscles are active in locomotion so exercise reduces soreness that may develop at the injection site. In the event of an abscess, infection in the thigh is constrained to a local area where it is easily lanced and drained.

Other Sites

Pectoral muscles are rarely used as

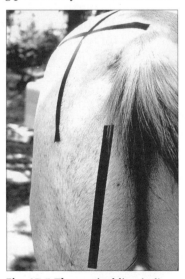

Fig. 17.5 The vertical line indicates the IM injection site for the thigh.

they tend to become swollen and sore. They are used if multiple anti-biotic injections are necessary for prolonged periods. These muscles are readily accessible and allow easy drainage should there be formation of an abscess.

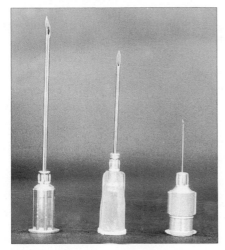

Fig. 17.6 There are different size needles available for every type of injection.

Size of the Needle

Equine muscle is thick and profusely laced with minute blood vessels. A needle should be long enough to penetrate deep into a muscle injection site to deposit the drug so the circulatory system can retrieve it from the muscle bed. A proper length of needle for most injections in the adult horse is $1\frac{1}{2}$ inches long, and 18 gauge or 20 gauge depending on the drug being used. Foals require no more than a 20 gauge, 1-inch needle.

Inserting the Needle

The needle should be inserted decisively, with a quick thrust, perpendicular to the skin. Pinch a fold of neck skin to momentarily distract the horse, then thrust the needle in just to the side of the pinched skin. Punching the horse several times on the hindquarters before poking in the needle only alerts it to the fact that it is soon to be pricked. A quick thrust of the needle, with no warning to the horse other than a soothing voice and hand, is all

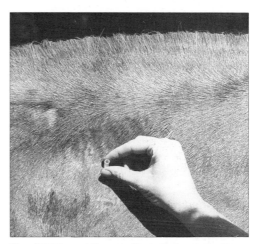

Fig. 17.7 Insert the needle and then attach the syringe.

that is required. Go for it, and do not hesitate.

Always insert the needle without the syringe attached. If a horse moves while a syringe is attached to the needle, its flopping further scares and irritates the horse. A moving needle lacerates surrounding blood vessels and muscle tissue. Once a needle is in place and the horse is standing quietly, attach the syringe.

Always pull back on the plunger before injecting the drug to be certain there is *no* blood in the hub of the needle. Accidental administration of vaccines or penicillin, as examples, into a blood vessel can result in an anaphylactic reaction (severe allergic reaction) and death. Always be sure no blood is leaking back through the needle. If a needle has penetrated a vessel or capillary and blood comes back, remove the needle, reinsert it, and start again.

If a needle is bent, throw it away and start with a fresh one. Otherwise the needle may break and become embedded in deep muscle during the second insertion.

Adverse Reactions

With careful selection of the compounds a horse receives, and with clean injection technique, over 80% of adverse drug reactions can be avoided. A new era finds more horse owners assuming the responsibility of their horse's care by administering vaccines and medicines. This do-it-yourself approach to health management is commendable, but it must be backed up with comprehensive education. Knowing the risks and taking the necessary precautions ensures the horse's safety.

Abscess

Despite taking all precautions, some horses still experience adverse reactions to IM injections. A localized, firm and tender swelling at the injection site may be a mild side effect, accompanied by muscle stiffness and soreness. However, if a swelling enlarges and softens, it may be developing into an abscess needing veterinary attention to lance, drain, and flush it. An abscess moves like a wave when touched, like a small water balloon, and is usually warm and sensitive to finger pressure.

Cellulitis

Whenever a needle penetrates skin, a horse receives a microscopic amount of bacteria. Normally, the local immune system surrounding this needle prick cleans up microorganisms that were introduced,

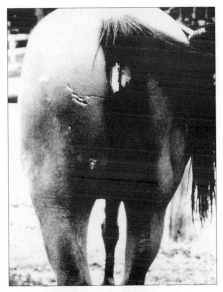

Fig. 17.8 An infected injection site can rapidly swell to huge proportions.

and only a very small localized swelling may result, if anything.

However, if an infection persists and is left to simmer within the muscle, *cellulitis* can develop. Inflammation and obstruction of circulatory and lymphatic drainage systems cause the tissues around the injection site to become hot, painful, and swollen. Swelling compromises blood and oxygen supply to the affected tissues, worsening the swelling and infection.

Careful monitoring of an injection site for several days reveals a problem before it becomes serious. Look for minute or excessive swelling, tenderness to finger pressure, lameness, or stiffness. More often than not, a mild reaction at the site of an injection resolves by itself within 3 – 4 days. Exercise, hot packs and massage can hasten recovery. If swelling worsens, or seems abnormally enlarged or painful, contact a veterinarian immediately.

Clostridial Bacteria

Localized cellulitis promotes *clostridial* bacteria that prefer an anaerobic environment (without oxygen). These bacteria are rapidly lethal to a horse due to an overwhelming toxin production. Clostridial spores abound in manure and soil, and exist normally on a horse's skin and gut. However, if clostridial bacteria that are normally in the digestive tract seed themselves in muscle, there is inflamed or dead tissue within 2–5 days. The site is overwhelmingly painful, far out of proportion to the actual amount of swelling. The area feels crackly like tissue paper *(crepitation)* due to gas bubbles trapped beneath the skin.

Fibrotic Myopathy

Whenever an infection occurs within a muscle mass, the inflamed tissue is ultimately replaced with scar tissue to varying degrees. If tissue within the thigh muscles scars to a large extent, it can result in a lameness syndrome called *fibrotic myopathy*. Forward extension of the hind leg is reduced due to mechanical constriction by fibrous scar tissue.

Fibrotic myopathy is commonly attributed to sudden sprint activities when a horse may tear muscle tissue. A horse that abruptly slams on the brakes, setting the hind legs far under it, can pull or tear a thigh muscle in the process. On rare occasions, however, this syndrome also develops from an infection after an IM injection.

Muscle Soreness

Remember that a horse has two sides to its body. If multiple injections are necessary, use as many different muscle groups as possible to limit soreness. A left-sided muscle group is used in the morning, and the right side at night. Remembering 'right at night' avoids confusion.

Because a dressage horse depends on engagement of the hindquarters to collect and perform symmetrical and rhythmic movements, most dressage riders prefer to give IM injections in the neck, away from the hind end. This method prevents loss of several days' training if a horse becomes stiff or sore from an injection.

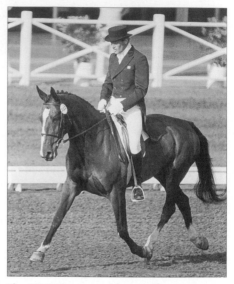

Fig. 17.9 Dressage riders prefer to give injections in the neck instead of the hind end.

Flu-like Symptoms

Sometimes a horse reacts adversely to an intramuscular vaccine by exhibiting flu-like symptoms, such as aching muscles, fever, depression or lack of appetite. If these symptoms appear, consult your veterinary surgeon. If the horse is known to be sensitive to vaccines, remind him or her of this when the next dose is due.

Sore Neck

Even more important, an injection into the neck can cause a horse to become so sore that it refuses to eat or drink—these efforts require stretching of a painful neck muscle. If a horse stops drinking, an impaction colic can develop, which is potentially life-threatening. A sore neck might discourage a foal from nursing, resulting in weakness and stress.

Anaphylactic Shock

The worst complication arising from any injection is an allergic reaction *(anaphylactic shock)* which can abruptly kill a horse. Penicillin, some vitamin injections, and many of the non-steroidal anti-inflammatory drugs are implicated in these reactions, although any drug can cause anaphylaxis. The immune system of an individual that has previously been sensitized to a particular drug can react within seconds or minutes after the drug is deposited in a muscle. An overwhelming immune response suddenly assaults the body. The accompanying airway spasm and throat swelling rapidly lead to asphyxiation and shock. Without immediate action the horse can lapse into cardiac arrest and die. If a horse is experiencing an extreme anaphylactic allergic reaction, it may roll or convulse violently. Epinephrine (adrenaline) opens the airways, allowing the horse to breathe can be injected anywhere by any injection method (IV, IM, subcutaneous, etc.) to achieve an instant result.

Warning Signs

Often a horse shows mild allergic symptoms before developing a full-blown anaphylactic reaction. Watch carefully for hives *(urticaria)* that may or may not itch and can be located anywhere on the body. Also, diffuse swelling of the limbs, head or abdomen, an elevated respiratory rate, or behavioural changes such as agitation or depression may signal an allergic response. Any combination of these problems may be warning signals that medication should be discontinued at once, and a veterinarian contacted. Profound hypersensitivity reactions can occur without warning; abrupt and fatal anaphylactic shock may be unavoidable.

Precautionary Measures

After administering a drug or medication to a horse, do not walk away immediately. Instead, stay around to watch for an adverse reaction which often peaks within 10 – 30 minutes.

To prevent adverse reactions from intramuscular injections:

- obtain a thorough drug history on each horse to identify previous allergic responses to certain medications

- affix a warning card on a horse's stall door to alert others of an allergy to specific drugs
- avoid mixing medications without first consulting a veterinarian
- properly dose a horse according to body weight and age to avoid excesses, and dose at appropriate time intervals
- read all labels to ensure that a drug is approved for administration
- throw away outdated or improperly stored medicines

Above all, *avoid indiscriminate use of medications!* If a drug is not really necessary or is not recommended by a veterinarian, do not give it. Substitute oral preparations for intramuscular medicines whenever possible, particularly with vitamins or non-steroidal anti-inflammatory drugs. It takes longer for a drug to be absorbed from the intestine than it would through a muscle, yet it may ultimately be safer.

INTRAVENOUS INJECTIONS

Besides intramuscular injection, intravenous (IV) administration of medications is the most common means of injection in the horse. The horse's jugular vein is large and well-defined in the jugular furrow (groove) parallel to the underside of the neck. It swells as blood flow is briefly obstructed with finger pressure along the vein.

Not only is the jugular vein an opportune location for injecting medication, but it is the common site for collecting blood for equine infectious anaemia testing, complete blood counts, chemistry panels, blood typing, and drug testing. A blood tube with a vacuum in it permits rapid extraction of intravenous blood for these tests.

Many liquid medications are formulated for exclusive use as intravenous injections, but many substances can be given either intramuscularly or intravenously depending on how rapidly the effect is desired. Many sedatives and tranquillizers can be administered either way, but an immediate result

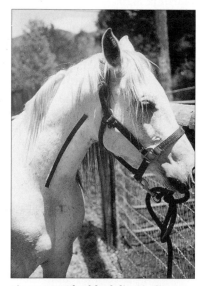

Fig. 17.10 The black line indicates the jugular furrow.

is seen with IV injection. Any injection given intravenously should be a sterile preparation intended for IV use.

Administering IV Injections

If an injection is to be given IV, the needle can be inserted facing either towards the head or towards the heart, but remember that, in the jugular vein, blood flows from the head to the heart. Once the needle is inserted into the vein, blood should only come back through the hub of the needle if the vein is compressed with finger pressure. If blood spurts vigorously from the needle without compressing the vessel, there is a strong possibility that it has been inserted into the carotid artery. *No medication should be administered in the carotid artery* because it would go directly to the brain and central nervous system and could result in instant death.

This route of injection should not be used without advice and training from a veterinary surgeon. Drugs given by the route must be injected *slowly* and great care must be taken to ensure the needle is in the middle of the vein.

If medication which should be given directly into the blood vessel leaks into surrounding tissue, serious skin irritation can lead to massive loss of skin in the area, and potentially to inflammation of the vein *(thrombophlebitis)*. Phenylbutazone, sodium iodide, tetracycline, and guafenisin (a general anaesthetic agent) cause this problem most often.

IV Catheter

If frequent IV medication must be given, or large volumes of electrolyte solutions are to be administered, an indwelling intravenous catheter is placed in the vein after clipping and scrubbing the insertion site. The catheter is a flexible plastic material that can safely remain in the jugular vein for up to 72 hours if these sterilizing procedures are followed for its placement.

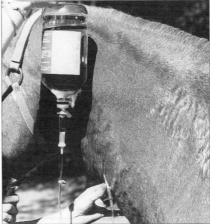

Fig. 17.11 An intravenous catheter for frequent IV administration.

SUBCUTANEOUS INJECTIONS

Most medications are designed to be injected deeply into the horse's muscle tissue, or directly into the vein. However, sometimes a therapeutic medication is given subcutaneously (subQ).

This method of injection should not be attempted without advice and training from a veterinarian.

The loose skin behind the horse's elbow makes an ideal location for a subQ injection. The needle is placed just under the skin, but not into muscle, and the material is slowly injected. If the spot swells too much, the needle can be fanned in a semicircle to spread the medication out over a larger area. Medication or fluids given under a horse's skin are absorbed slowly, so there will be a lump at the injection site for several hours.

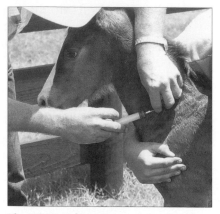

Fig. 17.12 Subcutaneous injections are given just under the skin.

Local anaesthetic is often placed subQ to numb an area for suturing or a scalpel incision. Fanning the anaesthetic into the subcutaneous tissues increases the area of effect. Heparin is sometime administered for the prevention or treatment of laminitis, and it can also be given subQ.

INTRADERMAL INJECTIONS

An intradermal (ID) injection involves placing a needle inside the uppermost layer of the skin. This method is even more difficult than subQ injections. It should not be attempted without first being advised and trained by a veterinarian.

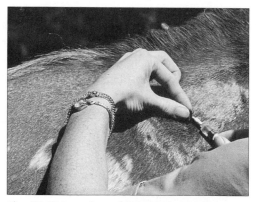

Fig. 17.13 Intradermal injections are given inside the skin.

406

In some instances local anaesthetic is injected intradermally. When corticosteroid is injected into nodular necrobiosis skin lesions, it is by intradermal infusion. Also, use of Bacillus Calmette-Guerin *(see Chapter 15 for more information on BCG and sarcoids)* to treat sarcoid tumours requires intradermal injection for best results.

18

NON-STEROIDAL ANTI-INFLAMMATORY DRUGS

Equine athletic pursuits often result in sore muscles, swollen limbs, or mild lameness. It is not unusual for a horse owner or trainer to open the medical kit and reach inside for a short-term anti-inflammatory solution to an ache or pain.

In theory, this practice seems sensible, and it is one we commonly apply to ourselves. Yet, our efforts to help a horse by numbing the problem with an anti-inflammatory drug may do more harm than good.

USE OF NSAIDs

The most overused and abused drugs available today are those belonging to the class of non-steroidal anti-inflammatory drugs (NSAIDs), particularly phenylbutazone ('bute') and flunixin meglumine (Finadyne®). Bute and Finadyne® are useful for a wide range of conditions. Other, less common NSAIDs include dipyrone, Ketofen® and naproxen.

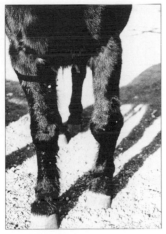

Fig. 18.1 NSAIDs can help a horse with chronic arthritis.

Benefits of NSAIDs

NSAIDs are powerful drugs, improving a horse's working capabilities. They are not stimulants. They simply allow a horse to perform up to normal capabilities, without lameness and pain. NSAIDs help control leg swelling, or reduce an out-of-control fever caused by infections. They can relieve spasms from muscle strain or a mild colic. They are helpful to the chronically arthritic horse to enhance its quality of life and the longevity of its performance career. Yet, NSAIDs should not be taken for granted and used indiscriminately.

Drawbacks of NSAIDs

Giving NSAIDs to a mildly lame horse while asking it for continued performance can aggravate an undiagnosed tendon or muscle injury. If a horse with beginning signs of colic receives a dose of Finadyne® or bute from a concerned owner, the pain seems to subside due to the anti-inflammatory effects of the drug. But the real problem goes unanswered. A horse only communicates via depression, lack of appetite, or pain, and the effect of the drug disguises these symptoms. Masking a serious colic condition, which may require surgery, permits the damage to intensify beyond repair.

Method of Action

When a horse is hurting from a wound, pulled muscle, colic, or arthritis, its body responds by producing substances called *prostaglandins.* Prostaglandins cause the cascade of events involved in the inflammatory process. Prostaglandins are short-lived molecules, and are only produced at or close to their site of action. They are produced upon demand and are not stored by the body. NSAIDs act as anti-inflammatory agents by inhibiting the normal production of prostaglandins.

At the site of action, prostaglandins stimulate contraction and permeability of the cells lining the blood vessels, causing leakage of fluids into surrounding soft tissues. This results in oedema, which is seen as swelling.

At the same time, prostaglandins cause the smooth muscle of the blood vessel walls to relax, leading to the pooling of blood in localized areas, which results in redness *(erythema)*.

Prostaglandins enhance the effects of other players in the inflammatory cycle, such as histamines and *bradykinin*. These chemicals attract white blood cells, and increase blood circulation to the inflammation site. Warmth is felt in the area due to increased blood flow and local blood pooling.

In addition to swelling, redness, and heat at a site of injury, prostaglandins make pain receptors super-sensitive, contributing to an exaggerated pain response.

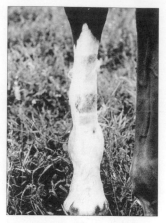

Fig. 18.2 Swelling of an injured site is caused by prostaglandins.

Therefore, as anti-inflammatory agents, NSAIDs act as anti-prostaglandins. By inhibiting production of prostaglandins, NSAIDs reduce the spiralling events that result in inflammation and swelling; pain subsides as well.

TYPES OF NSAIDs

Understanding the different pharmacological aspects of a drug is essential for its safe use. Manufacturers' labels and package inserts contain information about proper dosages and adverse side effects.

Different products within the NSAID drug class act better on some ailments than others. For example, bute is effective for musculoskeletal problems such as arthritis, a pulled muscle, or tendinitis. Flunixin meglumine is potent against gastrointestinal pain and endotoxaemia.

Phenylbutazone

One of the least expensive and more potent examples of the NSAIDs is phenylbutazone, or bute. Once an intravenous dosage of bute is administered, it requires about ½ hour to begin blocking prostaglandin production. If given orally in paste, powder, or tablet form, it takes 2 – 3 hours to be absorbed from the gastrointestinal tract.

NSAIDs have no effect on the prostaglandins already produced.

Therefore, once bute is administered, it does not take effect for 3 – 5 hours. This time lag is required for the body to break down enough of the previously manufactured prostaglandins. Total breakdown requires up to 12 hours. In the meantime, bute prevents additional prostaglandins from being produced.

If the blood level of bute is not maintained at a therapeutic level, prostaglandins begin to accumulate again and the inflammatory cycle repeats itself. Depending on the ailment, bute protects against inflammation for 12 – 24 hours.

Flunixin Meglumine

Flunixin meglumine (Finadyne®) is very useful for pain due to colic. It is also helpful against the effects of endotoxaemia caused by a retained placenta, an overdose of rich feed, or a pituitary disorder. *(See Chapter 4 for more information on endotoxins.)* Finadyne® is more potent than bute, and maintains its therapeutic effect for up to 30 hours.

Uses of NSAIDs	
Phenylbutazone	Effective against musculoskeletal injuries. Also effective against gastrointestinal pain.
Flunixin Meglumine	Effective against musculoskeletal injuries. Also effective against gastrointestinal pain and endotoxaemia.

Fig. 18.3

NSAID TOXICITY
Stomach

While NSAIDs inhibit production of prostaglandins involved in the inflammatory process, they also interfere with production of prostaglandins necessary to normal physiological function. Prostaglandin E2 protects the stomach lining by stimulating mucus production and the secretion of sodium bicarbonate by gastric cells to buffer the stomach's acid environment. Optimal blood flow to the stomach and intestinal tract is normally controlled by prostaglandin activity.

Without this protection, the stomach and intestines are prone to gastric ulcers. Ulcers are not only painful, but can be life-threatening.

Oral ulcers along the gums, palate and tongue may accompany gastric ulcers. These ulcers are more common in horses receiving excessive NSAIDs orally, that is as paste, tablets or powder. Mouth pain depresses appetite, and performance suffers.

Kidneys

Prostaglandins also are responsible for maintaining normal blood flow, function, and water resorption abilities of the kidneys. In a horse that is dehydrated (due to lack of water, excessive sweating, bleeding, or severe colic) prostaglandins act as a protective device to dilate and enhance the blood supply to the kidney.

Irreversible toxic effects may occur within 48 hours in dehydrated or blood volume-depleted horses that are given a single dose of an NSAID, particularly bute. The syndrome is known as *renal papillary necrosis*, and is fatal. Even if administered at recommended doses, bute can be a toxic product for a dehydrated horse.

Symptoms of NSAID Toxicity

Excessive amounts of NSAIDs damage the gastrointestinal lining with subsequent leakage and loss of proteins. Symptoms of NSAID-induced toxicosis and protein loss include diarrhoea, oedema of limbs and abdomen, blood loss in the faeces, and weight loss. Some horses exhibit depression, loss of appetite, or abdominal pain due to gastric ulcers or oedema of the intestinal lining.

A lower-than-recommended dose can cause toxicosis if given to a horse that is dehydrated, in pain, or stressed. Those horses respond to stress by producing internal corticosteroids. When internal corticosteroids are combined with an NSAID, steroid effects are amplified, resulting in toxicity.

Toxic effects occur with administration of excessive amounts of an NSAID over a short time (3 – 5 days), or by chronic dosing over months or years.

After more than a decade of use of many different non-steroidal anti-inflammatory drugs, equine practitioners have discovered that previously assumed safe doses in the horse can exert toxic effects if maintained at these levels too long. For example, 4 grams of bute a day for a 1000-lb horse should not be administered more than 4 days in a row, assuming normal kidney and liver function. Once the drug has achieved therapeutic levels in the bloodstream, that level is safely maintained at 1 – 2 grams per day.

Allergic Reactions

Long-term use of NSAIDs (sporadic or consistent) can hypersensitize a horse to any drug in its class, and result in allergic reactions. These reactions range from a mild case of hives, or facial or limb oedema, to a severe anaphylactic allergic reaction and death.

Some people may make a dangerous mistake: repetitive dosing with NSAIDs while applying a misguided theory that 'if a little bit works, a lot must be better'. An NSAID should never be repeated at less than 12-hour intervals unless specified by a veterinarian. Recommended dosing instructions per pound of body weight should never be increased.

Double Dosing

Another common mistake is to give an appropriate dose of one NSAID, followed immediately by an appropriate dose of another NSAID. Toxic effects are additive, and this practice simulates a double dose of any single NSAID. Toxicosis results from combining NSAIDs.

If relief is not achieved from the initial drug treatment, there is no reason to believe relief will come from an additional product with a similar mechanism of action. There is a time lag of several hours until clinical relief is seen. The prostaglandin cycle is blocked immediately, but existing prostaglandins need to be metabolized and removed from the system. Adding more NSAIDs will not alter or speed up this process.

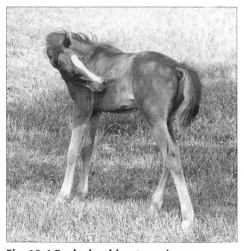

Fig. 18.4 Foals should not receive an NSAID except as recommended by a vet.

NSAIDs and Foals

Foals less than 6 – 8 months old are extremely susceptible to the toxic effects of NSAIDs. Under normal circumstances, newborn foals are never given NSAIDs. If it is a dire emergency, *a veterinarian* may decide to administer an NSAID.

The dangers of administration of NSAID medications to horses less than 1 year of age so far outweigh any possible benefits gained from anti-inflammatory or anti-pyretic effects, that a general rule-of-thumb should be followed: *never administer any NSAID to any horse under 1 year old.*

Professional Advice

Obtain professional veterinary advice before using NSAIDs. What 'worked' for one horse may have no application to another. What seems to be a mild problem may be serious, requiring medical attention and expertise. It is easy to pick up the telephone and get professional advice, and has a less damaging toll on a horse's health than guesswork.

WITHDRAWAL FOR COMPETITION

There are legal responsibilities involved with the use of anti-inflammatory agents. Drug levels are detectable in urine or blood. It is important that the requirements of the association and the rules of each competition be checked well in advance to ensure that the horse meets the drug withdrawal requirements.

PREPURCHASE EXAMS

Be cautious during prepurchase examinations. An unethical seller who wants to mask a mild lameness problem may 'after' the examination results by using NSAIDs or other drugs.

ALTERNATIVES TO NSAIDS

Before grabbing a tube or tablets of an NSAID, examine other therapeutic alternatives such as rest, or hot or cold soakings. Rub a swelling with DMSO (dimethyl sulphoxide), or massage sore muscles. Examine shoeing practices that might have changed a limb's biomechanics enough to bring on lameness. Re-evaluate training methods, and the rate of increase in difficulty. Look to management, parasite control, and feeding changes to decrease the incidence of colic.

Remember, horses were designed to live on grasses, water and salt. Anything else we put into their bodies must be evaluated for suitability and safety. The Veterinary Products Committee or the Veterinary Medicines Directorate approve drugs at specified dosages and frequencies to comply with research studies in safety and efficacy. *NSAIDs have a role in the horse world, **provided** they are used intelligently and in moderation.*

19

SAFE AND EFFECTIVE RESTRAINT

Building a partnership that is based on trust is a goal that takes time, but is full of reward. Unfortunately, not all events in a horse's life are free from unpleasantness or pain. Some examples are wound doctoring, routine vaccinations, and administration of medications. Eventually the inevitable occurs, and the horse objects to a procedure.

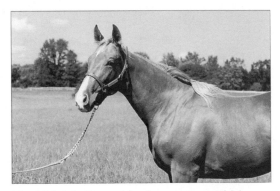

Fig. 19.1 A halter and lead rope are a mild form of restraint.

For some horses, administration of deworming pastes, use of electric clippers or horseshoeing are traumatic experiences. Other horses object to benign grooming procedures such as bathing, or pulling and plaiting the mane.

The objectives of restraint are:
- to avoid getting hurt
- to prevent injury to the horse
- to get the job done effectively

Restraint of a half-ton animal obviously requires more than sheer human strength. A rearing horse can suspend a 200-lb man from the end of a twitch, and a horse recovering from general anaesthetic can quickly flip two grown men off its neck. The brute strength of a horse should be addressed in a psychological arena, not in a physical showdown.

UNDERSTANDING HORSE BEHAVIOUR
Natural Instincts

By using our human mind we can outwit a horse at its own game of resistance. To do so, we must understand the motivating influences behind the horse's contrary behaviour. Horses evolved survival mechanisms to protect themselves from predators, such as the big cats. Their immediate response when threatened is to flee from the area. A flighty horse is only responding to natural instincts to run from a fearful situation. A response to a painful or scary event is to move away from the stimulus by backing up, lunging sideways, or rearing. If backed into a corner or prevented from fleeing, a horse then reverts to

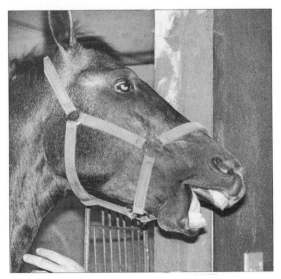

Fig. 19.2 Teeth can be used as a defensive weapon and also for aggression.

using its built-in defence weapons—its teeth and hooves. This fear translates to biting, kicking or striking, all of which are unacceptable behaviour from a human point of view.

By understanding normal equine behavioural instincts, we can capitalize on them and modify their behaviour to the task in hand. Horses evolved in a herd hierarchy, and they accept a single dominant herd member as the leader. Because a horse is able to distinguish between dominant and submissive individuals and respond accordingly, it is logical for humans to achieve dominance to successfully fulfil the objectives of restraint.

Learn to read a horse's behavioural cues, such as flattened ears, or bared teeth that indicate aggression, or a tightly clasped tail and hollow, tense back reflective of pain or fear. Other signals are more subtle, but perked ears, a relaxed posture, or droopy lip and eyes should be positively rewarded, because they are signs of cooperation.

CREATING CALMNESS

The temperament of an individual horse and its breed type are factors that may dictate a specific approach. However, certain fundamentals should be applied to restraint of any horse.

Environment

Make the situation appealing to the horse by working in a familiar environment that feels secure, and by using familiar equipment. Approach the horse quietly, and spend several minutes getting acquainted with its body language, and allowing it to become accustomed to the situation as well. Working off the near (left) side is comforting as most horses are accustomed to that. Talk to it in a quiet, calming tone of voice; a monotonous monologue can exert hypnotic effects upon the horse's psyche.

Reassurance

Take a few extra minutes to reassure the horse. The horse will then begin to build confidence. More trust is gained by not over-pressuring it, but proceeding when it is ready to accept the situation with some degree of reassurance. Reward any agreeable behaviour with praise, and stroke its neck and face. Many horses like to be rubbed around the eye or over the withers.

Confidence and Patience

Looking a horse in the eye commands its attention. Act decisively, because hesitation promotes the horse's suspicion and enhances its anxiety and distrust. Humans easily transmit fear and nervousness to a horse. Slow and deliberate movements build confidence. Be firm with commands, and discipline appropriately.

Many horses are not necessarily fearful of a procedure, but may only be spoiled. These horses will respect a firm reprimand. Human efforts at psychological domination are a positive learning experience for the spoiled horse. Using sensitivity and patience teaches a horse about the necessity and benefits of submission to human will. Not only does this method make ground work more enjoyable for the horse and its handlers, but the horse's response to riding or driving training also improves. With respect comes obedience and cooperation.

An essential ingredient in any restraint conflict is to restrain our own fits of temper. Above all, stay cool and calm, and use the rational mind to command the situation. This advice sounds simple, but many of us know that self-restraint is not always easy during a battle of wills. It is always better to back off, count to ten (or fifty if necessary), and start again rather than to embark upon a counterproductive physical match with the horse.

Psychology

A horse should always be reacting to the people, rather than the people reacting to the horse. This goal is *not* accomplished by threatening the horse verbally or physically; instead, be mentally one jump ahead of the horse. Anticipate what it will do. Before it has even started to make that move, take steps to counter it, converting the move to something else. Unwanted behaviour is diverted, and it also perplexes the horse so now its attention is focused on the person. The horse looks to that person for a lead, accepting him or her as the dominant leader in the 'herd'.

This method of training requires empathy to individual equine personalities, and often is a gift with which one is born. Certain techniques can be learned by reading or attending seminars and clinics, but it is best to trust to common sense and sensitivity. Recipes for psychological modification should only be used as guidelines. Each person should find what works with an individual horse and stick to it.

Restraint of a fractious horse is not about physical force. Instead it depends on the mental approach and understanding of each horse's unique response to any given situation. Figure out what makes the horse tick, and take strides to mould this knowledge into a plan of human design, without reacting to the horse.

HANDLING PROCEDURES
Safe Area

When approaching a situation that will be disagreeable to a horse, work in an area free of entrapments such as machinery, vehicles, rakes, wheelbarrows, low overhangs, nails and latches, and electrical cords. Find level ground with enough space for safe movement. Children, bystanders and pets (e.g. dogs and cats) should be asked to leave the working area. This practice ensures their safety, and prevents people from tripping over them while they work.

There should be at least two people involved in the procedure: the restrainer and the operator. The restrainer holds the horse while the operator performs the procedure. The restrainer should be a person who understands horses, and with whom it is easy to communicate.

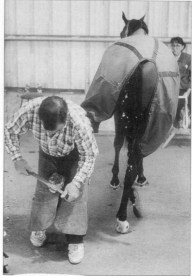

Fig. 19.3 A clear working area ensures the safety of the horse and handlers.

Dedicated Restraint

The restrainer must be confident and stay with the horse, not letting go at a jumpy reaction by the horse. If the restrainer lets go there is risk that the restrainer or operator could be hurt by a loose horse. Furthermore, letting go reinforces the adverse behaviour and the horse now knows how to extract itself from the situation. Rather than submitting to the procedure, the horse intensifies its efforts to get away.

Safe Equipment

Check the safety of all equipment, using intact, well-fitting halters and stout lead ropes. Be sure all buckles and snaps are functional, and are likely to remain so if stressed.

Always keep hands and fingers out of the halter, and never wrap a lead rope around the limbs or body. This practice prevents sprains, strains or lost fingers if a hand is entangled in a rope as a horse reacts suddenly.

Standing Position

The best place to stand during any procedure is close to the horse, just behind the shoulder so it cannot strike out with a leg. An operator who is standing close to the horse when it suddenly throws its weight feels far less impact than if he or she stood a few feet away.

Never stand directly in front of any horse while performing a procedure. In this position, there are many ways for the horse to cause a problem, such as lunging, pawing or rearing.

The restrainer usually stands on the same side as the operator, if possible. This position allows him or her to pull the horse's head towards the people, which automatically swings kicking hindquarters away.

METHODS OF RESTRAINT

Because a horse's instinct to flee is so intense, submissive behaviour is induced by removing the ability to flee. Restraint of a horse's flight instinct is accomplished by either physical or chemical methods.

Application of any form of physical restraint depends on psychological wit to ensure success. Learn which physical restraint method works best for the horse and recognize when the desired effect has been achieved. Some horses may object so violently to certain restraining measures, such as stocks or a twitch, that more cooperation may be achieved by quietly asking the horse to submit to a procedure without any physical restraint. Experience teaches which horses respond best to a 'least restraint' technique.

Physical restraint begins simply when we place a halter and lead rope on a horse. Assuming a horse knows how to lead, it will go where we go. Now that the horse is 'in hand', more physical restraint can be applied as necessary.

Placing a horse in a safe stall limits its ability to plunge and flee across a paddock or pasture. A horse can be backed into a corner where it feels more under the control of the handler.

Stocks

Use of 'stocks' confines a horse and severely limits its movements. Never be complacent about a horse in stocks because it is still able to kick or bite, or may attempt to jump out. A seat belt, snugly fit over the horse's withers, deters a tendency to leap upwards.

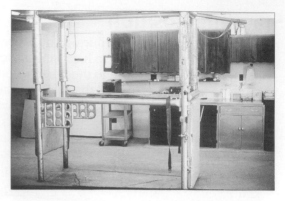

Fig. 19.4 Stocks with a restraining back strap made from a car seat belt.

Twitch

A *twitch* placed on the upper lip applies pressure to sensory nerves of the lip. It is uncomfortable enough to distract a horse's attention from other areas of the body. Evidence shows that endorphins are released by twitch application. Endorphins are narcotic-like substances produced in and released from the central nervous system, and they block referred pain from other parts of the body, causing the horse to relax.

An *easy twitch*, sometimes called a humane twitch, is a piece of steel or aluminium clamped over a horse's nose like a pair of pliers. A *chain twitch* is a device that winds a chain over the lip. A long handle is attached to the chain for increased leverage. If a horse throws its head and the twitch gets away from the restrainer, a chain twitch can become a flying missile capable of seriously injuring the restrainer,

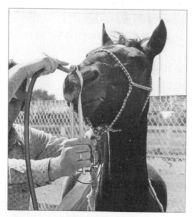

Fig. 19.5 An easy twitch.

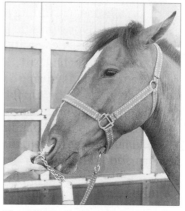

Fig. 19.6 A chain twitch.

operator or bystanders.

An applied twitch should be held vertical to the ground, as twisting it sideways or upside down is painful enough to elicit violent reactions from a horse. Do not pull on it or use it to lead a horse. For some horses, a twitch is a fearsome device; a normally tractable horse may strike out.

Lip Chain

The horse that fears and abhors twitches may respond positively to the use of a *lip chain*. A lip chain is placed over the upper gum just under the lip, and serves as a self-punishing device capable of training the horse. The lip chain is less intimidating than a twitch.

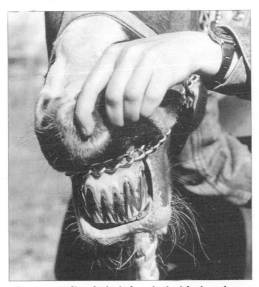

Fig. 19.7 A lip chain is less intimidating than a twitch.

Before applying the chain, running the fingers under the upper lip and along the gums provides a horse with a familiar taste of salt from the fingers and encourages confidence. Then the chain is quietly and smoothly slipped into place. If a horse exhibits undesirable behaviour, the chain tightens over the gum and is painful, but as soon as the horse responds appropriately, it is instantly rewarded by release of pressure and pain. Rapid jerks on the chain by the restrainer are counterproductive and can result in rearing. A light, steady pressure is all that is necessary to keep the chain in place. The horse's response automatically tightens or loosens it.

Stud Chain

Instead of placing the chain under the lip, it can be applied over the nose as a *stud chain*. A firm jerk on a chain in this position causes pain to the nose, enforcing a verbal reprimand.

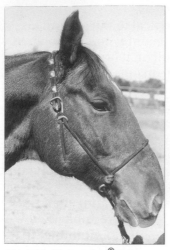

Fig. 19.8 A Be-Nice® halter.

Be-Nice® Halter

A Be-Nice® Halter works effectively on horses that react negatively by throwing their heads or rearing. The weight of the halter tightens the nose piece and pulls down on the poll section. If the 'prongs' are placed downwards in contact with the poll, negative reinforcement is asserted when the horse raises its head. Dropping its head (and body) causes the pain to cease. A Be-Nice® halter can self-train by punishing and rewarding a horse instantly at the time of the behaviour.

Blindfold

Blindfolding also prevents a horse from fleeing. It is now completely subservient to the restrainer because it has no idea of where to move. Occasionally, it is necessary to blindfold a horse to apply another physical restraint method such as a twitch. This can be a simple but useful method of restraint. A towel is a suitable blindfold and can be easily tucked into the head collar.

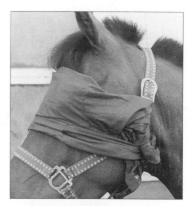

Fig. 19.9 A blindfold may be helpful when applying a twitch.

Hobble

Another means of removing a horse's ability to escape is to tie one leg in a hobble. The leg is flexed at the knee, and a leather strap or soft cotton rope is placed around the forearm and pastern. If one leg is held off the ground, a horse feels 'crippled'. Its other limbs mildly fatigue. Many horses hop around in confusion as they try to free their leg. Occasionally, a horse overreacts by throwing itself to the ground. Others become subdued. This should only be carried by an experienced horseman as there may be danger for the human and the horse if the horse reacts violently.

The goal is achieved when the horse recognizes the human as the 'saviour' who removes the hobble from the leg. Now the human is

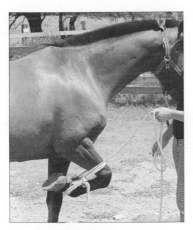

Fig. 19.10 A hobble makes the horse feel 'crippled'.

The Good Guy who presents the horse with the lesser of two evils: it can submit quietly with all four legs on the ground, or lose the use of one of its legs with a hobble.

Backing the Horse

Some horses prefer to back up to flee from an unpleasant situation. Unless there is a safe obstacle for them to back into, this flight behaviour is incredibly frustrating. Forcing such a horse to rapidly back around and around a paddock may sufficiently fatigue its muscles so it willingly stops backing and allows the procedure. At the same time, the restrainer has achieved psychological domination over the horse. Such a procedure is not without its dangers.

Distracting Noises

Sometimes jiggling a halter distracts a horse's attention as it listens to the jingling buckles. Knocking on its forehead in a non-rhythmical pattern also diverts its attention to the feel and sound. Knock in a random pattern so it does not know when the next tap sequence is coming. The horse may temporarily tune in to this distraction, long enough to give an injection or apply a bandage.

Earing Down (Ear Twitch)

Gently grabbing an ear and firmly pulling downwards is another method of distraction. An ear should not be twisted or jerked as that can injure it. Downward traction is all that is required to achieve the necessary response. If performed properly, 'earing' a horse rarely makes it head-shy afterwards. However, it is often difficult to grab hold of an ear on an already head-shy horse. A similar distracting method is to grab a fold of skin on the horse's neck and pinch it.

Cross-Ties

Cross-ties are a poor means of restraining a horse. Not only can a person be entangled in the cross-tie ropes, but a violently thrashing horse can rear up and flip itself over in the cross-ties, fatally injuring its head or neck. If cross-ties are the only available holding device, connect them with a quick-release buckle, and never leave a horse unattended in cross-ties.

Foal Restraint

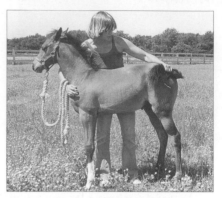

Fig. 19.11 Proper foal restraint.

Restraint of a foal requires a different technique from those used on grown horses. Foals often quieten down if the re-strainer encircles the foal's chest with an arm, and runs the other arm around behind the buttocks. The tail can be pulled up gently, with no adverse ef-fects, to stabilize the foal. Be sure the forward arm is not too high up on the neck so air flow through the trachea is not impeded. Pushing a foal against a safe wall, and placing a knee firmly into its flank while encircling it with the arms usually holds it steady so the operator can perform the necessary chore. Do not be fooled by a foal's size; the smallest newborn can crack someone's ribs or dent a head or shin. Be firm, but patient, with foals.

Chemical Tranquillizers

For horses that do not comply with any form of physical restraint and threaten to injure a person or themselves, or for a horse that must be subjected to a painful procedure such as wound suturing, chemical re-straint may be necessary. In this era of modern medicine it is no longer necessary to resort to the use of casting ropes that yank a horse off its feet and then submit it to having its feet tied together. Chemical tran-quillizers and sedatives diminish stress to both the horse and operator and prevent a horse from injuring itself.

Adverse Reactions

Tranquillizers and sedatives should be used under veterinary supervision, for although adverse reactions to these drugs are un-common, they can occur. The horse's heart should be monitored with a stethoscope to check for any murmurs or arrhythmias. Sedatives or tranquillizers exert cardiovascular effects that can adversely affect a poor heart condition.

Many mortality insurance policies do not cover fatal accidents that occur from medication or drugs given without veterinary supervision.

Methods of Administration

Sedatives or tranquillizers can be administered either intravenously (IV) or intramuscularly (IM). If given into the vein, the effects are fairly immediate (within several minutes), but not as long-lasting as they are when given IM. An IM injection requires at least 10 minutes before the head drops and the horse's body relaxes.

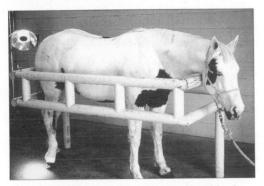

Fig. 19.12 A lowered head and relaxed body indicate sedation.

Different dose levels are calculated depending on whether the IV or IM route is used. Always discuss with a veterinarian how much and in what manner a drug should be given to avoid disastrous consequences. Learn about side effects for any drug given to a horse.

Excitement Prevents Tranquillizing

It is essential to keep the horse quiet before giving the sedative drug and during the time it takes to act. If a horse is excited and adrenaline is flowing before administration of a sedative or tranquillizer, the beneficial depressant effects of the drug may not be achieved. Adrenaline speeds up the heart rate and blood flow through the body, and results in flushing of the drug through the system too rapidly to affect the central nervous system.

Try to anticipate whether it would be advantageous to start with chemical restraint rather than getting the horse excited first. Once a horse is excited and a decision is made to try a chemical approach, it is best to wait 20 – 30 minutes for everyone to calm down before administering the drug. This method achieves an effective and less stressful result.

ALTERNATIVE SOLUTIONS

If a tactic is not working sufficiently, then stop and regroup. Think the situation over. Try to figure out what exactly is troubling the horse. Remember, the best approach is to use the *least* restraint necessary. Overpowering a horse mentally and physically elicits more of a fight. The objective is to convince a reluctant horse to *cooperate*. Cooperation does not mean that it willingly complies. Sometimes, just standing still is a sign of submission. Accept small winning steps, and reward cooperation. If necessary, seek professional help from a veterinarian.

Ideally, the goal is to train a horse to accept and tolerate a disagreeable event. Horses do not lie down, roll over, and just say, 'Here, do what you will'; that will never happen. Be satisfied with incremental successes, and build on these. Maintain a bright, optimistic outlook, and this attitude will be transmitted to the horse.

Above all, stay rational and do not prematurely admit defeat. By drawing on reservoirs of psychological, physical and chemical restraint, there is always a way to get the job done, both effectively and safely.

20

MANAGING THE CONFINED HORSE

Due to showing, racing, limited land resources, and for various other reasons, many horses are confined to paddocks, runs or stalls.

Stalls are a practical means of housing a large number of horses in a limited space, maximizing use of land and pasture resources. At horse shows and racetracks, a stall is usually the sole facility in which a horse is kept during its stay.

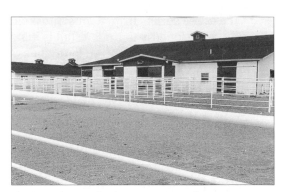

Fig. 20.1 For various reasons many horses must be confined to stalls or pens.

429

HERD INSTINCT

Studies reveal that under natural, free-ranging conditions, horses spend approximately 60% of their time grazing, preferably with the herd. Not only does frequent grazing satisfy a physiological need for

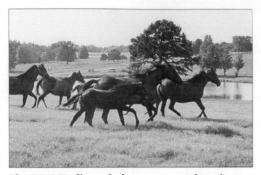

roughage and a psychological need to chew fibre, but grazing involves a fair amount of wandering and exercise during the course of a day.

As herd animals, horses enjoy the company of other horses. Grooming behaviour, frolic and play are just a few examples of social interactions between individuals within a herd. Horses like to

Fig. 20.2 Frolic and play are examples of social interactions within a herd.

touch, smell and taste each other. A pecking order, or social hierarchy, is established through social interplay as each horse assumes a comfortable and secure social position within the herd.

REASONS FOR CONFINEMENT

There are other circumstances, other than lack of acreage, which may cause an owner to prefer confining a horse indoors. Stalls provide shelter from wind and cold, rain or snow. Stalling a horse out of the sun also prevents sun bleach of a sleek and lustrous hair coat, giving a competitive advantage in the show ring.

If a horse suffers from a musculoskeletal injury requiring confinement for a lengthy period, a stall is instrumental in ensuring rest. A stall restricts movement, so bandages or limb casts stay clean and dry inside a well bedded stall, hastening the healing process.

Some horses tend to self-destruct if left to run loose in a pasture or paddock. Nervous horses may unceasingly gallop a fence line, risking strain and exhaustion.

Mares in heat or hormone-driven stallions may injure themselves or other horses during disputes across a pasture fence. Individuals that are too aggressive in the herd must be kept separate from other horses. For nervous or combative horses, housing within the quieting confines of a stall may prevent unnecessary mishaps. Dim indoor lighting and seclusion calm belligerent or nervous behaviour.

Still other reasons induce us to stall our horses. A horse requiring a special diet can be fed appropriately without competition from a herd. Stalling a mare under lights during late winter or early spring hastens the onset of oestrus so she can be bred earlier in the season. A mare due to foal is brought into a large foaling stall to provide a clean and sheltered environment that is easily monitored and safe from predators or dominant herd horses.

PSYCHOLOGICAL STRESS

What psychological stresses are imposed when we pull horses away from their social life, and isolate them? What happens when we remove access to grazing and movement by locking our horses inside a boxstall? They become dependent upon humans for feed, exercise and companionship. Food may show up regularly two or more times a day, and in some cases free choice hay is available at all times. Yet, exercise and human companionship is only forthcoming for an hour or two a day.

For horses permanently stalled, 23 or 24 hours a day is a long time in which to do nothing, day after day. A lucky few have a door or window that opens to the outside, so they can stick their heads out of the opening, and look at the world around them. Visual stimuli and sunlight are welcome diversions from

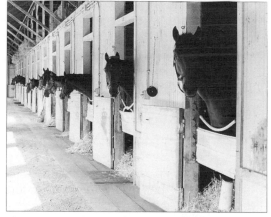

Fig. 20.3 Windows reduce boredom.

overwhelming boredom. Horses provided with free choice hay have the luxury of fulfilling a powerful need to chew fibre. But because a horse can only consume 2–3% of its body weight per day, it can only eat so much before becoming full of easily obtainable and highly nutritious hay. There is a lot of time left over for 'hanging about' with no way to vent its pent-up energy. This may also be manifested by excessive drinking of water.

Other stalled horses are fed a limited amount of hay twice a day, and may have no window or door through which to gaze upon the outside world. A belligerent horse or a stallion may be enclosed by

431

metal bars or mesh fencing that prevents hanging a head out into the aisle of a barn. Such horses experience no stimuli, no physical contact, and little or no exercise. Under such conditions, what do horses do?

Stall Vices

Not all horses fare well in the restrictive confinement of a stall. Removing a horse from a natural habitat (in which it could roam, graze, and interact within a herd) is an extreme form of stress. It is no wonder stall vices develop when a horse is confined.

A stall vice is a behaviour developed as a result of stress. Once a behavioural pattern emerges, it is difficult to break the habit. If a problem is recognized in the beginning stages, measures can be taken immediately to alter the horse's environment. Initially, an unhappy horse may exhibit subtle behavioural changes while being saddled or ridden, or it may display uncharacteristic aggressive tendencies towards other horses or people. Ground manners may change: for example, a horse may present a rear end as a person enters the stall, and lay its ears back in agitation. To a sensitive owner, such warning signals may be glaringly obvious, but the reason behind them can remain elusive.

Start by asking what has changed in a horse's routine, including:

- Has it been moved from a paddock to a stall?
- Is it stalled in a different location than before?
- Has a companion horse left the premises, or a new arrival moved in next door?
- Have new employees assumed cleaning and feeding chores in the barn?
- Have feeding times been changed?
- Is the food quality different?
- Is it breeding season, a time that hormonally alters the behaviour of mares and stallions?
- Have exercise levels changed?

If the horse could talk, it might say what is bothering it. In its own simple way it is communicating distress by body language and mood. When people listen with all of their senses, they usually find the underlying cause.

Wood Chewing and Cribbing (Crib-biting)

Horses have a natural urge to chew. Wood chewers eat the insides of wooden stalls in an insatiable demand for fibre. It may also be due to boredom or lack of minerals. This behaviour may result in splinters in the mouth. Swallowed splinters can lodge in the throat, or irritate or puncture an intestine, with serious consequences. Good quality pasture, and free-choice hay and salt will help prevent wood chewing.

Boredom may also spur a horse to latch its teeth on to an edge of the stall, a water container or a feed bucket and swallow air. *Cribbing* is an incessant behaviour pattern. It is speculated that cribbing activates narcotic receptors within the central nervous system, causing an addiction.

A horse that has been a cribber for very long can be identified by its teeth: the upper, front incisors are worn. They may also be hard keepers because they will turn away from food to nurture the habit. In addition, cribbers are predisposed to gaseous colic. *(See Chapter 13 for more information on colic.)* Cribbing can be controlled by feeding more often, providing more exercise and/or free time outside, or through the use of a neck brace, neck strap or muzzle.

Abnormal Movement

Other stall vices are based on weird movement behaviour, such as pacing, or weaving back and forth while standing in one place, re-mindful of the rocking motion used to calm an infant. Some horses dig holes of considerable depth in their stalls, while others kick at the walls with front or hind limbs, or both.

Stall Kicking

One of the more destructive stall vices is the habit of stall kicking. Not only does damage to a stall cost money to repair, but a horse can inflict serious damage upon itself. Splintered wooden walls and doors, bent metal components, and razor sharp edges result from damage to the structural integrity of the stall—and pose a serious hazard to a horse's vulnerable legs and face. If a door is kicked off its tracks or bent outwards, a foot can get caught in a newly made opening before the hazard is discovered.

The trauma on a horse's limbs as it kicks or paws at walls can strain or sprain ligaments, tendons or muscles.

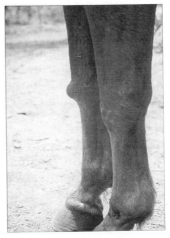

Fig. 20.4 A hygroma from constant stall kicking.

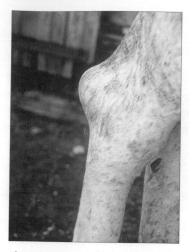

Fig. 20.5 Capped hock due to stall kicking.

Areas like the front of the knee *(carpus)*, fetlock, or back of the hock are particularly vulnerable to bruising and abrasion. Capped hocks or hygromas of the knee are caused by continuous trauma to bursal sacs underlying superficial tendons. Such blemishes are usually only of cosmetic significance, but if repeatedly aggravated, can develop into functional problems and impede performance.

Bruised muscle or connective tissue can develop serum or blood pockets, or an overwhelming inflammatory response known as *cellulitis*, which is accompanied by intense pain and swelling in the affected limb. Powerful impacts to the bottom of a foot as a horse kicks at a rigid wall can injure the coffin bone inside the hoof. The coffin (pedal) bone can even fracture if an intense blow is sustained.

If a wooden structure is weakened by continual kicking, a solid impact can blow it apart, with a limb shooting through splintered wood. Serious lacerations can result.

Reasons for Stall Kicking

Anxiety and Frustration

What causes horses to kick or paw in a stall? Frustration at restriction of movement creates anxiety, leading to displacement activities such as pawing and kicking. Transfer of pent-up energy also assumes the form of kicking or striking out at confining walls. If a horse sees other horses running at play, its frustration is intensified because it wants to join the frolicking herd.

Feeding Time

Some horses anticipate arrival of breakfast or dinner as soon as they spot the feeding person arrive at the barn. A horse displays an eager appetite by striking on a wall or door with its leg. What may start out as a small signal of impatience can escalate into an irrepressible habit.

Horses fed concentrated feed pellets finish their meal in less than an hour or two a day. Considering that, in a range habitat, a horse intermittently grazes for about 16 hours a day, a stalled horse on a pelleted likely to become diet is remarkably bored. It may begin banging on the sides of its stall to get attention, or just to have something to do. This type of problem is readily resolved by feeding a grass hay diet to accommodate a need to chew roughage throughout the day.

Space and Relationships

Certain horses are extremely territorial about their space, and may be particular about a neighbour next door. Once pleasant relationships are established between horses, try to house them side by side. Keeping friendly horses in sight of each other reduces stress. Although they are unable to make physical contact, the visible presence of a friendly horse has a strong calming influence.

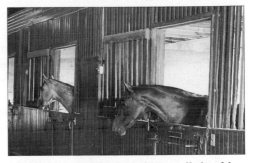

Fig. 20.6 Horses that get along well should be stalled next to each other.

Isolation Stress

Horses thrive with physical contact. A companionable horse who cannot nuzzle and smell a neighbour by sticking its head out of a door or over a partition may strike at the walls in frustration. Isolation for a normally social animal is a cause of anxiety. Individuals craving contact or companionship may relax with the introduction of a gentle goat or chicken, that lives in the stall with the horse. Herd relationships and bonding are established between a horse and any living creature. All it takes is a little imagination, and finding a suitable animal.

Loners

Certain horses prefer to be by themselves, perhaps because that is how they were raised and they are used to it. If a horse next door reaches towards the stall of a 'loner', the loner horse may feel its space has been violated. In frustration and territorial intent, a loner horse kicks and strikes at an offending neighbour even if the friendly horse only glances its way.

New Surroundings

If a horse is moved to a new barn or is stabled at horse shows, not only are the surroundings new and different, but so are the other horses housed next to and across from it. Not all horse personalities get along in such enforced conditions, and the only separation may be a wooden partition with mesh fencing at the top. Feeling trapped and enclosed, a horse exhibits stress by striking or kicking out at a neighbour. Walls of the stall take the brunt of the blows, but this activity may be the start of a terrible habit when a horse returns home.

Mares in heat or stallions stalled next to stallions or cycling mares may pound on the walls from a breeding-related or physical dispute.

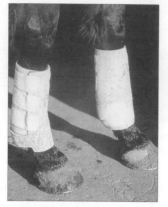

Fig. 20.7 Protective boots prevent injury.

Protection for Stall Kickers
Boots and Padding

Methods to protect a horse from wreaking physical damage to itself from stall kicking include armouring it with hock boots, fetlock boots, shin boots, or knee pads to protect these areas from trauma. Vinyl-covered foam padding on walls and doors reduces abrasions and trauma caused by striking a surface. Continual upkeep of padding is time-consuming and costly. Lining a stall with straw bales reduces the impact of hoof blows, but further limits the internal space within a stall, increasing a sense of claustrophobia and restriction of movement.

RELIEF FROM BOREDOM
Toys

Toys in a stall can relieve boredom and help prevent all types of stall vices. Hanging rubber or plastic balls give a horse something to bang or chew on without risk of injury. Gallon water jugs can be hung from the rafters to create the same effect. Commercially available hanging plastic 'apples' and 'carrots' also serve as playthings for bored or restless horses.

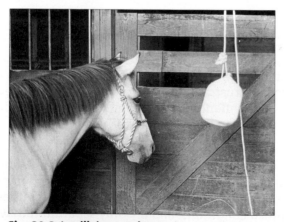

Fig. 20.8 A milk jug can be used as a stall toy.

Self-Exercise

When a horse is confined in a stall, it finds ways to wear off pent-up energy. Pacing, weaving, kicking and pawing are all manifestations of a need to move. A horse that is stalled for most of the day should be allowed daily self-exercise in a large turn-out area or paddock. In this way it can vent its fire, buck and kick, and romp. If turn-out is not an option, then a stalled horse should be put on a 'walker' or hand walked for at least an hour per day. An occasional break in hand walking for a relaxing graze of

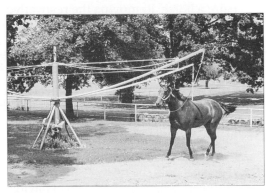

Fig. 20.9 A walker is an outlet for energy.

fresh grass is also a benefit. Horses stabled or boxed following injury should be walked out for exercise and to relieve boredom. Failure to do this may lead to the horse's causing itself further damage by 'wheeling round' or 'pacing' the box.

Performance Exercise

Of course, the performance horse should be exercised properly for its particular event. However, calm easy riding occasionally in place of daily training helps to relieve stress. A horse should not feel that each time it is saddled it will be put under mental and/or physical pressure.

CHANGING THE ENVIRONMENT
Moving Outside

Along with exercise, perhaps the best cure for an anxious horse exhibiting stress behaviour or a stall

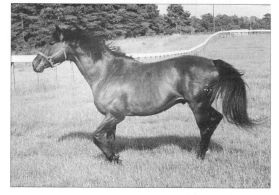

Fig. 20.10 Fresh air and sunshine help to calm a stressed horse.

vice is to move it into the Great Outdoors. If possible, enlarge the spatial dimensions of an outdoor paddock relative to the previous size of its stall. Outside fence panels are used to restrict the area of movement if a horse is recuperating from an injury. Fresh air and sunshine, long distance views, and seeing other horses significantly calm a horse. Removing the restrictive walls of a stall also removes a rigid surface for a horse to kick.

Adjusting for Personality Conflicts

Recognizing personality conflicts between horses and physically moving horses around until proper relationships are established reduce a horse's anxieties. It is also important to monitor how stable employees interact with a horse. An owner or trainer may find this interaction difficult to evaluate unless he or she arrives at the stables in time to watch reactions from the relationship. A horse may dislike a specific handler, groom or helper. Anticipation at having to interact with a disliked person adds to a horse's stress level, with abnormal behaviours surfacing from underlying tension.

Changing Handlers or Location

If a once-happy horse starts stall vices or adverse behavioural patterns, it may be time to consider changing handlers or location. Possibly there is no specific reason for a horse's neurotic behaviour other than a dislike of the surroundings or discomfort with a farm's routine. It may be worthwhile to move a distressed horse around on a property in an attempt to rule out certain neighbouring animals, visual stimuli, noises and physical locations before entirely moving a horse off the property.

Sometimes, no matter where a horse is located on a particular farm, it remains stressed and unhappy. As soon as it is moved to a different facility, or to a new geographical location, it resumes a calm and quiet behaviour by which the handlers have known it for years. Many of us can commiserate with specific geographical preferences. Most people at one time or another have personally encountered an uncomfortable situation. People exhibit spatial preferences; some people elect to sit on an aisle or in the back of a crowded auditorium, while others thrive in a crowd. In working environments, some people prefer a secluded cubby hole, and others want to be in the middle of the hubbub.

Horses are no different in seeking spatial arrangements to suit individual temperaments. Yet, their choices are limited by human arrangements of a limited land resource. By eliminating a natural, free-ranging habitat, people remove a horse's ability to seek its place in a geographical and social context. Placing walls around its restless spirit, and curbing its eating behaviour to suit humans, reshape a horse's mental and physical state into something different from its natural predisposition.

Even within a restricted urban environment, people can listen to the message a horse conveys through its manners and actions. Fine tuning an environment and eliminating stresses channel a horse's energies into more useful applications than stall vices. Powers of concentration and learning abilities are improved in a happy horse, enabling it to give splendidly in athletic performance.

21

SAFE TRAVEL FOR THE EQUINE ATHLETE

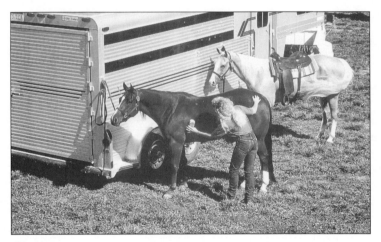

Fig. 21.1

TRAVELLING STRESS

For many people, travelling is stressful, upsetting the balance of everyday routine. Eating habits, sleeping patterns and usual daily procedures are disturbed. When a horse's routine is disturbed, it may suffer from stress as well. However, the stresses on equine health can be minimized. Many studies provide useful information about how horses respond to long distance travel. Whether the horses are enclosed in a van, a trailer, or in a cargo hold on an aeroplane, they are a large animal confined within a small metal tube. Such confinement leads to both mental and physical stress. Even in this era of supertechnology, 6% of horses transported long distances become seriously ill. Records from the turn of the century reveal similar figures, indicating that in almost 100 years there has not been much reduction in life-threatening illness from transport stress.

Effects of Travelling Stress
Colic
Similar to people, horses are creatures of habit. They are happiest when familiar events occur each day on a consistent routine. It is known that feeding horses on a regular time schedule benefits intestinal health. When a horse expects a meal to appear, its stomach juices and saliva production increase. If the meal fails to arrive, the effects on a sensitive metabolism can cause spasmodic or gaseous colic because the body was geared up for an event that did not happen. Travelling stress can also cause intestinal upset and colic. Some horses regularly have a mild colic attack, which is like 'butterflies' in the tummy', with any excitement.

Monitoring the Long Distance Traveller
In one study of horses travelling by air half-way around the globe, specific health indicators such as heart rates were evaluated. Researchers hoped to find a way to monitor horses transported long distances. By using the information obtained from the aeroplane study, horse owners or trainers can minimize stress on travelling horses and provide healthier conditions while a horse is in transit.

Increased Heart Rate
Fright is a form of stress and it can be evaluated by monitoring a horse's heart rate. On a long distance air flight of over 27 hours, horses' heart rates that averaged 52 beats per minute (bpm) before movement soared to 162 bpm at the first take-off. The average heart rate at the second take-off was 152 bpm, while the third resulted in heart rates averaging 130 bpm.

These results resemble the effect of conditioning: the horses gained experience and responded more favourably to each repetition of the experience. Conditioning horses to travel in a confined space such as a horse trailer, similarly diminishes stress from fear and anxiety.

Suppressed Immune System

Fear or stress increases the circulation of *cortisol* produced by the body. For a short trip, the cortisol response is minimal, but cortisol levels rise with longer transport, because the horse is under increased stress. Cortisol has an adverse impact on the immune system.

Transportation within a short distance causes no change in a horse's immune status. However, when horses travel long distances, the immune system is compromised. It cannot efficiently respond to challenge from microorganisms.

A study at Washington State University showed that horses travelling 700 miles over a 36-hour period had a depressed immune response. Not only is there a reduction in numbers of white blood cells to scavenge harmful microorganisms, but they are less effective at it. This suppression of the immune response predisposes a horse to infections.

Weight Loss

Another parameter that gives invaluable insight into transport stress of an individual horse is its body weight before and after transport. Within 12 hours, normal horses lose up to 33 lb, or about 3% of body weight. Some of this weight loss is caused by varying degrees of dehydration. Horses that develop shipping fever lose about 51 lb. The correlation of weight loss with development of infection is significant. Weighing horses before and after a long trip is useful for deciding if preventative care should be initiated.

Respiratory Disease

Environmental factors also have a profound effect on infection rates in horses. For example, as an aeroplane is in motion, air exchange occurs three times each minute. Air exchange greatly reduces the bacterial contamination of the environment, although continued environmental exposure to manure and urine eventually heightens bacterial counts. The number of colony forming units (cfu), both bacterial and fungal, number around 200 on a plane in flight. More than 5000 cfu flourish when a plane is stationary and loaded with horses.

Not only do the number of microorganisms increase when a plane is stationary, but temperature and relative humidity also are affected. In flight, temperature remains around 64° F. When a plane sits on the ground with long delays, the airline is only responsible for keeping the temperature between 45 and 85° F. Relative humidity escalates from an acceptable 47% while in flight to 90% when on the ground.

High temperature and humidity promote bacterial and fungal

growth, increasing exposure of the lungs to microbes. Coupling these factors with a suppressed immune system due to stress develops a situation ripe for disease, particularly of the respiratory tract.

The greatest cause of loss in performance from illness or death is due to complications from respiratory disease. Over 50% of 'shipping fever' related illnesses occur *after* a horse arrives at its destination. Travel may also expose a horse to allergens, with subsequent allergic respiratory disease problems.

Elevated White Blood Cell Count

Before and after transit, blood samples are useful to evaluate impending infection. Cellular counts for horses that remain in good health have been compared with those that develop shipping fever. After transport, white blood cells do not elevate in normal horses whereas, within 2 days of arrival, horses developing shipping fever show an increase in total white blood cells.

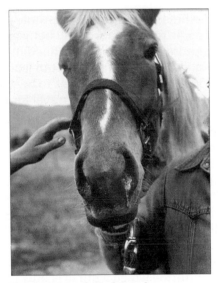

Fig. 21.2 Nasal discharge is a symptom of respiratory disease.

Pre-Existing Respiratory Disease

Pre-existing respiratory disease predisposes a horse to serious respiratory disease from transit stress. In a horse with a pre-existing respiratory disease, the normal airway clearance mechanisms (such as coughing) are overwhelmed by increased temperature and humidity. A horse experiences more stress on its journey due to an overwhelming exposure to microorganisms, dehydration (correlated to weight loss), and delays in transit that prevent adequate air circulation and quality. These factors tip the scale of health and disease towards development of disease.

The best way to manage a travelling horse is to minimize stress. Common sense and humane practices during long distance transport of horses will improve the standards of health for equine travellers. Although a horse may not appear sick upon arrival to a far-off destination, performance may suffer slightly, removing the winning edge in a competition. Careful monitoring of attitude, rectal temperature, body weight and feed and water consumption can detect problems early on.

LONG DISTANCE TRAVEL PREPARATION

Although few horses are subjected to long distance air transport, similar principles can be applied to long distance travel between regions and countries. With competitions or breeding farms spaced hundreds of miles apart, multiple-day trailer trips are not uncommon. Certain steps can be taken to promote a more stress-free journey, and to control the continued health of the horses so they arrive in the best shape.

Physical Examination

A careful evaluation of each horse before shipment is of primary importance. A health certificate may be required for travel between countries. Advice on the current requirements can be obtained from the state veterinary service. In most cases there is a minimum lead-time with the requirement for blood and for other samples to be examined. Allow at least 2 if not 4 weeks before the date of travel for the tests to be completed, to allow issue of the health certificate. For example, even if a second veterinary visit is required, the necessary Coggins test (for equine infections anaemia) paperwork must be available in time for shipping. Health certificates are meant to screen out horses that are carrying a transmissible disease such as lice, fungal dermatitis, *vesicular stomatitis* (caused by a virus), or viral respiratory illness, to name a few. Yet, a health certificate is also a safety precaution to identify a marginally or overtly sick horse that is about to be transported.

Not all illnesses are identified at the time of health inspection because there is an incubation period during which a horse is infected with disease but has not developed clinical symptoms. Some horses will slip through even the most arduous screening process. However, careful examination of a horse just before transport improves the possibility of discovering a marginally ill horse.

With the additional stress of shipping, what may have normally developed into a mild upper respiratory viral infection can become sudden, severe pneumonia, leading to permanent respiratory damage or death. It is to a horse's advantage to be examined within several days of transport, rather than a protracted 2 – 4 weeks before.

Identification Inspection

Check to establish laws pertaining to travelling away from home with a horse. Often an inspection of the marking, or other form of identification such as a brand or identichip, is required for horses. A permanent passport card can be issued for the horse's lifetime unless it is sold to a new owner. Each time a horse is purchased, the change of ownership is rewarded.

Vaccinations

The vaccination status of a horse should be current and appropriate not only for the environment from which the horse originates, but for where it is going. To develop an adequate immune response to viral respiratory vaccines, boosters should be administered at least 2 weeks before travel. A veterinarian can administer vaccines at this time and obtain a blood sample for a Coggins test during the same visit. Then the next visit for a general physical exam and health certificate is scheduled for just a few days before a horse is expected to leave.

Unnecessary Antibiotics

Resist the impulse to start a horse on a preventative course of antibiotics before long distance travel. The problems that most commonly confront travelling horses stem from respiratory *viruses* for which there is no direct treatment; they must run their course. Yet once a viral infection is identified and diagnosed, a course of antibiotics may prevent bacterial infections that lead to pneumonia.

It used to be standard practice to give a horse a one-time injection of procaine penicillin just before shipping. This practice encourages development of bacterial resistance to antibiotics. A single injection does not instill a high blood level of antibiotic in the horse, nor does it persist long enough to effectively kill bacteria. There is no point in a single injection, and this practice should be discontinued.

Mineral Oil

A horse that is a nervous traveller and going a long distance may benefit from a stomach tubing with a gallon of mineral oil just before departure. Mineral oil serves as a laxative to sustain intestinal motility, and it diminishes the build-up of gas within a nervous or stagnant bowel. Mineral oil also prevents absorption of endotoxin from the gut that can cause laminitis. Incidence of colic and associated laminitis are reduced by this practice, but only flighty individuals going long distances need mineral oil.

Maintain Air Quality

The environment in which a horse travels is of utmost importance to respiratory health. Good air quality and

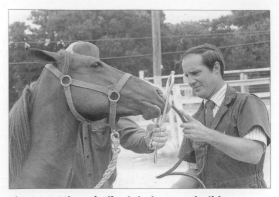

Fig. 21.3 Mineral oil minimizes gas build-up which can lead to colic or laminitis.

adequate ventilation are essential to keep temperature and relative humidity at safe levels. For horses hauled in trailers, exhaust pipes should be directed away from the intake air for the horses.

If a trailer or van stops moving for long periods, particularly in the summer, open the doors to allow circulation of fresh air through the horse stalls, or unload the horses and tie them outside. During stops, clean urine-soaked bedding and manure out of the trailer. Cleaning the area decreases bacterial and fungal contamination so numbers of microorganisms remain below an infective threshold.

Avoid long delays at international border crossings, ferry connections and refuelling stops. The longer horses are kept in a small, enclosed space with limited air circulation, the more the temperature and humidity rise, and the greater the exposure to microorganisms that challenge the respiratory tract.

Dust-Free Feeding

Always clean the mangers of stale hay and dust, and restock them with fresh, non-dusty hay. Fungal spores circulating in a trailer are decreased even more by providing vacuum-cleaned hay.

For respiratory tract clearance, horses should not be tied with their heads up high. If hay nets are tied low enough to encourage safe, head-down feeding, they allow small particles to fall down, away from a horse's airways. Nets should not be affixed so low that a horse can get a leg entangled in them.

Water and Electrolytes

Water should be offered at rest stops, at least every 4 hours. Electrolytes can be provided by oral paste or free choice to improve gastrointestinal function, and to stimulate natural thirst. Horses that do not drink strange water are at risk of serious dehydration. It is sometimes helpful to bring 5 –10 gallons of water along from home.

Provide Companionship

To further minimize the stress of trailering, some horses settle into a better routine if accompanied by a calm equine companion experienced in such trips. The more times a horse undergoes an experience, provided it has not been alarmed or frightened, the more it is conditioned to travelling, and the less stress response it exhibits. Its immune system functions more efficiently, and is more capable of warding off the challenge of infection. Some horses travel better with a companion such as a pony or even a goat or a dog.

Travelling Backwards

Research at Texas A & M determined that the direction a horse faces is a more important factor than the distance travelled. Considerable muscular effort is required to retain balance while in motion. Horses that travel *facing the rear* of a trailer or transport vehicle are less affected by transit stress than are horses that are confined facing forwards. In journeys further than about 20 miles, analysis of blood samples shows an increase in muscle enzymes, reflecting the physical work that is required by a horse to maintain balance. A horse facing forwards is unable to optimally use its hindquarters to diffuse the sway. By facing rearwards as a trailer, van, aircraft or boat travels with jerky starts and hesitations, a horse easily shifts its weight to the haunches and maintains its balance with less effort. With a trailer the weight distribution is also improved.

PROTECTIVE BANDAGES

Whether or not to put leg wraps on a horse is a heated controversy. However, from a veterinarian's point of view, horses wearing proper shipping bandages are rarely seen for trailer-inflicted injuries. Bandages must be properly fitted with adequate underlying Gamgee® or cotton wool.

No matter how well a horse loads or rides, anything can happen. Suppose an adjacent horse with iron shoes loses its balance and steps on the horse's leg. Or, a horse can step on its own legs as it scrambles in the trailer due to sudden braking or a sharp curve.

Loading and unloading are the most dangerous times for legs.

Trailer wraps provide a barrier between metal and flesh, and ground and flesh, particularly when loading or unloading a fractious, resistant horse. Moreover, if the flooring or ground is damp, a horse can slip and catch a leg on a ramp or on another limb, or a leg can slide underneath a step-up trailer.

Backing off a ramp is a shaky experience for a nervous or inexperienced horse. A leg can slip off the ramp, and with a convulsive jerk to regain footing the horse can lacerate its leg on a sharp edge. If a foot wedges under the

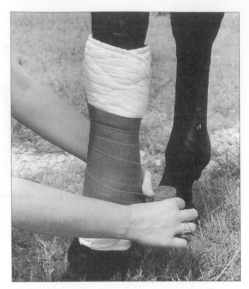

Fig. 21.4 Proper bandaging protects the legs from cuts and bruises.

ramp, self-inflicted wounds or fractured limbs can result as a horse struggles to free its entrapped leg.

Some horses explode backwards when asked to load. If not armoured with leg wraps, skidding across the pavement or gravel abrades and cuts thin skin.

Shipping Boots

There are many ways to apply shipping boots and bandages. It is important to cover the heel bulbs and pasterns as these areas are most likely to be injured. Wrapping the tendons and cannons is a good start, but if the bandages do not extend low enough, using bell boots will protect the heel bulbs. Then, a hind foot cannot lacerate a front limb. Bandages put on from the hoof to the top of the cannon bone will also provide support.

Fleece-lined shipping boots with Velcro® closures take only moments to apply to all four legs although they are not as substantial as wrapping the legs with cotton quilting and 'track bandages'. Thick batting under the bandages pads the legs and is secured snugly into place, keeping the wraps from slipping.

For a short trip or in an emergency, use disposable nappies or cotton pads under a stable bandage. Be careful not to pull the stable bandage too tight or it will constrict the tendons.

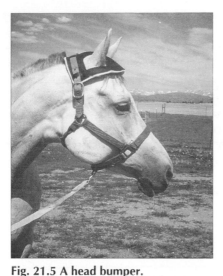

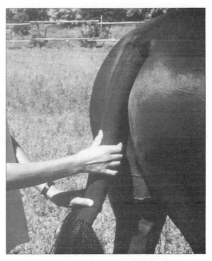

Fig. 21.5 A head bumper.   Fig. 21.6 A neoprene tail wrap.

Head Bumper and Tail Wrap

A head bumper protects the poll of a fractious horse in case it rears up and hits its head on the edge or top of the trailer.

A tail wrap prevents abrasion at the dock that can rub a horse's tail down to raw flesh. Commonly used are commercial neoprene tail bandages, or a track wrap or polo fleece. Be sure the tail wrap is not applied so tightly as to constrict blood flow through the tail, and not so loosely that it slips and falls off.

Another way to protect the tail from rubbing on the door or butt bar is to fasten thick foam padding with duct tape over the butt chain. Also, place the horse's tail inside the trailer so it is not hanging loose and flying in the breeze. The tail can hook on a protrusion, frightening and seriously injuring the horse.

Bandaging the horse will probably take 20 minutes the first few times. With practice the whole exercise consumes no more than 5 minutes and may save the horse from a crippling injury. At the very least those few extra minutes may save on expenses for veterinary care, emotional hassle, and time nursing an injured horse.

SAFETY MEASURES
Training

A horse that is inexperienced in trailering can be conditioned to load and ride with a sense of confidence. Taking the time to accustom the horse to load and unload quietly minimizes injuries, and makes a more pleasurable experience for all. This conditioning can be accomplished by practising loading and unloading with an experienced horse already in the trailer. Or, the novice horse can be fed in the trailer to give it a positive experience.

Once the horse confidently enters and backs out on command, take it on short rides to accustom it to the feel of movement. Again, a calm companion horse instils confidence into the learner. Longer trailer rides are introduced after the horse is conditioned to travel quietly. Each positive experience reinforces excellent trailering behaviour.

A loading bay is a good investment for a yard. It is great help in training the novice and with nervous horses.

Keep Doors Closed

Once a horse is loaded, a common mistake is to leave manger or escape doors open so the horse can look around while waiting to depart. This practice results in face and head lacerations and eye injuries. It only takes a spooky monster such as flying paper or a tractor driving by to cause a horse to jerk its head back through the open hatch. Occasionally a horse catches its head on a low door sill, which not only cuts the head, but panics it further.

The lesson here is simple. A horse spends most of its life with the freedom to look at the world around it. A few more minutes of gazing from the inside of a trailer is not worth the potential hazard. Close the manger and escape doors as soon as the horse is in the trailer.

Some horses are terrified of being in the trailer, and an open manger or escape door is perceived as an escape route. For such individuals, these doors should be closed even before the horse is loaded in the trailer.

Tying the Horse in the Trailer

It is best to tie the head to the manger loop, or to an overhead tie loop. A horse with its head free in the trailer may try to turn around. The horse is then tightly wedged in a potentially life-threatening position.

A frightened horse without its head tied can also launch itself into the feeder. A poor traveller can inflict leg injuries on itself, and once it finds its front leg and head tightly wedged in the feeder it is no longer a mildly reasonable animal.

When tying a horse's head, give it enough rope that it can comfortably move its head side to side, but cannot turn it backwards. The rope should not be so long that it can tangle in a leg or wrap around the head.

Commercially available 'quick-release' snaps are the ideal way to tie a horse. The snap is easily released in an emergency with a quick snap of the special buckle, and it is difficult to snare fingers in the safety snap.

Always attach the butt bar or butt chain and close the door before tying a horse. When unloading, always untie a horse before opening the trailer. A horse that is prone to bolting backwards can quickly pull on a lead rope, causing numerous problems.

A Butt Bar or Chain

A butt bar or butt chain adds a stop-gap for the unwelcome possibility that the back door of a trailer might fly open while it is moving.

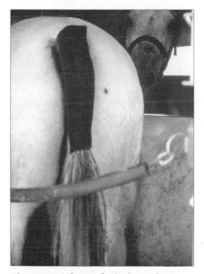

These doors are known to fly open for a number of reasons, namely the loosening of bolts that hold down the door handles. Road vibration works nuts and bolts loose over time, so these areas should be inspected frequently. A horse kicking at the trailer door can kick it open with explosive force.

A butt bar or chain may keep the horse inside the trailer long enough for a flapping rear trailer door to be discovered. Also, it prevents a horse from leaning on the back door. A thousand pounds (or more) of weight pushing on the door weakens the hinges and door bolts over time, creating conditions for potential mishaps.

Fig. 21.7 A butt chain is an important safety device.

First Aid Kit

Whenever it is necessary to journey away from home with horses, take along a first aid kit expressly for them. The following list is a good starting place from which to build such a kit. A veterinarian may add to these supplies and provide information on how best to use them.

- Table salt and a clean container: mix ½ tablespoon salt per quart of water for saline rinse
- Tamed iodine antiseptic scrub
- Sterile gauze sponges
- Dermisol® cream or Savlon® cream
- Clean stable bandages
- Conforming roll gauze and sterile surgical pad
- Bandage (self-adhesive stretch tape)
- Bandage scissors
- Non-steroidal eye ointment for injury from branches, wind, dirt
- Easy Boot® in case a shoe is lost
- Thermometer

While on a long distance trip it is a good idea to stop every 3 – 4 hours to check on the state of affairs in the horse trailer and to offer the horses fresh water. It is hard work for some horses to ride in a trailer, as they struggle to stay balanced through the twists and turns of the road and the sway of the trailer. A half-hour rest stop allows horses to relax taut muscles while remaining tied in the trailer.

Recovery Time

Once a horse arrives at its destination after a long journey, monitor body temperature twice a day. A fever often develops 2 – 3 days after arrival in horses that have contracted an infection. With prompt diagnosis, aggressive therapy can dramatically alter the duration and severity of a disease. The faster a problem is recognized, the more quickly a horse responds to treatment, and the more likely that permanent effects will be prevented.

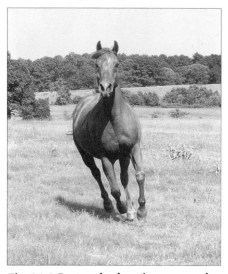

Fig. 21.8 Rest and relaxation are good for a horse after a long trip.

People expect their equine companions to understand where they are going and what is expected from them, and to immediately go to work upon demand. However, it is advantageous to plan a few extra days at the end of a journey to allow a horse to acclimate to a new environment, and to recover from the stress of transit.

TRANSPORTING BROODMARES

Another performance horse, besides the athlete, is the broodmare that is transported to the breeding farm and back home again. After all the effort required to get a mare in foal, it is a shame to lose a foetus to the effects of transit stress. The greatest incidence of early embryonic death (EED) before 50 days of gestation occurs between days 15 – 20 and days 30 – 35.

A study at Colorado State University analysed the effects of trailering on newly pregnant mares. During days 14 – 18, the mare's body must recognize the embryo for it to survive. Once it has passed this obstacle, at day 35 the embryo firmly implants in the uterus, and endometrial cups form to secrete progesterone hormones, which maintains the pregnancy.

Three groups of mares were studied. The 24 pregnant 'control' mares remained at home between days 16 – 33 and had free access to food and water. A second group of 15 pregnant mares was trailered between days 16 – 22 of gestation for a 9-hour ride with no food or water. A third group of 15 pregnant mares experienced a similar 9-hour trailer journey between days 32 and 38 of gestation.

Hormonal assays of progesterone and cortisol were obtained on each mare. Progesterone is a hormone necessary to maintain pregnancy, and low levels are highly correlated to early embryonic death. Progesterone concentrations increased in the two groups of trailered mares as compared with the controls left at home, and progesterone levels in Groups 2 and 3 remained higher for a time upon return with the farm.

Of the 24 control mares, 3 lost their embryos. Another 3 of the 15 mares that were trailered between days 16 and 22 lost their embryos, and 1 of 15 mares trailered between days 32 and 38 lost her embryo. Therefore, there was no real statistical difference between any group of mares in this study. The mares that did abort started with lower progesterone levels, which may explain the loss of the embryo.

The study concluded that trailering mares during a critical time between days 16 and 33 has no influence on maintenance of pregnancy, and that transportation at that time poses a minimal risk for pregnant mares.

Endotoxin Study

Another study conducted at the University of California at Davis surveyed a different slant on early embryonic death. If a mare experiences any surge in endotoxin release before day 50 of gestation, this stimulates release of prostaglandin F_2-alpha. This particular prostaglandin interferes with function of the *corpus luteum* on the ovary that is responsible for progesterone secretion until about day 50 of gestation. By day 50, progesterone is secreted from other sources to maintain a high enough level for pregnancy to persist.

Endotoxin release accompanies stress-related syndromes such as colic, diarrhoea, or other gastrointestinal disorders. It is of prime importance, then, that early term pregnant mares trailered for long distances receive ample food, water and electrolytes while on their journey. This practice minimizes intestinal compromise that results in release of endotoxins.

Progesterone Supplements

To minimize the risk of early embryonic death from endotoxin in an early term pregnant mare during transport, the mare can be placed on a supplemental source of progesterone, such as Regumate®. This supplement is fed daily until day 50 or 60 of pregnancy. Oral Regumate® provides ample progesterone to maintain pregnancy even if the function of the corpus luteum is compromised by stress-induced endotoxin release.

BASIC TRAILERING TIPS

It is wise to have a mechanic do a complete check and maintenance on the trailer every year. Then, before every trip, running through the checklist and inspecting the mechanical features of electrical connections, brakes, tyres, hitch, and bumper takes only a few minutes.

Always check the connections between the truck and trailer:

- ensure that the trailer ball is the right size
- make sure that locking pins are secure
- safety chains or cables should be strong enough to hold the trailer if the hitch comes off the ball
- check that the trailer ball is bolted on properly
- be sure the draw bar is strong enough to pull the trailer, and that it is securely affixed

Check the electrical connections, making sure the plug fits the socket and that the wiring is correct. When driving in hilly areas, electric trailer brakes reduce wear and tear on the truck brakes and provide full braking power if needed.

Check the pressure of all tyres (truck and trailer). Fully inflating tyres to manufacturer's recommendations also reduces tyre wear,

and achieves the minimum fuel consumption for the vehicle by reducing road friction. Take along spare tyres (and a jack and lug
wrench), for the truck and trailer.

Make sure that the registration plate is fitted in such a position that
the horse does not get injured.

Clean out the trailer after every ride to remove manure and urine-
soaked bedding and debris. Also pull out the trailer mats to allow the
floor boards underneath to dry. Constant exposure to wet manure
and urine inevitably rots the floor boards. Pulling up the mats and
sweeping or hosing out the soiled bedding prolongs the life of the
flooring and allows it to be inspected for weakness or rot.

The mangers should be swept clean after each trip. Otherwise, hay
and grain will accumulate and become mildewed. Since most mangers are at nose level, mould spores and hay dust are inhaled into a
horse's respiratory tract, possibly stimulating an allergic reaction
and respiratory disease. Problems develop when a trailer is tightly
enclosed without air exchange, or when a breeze stirs up dust from
the manger.

Using a Trailer As a Hitching Post

It is often convenient to use the horse trailer as a hitching post. At a
horse show, trailers may need to be parked on a treeless lot leaving
little choice where to tie a horse. At an endurance or long distance
competition, horses are restrained next to a trailer off and on for several days during the course of a competition. Because of such provi-
sions, a trailer becomes the sole means of confinement. It is
important for the trailer to have safety features similar to those of a
stall, paddock or pasture.

After parking and before opening the trailer doors, survey the
area. It should be flat and free from dangerous obstacles all
around. If the trailer is parked too close to an embankment, the
horse will be standing on an incline. Watch out for dangling overhead tree branches the horse might get tangled in.

If possible, analyse the direction the sun will travel through the
sky, so the trailer will not receive too much sunlight during the
day. Park so that horses are tied in the shade of a trailer to provide
relief from direct sunlight.

Once the rig is parked, place some hefty rocks or wooden blocks in
front of and behind a couple of tyres as insurance that the trailer will
not move.

Remember to untie the horse's head before releasing the butt bar
or chain, so there will be no accidental bolting backwards while a
horse is still tied. If more than one horse is along for the ride, it is

always a good idea to unload a green horse first so it is not left behind as its companions are removed to the side of a trailer out of sight. If an inexperienced or nervous horse is left until last, it might work it-self into a frenzy. It may paw vigorously to be let out, or strain on the butt bar, making it difficult to unload.

Unhitching the Trailer

When using a trailer as a hitching post, *never* disconnect a trailer from the truck. A frightened horse can easily pull an unhitched trailer which further panics the horse. Leaving a rig hooked up and placing rocks or wood blocks behind tyres prevents these disasters. All doors and ramps should be closed before tying a horse to the trailer. An open manger, escape, or tack compartment door invites injury to a horse's face or legs. Usually these doors have sharp edges capable of lacerating the horse, so it is best to close them. Back doors or ramps should also be closed if a horse is tied near them. Some horses will try to load themselves, leading to a very tangled and frightened animal.

Safe Tying Methods

Tying two or more horses randomly to a trailer causes many prob-lems. Only compatible horses should be tied side by side to prevent unruly behaviour and potential injury. It is important to discourage conflicts between horses outside the trailer.

Lead ropes should be short enough so a horse will not entangle its leg or head or its buckets in the line, but long enough that it can comfortably reach hay and water. A horse should have just enough lead to move side to side so it is not stuck in one spot. Ex-cessively long lead lines can catch on the door of many trailers. Tie horses away from door handles to prevent a rope from getting caught. A tennis ball that has been cut open and placed over the door handle also prevents snagging of a lead rope.

To attach a lead rope on to the tie-in spot on a trailer, tie a quick-release safety knot that pulls loose with a swift tug on the dangling end in case of an emergency. Safety knots do not always pull free if a frightened horse heaves back on the line and tightens the knot. As an alternative, quick-release buckles, as used to tie a horse in the trailer, provide a safer way to fasten a halter buckle and a better guarantee of effective release.

Carry a sharp pocket knife at all times to cut a rope if a knot is too tight to release. A panicked and entangled horse does itself consider-able damage if left to struggle for too long. A pocket knife quickly frees the horse from entrapment without endangering humans.

If a flighty or devious horse lunges backwards with a violent tug on a lead line, considerable damage can be done. Not only will a horse endanger itself as it sits back on its haunches, threatening muscle strain from the effort, but stretching its head and neck can also result in injury. If a rope or halter breaks at this moment, a pulling horse can catapult backwards into another object or horse, or it can flip or fall down with impact. Serious injury to head or limbs may occur from such behaviour.

Bring along a spare halter and lead rope in case they are damaged or broken. It is a serious inconvenience if this equipment is lacking.

Even a well behaved horse is frightened if a stirrup iron, saddle or other piece of tack snags on trailer bumpers. Never leave a tacked horse unattended while tied next to a trailer. Dangling martingales, tie-downs, breast collars, stirrup leathers and reins should be removed if someone cannot watch the horse.

When ill-behaved or frightened horses pull and fight being tied, other horses tied to the trailer are frightened as it rocks and vibrates.

Caring for the Tied Horse
Feeding and Watering

Before attending to personal needs, set up hay nets and water buckets for each horse. Do not hang a hay bag or net too low or a

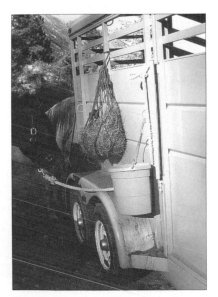

horse can get tangled in it. Since a fair amount of hay generally falls out of a hay net on to the ground, be sure lead ropes are not so long that an unattended horse is tempted to rescue stray hay pieces off the ground. A long rope that is wound around a leg can cause serious physical damage. Too long a rope also allows a horse's head to lower where a halter can catch on a bumper or other projection, resulting in fright and injury.

Plastic or rubber water buckets are easily hung from a trailer using chains or nylon ropes with quick-release buckles. Buckets so suspended should be no lower than the horse's shoulder height

Fig. 21.9 A rope caught around a water bucket can create a problem.

so it has easy access to water or grain without snagging a rope around the bucket. A rope tangled with a bucket dumps out the contents and shortens a horse's line, possibly scaring it into an unpredictable reaction.

Water should be available at all times so a horse does not become dehydrated. Water is essential for muscular work and digestive processes. An average horse drinks 7–20 gallons each day, depending on climate and exercise. Refills of fresh, clean water encourage adequate water intake to prevent colic, tying-up or heat stress.

Some horses are finicky about strange water supplies, and subsequently do not drink well. Lightly treating water with cider vinegar or sugar disguises the strange taste, making the water more palatable. This trick is especially effective if a horse is conditioned to vinegar or sugar in the drinking water back home before the trip. Or, familiar water from home can be brought along for a finicky horse.

Electrolytes

It is difficult to provide free choice salt blocks to horses tied to a trailer. Supplementing with 1 – 2 tablespoons of a salt mixture in grain each day of the journey replaces essential electrolytes lost in sweat. This factor is particularly important if a horse is used for rigorous athletics or if subjected to high temperatures or humidity. A good mixture is produced by mixing one part potassium chloride (Lite® salt) with two parts sodium chloride (table salt). When supplementing a diet with salt in this manner, it is important that the horse is drinking well. A proprietary electrolyte solution can also be purchased.

Rugging

When horses are tied to a trailer for extended periods, they are unable to move about to warm muscles and maintain suppleness of tendons and ligaments. If night air is cold or breezy, it might be advantageous to rug the horse, with either a sheet or heavier blanket appropriate for the weather. Rugging keeps muscles warm, and provides a windbreak, if no shelter is

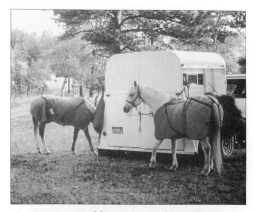

Fig. 21.10 A tied horse in cool weather should be rugged to keep muscles warm.

provided by the trailer. If a horse has an ample hair coat and is used to the rigours of the environment, it may not be necessary to rug. In the event of a driving rain or hail storm, horses can be loaded briefly into the trailer for respite from the elements. A horse that has exerted a tremendous athletic effort during an endurance or long distance competition may also benefit from a protective sheet or blanket to retain warmth in the muscles.

Horses do not need to lie down in order to sleep. A unique anatomical arrangement called the *check apparatus* 'locks up' the legs and keeps them from buckling as a horse sleeps. It is less dangerous to keep a horse tied so that it cannot lie down, than to lengthen its lead. If it has enough length of rope to lie down, it can also get entangled in it.

Hand Walking

It is more important than usual to adequately warm up and cool-down any horse engaging in exercise after and before being tied to a trailer for a long period. Warm-up and cool-down time loosens kinked joints, tendons, ligaments and muscles, providing circulation to adequately oxygenate tissues and remove toxic by-products. Suppleness improves as does performance, and tissue strain and fatigue are lessened.

A horse cannot move about at will when tied. Hand walk it at intervals after a day's athletics. Walking removes accumulated toxic by-products from muscle tissue, and improves circulation in the limbs so windgalls do not develop overnight.

Alternatives to Tying

If it is unknown whether an inexperienced horse has been trained to tie for long periods, consider what it might do if startled. Depending on how they were trained, not all horses are excellent candidates for tying to anything. Some horses explosively fight such restraint when they discover they cannot get loose. Other horses have learned that if they pull hard enough, the rope or halter will break, freeing them completely.

Temporary Paddock

There is a solution to the problem of confining a horse that has not been trained well and poses a danger to itself and others. Build a temporary paddock out of fence panels or PVC pipe. Fence panels, strapped to the side of the trailer for transport, are cumbersome, expensive, and time-consuming to assemble. Yet, they provide a safe solution to the problem. Rope can be used to fashion a paddock. However, it is not as secure and can loosen or droop, inviting a horse to jump out.

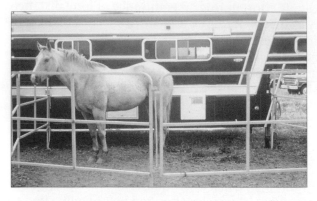

Fig. 21.11 Temporary paddocks made of fence panels are a safe solution to confining horses while on the road.

If there is more than one trailer on a journey, a small holding paddock can be fashioned by rigging panels, plastic pipe or rope between the sides of the two trailers. A horse can move around freely, and lie down at will. Feed and water buckets are placed on the ground if desired or hung from the side of the trailer. Trailer bumpers should be covered with chrome or rubber protector strips so the horse cannot cut itself. Remove the halter so the horse cannot snag it on anything.

If there are no other large vehicles or trailers to build a holding pen, another option is to purchase commercially available electric fence chargers that operate on solar power. These can create a temporary holding pen using fence stakes and electric wire. If remaining in one spot for a while, it may be necessary to build such an enclosure.

22

PREPURCHASE
EVALUATION

SELECTION CRITERIA

Certain criteria should be considered when choosing a horse. Because demands on an athletic horse are so varied, some characteristics will be more important than others. Each horse must be judged according to its own merits.

Consult a trainer or reputable horseperson for an educated opinion about a horse's capabilities and level of training. A determined screening process weeds out candidates that, despite being fabulous horses, may not be athletic enough for the required tasks. A testing period also reveals horses that are soured to a specific athletic endeavour due to negative experiences.

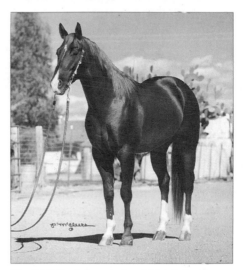

Fig. 22.1 Each horse should be judged on its own merits and the buyer's goals.

Age

An important consideration when purchasing a horse is its age. A young and green horse must be brought slowly through the ranks and schooled at the basics. Due to the rigorous demands of certain athletic pursuits and the differences in breed maturity, some horses should be allowed to mature to at least 5 years of age. This time allows for musculoskeletal maturity and development of mental concentration.

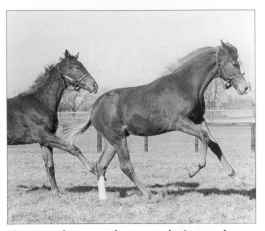

Fig. 22.2 The young horse needs time to develop musculoskeletal and mental agility.

There is always a beginning when every horse *and* rider are in the basic stages of learning. A novice rider should consider purchasing an experienced horse that can perform the intended task without compromising the safety of the rider.

An older horse, although initially lacking experience in a specific sport, is usually able to learn faster due to prior achievements. Physical maturity also provides the horse with the strength and stamina necessary for training and competing. A mature horse can be entered into a higher level of competition sooner than a youngster, provided it has mastered the basics of training. Of course if a horse is much older when beginning a performance sport, it may arrive at advanced levels too old to remain actively competitive.

Breed

Some breeds are genetically predisposed to excellence in certain athletic pursuits. The Arabian is bred for endurance and long distance competitive races. The Thoroughbred's speed makes it exceptional on the racetrack or as an event horse. The strong hindquarters of the Quarter Horse or Appaloosa promote their popularity in sprint sports. The Standardbred displays exceptional speed at trotting and pacing. Warmbloods shine in dressage, jumping, eventing and combined driving. Yet, there are horses with natural athletic talent which allows them to rise above breed prejudices and make their mark as versatile competitors.

Temperament

Brilliance in movement is not essential for athletic success. Scoring may depend on accuracy and obedience, flexibility and agility. The mind of the horse has as much to do with its performance as an inborn 'way-of-going'. Too often horses are purchased because of their beauty or athletic prowess. Without a sensible and accepting mind to 'operate' these physical endowments, a gorgeous horse may be unsuitable for competition.

An excessively nervous horse may not hold up well under the stress of travel, training and competition. It may also be prone to gastrointestinal disorders such as diarrhoea or colic. A calm, observant attitude enables a horse to cope better with the bombardment of multiple stimuli as it campaigns. Also, observing a horse in the pasture or stable identifies serious vices such as cribbing, wood chewing, stall walking, weaving or stall kicking.

Test Under Saddle

An essential criterion in assessing any horse is the potential for a partnership with the horse. Teamwork and trust are necessary elements to successful campaigning. A horse must be kind and forgiving. Judgement errors by a rider will occur on occasion, but the horse should continue to rely upon the rider for instruction. A temperamental and unpredictable character is dangerous, no matter how athletic the horse.

If possible, ride the horse being considered to determine the connection between horse and rider. Are its gaits enjoyable? Is it respectful and responsive? If the horse is experienced in a specific sport, ride it at its level of expertise or have a professional trainer or the owner do so. Note any quirks that may only show up under saddle.

Much information can be gained by trying out a prospect on more than one occasion. In this way, talent and temperament are more accurately assessed.

Intelligence and Attitude

A sport horse should be eager to learn, and intelligent so that it is able to learn. It should be able to think its way out of a crisis. This ability is often born as an innate cleverness, but also comes from experience and training. The horse should possess the inclination of 'try' that encompasses courage, enthusiasm and heart. Its attitude should be willing and bold, yet not reckless. The horse must accept discipline in all phases of training and competition.

So is this a description of the perfect horse? Individuals like this do exist, but as often happens, a horse can have all the desired characteristics in temperament, yet have an unsound limb, a heart condition, or chronic respiratory disease, making it unfit for consistent performance.

Conformation

Conformational defects should be analysed carefully to assess the possibilities of a physical breakdown. Such a breakdown can put a horse out of work, or worse can pose a hazard to both horse and rider. Safety accompanies soundness. Ideal qualities include:

- big, solid, straight bones
- strong, uninjured tendons and ligaments
- flexible, pain-free joints
- strong, well proportioned feet

Health Problems

When choosing a horse, consider the long-term effects if the horse has low-grade pain from foot soreness or mild arthritis. Will this pain interfere with stamina and willingness of the horse? Could the condition cause it to stumble and fall, or hesitate when asked to do something demanding? Will a currently mild problem progress to a crippling injury as greater athletic demands are placed on the horse?

A chronic respiratory problem may interfere with exercise tolerance at the desired level of training. The horse should be able to achieve rapid heart and respiratory recoveries after an exertion, so as not to compromise its metabolic status. Also, a known history of tying-up may preclude its purchase.

The rigours of athletic training place fantastic demands on the metabolic and musculoskeletal systems of a horse. If possible, start without any physical liability that may later interfere with active and safe participation in the chosen sport. Have a thorough prepurchase exam performed by a competent veterinarian who is well versed in the athletic demands of the sport.

The Overview

It is helpful to make a list comparing the pros and cons of the horse. Put the price at the top of the list. Are the shortcomings on the 'con' side acceptable when compared to the assets on the 'pro' side? There will always be some less-than-perfect characteristics in the unproven individual that may work for one owner, but not for another.

Try not to set expectations too high, as it often leads to disappointment. View the purchase realistically, and be patient with the training process. Often it is impossible to fully appreciate how well a horse will respond to training until after purchase. If that individual does not respond well after a reasonable period, sell it and move on to another prospect rather than wasting time, emotional energy and money on an unsuitable prospect.

PREPURCHASE EXAM

Regardless of whether a novice rider or a seasoned trainer is purchasing a horse, it is always prudent to ask a veterinarian to evaluate the horse before purchase. Even if monetary outlay for a horse is negligible, it is advisable to hire a skilled professional.

Thorough assessment of a horse reveals disabilities that can halt an athletic career before it begins.

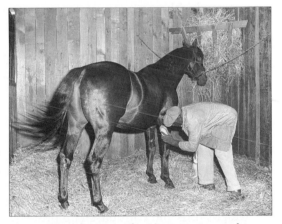

The cost of a thorough prepurchase exam should be factored into the initial purchase price. A veterinary prepurchase exam points out potential problems that one should be aware of before committing to an investment in a horse. Also, a veterinary

Fig. 22.3 Feed, care and maintenance must be remembered as part of the cost of a horse.

nary exam is useful before leasing a horse to identify specific problems prior to assuming full responsibility and personal involvement with another person's horse.

During the search for a horse, a process of elimination finally reveals a suitable equine prospect. Try to maintain an objective distance until a prepurchase exam has been completed. If the decision is subconsciously made before a complete veterinary analysis, it is easy to ignore important facts that can spell disaster. It is difficult to divorce oneself from expectations and visions about the animal before a prepurchase exam. Then, if lameness or other unsound characteristics are discovered by a veterinarian, it is harder to walk away from a purchase, especially if a deposit has already been made.

The danger in ignoring veterinary advice is that the buyer ends up with a horse that has a crippling disability. Expenses continue to mount, and it is difficult to resell the horse and regain the initial investment.

The Role of the Veterinarian

A veterinarian does *not* offer a 'pass/fail' judgement on a horse. Normal procedure is for a veterinarian to carefully examine all visible features of a horse along with:

- a comprehensive motion evaluation
- flexion stress tests of the limbs
- analysis of respiratory and heart rate recovery with exercise
- diagnostic tests when appropriate

Armed with complete information, a veterinarian describes for the buyer the good points and faults of an animal. A veterinarian describes the significance of the faults to the chosen sport. It is then the buyer's responsibility to decide if the imperfections or permanent injuries are acceptable. Some problems may only be cosmetic, while others may functionally impair athletic or breeding performance throughout a horse's lifetime.

Often, complaints arise that a prepurchase exam is non-committal on the part of the veterinarian. It is imperative that a buyer appreciate the role a veterinarian plays in the process. A veterinarian states facts discovered at the time of the prepurchase exam. It is a veterinarian's prerogative to speculate about future soundness and health of a horse, but there is no way one can really know. The buyer weighs pros and cons based on professional advice from a veterinarian and trainer. *The buyer assumes full responsibility for a decision to buy.* This determination is based not only on the findings of a veterinary exam, but also on the suitability of a horse for a buyer's personal goals as evaluated by the buyer.

Understanding the Prepurchase Exam

There are some points that should be clarified about what a prepurchase exam accomplishes, and how the buyer can help a veterinarian derive the most information from an exam.

Inherent in the purchase of any horse is a long-term commitment and responsibility to that animal. Such a decision should not be made on the spur of the moment. It is a mistake for a buyer to be pressured by a seller to quickly complete a deal. Schedule adequate time with a veterinarian to conduct a thorough exam. Enough pressure is placed on a veterinarian to present a buyer with a complete assessment without also encountering urgency for immediate results.

Prepurchase exams require at least a couple of hours to complete. A buyer or agent for the buyer should be available during the entire exam, not only to handle the horse during examination procedures, but also to ride the horse, if necessary.

Ideally, all three parties (buyer, seller or agent, and veterinarian) should be present during the exam for full communication between all individuals, and to obtain information about the horse. This arrangement is not always feasible, but should be made whenever possible.

Avoiding a Conflict of Interest

It is important that all parties understand for whom the veterinarian is working. Usually, the person paying the veterinary fee is the buyer. That individual has, in fact, hired a veterinarian to act on his or her behalf. Therefore, the veterinarian is protecting the buyer's interests.

If a veterinarian usually works for both buyer and seller, hiring a different, impartial veterinarian to evaluate the horse eliminates a conflict of interest. This practice prevents accusations that a veterinarian has a vested interest in either the seller or the buyer that might prejudice the examination results. Hiring another veterinarian to do the prepurchase exam also avoids hard feelings.

If the buyer and seller both insist that their same, usual veterinarian perform the exam, no offence should be taken by a seller when problems with the horse are identified. At the same time, a buyer must trust that the veterinarian will be fair and maintain an objective viewpoint.

Medical Confidentiality

All reports of findings, diagnostic procedures, and radiographs belong as a legal medical record to the veterinarian. If a prepurchase exam has previously been performed on a horse, do not expect to call that veterinarian and obtain blanket information over the telephone. Under the ethics of medical confidentiality, none of this information can be released to another party without con-

sent from the person who originally hired the veterinarian to perform the exam. A veterinarian must also contact the horse owner
for consent to divulge medical history to a prospective buyer.

Disclosure Statement

Often at the time of a prepurchase exam a veterinarian or buyer
will request a *disclosure statement* from a seller or agent to provide
an historical background about the horse. The age of the horse,
previous use, and current level of exercise or training give valuable information to a buyer and a veterinarian. If a horse has been
retired to pasture for several months or years, a rest period may
positively influence how 'sound' an injured animal moves.

Information obtained from a disclosure statement includes a
complete medical history, deworming and vaccination schedules,
history of colic, prior surgery, and disclosure of any medication or
drugs a horse has previously received or is currently receiving.
This last item is a delicate issue as anti-inflammatory medications
can mask problems of utmost concern to the animal's performance capabilities. A tranquillizer or sedative can alter a horse's
disposition and behaviour. All medications should be withheld at
least 5 – 10 days before an examination.

Before the exam, it is also helpful for the veterinarian performing a prepurchase exam to receive a copy of the horse's medical
record from the seller's veterinarian. Disclosure statements are
not necessarily standard procedure, but are recommended to ensure fair representation of the horse by the seller.

Benefits of a Complete Exam

Some people are not interested in a complete prepurchase exam
due to the cost involved. Requests such as 'I just want you to look it
over, Doc, and tell me if you see anything wrong' put a veterinarian
in an impossible situation. It is impractical to expect a veterinarian to
perform a 'partial exam' not only because very little information is
obtained in an exam lacking thoroughness, but also due to legal implications involved in a prepurchase examination.

Compare buying a horse to purchasing a car. If a person second-
hand glances at a vehicle on a lot, or watches it drive on to the
forecourt, all that can be said of that car is that it looks all right, and
moves under power of its engine. On that basis, how can one tell if
the brakes work, if the transmission is sound, or if the engine knocks
and bangs? A cursory view does not determine if the frame or axles

are bent, or if reconstructive body work has been done. Much the same can be said of an incomplete inspection of a potential equine athlete.

Detecting Problems

It is impossible to identify cardiac arrhythmias or murmurs without a stethoscope. Ophthalmic examination identifies corneal scars, cataracts, or vision problems. Use of hoof testers helps identify internal foot problems. Without placing a horse under a battery of tests which include manipulation of joints, tendons, ligaments and muscles of the limbs, along with careful motion evaluation at all

gaits, all a person can say about a horse standing at rest is that it looks okay. Perhaps a particular blemish or suspect musculoskeletal problem can be pointed out, but anything else about a horse's capabilities is pure speculation.

If possible, have the exam done at a location where there is access to both a hard-

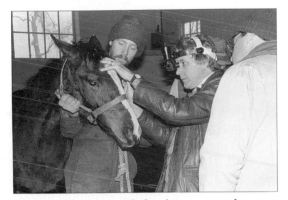

Fig. 22.4 An eye exam helps detect corneal scars, cataracts and vision problems.

pack surface and a softer surface such as grass or sand. A level surface enables a veterinarian to analyse foot placement and abnormal limb motion (winging, paddling) that may influence athletic soundness. An area with a slight incline is particularly helpful to identify a very subtle lameness.

The horse handler should be prepared to trot the horse in hand, and to lunge the horse both directions. The horse should not be exercised prior to the motion exam so as not to obscure problems that may improve as the horse warms up.

Not all lameness problems are obvious until a horse is asked to perform the task for which its purchase is intended. Asking a jumping candidate to jump or a dressage horse to perform at its current level of training is desirable. While a horse is performing under the stress of these activities, subtle problems in the back, withers or limbs may become visible to a skilled veterinarian.

Exercise may reveal other problems such as 'roaring' (laryngeal

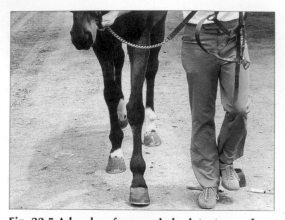

Fig. 22.5 A level surface can help detect poor foot placement.

hemiplegia), which is a serious impairment to airflow through the upper respiratory tract. In a mild case, the horse does not make a 'roaring' noise, and the only way to identify paralysis of a cartilage in the throat is with an endoscopic exam.

For broodmares or breeding stallions, a fertility evaluation at the time of a prepurchase exam prevents disappointing surprises in the future.

Further Diagnostic Tests

Further diagnostic procedures include radiographic exam of specified areas of a limb, ultrasound exam of tendons, a complete blood count, blood chemistry tests, and drug tests.

A buyer and seller should expect a time lag for diagnostic tests upon which a sale may depend. Drug testing, blood work, and radiographic evaluation require a short period for results to be returned to and analysed by the veterinarian. Some tests rely on outside laboratories which causes further delay.

Drug Testing

A drug screening test does not detect medication injected into a joint, nor does it identify all systemic medications that are available to suppress pain. To be completely certain that a horse has been off medication for at least several days prior to the scheduled exam, the horse can be moved to the buyer's boarding facility. Insurance policies can be purchased for a short time to cover accidental mishaps or illness while the horse remains in the prospective buyer's possession.

X-Ray Films

A single X-ray film of an area of concern on the leg does not provide complete information. To analyse a particular area on a limb, it is necessary to radiograph each joint separately, with four to five different directional views per joint.

A prepurchase exam identifies areas of concern that may require further evaluation with X-ray films, or in an unusual case, with diagnostic nerve blocks. A client should be prepared to spend as much money as is reasonably necessary to complete extra diagnostics. If not, a buyer is compelled to weigh a veterinarian's assessment without concrete radiographic evidence, possibly allowing an important defect to escape discovery. Clinical impressions are offered, but without X-ray films of suspect areas it is difficult to determine if degenerative joint disease or osteochondrosis lesions are present in a joint. Permanent damage from previous infection or trauma in a bone is also difficult to identify without X-ray films. Radiographic examination of the foot often requires removal of the horse's shoes. The seller should be advised of this possibility and permission obtained ahead of time. Then the seller can make arrangements with the farrier to replace the shoes.

The Untrained Horse

If a horse has not yet been trained to the prospective desires of a buyer, it may be difficult to evaluate its ability for specific athletic pursuits. Yet, if trained under saddle, a horse should be ridden by the buyer, trainer, or seller during the examination.

It may be somewhat difficult to evaluate an untrained horse that is incapable of leading in hand, or unused to having its legs or body handled by humans. As a young horse jerks and fidgets, interpretation of results from limb manipulations or hoof testers may be confusing. Arrangements should be made to exercise a green horse freely in a confined arena. A buyer should be aware of limitations of a prepurchase exam under constraints where a veterinarian cannot perform a thorough, hands-on evaluation.

Looking Into the Future

Once obtained, results of diagnostic procedures are not always clear-cut. A predominant problem in the equine industry is use of X-ray films to determine if a horse suffers from a lameness that currently shows no physical symptoms. Commonly, veterinarians are asked to predict if a horse will continue to be 'sound' and of athletic use in the *distant* future based on clinical findings and X-ray films taken on the day of an exam. Often the buyer also wants to know if a horse will retain its worth upon resale. It is expected that a veterinarian can clearly see into the future!

All a veterinarian can provide is an answer based on a clinical impression bolstered by past experience. As with any law of averages, some judgements can be wrong. Many issues cannot be factored into a professional opinion at the time of a sale. Some examples are:

- the type of work the horse will be asked to do
- how well a conditioning programme develops the musculoskeletal system
- the terrain on which the horse will be exercised
- the expertise of the farrier
- age-related breakdowns

Navicular Radiographs

The deepest quagmire for prepurchase exams comes from radiographic evaluation of navicular films. For example, at a convention of the American Association of Equine Practitioners it was commented that 43% of legal problems over prepurchase exams stem from navicular X-ray films.

Navicular films alone are *not* a basis for diagnosing navicular disease. All information compiled from clinical history, clinical exam during exercise on different ground surfaces, hoof tester results, flexion tests, diagnostic nerve blocks, and navicular X-ray films must be gathered before arriving at a diagnosis.

Yet, great importance has been attached to the sole use of navicular films during a prepurchase exam. Buyers expect the films will predict the likelihood that a horse is currently afflicted with navicular disease or will develop it some time in the future. Scientific evidence shows that navicular X-ray films do not completely correlate with clinical disease.

A horse may mimic navicular syndrome while simply suffering from bruised heels or imbalanced shoeing, although none of the navicular apparatus is abnormally affected. This horse may be incorrectly diagnosed as 'navicular' without being given a chance to heal and show its true ability.

Not all horses with a true navicular disease syndrome have radiographic changes in their navicular bones. This lack of change may be because soreness comes from the soft tissue structures of the deep digital flexor tendon or the navicular bursa rather than from the bone itself. After a long lay-off and on a good day the horse may show no lameness and can slip through a lameness evaluation, complete with X-ray films, without identifying the problem.

On the other hand, many horses, especially athletes past 10 or 12 years, may show definite signs of wear-and-tear of the navicular apparatus on X-ray films without having any symptoms or history of lameness. Basing a judgement of navicular disease solely on radiographic findings is flawed and unjustified.

Liability for the Future

X-ray films of the feet need to be analysed with utmost care, and not too much read into them. Veterinarians have been placed in a position where they are held liable for the future soundness of a horse while basing judgements and opinions on information gained over the course of a several hour exam. Such legal precariousness forces a veterinarian to be overly conservative and pessimistic in rendering an opinion.

Not only is this predicament an injustice to a veterinarian, but all too often a 'pre-navicular' diagnosis is placed on a horse, condemning a horse and owner. For starters, a horse's value is diminished considerably, financially harming the seller. Secondly, it becomes increasingly difficult to find a buyer for that animal once word gets around. Thirdly, few insurance companies will insure a navicular horse for mortality.

Information for Assistance

In the old days people relied primarily on a philosophy of 'buyer beware', but now with sophisticated instruments and a sophisticated level of education and expertise, veterinarians can help protect a buyer's interests. Arduous years of schooling and clinical experience develop trained eyes and skilled minds of equine doctors. These skills enable a veterinarian to identify problems during a prepurchase exam, but do *not* provide a crystal ball to see into the future.

The following points should be carefully considered:

- It is *the buyer's* decision to hire a veterinarian and to place trust in that person.
- Veterinarians are capable of human error.
- Through use and time, any horse may break down.
- There is no such thing as a guarantee on the health and soundness of any living being.
- No horse will be as perfect as those in our imaginations.
- The buyer makes the final decision on purchasing.

By knowing what to expect from a prepurchase exam, and by recognizing human limitations to make long-range predictions, a veterinary prepurchase exam enables a buyer to make an *informed decision* whether to purchase the horse.

For a horse that is basically sound in mind and body, a prepurchase exam is also a starting point from which a buyer can build a sound conditioning and feeding programme. Noted weaknesses in conformation alert the buyer to areas that should be closely monitored during training. Problems with shoeing or imbalance of the feet are identified, and arrangements made to begin correction. This information gives a potential owner an intelligent foundation on which to develop an athletic prospect.

23

BREEDING THE PERFORMANCE HORSE

There may be times in the life of an equine athlete when it is unable to actively perform. During training or competition, a horse may sustain a musculoskeletal injury, requiring a lay-up of many months. If the idle horse is a mare, the down time may be used to advantage by breeding her.

Of all domestic farm animals, mares have the lowest reproductive efficiency; less than 60% of mares bred each year produce live foals. As with a performance athlete, sound management of the broodmare encourages her to perform to potential. Thoughtful planning and a prebreeding veterinary examination improve a mare's chances for conception and birth of a healthy foal.

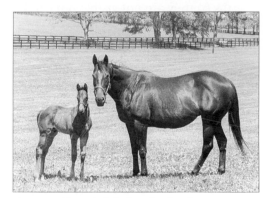

Fig. 23.1 Thoughtful planning leads to a healthy future athlete.

PREPARING FOR BREEDING

A mare cannot be pulled out of rigorous athletics and expected to

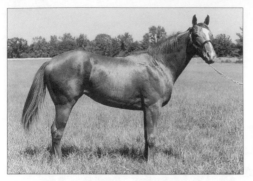

Fig. 23.2 An athletic mare should stop work at least 2 months before breeding.

immediately conceive. If a mare is engaged in competitive athletics or on the show circuit, pull her out of work *at least 2 months* before breeding. This 'let-down' period reduces her stress load and allows her reproductive pattern to settle into a regular cycling interval. Over several months her psychological state also adjusts to the relaxed environment.

Likewise, the stress of competition reduces the fertility of a stallion. A let-down period of several days may be necessary for him, to improve the chance for conception on the first attempt.

Weight Problems

As an athletic mare is pulled out of performance, she may be too thin to encourage normal reproductive cycling. Once her athletic activity is minimized, she should begin to gain weight. Mares that are on a steady weight gain programme *(flushing)* before the breeding period attain oestrus 1 month sooner than mares that are not gaining weight. The fit breeding mare has a thin layer of flesh covering her ribs so they are not visible but can be felt as the hand is run lightly across the body.

A halter horse pulled from the show circuit may have the opposite problem from the athlete—it may be too fat. High energy rations should be removed immediately from the diet of a halter horse intended for breeding. It should be placed on a balanced maintenance diet with ample roughage and minimal grain. *(See Chapter 7 for more information.)*

THE MARE
Abnormal Oestrous Cycles
Performance

Often, the stress of intense competition temporarily alters normal reproductive cycling. Some mares stop cycling altogether, or may display erratic heat cycles. A racetrack mare may have difficulty conceiving a foal during the first season after she has stopped racing.

Steroids

Anabolic steroids are sometimes used to 'improve' a horse's body condition, growth and muscling. Anabolic steroids have adverse effects on a mare's endocrine system. The mare that is influenced by the male sex hormone properties of these drugs has inconsistent or absent oestrous cycles. If given repetitively, anabolic steroids can cause a mare to display stallion-like behaviour. Once administration of the drug is stopped, the effects are reversible but may require several months for a mare to return to normal oestrous cycles.

Pain

The performance horse that suffers from a serious injury that involves intense pain may have difficulty conceiving. Intense pain interferes with hormone production and may interrupt a normal oestrous cycle.

The Mare's Reproductive Cycle

The mare is *seasonally polyoestrus*, meaning that she cycles many times during the breeding season. Her optimal fertile period is between April and August (in the Northern Hemisphere), although many mares are bred earlier. Most mares stop cycling in the winter months *(anoestrus)* between November and February. In February and March she enters a *transitional period*. Pituitary hormones controlling the reproductive cycle respond to longer daylight hours, stimulating the activity of the ovaries. The ovaries start producing follicles that eventually mature. Rupture of a mature follicle releases an egg for potential fertilization.

During the transitional period, oestrous cycles are erratic, and may be prolonged without the production of an actual egg. Normally, during April through August, a mare cycles every 21 days, with visible signs of oestrus (winking of the vulva, tail lifting, or frequent urinations) present for about 5 days.

Nature protects the survival of the species by maximizing fertility of both the mare and the stallion during the warmer times of the year. Then, a gestation period of 11 months allows a foal to be born into a welcoming and nutrient-rich environment for both mare and foal. By evaluating a mare's reproductive capabilities before the optimum breeding period, health problems can be addressed and resolved before the breeding season.

Each time a mare is bred, there is a risk of injury or uterine infection. If her fertility is coordinated with the proposed breeding date she will become pregnant with fewer breedings, avoiding these situations.

Hormonal Manipulation

Techniques to synchronize follicle maturation with the proposed breeding date include use of specific hormones or hormonal analogues, such as progesterone, prostaglandins, or human chorionic gonadotropin (HCG). However, hormonal manipulation of a mare is not practical until her ovaries are active and cycling.

If she is in the quiescent, winter anoestrus, or just entering the transitional period around February or March, hormonal drug therapy may be ineffective in coordinating the timing for breeding. Only 20–30% of mares cycle and ovulate at regular intervals during February and March, whereas over 80% do so by April or May.

Artificial Lighting

To encourage mares to cycle earlier in the year, the erratic 2-month transitional period can be advanced by manipulating natural hormonal surges with artificial lighting. The photoreceptors of the eyes

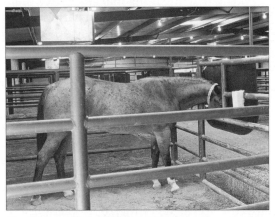

detect light, which sends a message to the *pineal gland* located behind the *hypothalamus* in the brain. The message mimics longer daylight hours of springtime, stimulating hormonal activity by the hypothalamus. As hormone secretions respond to the light, ovarian tissue is activated, and follicles form, mature, and ovulate. Each

Fig. 23.3 Artificial lighting stimulates the mare's body to cycle earlier in the year.

oestrous cycle reoccurs approximately every 3 weeks to provide the breeder with many opportunities to get the mare in foal.

Recommendations

For this method to work best, 16 hours of 'daylight' are required.

The type of light is not as important as the number of hours the mare is exposed to it. Incandescent, fluorescent, mercury vapour, and tungsten lights are all successful in stimulating a mare's reproductive activity. It is necessary to provide 2 months of lengthened daylight to enhance ovarian activity; a month later, follicles mature and ovulate. To maximize the use of artificial lighting, begin the programme on 1 December, with anticipated start of breeding to be 1 March.

Lights should be turned on from 4:30 p.m. until 11 p.m. This schedule ensures a total of 16 hours of both natural and artificial light. A 200-watt incandescent bulb or two 40-watt fluorescent bulbs are placed 10 feet above the mare in a 12×12 foot stall. There should be enough light to read a newspaper in the stall at eye-level with the mare. The mare should not be able to remove her head from the light source. If she does, the pineal gland is not stimulated by light.

As an energy-saving alternative, recent studies indicate that 1 – 2 hours of artificial light applied 8 – 10 hours after sunset may be sufficient to stimulate the pineal gland. Turning the lights on between 1 – 4 a.m. hastens the transitional period.

Rugging and Food

A mare that is put under lights is also stimulated to shed out her winter coat. In a cold climate, premature shedding requires rugging and shelter. The mare may require extra food to maintain good body condition. Remember, if an early breeding schedule is implemented in colder climates, indoor housing must be available to a mare foaling in January, February or March to avoid climatic stress on the foal.

Preventative Medicine

A preventative medicine programme, if not already in place, should be instituted before breeding. This programme includes:

- deworming every 2 months with products approved for pregnant mares
- a rhinopneumonitis vaccine before breeding, and boosted at 5, 7 and 9 months of pregnancy to reduce the risk of viral abortion
- regular tetanus and influenza boosters at appropriate intervals as determined by a veterinarian

The Mare's Prebreeding Exam

Ensuring the reproductive health of a mare from the onset avoids wasted time during the crucial breeding season, as well as unnecessary and repeated expenses that result in extreme frustration and financial loss. A veterinary prebreeding examination may detect external and internal abnormalities of a mare that can lead to reproductive failure.

General Physical Exam

To start, a general physical exam is performed to ensure the health of the heart and lungs, and the soundness of limbs and feet. Heart murmurs or arrhythmias reduce metabolic efficiency. Chronic lung disease interferes with the oxygen supply so important to placental and foetal health. A chronic cough from obstructive pulmonary disease (heaves) can cause enough straining to develop a 'windsucking' vagina *(pneumovagina)* that pulls bacteria into itself, resulting in inflammation or infection.

Severe, chronic pain caused by arthritis, laminitis or other limb problems can stress a horse enough to reduce her chances not only of conception but of carrying a foal to term. A mare with chronic laminitis poses an added reproductive risk. If the laminitic mare has difficulty with birthing or develops a uterine infection *(metritis)* after the birth, endotoxins may be absorbed into the bloodstream. Endotoxins may worsen an already crippling foot condition of laminitis.

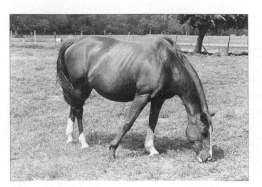

Fig. 23.4 This broodmare has a good body condition with her ribs barely showing.

Without good teeth, a mare is unable to meet nutritional needs important to maintaining pregnancy, foetal development, and lactation. Body condition is examined during the prebreeding exam so that appropriate nutritional adjustments can be discussed. Ideally, the mare's ribs should barely be visible. Therefore, a slow, controlled weight gain programme can be implemented 1 – 2 months before the breeding season. Obesity is detrimental to conception and reproductive health however, a malnourished horse is also at risk for infertility.

Examining the hair coat indicates the success of parasite control programmes, and hormonal regularity. A rough coat may reflect internal health problems or an intestinal parasite load. A mare that is late in shedding her winter coat may also lack an appropriate hormonal response to the long daylight hours of the breeding season.

Maturity

A mare should not be bred until she is sexually and skeletally mature to prevent additional stresses and demands on her own growing body. The period of greatest foetal demand occurs in the last trimester (8 – 11 months) of pregnancy. A mare should not be bred any earlier than 3 years old. A mare bred as a 3-year-old approaches her fourth year before the foal taxes her system with rapid developmental growth and the subsequent energy demands of lactation.

External Exam of the Reproductive System

A common reason for failure to conceive, or for early embryonic death, is infection of the uterus (metritis). The unique anatomy of the *perineum*, which is the area around the anus and vulva, provides the first line of defence in protecting the uterus from bacterial invasion.

The Perineum

A normal mare has a vertical vulva with full *labia* (lips of the vulva) that are tightly aligned in a snug fit so that neither air nor faeces can enter the vagina. In a normal mare, about 80% of the vulva is positioned below the pelvic brim, with the anus positioned very slightly behind or directly above the vulva so faeces do not fall on to the labia.

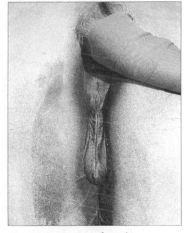

Fig. 23.5 A normal perineum.

Tilted Vagina

In a mare with a tilted vagina, the labia sit high above the pelvic brim, the anus is pulled forwards, and the vulva tilts horizontally. With the vagina tipped forwards and the anus recessed inwards, faeces fall directly on to the labia. The labia may gap, and then windsucking pulls air and faeces into the reproductive tract. To check for windsucking, place the flat surface of the hands on each labial lip, and gently part them. In a windsucking mare, air is aspirated into the vulva as the labia are manually parted, resulting in a sucking sound. In many older mares, or in very thin horses, the position of anus and vulva is altered due to loss of muscle tone.

Vestibular Seal

The next barrier to uterine contamination is the *vestibular seal* created by the back portion of the vagina, the hymen if present, and the pelvic floor. If the vulva is tilted horizontally, constrictor muscles of the vulva and vestibule cannot prevent contamination of the reproductive tract.

Not only does a tipped vulva develop from age-related conformational changes or severe weight loss, but it can also be caused by an inherited defect from birth. Such fillies should be identified early so corrections can be made to enhance their future fertility. Keep in mind that conformation is heritable, and undesirable traits may be passed down from mare to foal. Normally, Mother Nature accounts for this problem by making poorly conformed mares unbreedable, but advances in scientific techniques encourage continued fertility and breeding of many of these mares.

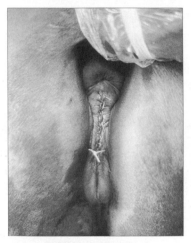

Fig. 23.6 This mare has had a Caslick's surgery.

Caslick's Surgery

Contamination to the reproductive tract may result in infertility from infection and subsequent scarring of the uterus. Once a mare with a forwardly tipped vagina has been bred and 'settled', a *Caslick's* surgery *(episioplasty)*, performed by a veterinarian, closes the lips of the vulva to prevent contamination. Local anaesthetic is placed along the borders of the vulva, tissue is trimmed away, and the two lips are sutured together to join as they heal. Several weeks before foaling, the Caslick's should be opened to allow normal birth of the foal without tearing.

Third Degree Perineal Laceration

Sometimes a foal is delivered with an improperly aligned leg, which tears the perineum. These mares should have the perineum reconstructed well ahead of the next breeding time to adequately clear a uterine infection from the system. In severe *third degree recto-vestibular lacerations*, as these are called, torn flesh between the rectum and the vagina allows faeces to fall directly into the vagina. This condition requires three phases of surgical repair. Up to a year of healing time is necessary before breeding the mare again.

Udder Evaluation

In a prebreeding evaluation, the udder is examined for abnormali-

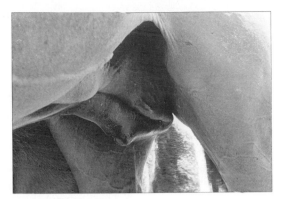

Fig. 23.7 A mare with mastitis.

ties in size or consistency, tumours or scar tissue, or evidence of previous or current *mastitis*. Mastitis is an inflammation of the udder. The thighs and underside of the tail are also examined for evidence of an abnormal vaginal discharge.

Internal Exam of the Reproductive System

Rectal Exam

Once the mare's overall body health and external genitals have been thoroughly evaluated, examination of the internal reproductive tract can begin. Initially, a *rectal examination* is performed with the veterinarian inserting an arm covered by a lubricated, plastic sleeve into the rectum. The veterinarian then manually palpates the ovaries, uterus and cervix to assess general health, activity and abnormalities. Size of the ovaries is determined, while the amount of follicular activity present on each ovary ascertains if the mare is currently cycling. The tone and size of the uterus and cervix establish if fluid, tumours or abscesses, adhesions, or scar tissue are present. A flaccid and doughy-feeling uterus may signal infection within or abnormal endocrine function.

A *maiden mare* that has never been bred should be examined rectally to determine if all appropriate reproductive 'equipment' is present; that is, two ovaries, a cervix, and a normally shaped and positioned uterus. On rare occasions, abnormalities such as lack of an ovary, tumour of an ovary, or a split cervix may be felt.

Vaginal Exam

After thoroughly washing the perineum and wrapping the tail to prevent pulling debris inwards, the next step is a *vaginal speculum exam* to visually inspect the vagina for:

- inflammation
- vaginal cysts
- congestion
- abnormal discharge
- vaginal or vulvar tearing from prior births
- cervical lacerations or adhesions

The *cervix* is the third barrier to uterine contamination, and its integrity is important to reproductive health. In a maiden mare, a *hymen* may be present, and can be broken down at this time. Blood is spermicidal and interferes with semen fertility, therefore, it is best to open the hymen before breeding.

The colour and moistness of mucous membranes within the vagina reflect vaginal health and endocrine function. Air bubbles may indicate chronic windsucking, while a collection of fluid on the vaginal floor warns of other serious problems.

Urine Pooling

An important cause of infertility in some mares is a syndrome known as urine pooling *(vesiculo-vaginal reflux,* or VVR) on the floor of the vagina. Urine is not only spermicidal, but it is an irritant which can cause inflammation of the vagina *(vaginitis)*, inflammation of the cervix *(cervicitis)*, and inflammation of the uterus with subsequent infertility. If urine is not entirely voided clear of the reproductive tract, small, residual amounts drain forwards to collect on the vaginal floor. The veterinarian can see the urine (when the speculum is in place) with a flashlight. Suspect fluid can be analysed biochemically to confirm that it is urine.

A mare with a tipped vulva is particularly susceptible to urine pooling. In a normal vulva, entry into the vagina requires an upward path, ensuring that urine is drained down and out. A tipped vulva directs the entry downwards, therefore, urine tends to flow into the vagina. It occurs very slightly during oestrus when the reproductive tract relaxes, or if a Caslick's surgery is improperly sewn.

Surgery

To correct urine pooling, *urethral extension surgery* 'builds' a urethral tunnel from pre-existing shelves of tissue within the vagina. Urine travels outwards through the tunnel, and cannot collect within the vaginal cavern. In one study, this surgery resulted in a conception rate of 92% of mares with previous urine pooling, and 65% carried foals to term.

Maiden Mare

A maiden mare is a mare of any age who has never been exposed to semen. Once she has been 'bred,' whether she conceives or not, she is no longer a maiden. The untouched uterus is a sterile environment. In a maiden mare, the reproductive exam often stops after rectal palpation and a vaginal exam. There is no reason to assume any possible uterine infection unless conformation of the vulva appears suspect, or if vaginal inflammation or urine pooling has been confirmed.

For a mare that has been bred, with or without conception, or for a poorly conformed maiden mare, the prebreeding exam continues.

Bacterial Culture of the Uterus

A bacterial culture is obtained directly from the uterus to determine whether there is an infection of the uterine lining. A very long cotton swab is passed through the cervix, guarded in a plastic sheath. A protective cap on the end of the sheath is pushed open once in the uterus, and uterine secretions soak into the swab for 30 seconds. The swab is pulled back into the sterile protective sheath and removed from the reproductive tract. The sample is sent to the lab to be checked for bacterial growth over the next 48 hours. If bacterial growth does occur, the lab can determine the antibiotic to which the bacteria are susceptible.

Effectiveness of Bacterial Culture

By itself, bacterial culture of the uterus has a poor correlation with the presence of actual disease. As many as 61% of mares with infection of the uterus do not show significant bacterial growth when a culture is taken. Other mares may have non-harmful bacteria resident in the uterus, with no accompanying disease. Bacteria are detected in the uterine linings of 80% of mares up to 3 days after breeding, and up to 30 days after foaling. A normal mare's immune system quickly clears them from the reproductive system.

However, bacterial culture and antibiotic sensitivity testing of the superficial uterine lining are helpful in confirming other diagnostic findings, such as:

- an abnormal-feeling uterus
- presence of fluid or urine pooling
- continued infertility
- results from uterine biopsies and cellular evaluation *(cytology)*

Specific bacteria, such beta-haemolytic streptococci, *Klebsiella, Pseudomonas* and *E. coli,* and yeasts, are significant if found on the culture. An infected uterus needs to be treated with local antibiotics and/or antibiotic injections before breeding.

Cellular Evaluation of the Uterine Lining

The swab used to gather secretions from the uterus also collects cells from the uterine lining. In the lab, the swab is rolled on to a glass slide, stained, and examined under a microscope for inflammatory cells, debris, or bacteria. The presence of specific inflammatory cells provides warning signals about the duration and severity of an infection.

Uterine Biopsy

The most informative diagnostic tool for analysing the viability, health, and structure of the equine uterus is the *uterine biopsy*. A special instrument is inserted through the cervix into the uterus, and its movable jaws are closed to tear off a deep tag of tissue. The uterine lining *(endometrium)* of the mare, unlike that of humans, has no nerve endings, therefore a horse does not feel the tug or tearing of tissue as the biopsy is taken. The tissue sample is prepared at the laboratory by slicing it microscopically thin for examination under a microscope. A random sample provides adequate information about overall uterine health.

Infertility Due to Uterine Infections

Often, infertility is caused by uterine infections in the deep tissue layers. These can only be inspected by biopsy of the tissue. Microscopic evaluation identifies infection, inflammation or scarring *(fibrosis)* of the glands that support uterine nutrition. There is a direct correlation of biopsy findings with fertility, which makes this procedure an invaluable diagnostic tool. A Kenney classification system categorizes the degree of uterine *pathology*, or disease, and predicts the mare's chance of success.

Kenney Classification System

Grade I Uterus

A Grade I uterus has at least an 80% chance of conception, with minimal or no pathological changes (infection, inflammation or gland scarring) present in the endometrium.

Grade II Uterus

A Grade II describes moderately severe inflammation and gland scarring that interfere with the ability of the endometrium to adequately support a foal to term. A Grade IIA uterus is associated with a 50–80% chance of success of maintaining a pregnancy. A mare with this classification has a reasonably good possibility for return to Grade I status with appropriate treatment. A Grade IIB uterus has more widespread abnormalities in the endometrium, and will have limited success (10–50%) of carrying a foal to term.

Kenney Classification System		
GRADE	**CHANCE OF CONCEPTION**	**PATHOLOGY**
Grade I Uterus	at least 80%	minimal or none

Grade II Uterus
    Grade IIA
    Grade IIB
	50% – 80%
	10% – 50%
		moderately severe: may reverse with treatment

Grade III Uterus	less than 10%	irreversible, widespread damage

Fig. 23.8

Grade III Uterus

A Grade III classification is the most severe, with irreversible, widespread inflammatory changes and periglandular scarring, providing less than a 10% chance of conception and carrying a foal to term. Widespread scarring in the uterus decreases uterine motility during a critical period when normal motility is essential for continued pregnancy.

With diminished uterine motility, an embryo may not migrate throughout the uterus during days 5 – 15 after conception. Embryonic migration stimulates chemical signals which block the release of prostaglandins from the uterus. Without embryonic migration, prostaglandins are released. Prostaglandins cause a premature reduction of the hormone, progesterone, which is necessary for maintaining early pregnancy. The foetus is then lost. Extensive scarring of the uterus, and particularly of the glandular areas, also reduces nutrient supplies essential to support a developing embryo.

Breeding For Excellence
Scientific Interference

The days of spontaneously breeding a mare in a whimsical moment have pretty much vanished, as quality stallions and mares must schedule time for propagation of the species. With human interference and manipulation of reproductively less efficient animals, we may, in fact, perpetuate the necessity of scientific manipulation. Mother Nature no longer selects for reproductively sound horses that breed and foal without human assistance. Many other variables arise as we breed for athletic performance and beauty, and remove the natural selection process for reproductive efficiency. A poorly conformed, slanting vagina, urine pooling, or an infected uterus often are medically or surgically repaired. These problems are genetically passed to the foal, allowing continued propagation of problems that would never have remained under normal circumstances.

Promoting Genetic Improvement

Only with conscious recognition of undesirable traits and a concerted effort to eradicate these characteristics will a breeder promote continued improvement of horses. Discuss suspected flaws with a veterinarian and other breeders. Be hypercritical of a mare.

Before breeding, carefully assess the contribution the mare can make to the horse population. Breeding a mare that is crippled due to conformational defects does little to improve the equine world at large, and may produce a foal with similar problems.

Breeding an excellent mare to a poor stallion, or vice versa, is a huge mistake. Do not cut corners by diluting good stock. The initial cost of breeding the mare is only a small part of raising a foal to performance age. Therefore put money into the initial investment by selecting an excellent quality mare *and* stallion. Selecting an excellent stallion ensures improvement of the genetic pool. Analyse the performance of the sire and his offspring, and the compatibility of conformational aspects between the stallion and mare.

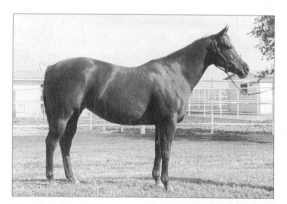

Fig. 23.9 Carefully assess the contribution a mare can make if she is bred.

THE STALLION

A breeding stallion has a unique place in the performance world. Not only is it possible to ride him as a performance horse, but his genetic characteristics will be passed on to future generations. Because of this lasting influence, a stringent selection process should be applied to the stallion by both the potential stallion owner and the broodmare owner looking for the perfect complement to the mare.

The stallion's disposition and temperament are vital to the enjoyment of the stallion and his progeny. A bad-tempered stallion is hazardous to his handlers, to farm personnel, and to broodmares. A bad disposition is potentially passed to the foal. It is wise to geld a dangerous stallion rather than risk passing this genetic tendency on to future offspring.

Before investing in a breeding stallion, evaluate the stallion's performance results. If he has progeny old enough to compete, track their performance results, both successes and failures. Examine the offspring to see if the desired characteristics are passed to succeeding generations. Pedigree may suggest potential, but recent generations of offspring prove or disprove the athletic value of a specific genetic line.

When considering a stallion, match him to a mare with a complementary body type and strength. Find a stallion with similar desirable characteristics to reinforce them in the foal, and with characteristics that improve or correct the weak components of the mare. If the mare has too many faults, consider breeding a different mare rather than risk passing her conformational defects to the foal. A mare or stallion that has been retired due to lameness caused by conformational problems should not be considered as a breeder. There is no sense in breeding the mare or stallion only to create a foal with a similar unsoundness.

Breeding Performance

Not only do good looks, strong conformation, and an impressive athletic record make a stallion excellent for propagating these desirable traits, but he must be able to perform his duties as a breeding horse.

To adequately evaluate a stallion's reproductive capacity, his semen should be collected and analysed. In the process of collecting semen, information is also gained regarding the stallion's libido and breeding behaviour. Some stallions are intimidated by the breeding process due to bad experiences. It is valuable to discover if the stallion is aggressive and difficult to handle when presented with a mare in heat, or if he has trouble attaining and holding an erection, mounting the mare or dummy, or achieving ejaculation. However, it is premature to make too many assumptions about the performance of an inexperienced stallion in his first attempts.

The breeding stallion must be able to rise on his hind legs to mount a mare or a phantom breeding dummy. Some breeding sheds in Kentucky have created special facilities to place a mare in a low point on the ground to allow an arthritic stallion easier access to her. Such management considerations by the breeding farm are as important as the overall health of the stallion because they ensure the success of live coverage.

A thorough exam evaluates the soundness of the stallion's breeding capabilities. A breeding exam starts with a thorough history and general physical examination of the stallion's overall health. Deworming and vaccination schedules are reviewed, and prior experience or problems associated with breeding are discussed. A complete history of medical or surgical events should be disclosed at this time to determine if a past problem is injurious to a stallion's career as a breeding horse.

General Physical Exam

The breeding stallion should be in good flesh, neither too fat nor too thin. His teeth should be fully checked for problems that can interfere with his continuing good condition. His heart and lungs should be examined at rest and with exercise to detect abnormalities. A broodmare owner with the intent of using a stallion at stud also should carefully assess the stallion's straightness of limbs, size and health of feet, and general body proportions to determine if the stallion will complement the mare. Remember that the stallion contributes half the genetic information, therefore his defects can be passed on to the offspring.

Heritable Abnormalities

It is important to identify the existence of undesirable, heritable traits such as a retained testicle (cryptorchidism), a scrotal or umbilical hernia, parrot mouth, combined immunodeficiency disease (CID), or eye cataracts. These abnormalities are all passed down in a genetic link, and the presence of one or more of such heritable traits renders a stallion unfavourable for breeding.

Other syndromes that are not entirely linked to genetics but may have a heritable tendency are developmental abnormalities such as angular limb deformities, osteochondrosis, or cervical spinal malformation which can lead to *wobbler syndrome*. Ascertain if the stallion has a history of such problems in his lineage or in his offspring.

Investigate soundness problems that have developed in the stallion or his offspring. Identify conformational abnormalities that interfere with continual soundness, such as angular limb deformities, too long a pastern slope, or post-legged hindquarters. The mare contributes half of the genetic information to the foal, therefore not all problems can be traced exclusively to the stallion.

Reproductive Exam

Examination of both the internal and external genital structures is an important part of a stallion's breeding exam. The prepuce is checked for injuries, scars or tumours. Both testicles are measured with callipers across the widest part of the scrotum, and their consistency is determined by manual palpation.

The Testicles

The testicles should feel firm, whereas a soft, mushy or hard consistency may indicate degeneration or disease. A rectal exam or internal ultrasound exam evaluates the health of the internal genital glands.

Testicular size is highly correlated to the amount of sperm output, which determines fertility. Although a young colt may begin producing viable semen by 13 months of age, most stallions are not purposely put to stud until they are 2 – 3 years old. A 2-or 3-year-old stallion should have testicles that each measure 5 centimetres or more. Size of the testicles depends on the age of a stallion, with maximum size attained by age 6. Testicular size is heritable; if a stallion has undersized testicles, not only is he potentially a poor sperm producer, but small testicles could be passed on as an undesirable trait.

The size of the testicles does decrease with a horse in training, the stress of competition (especially racing), and with medication such as anabolic steroids.

The Penis

After the stallion is lightly teased, his penis is examined for skin lesions consistent with melanomas, squames, sarcoids, warts or summer sores. Evidence of inflammation around the urethra may signal a mild infection or a venereal disease.

Venereal Disease Testing
EIA and EVA
As part of a general physical exam, the stallion should be blood tested for equine infectious anaemia (EIA) and equine viral arteritis (EVA). Both viral diseases are potentially passed venereally to the mare. EVA can be passed to other mares by the respiratory route. Not all stallions shed EVA virus in their semen but the semen should be evaluated as this virus can cause abortion. Any mare to be bred to a stallion that has tested positive for EVA should be vaccinated before breeding.

Another venereal disease is caused by yet another virus, equine herpes virus-3 or *equine coital exanthema*. Stallions or mares may be asymptomatic carriers, but horses with active herpes lesions should not be bred by live coverage, although the virus does not interfere with conception rates.

CEM
A stallion that is imported must be quarantined for *contagious equine metritis* (CEM), a bacterial infection caused by *Taylorella equigenitalis*. The stallion only carries the bacteria as a surface con-

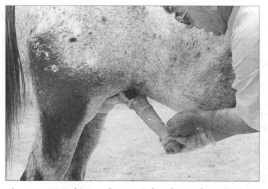

Fig. 23.10 Taking a bacterial culture for CEM.

taminant on his penis, whereas infection of a mare persists in her reproductive tract. A stallion's immune system does not respond to the disease by building antibodies that circulate in the blood. Therefore, blood testing a stallion for exposure to the bacteria does not identify a carrier stallion. The only way to determine CEM infection is by taking repeated bacterial cultures swabbed directly from the penis.

Bacterial Culture
Both before and after ejaculation, a bacterial culture is taken by gently inserting a cotton swab into the urethra. Then the swab is taken to a lab which can determine the presence of other bacterial organisms that can be transferred from the stallion to the mare

through the semen. Some bacteria can cause an infection in the mare serious enough that it will prevent conception or induce spontaneous abortion.

Semen Evaluation

The semen is evaluated for its quality by collecting samples on successive days until the semen quality has stabilized. Evaluating the semen in this manner gives a realistic picture of how much sperm a stallion can produce, its colour and structure, and how vital the sperm is.

Colour

The colour of the semen is examined for blood *(haemospermia)* or urine; both substances damage fertility by killing sperm cells.

Motility

One of the most important aspects of semen fertility is the *motility* of the sperm, which is the ability of the sperm to move. The activity of the sperm and its propensity to swim in a forward direction is called *progressive motility*. A drop of semen is placed on a warm slide and examined under a microscope immediately after collection to determine the percent of sperm that are motile compared with those that are inactive. An ideal sample would be one with over 80% of sperm showing active progressive motility, but over 50% motility is considered acceptable. Raw semen of fertile stallions retains over 10% motility for 6 hours. If semen motility is diminished to less than 10% in under 2 hours, conception rates are poor.

Structure

The structure *(morphology)* of individual sperm cells is important to their effective motility. Sperm with defective tails are unable to swim forward, and may travel in circles or in reverse. The head of the sperm must be perfect for the *acrosome* of the head eventually penetrates the waiting egg. Even if a sperm is able to swim to its destination, a defective acrosome would prevent it

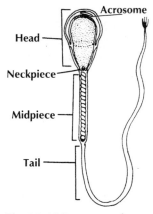

Fig. 23.11 Structure of a sperm.

493

from fertilizing the egg. Ideally, more than 60% of the sperm cells should be normal with less than 10% major structural defects.

Concentration

The *concentration* of sperm is important to a stallion's fertility. This figure is obtained by a spectrophotometer that counts the total number of sperm cells in a measured sample. The minimum concentration necessary to ensure conception of a mare is estimated at 5×10^8 (500 million) sperm cells per inseminated dose.

Other Factors Affecting Fertility

Stress Level

The stress of competition reduces the fertility of a stallion and has a marked effect on his breeding performance. This fact should be considered if a mare is booked to a stallion that is actively campaigning between breeding dates. Semen that had ample potency on collection may be infertile at insemination 12 or more hours later. This is particularly significant if semen is to be transported long distances.

Semen Extenders

Semen extenders that provide the sperm with adequate energy and nutrients are a vital aspect of the longevity of shipped semen. An extender must be matched for compatibility with each stallion's semen. An ideal semen extender will increase the conception rates of mares receiving transported semen.

Season

The season the stallion is bred also affects his fertility. April through August is the normal breeding season in the Northern Hemisphere. These summer months offer the optimum fertile period for breeding, not only for the stallion, but also for the mare.

Siring Records

The potency of a stallion with a past breeding history can be put to the test by examining his siring records. This is particularly helpful when selecting a stallion for transported semen, as the costs of semen collection, air transport and insemination can oescalate with each oestrous cycle if the mare does not conceive. If a stallion has a history of standing to stud, it is possible to categorize him as a satisfactory, questionable, or unsatisfactory breeder.

Satisfactory Breeder

The satisfactory breeder achieves at least a 75% conception rate during a single breeding season. A satisfactory breeder can potentially accommodate a large booking for the season if the season is extended from mid February to mid August, and the mares are presented to him at staggered cycles. It is possible for a fertile stallion to be booked to as many as 45 mares for natural cover, or to 125 mares for artificial insemination if his semen quality is consistent throughout the breeding months.

Questionable Breeder

A stallion would fall into the questionable category if he has problems with libido or effective ejaculation, or if his semen quality is marginal.

Unsatisfactory Breeder

The unsatisfactory breeder is the stallion that has poor semen quality leading to low fertility. A stallion with heritable defects or venereal disease is excluded as breeding stock, and by definition is unsatisfactory.

Maintaining a Stallion's Health

The breeding stallion is a performance horse that can continue in his duties well into his twenties if he is properly cared for and conditioned. An idle stallion becomes obese and unhealthy, and is prone to laminitis, colic and heart failure. A stallion's body condition score should be carefully monitored to ensure the quality of his diet. A stallion that is exercised on a regular programme has greater longevity in the breeding sheds. Turning

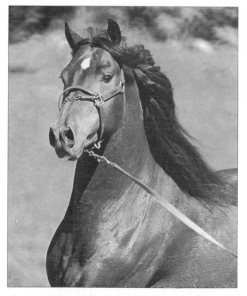

Fig. 23.12 Exercise and nutrition ensure a stallion's health and reproductive longevity.

the stallion into a paddock or pasture each day is primarily good for his mental state, but forced exercise for 30 – 60 minutes a day is required to keep him fit and in prime metabolic condition.

ARTIFICIAL INSEMINATION

This era of advanced supertechnology has enhanced the options on how to have a mare bred, and to whom. If alternative methods of breeding such as artificial insemination (AI), shipped cooled or frozen semen, or embryo transfer are employed, carefully research the stallion. Major, unrecoverable expenses can be incurred in collecting a stallion and shipping semen that has low fertility or viability. For long distance breeding methods or for embryo transfer, plan ahead to work out problems such as airline schedules, show schedules, or synchronizing ovulation for embryo transfer candidates. Check with the breed registry if methods other than live cover *are allowed* so the foal can be registered.

Artificial insemination may be used on mares at the breeding farm, or for mares living long distances from a stallion. Costs incurred by using artificial insemination include semen collection, transport of cooled or frozen semen to the mare at home, along with veterinary fees to collect the stallion and to inseminate the mare.

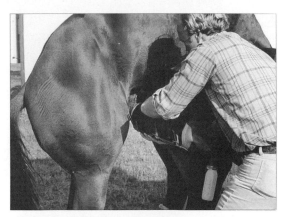

Fig. 23.13 Collecting semen for AI.

Advantages of AI

Artificial insemination is beneficial not just to the mare owner, but also to the stallion owner. Because one collection of semen can be divided into multiple inseminations, more mares can be bred than with natural cover.

Breeding Several Mares at Once

It is common practice to collect semen from a stallion on the premises, and having synchronized several mares to the same oestrous cycle, all the mares can be bred at the same time. Not only does the stallion have to perform as stud fewer times to breed all the mares, but this facilitates management 11 months later when it is time to monitor the mares for foaling.

Reduced Risk of Injury

There is less risk of physical injury to both the mare and stallion if the stallion does not have to approach or mount a mare to breed her. AI reduces the chance of infecting a mare with a hidden bacterial venereal disease, especially if antibiotics are added to a semen extender used for shipping semen to a distant location.

Breeding Mares With Foals

If a mare has a foal by her side it is often easier and safer to use AI. The mare accepts the breeding without having to protect her foal, and the mare and foal need not be shipped to the stud farm.

Breed Registries and AI Regulations

It is strongly recommended that persons intending to use artificial insemination consult with the breed registries and their veterinary surgeon. Not all breed registries approve artificial insemination. It is wise to have all the appropriate paperwork in hand and registry fees paid before breeding expenses begin to add up. The registry may require blood typing to ensure that the foal is truly the offspring of the stated mare and stallion.

It is usual for the use of artificial insemination to be overseen by each individual breed society with the exchange of semen between countries governed by national regulations. In many cases this is fresh semen, but liquid and frozen semen may be used.

Where AI Is Forbidden

The Thoroughbred industry does not permit any form of AI, nor for example do the American Miniature Horse Association or the Standard Jack and Jennet Registry of America.

British Horse Database

The prime objective is to promote selective breeding by collecting breeding and performance data, and collating the information to identify superior stock. The register at Wallingborough, Northants is open to all horses and ponies – those registered with breed or breeding societies and the many others that are unregistered.

BREEDING MANAGEMENT

Whether breeding is accomplished by natural mating at a breeding farm, by artificial insemination, or by cooled or frozen, shipped semen, expenses can run quite high before a mare is declared 'in foal.'

First, there is a stud fee. Then, there is the cost of daily 'mare care' while a mare remains at the breeding farm. The cost of transportation to deliver her to the breeding farm and home again must also be considered.

Breeding Contract

Usually, a written contract is executed between stallion breeder and mare owner. Read the contract thoroughly; make sure all wording is understandable. Discussion of mare care and liability for veterinary services while the mare is at the breeding farm should be included in the contract to avoid misunderstandings.

Find out if the stud fee includes semen collection charges if transported semen is to be used. If not, veterinary expenses can add up if the stallion must be repeatedly collected for a mare that fails to conceive on the first cycle she is bred.

Many stud farms require a uterine biopsy and bacterial culture of the mare's uterus before entering into a breeding contract. The costs of a prebreeding evaluation for the mare must be further considered when determining the financial feasibility of breeding a mare.

Most stud fees include a *live foal guarantee* (LFG), meaning that if the mare fails to conceive, aborts, or gives birth to a dead foal, the mare owner is not liable to pay the stud fee or is promised a breeding the following season at no charge. Review the contract for a clause stating a live foal guarantee, or the stud fee and related expenses may be lost.

Teasing Programmes

It is essential to find a reputable breeding facility that manages a competent breeding operation. Valuable time is lost without proper teasing techniques, teasing frequency, and record-keeping.

Interview the stallion manager about the farm's record-keeping and a consistent daily teasing programme to detect when a mare is on heat. One of the largest causes of 'infertility' is management's failure to identify if a mare is in oestrus and ready for breeding. An excellent teasing programme is a key to success so a breeder can identify when a mare is in heat. This identification may be difficult for mares with 'silent' heats who refuse to show to any stallion, or

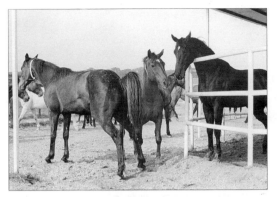

Fig. 23.14 Valuable time is lost without proper teasing techniques.

who show to only one particular stallion. In these cases, daily rectal palpation or ultrasound may be necessary to identify breeding time if not using natural coverage.

Careful attention to teasing records also minimizes the number of times a stallion is required to inseminate a mare. The fewer times he must breed her or be collected reduces the chances for injury and infection, and increases the number of mares he can breed in a season.

Booking to a Stallion

Long before it is time to breed a mare, arrangements should be made with the stallion manager to 'book' the mare in time for the breeding season ahead. A stallion can only breed so many mares each season, especially if he is involved in a show or performance schedule. To avoid profound disappointment at finding a stallion's bookings filled, plan as much as a year in advance.

APPENDIX

Parts of the Horse

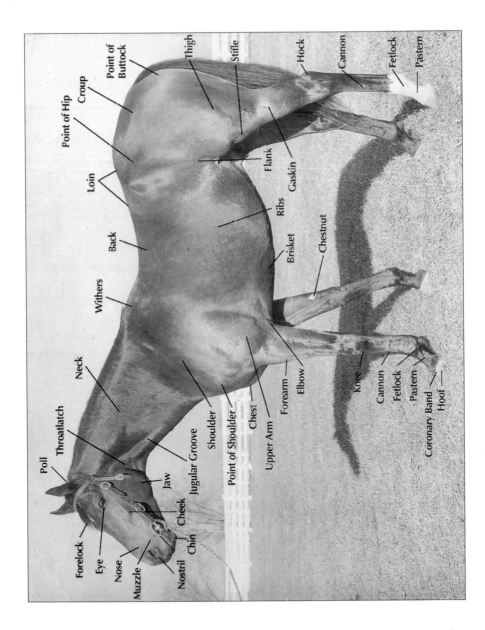

Bones of the Horse

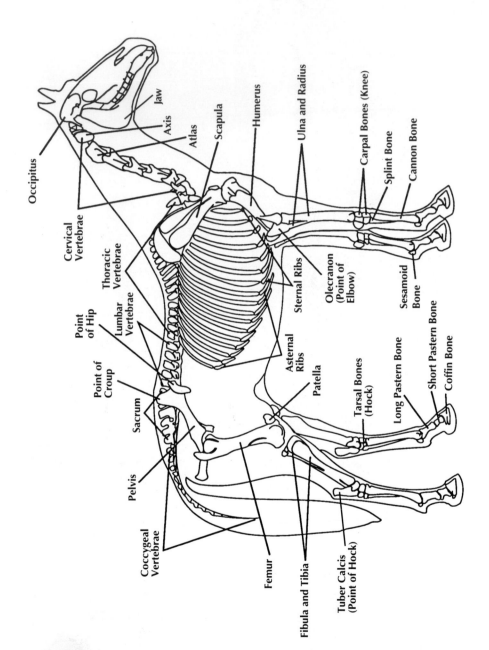

Muscles of the Horse

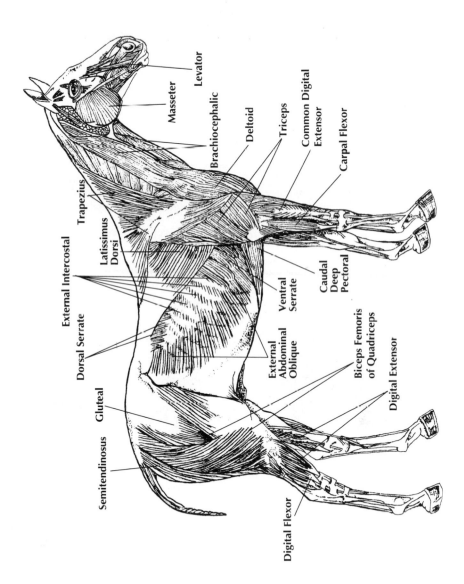

Bibliography

Alsup, E.M. "Dimethyl Sulfoxide." *Journal of the American Veterinary Medical Association*, Vol. 185, No. 9 (November 1984), pp. 1011 – 1014.

Antikatzides, T.G. "Soft Laser Treatment of Musculoskeletal and Other Disorders in the Equine Athlete." *Equine Practice*, Vol. 8, No. 2 (February 1986), pp. 24 – 29.

Asquith, R.L., E.L. Johnson, J. Kivepelto, and C. Depew. "Erroneous Weight Estimation of Horses." *Proceedings of the American Association of Equine Practitioners* (1990), pp. 599 – 607.

Austin, S.M., J.A. DiPietro, J.H. Foreman, G.J. Baker, and K.S. Todd. "Parascaris Equorum Infections in Horses." *Compendium on Continuing Education*, Vol. 12, No. 8 (August 1990), pp. 1110 – 1118.

Baker, D.J. "Rationale for the Use of Influenza Vaccines in Horses and the Importance of Antigenic Drift." *Equine Veterinary Journal*, Vol. 18, No. 2 (1986), pp. 93 – 96.

Balch, O.K., M.H. Ratzlaff, M.L. Hyde, and K.K. White. "Locomotor Effects of Hoof Angle and Mediolateral Balance of Horses Exercising on a High-Speed Treadmill: Preliminary Results." *Proceedings of the American Association of Equine Practitioners* (1991), pp. 687 – 705.

Banks, William J. *Applied Veterinary Histology.* Williams and Wilkins, Baltimore, 1981, pp. 245 – 261.

Barber, S.M. "Second Intention Wound Healing in the Horse: The Effect of Bandages and Topical Corticosteroids." *Proceedings of the American Association of Equine Practitioners* (1989), pp. 107 – 116.

Baucus, K.L., S.L. Ralston, et al. "The Effect of Copper and Zinc Supplementation on Mineral Content of Mare's Milk." *Equine Veterinary Science*, Vol. 9, No. 4 (1989), pp. 206 – 209.

Baucus, K.L., E.L. Squires, S.L. Ralston, and A.O. McKinnon. "The Effect of Transportation Stress on Early Embryonic Death in Mares." *Proceedings of the Equine Nutrition and Physiology Symposium* (1987), pp. 657 – 662.

Baxter, G.M. "Equine Laminitis." *Equine Practice*, Vol. 14, No. 4 (April 1992), pp. 13 – 22.

Baxter, G.M. "Wound Healing and Delayed Wound Closure in the Lower Limb of the Horse." *Equine Practice*, Vol. 10, No. 1 (January 1988), pp. 23 – 31.

Bayly, W.M., H.D. Liggitt, L.J. Huston, and W.W. Laegreid. "Stress and Its Effect on Equine Pulmonary Mucosal Defenses." *Proceedings of the American Association of Equine Practitioners* (1986), pp. 253 – 262.

Beeman, M. "Conformation: The Relationship of Form to Function." *Quarter Horse Journal* Reprint.

Bennett, D. "Principles of Conformation Analysis." Selected Articles from *Equus* 117 – 177.

Bertone, J.J., J.L. Traub-Dargatz, R.W. Wrigley, D.G. Bennett, and R.J. Williams. "Diarrhea Associated With Sand in the Gastrointestinal Tract of Horses." *Journal of the American Veterinary Medical Association* (December 1988), Vol. 193, No. 11, pp. 1409 – 1412.

Blagburn, B.L., D.S. Lindsay, C.M. Hendrix, and J. Schumacher. "Pathogenesis, Treatment, and Control of Gastric Parasites in Horses." *Compendium on Continuing Education,* Vol. 13, No. 5 (May 1991), pp. 850 – 857.

Boden, E., ed. *Equine Practice,* Vol. 1. Baillière Tindall, London, (1991).

Boden, E., ed. *Equine Practice,* Vol. 2. Baillière Tindall, London, (1993).

Booth, N.H. and L.E. McDonald, eds. *Veterinary Pharmacology and Therapeutics.* Fifth Edition. Iowa State University Press, Ames, 1982.

Bradley, R.E., T.J. Lane, R.F. Jochen, B.P. Seibert, and K.M. Newcomb, "Distribution and Frequency of Benzimidazole Resistance in Equine Small Strongyles." *Equine Practice,* Vol. 8, No. 2 (February 1986), pp. 7 – 11.

Bramlage, L. and Editorial Staff. "Surgical Repair of Bowed Tendons." *Thoroughbred Times* (February 1992), pp. 22 – 24.

Bramlage, L.R., N.W. Rantanen, R.L. Genovese, and L.E. Page. "Long-term Effects of Surgical Treatment of Superficial Flexor Tendinitis by Superior Check Desmototomy." *Proceedings of the American Association of Equine Practitioners* (1988), pp. 655.

Bridges, C.H. and E.D. Harris. "Experimentally Induced Cartilaginous Fractures (Osteochondritis Dissecans) in Foals Fed Low-Copper Diets." *Journal of American Veterinary Medical Association,* Vol. 193, No. 2 (July 1988), pp. 215 – 221.

Bryans, J.T. "Control of Equine Influenza." *Proceedings of the American Association of Equine Practitioners* (1980), pp. 279 – 285.

Buffa, E.A., et al. "Effect of Dietary Biotin Supplement on Equine Hoof Horn Growth Rate and Hardness." *Equine Veterinary Journal,* Vol. 24, No. 6 (1992), pp. 472 – 474.

Burch, G.E. "Transcutaneous Electrical Stimulation." *Equine Practice,* Vol. 7, No. 9 (October 1985), pp. 6 – 11.

Carleton, C.L. "Basic Techniques for Evaluating the Subfertile Mare." *Veterinary Medicine* (December 1988), pp. 1253 – 1261.

Carlson, G.P. "Medical Problems Associated With Protracted Heat and Work Stress in Horses." *Compendium on Continuing Education,* Vol. 7, No. 10 (October 1985), pp. 542 – 550.

Clabough, D. "Streptococcus Equi Infection in the Horse: A Review of Clinical and Immunological Considerations." *Equine Veterinary Science, Vol. 7,* No. 5 (1987), pp. 279 – 283.

Clarke, A.F. "Stable Design and Management." *Veterinary Annual,* Blackwell Science, Oxford, (1993).

Clarke, A.F., T.M. Madelin, and R.G. Allpress. "The Relationship of Air Hygiene in Stables to Lower Airway Disease and Pharyngeal Lymphoid Hyperplasia in Two Groups of Thoroughbred Horses." *Equine Veterinary Journal,* Vol. 19, No. 6 (1987), pp. 524 – 530.

Clayton, H.M. "Comparison of the Stride of Trotting Horses Trimmed With a Normal and a Broken-Back Hoof Axis." *Proceedings of the American Association of Equine Practitioners* (1988), pp. 289 – 298.

Clayton, H.M. "Time-Motion Analysis in Equestrian Sports: The Grand Prix Dressage Test." *Proceedings of the American Association of Equine Practitioners* (1989), pp. 367 – 373.

Clayton, H.M. *Conditioning Sport Horses.* Sport Horse Publications, Saskatoon, Saskatchewan, Canada, 1991.

Coffman, J.R. "Muscle Fibers: Coupling and Contraction and Energy Metabolism." *Equine Sportsmedicine,* Vol. 3, No. 2 (1984), pp. 1 – 3.

Coffman, J.R. "Stress and the Racehorse." *Equine Sportsmedicine,* Vol. 3, No. 4 (1984), pp. 1, 7 – 8.

Colles, C.M. "A Technique for Assessing Hoof Function in the Horse." *Equine*

Veterinary Journal, Vol. 21, No. 1 (1989), pp. 17 – 22.

Colles, C.M. "The Relationship of Frog Pressure to Heel Expansion." *Equine Veterinary Journal*, Vol. 21, No. 1 (1989), pp. 13 – 16.

Collier, M., et al. "Electrostimulation of Bone Production in the Horse." *Proceedings of the American Association of Equine Practitioners* (1981), pp. 71 – 89.

Collins, L.G. and D.E. Tyler. "Phenylbutazone Toxicosis in the Horse: A Clinical Study." *Journal of the American Veterinary Medical Association*, Vol. 184, No. 6 (March 1984), pp. 699 – 703.

Colquhoun, K.M., et al. "Control of Breeding in the Mare." *Equine Veterinary Journal*, Vol. 19, No. 2 (1987), pp. 138 – 142.

Cook, W.R. "Diagnosis and Grading of Hereditary Recurrent Laryngeal Neuropathy in the Horse." *Equine Veterinary Science*, Vol. 8, No. 6 (1988), pp. 431 – 455.

Cook, W.R. "Recent Observations on Recurrent Laryngeal Neuropathy in the Horse: Applications to Practice." *Proceedings of the American Association of Equine Practitioners* (1988), pp. 427 – 478.

Cook, W.R. "Some Observations on Form and Function of the Equine Upper Airway in Health and Disease: 1. The Pharynx." *Proceedings of the American Association of Equine Practitioners* (1981), pp. 355 – 391.

Cook, W.R. "Some Observations on Form and Function of the Equine Upper Airway in Health and Disease: 2. The Larynx." *Proceedings of the American Association of Equine Practitioners* (1981), pp. 393 – 451.

Cook, W.R. *Specifications for Speed in the Racehorse: The Airflow Factors*. The Russell Meerdink Company, Ltd., 1993.

Cook, W.R., et al. "Upper Airway Obstruction (Possible Asphyxia) as the Possible Cause of Exercise-Induced Pulmonary Hemorrhage in the Horse: An Hypothesis." *Equine Veterinary Science*, Vol. 8, No. 1 (1988), pp. 11 – 26.

Cox, J.H. and R.M. DeBowes. "Colic-like Discomfort Associated With Ovulation in Two Mares." *Journal of the American Veterinary Medical Association*, Vol. 191, No. 11 (December 1987), pp. 1451 – 1452.

Cox, J.H. and R.M. DeBowes. "Episodic Weakness Caused by Hyperkalemic Periodic Paralysis in Horses." *Compendium on Continuing Education*, Vol. 12, No. 1 (January 1990), pp. 83 – 88.

Crawford, W.H., R. Vanderby, Jr., et al. "The Energy Absorption Capacity of Equine Support Bandages." *V.C.O.T.*, Vol. 1 (1990), pp. 2 – 9.

Crowell-Davis, S., W. Crowell-Davis, and A. Caudle. "Preventing Trailering Problems: Part II." *Equine Practice*, Vol. 9, No. 1 (January 1987), pp. 32 – 33.

Cunha, A. *Horse Feeding and Nutrition*, 2nd edn. Academic Press, New York, pp. 325 and 381.

Currey, J.D. "The Mechanical Consequences of Variations in the Mineral Content of Bone." *Journal of Biomechanics*, Vol. 2 (1969A), pp. 2 – 11.

Currey, J.D. "The Relationship Between Stiffness and the Mineral Content of Bone." *Journal of Biomechanics*, Vol. 2 (1969B), pp. 477 – 480.

Custalow, B. "Protein Requirements During Exercise in the Horse." *Equine Veterinary Science*, Vol. 11, No. 1 (1991), pp. 65 – 66.

Cymbaluk, N. "Water Balance of Horses Fed Various Diets." *Equine Practice*, Vol. 11, No. 1 (1989), pp. 19 – 24.

Derksen, F.J., et al. "Chronic Obstructive Pulmonary Disease Roundtable Discussion." *Equine Practice*, Vol. 13, No. 5 (May 1991), pp. 25 – 28. *Equine Practice*, Vol. 13, No. 7 (July/August 1991), pp. 15 – 19.

Derksen, F.J. "Physiology of Airflow in the Athletic Horse." *Proceedings of the*

American Association of Equine Practitioners (1988), pp. 149 – 158.

DiPietro, J.A. and K.S. Todd. "Anthelmintics Used in Treatment of Parasitic Infections of Horses." *Equine Practice*, Vol. 11, No. 4 (April 1989), pp. 5 – 15.

DiPietro, J.A., T.R. Klei, and D.D. French. "Contemporary Topics in Equine Parasitology." *Compendium on Continuing Education*, Vol. 12, No. 5 (May 1990), pp. 713 – 720.

Divers, T.J. and D. Dreyfuss. "Evaluating the Horse With a Poor Racing Performance." *Veterinary Medicine* (May 1990), pp. 522, 529.

Drudge, J.H. and E.T. Lyons. *Internal Parasites of Equids With Emphasis on Treatment and Control.* Hoechst-Roussel Agri-Vet Company, 1986.

Drudge, J.H. and E.T. Lyons. *Internal Parasites of Equids With Emphasis on Treatment and Control,* Revised 1989. Hoechst-Roussel Agri-Vet Company.

Drudge, J.H., E.T. Lyons, and S.C. Tolliver. "Strongyles—An Update." *Equine Practice*, Vol. 11, No. 4 (April 1989), pp. 43 – 49.

Duren, S., C. Wood, and S. Jackson. "Dietary Fat and the Racehorse." *Equine Veterinary Science*, Vol. 7, No. 6 (1987), pp. 396 – 397.

Dwyer, Roberta M. "The Practical Diagnosis and Treatment of Metabolic Conditions in Endurance Horses." *Equine Practice*, Vol. 8, No. 8 (September 1986), pp. 21 – 33.

Dyer, Robert M. "The Bovine Respiratory Disease Complex: A Complex Interaction of Host, Environmental, and Infectious Factors." *Compendium on Continuing Education*, Vol. 4, No. 7 (July 1982), pp. 296 – 307.

Dyson, S. "Potential Value of Diagnostic Ultrasonography for Assessment of Equine Superficial Digital Flexor Tendon." *Veterinary Annual.* Blackwell Science, Oxford, (1993).

Editorial Staff. *Dynamics of Equine Athletic Performance. Proceedings of the Association of Equine Sports Medicine* (1985), Veterinary Learning Systems Co., Inc.

Editorial Staff. "Conformation." *Practical Horseman* (May 1992), pp. 54 – 60, 90 – 91.

Editorial Staff. "Round Table on Interval Training." *Thoroughbred Times* (February 1992), pp. 14 – 21.

Editorial Staff. *Proceedings of a Roundtable on Equine Influenza* (December 1987), Coopers Animal Health, Inc.

Editorial Staff. "Hyperkalemic Periodic Paralysis Presents Medical and Ethical Challenge." *Journal of the American Veterinary Medical Association*, Vol. 202, No. 8 (April 1993), pp. 1203 – 1209.

Edwards, Gladys Brown. *Anatomy and Conformation of the Horse.* Dreenan Press, Ltd., Croton-on-Hudson, New York, 1980.

England, J.J. "Veterinary Virology, Part II: Pathogenesis of Viral Infections." *Compendium on Continuing Education*, Vol. 6, No. 2 (February 1984), pp. 145 – 154.

Equine Respiratory Medicine and Surgery. *Equine Veterinary Journal*, Vol. 19 (September/October 1987), No. 5.

Erickson, B.K., Erickson, H.H., and Coffman, J.R. "Exercise-Induced Pulmonary Hemorrhage During High Intensity Exercise: Potential Causes and the Role of Furosemide." *Proceedings of the American Association of Equine Practitioners* (1989), pp. 375 – 379.

Essen-Gustavsson, B., D. McMiken, et al. "Muscular Adaptation of Horses During Intensive Training and Detraining." *Equine Veterinary Journal*, Vol. 21, No. 1 (1989), pp. 27 – 33.

Eustace, R. A., *Explaining Laminitis and Its Prevention,* EFS20, Bristol, (1992).

Ewert, K.M., J.A. DiPietro, J.H. Foreman, and K.S. Todd. "Control Programs for Endoparasites in Horses." *Compendium on Continuing Education*, Vol. 13, No. 6 (June 1991), pp. 1012 – 1018.

Fadok, V.A. and P.C. Mullowney. "Dermatologic Diseases of Horses, Part 1: Parasitic Dermatoses of the Horse." *Compendium on Continuing Education*, Vol. 5, No. 11 (November 1983), pp. 615 – 622.

Foil, L.D. and C.S. Foil. "Dipteran Parasites of Horses." *Equine Practice*, Vol. 10, No. 4 (April 1988), pp. 21 – 38.

Foil, L.D. and C.S. Foil. "Arthropod Pests of Horses." *Compendium on Continuing Education*, Vol. 12, No. 5 (May 1990), pp. 723 – 730.

Foil, L.D., et al. "The Role of Horn Fly Feeding and the Management of Seasonal Equine Ventral Midline Dermatitis." *Equine Practice*, Vol. 12, No. 5 (May 1990), pp. 6 – 14.

Fox, S.F. "Management of Thermal Burns—Part 1." *Compendium on Continuing Education*, Vol. 7, No. 8 (August 1985), pp. 631 – 639.

Fox, S.F. "Management of Thermal Burns—Part 2." *Compendium on Continuing Education*, Vol. 8, No. 7 (July 1986), pp. 439 – 444.

Frape, D.L. *Equine Nutrition and Feeding.* Longmans, London, (1986), pp. 147-149

Frape, D.L. "Dietary Requirements and Athletic Performance of Horses." *Equine Veterinary Journal*, Vol. 20, No. 3 (1988), pp. 163 – 172.

Frazier, C. "Cardiac Recovery Index." *AERC Endurance News* (September 1992), pp. 4 – 6.

Frazier, D. "Equine Dietary Adaptation: Cardiac Recovery Index." *AERC Endurance News* (November 1992), pp. 10 – 15.

Fredriksson, G., H. Kindahl, and G. Stabenfeldt. "Endotoxin-Induced and Prostaglandin-Mediated Effects on Corpus Luteum Function in the Mare." *Theriogenology*, Vol. 25 (1986), pp. 309 – 316.

Freestone, J.F. and G.P. Carlson. "Muscle Disorders in the Horse: A Retrospective Study." *Equine Veterinary Journal*, Vol. 23, No. 2 (1991), pp. 86 – 90.

French, D.D. and M.R. Chapman. "Tapeworms of the Equine Gastrointestinal Tract." *Compendium on Continuing Education*, Vol. 14, No. 5 (May 1992), pp. 655 – 661.

French, D.D., T.R. Klei, and G.E. Hackett. "Equine Parasites: Dollars and Sense." *Equine Practice*, Vol. 10, No. 5 (May 1988), pp. 8 – 14.

Fricker C., W. Riek, and J. Hugelshofter. "A Model for Pathogenesis of Navicular Disease." *Equine Veterinary Journal*, Vol. 14 (1982), pp. 203 – 207.

Gach, J. "Trailer Studies Reveal Fewer Harmful Effects Than Expected." *Equus* 120 (1987), pp. 12 – 16.

Genetzky, R.M. "Chronic Obstructive Pulmonary Disease In Horses — Part 1." *Compendium on Continuing Education*, Vol. 7, No. 7 (July 1985), pp. 407 – 414.

Gerring, E.L. "All Wind and Water: Some Progress in the Study of Equine Gut Motility." *Equine Veterinary Journal*, Vol. 23, No. 2 (1991), pp. 81 – 85.

Getty, Robert, ed. *Sisson and Grossman's The Anatomy of the Domestic Animals.* Volume 1. WB Saunders Company, 1975.

Gillespie, J.R. and N.E. Robinson, eds. *Equine Exercise Physiology 2.* ICEEP Publications, Davis, California, 1987.

Gillis, C. and D. Meagher. "Tendon Response to Training." *The Equine Athlete*, Vol. 4, No. 5 (September/October 1991), pp. 26 – 27.

Ginther, O.J. *Reproductive Biology of the Mare.* McNaughton and Gunn, Inc., Ann Arbor, Michigan, 1979.

Glade, M.J. "Feeding Innovations for the Performance Horse." *Equine Veterinary Science*, Vol. 4, No. 4, pp. 165 – 166.

Goetz, T.E., C.H. Boulton, and G.K. Ogilvie. "Clinical Management of Progressive Multifocal Benign and Malignant Melanomas of Horses With Oral Cimetidine." *Proceedings of the American Association of Equine Practitioners* (1989), pp. 431 – 438.

Goetz, T.E., G.K. Ogilvie, et al. "Cimetidine for Treatment of Melanomas in Three Horses." *Journal of the American Veterinary Medical Association*, Vol. 196, No. 3 (February 1990), pp. 449 – 452.

Goodman, N., et al. "An Equine Roundtable Discussion on Lameness." *Equine Practice*, Vol. 12, No. 8 (September 1990), pp. 28 – 33.

Gorham, S. and M. Robl. "Melanoma in the Gray Horse: The Darker Side of Equine Aging." *Veterinary Medicine* (May 1986), pp. 446 – 448.

Grant, B.D., L.J. Smith, et al. "Hill Training for High-Speed Performance Horses." *The Equine Athlete*, Vol. 1, No. 1 (December 1988), pp. 6 – 7, 15 – 16.

Green, E., et al. "Endotoxemia Roundtable Discussion." *Equine Practice*, Vol. 14, No. 9 (October 1992), pp. 7 – 12. *Equine Practice*, Vol. 14, No. 10 (November/December 1992), pp. 13 – 18. *Equine Practice*, Vol. 15, No. 1 (January 1993), pp. 7 – 14.

Griffiths, I.R. "The Pathogenesis of Equine Laryngeal Hemiplegia." *Equine Veterinary Journal*, Vol. 23, No. 2 (1991), pp. 75 – 76.

Hackett, G.E., C. Uhlinger, R. Mitchell, F.B. McCashin, and S. Conboy. "Continuous Deworming Programs: Roundtable Discussion." *Equine Practice*, Vol. 14, No. 7 (July/August 1992), pp. 13 – 18. *Equine Practice*, Vol. 14, No. 8 (September 1992), pp. 27 – 33.

Halldordsottir, S. and H.J. Larsen. "An Epidemiological Study of Summer Eczema in Icelandic Horses in Norway." *Equine Veterinary Journal*, Vol. 23, No. 4 (1991), pp. 296 – 299.

Hamm, D. and E.W. Jones. "Intra-Articular and Intramuscular Treatment of Noninfectious Equine Arthritis (DJD) With Polysulfated Glycosaminoglycan (PSGAG)." *Equine Veterinary Science*, Vol. 8, No. 6 (1988), pp. 456 – 459.

Harkins, J.D. and S.G. Kamerling. "A Comparative Study of Interval and Conventional Training Methods in Thoroughbred Racehorses." *Equine Veterinary Science* (January/February 1990), pp. 45 – 51.

Harkins, J.D. and S.G. Kamerling. "Effects of Induced Alkalosis on Performance in Thoroughbreds During a 1600 Meter Race." *Equine Veterinary Journal*, Vol. 24, No. 2 (1992), pp. 94 – 98.

Harman, J. "Acupuncture for Horses." *AERC Endurance News* (August 1991), pp. 8 – 9.

Harper, Frederick. "Control of the Broodmare's Reproductive Cycle." *Equine Veterinary Science*, Vol. 9, No. 2 (1989), pp. 112 – 115.

Harris, P.A. "Differential Diagnosis of Equine Rhabdomyelyosis Syndrome." *Veterinary Annual*, Blackwell Science, Oxford, (1993)

Harris, P. and D.H. Snow. "Plasma Potassium and Lactate Concentrations in Thoroughbred Horses During Exercise of Varying Intensity." *Equine Veterinary Journal*, Vol. 23, No. 3 (1992), pp. 220 – 225.

Hart, C. "Equine Conformation of the Top Endurance Athlete." *AERC Endurance News* (August 1990), pp. 10 – 11.

Hayes, Horace M. *Points of the Horse.* Arco Publishing Company, Inc., New York, 1969.

Haynes, Peter. "Obstructive Disease of the Upper Respiratory Tract: Current

Thoughts on Diagnosis and Surgical Management." *Proceedings of the American Association of Equine Practitioners* (1986), pp. 283 – 290.

Henneke, D.R. "A Condition Score System for Horses." *Equine Practice*, Vol. 7, No. 8 (September 1985), pp. 13 – 15.

Herd, R.P. "Epidemiology and Control of Equine Strongylosis at Newmarket." *Equine Veterinary Journal*, Vol. 18, No. 6 (1986), pp. 447 – 452.

Herd, R.P. and A.A. Gabel. "Reduced Efficacy of Anthelmintics in Young Compared With Adult Horses." *Equine Veterinary Journal*, Vol. 22, No. 3 (1990), pp. 164 – 169.

Hickman, J. *Horse Management*, Academic Press, London, (1984).

Hickman, J. *Equine Medicine and Surgery*, Vols 1 & 2, Academic Press, London, (1985 and 1986).

Hickman, J. "Navicular Disease—What Are We Talking About?" *Equine Veterinary Journal*, Vol. 21, No. 6 (1989), pp. 395 – 398.

Hintz, H.F. "Factors Which Influence Developmental Orthopedic Disease." *Proceedings of the American Association of Equine Practitioners* (1988), pp. 159 – 162.

Hintz, H.F., et al. "Effects of Protein Levels on Endurance Horses." *Journal of Animal Science*, Vol. 51 (1980), p. 202.

Hintz, H.F. "Biotin." *Equine Practice*, Vol. 9, No. 9 (October 1987), pp. 4 – 5.

Hintz, H.F. "Effect of Diet on Copper Content of Milk." *Equine Practice*, Vol. 9, No. 8 (1987), pp. 6 – 7.

Hintz, H.F. "Protein Needs of the Equine Athlete." *Equine Practice*, Vol. 8, No. 6 (1988), pp. 5 – 6.

Hintz, H.F. "Some Myths About Equine Nutrition." *Compendium on Continuing Education*, Vol. 12, No. 1 (1990), pp. 78 – 81.

Hintz, H.F. "The 1989 NRC Estimates of Protein Requirements." *Equine Practice*, Vol. 11, No. 10 (1989), pp. 5 – 6.

Hintz, H.F. "Weighing Horses." *Equine Practice*, Vol. 10, No. 8 (1988), pp. 10 – 11.

Hodgson, D.R. "Exertional Rhabdomyolysis." *Current Veterinary Therapy 2*, WB Saunders Co., Philadelphia, 1987, pp. 487 – 490.

Hodgson, D.R. "Myopathies in the Athletic Horse." *Compendium on Continuing Education*, Vol. 7, No. 10 (October 1985), pp. 551 – 556.

Honnas, C.M., J. Schumacher, and P.W. Dean. "Laryngeal Hemiplegia in Horses: Diagnosis and Surgical Management." *Veterinary Medicine* (October 1985), pp. 752 – 763.

Houpt, K.A. "Thirst in Horses: The Physiological and Psychological Causes." *Equine Practice*, Vol. 9, No. 6 (June 1987), pp. 28 – 30.

Houston, C.S. *Going Higher: The Story of Man and Altitude*. Little, Brown, and Company, Boston, 1987.

Huddleston, A.L., P. Rockwell, D.N. Kulund, and R.B. Harrison. "Bone Mass in Life-Time Tennis Athletes." *Journal of the American Medical Association*, Vol. 244 (1980), pp. 1107 – 1109.

Hurtig, M.B., S.L. Green, H. Dobson, and J. Burton. "Defective Bone and Cartilage in Foals Fed a Low Copper Diet." *Proceedings of the American Association of Equine Practitioners* (1990), pp. 637 – 643.

Hustead, D. "Vaccines: What's Ahead?" *Large Animal Veterinarian* (March/April 1990), pp. 8 – 11, 36 – 37.

Ivers, T. "Osteochondrosis: Undernutrition or Overnutrition?" *Equine Practice*, Vol. 8, No. 8 (September 1986), pp. 15 – 19.

Ivers, T. "Cryotherapy: An In-Depth Study." *Equine Practice*, Vol. 9, No. 2

(February 1987), pp. 17 – 19.

Jacobs, D.E. *Equine Parasites*, Grove Medical Publishing, New York (1986).

Jeffcott, L.B. "Osteochondrosis in the Horse—Searching for the Key to Pathogenesis." *Equine Veterinary Journal* (1991), Vol. 23, No. 5, pp. 331 – 338.

Jennings, S., T.N. Meacham, and A.N. Huff. "Management of the Brood Mare." *Equine Practice*, Vol. 9, No. 1 (January 1987), pp. 28 – 31.

Johnston, A.M. *Equine Medical Disorders*. 2nd Edn, Blackwell Science, Oxford, (1994).

Jones, W.E. "Muscular Causes of Exercise Intolerance." *Equine Veterinary Science* (1987), Vol. 7, No. 5, pp. 312 – 316.

Jones, W.E. *Equine Sports Medicine*. Lea and Febiger, Philadelphia, 1989.

Jones, W.E. *Sports Medicine for the Racehorse*. Second Edition. Veterinary Data, Wildomar, California, 1992.

Jones, W.E., ed. *Nutrition for the Equine Athlete*. Equine Sportsmedicine News, Wildomar, California, 1989.

Kiley-Worthington, M. "The Behavior of Horses in Relation to Management and Training—Towards Ethologically Sound Environments." *Equine Veterinary Science*, Vol. 10, No. 1 (1990), pp. 62 – 71.

King, J.N. and E.L. Gerring. "The Action of Low Dose Endotoxin on Equine Bowel Motility." *Equine Veterinary Journal*, Vol. 23, No. 1 (1991), pp. 11 – 17.

Knight, D.A., A.A. Gabel, et al. "Correlation of Dietary Mineral to Incidence and Severity of Metabolic Bone Disease in Ohio and Kentucky." *Proceedings of the American Association of Equine Practitioners* (1985), pp. 445 – 461.

Knight, D.A., A.A. Gabel, et al. "The Effects of Copper Supplementation on the Prevalence of Cartilage Lesions in Foals." *Equine Veterinary Journal*, Vol. 22, No. 6 (1990), pp. 426 – 432.

Knight, D.A., S.E. Weisbrode, L.M. Schmall, and A.A. Gabel. "Copper Supplementation and Cartilage Lesions in Foals." *Proceedings of the American Association of Equine Practitioners* (1988), pp. 191 – 194.

Knottenbelt, D. and Pascoe, R. *Colour Atlas of Diseases and Disorders of the Horse*, Wolfe Publishing, London, (1994).

Kohnke, J. "Liquid Vitamin Supplements." *Equine Practice*, Vol. 8, No. 10 (1986), pp. 7 – 9.

Kopp, K. "Do Horses Bend?" *Equus* 115, pp. 31 – 38, 110.

Koterba, A. and G.P. Carlson. "Acid-Base and Electrolyte Alterations in Horses With Exertional Rhabdomyolysis." *Journal of the American Veterinary Medical Association*, Vol. 180, No. 3 (February 1982), pp. 303 – 306.

Kronfeld, D.S. "Symposium Sheds New Light on Equine Ventilatory Adaptations, Muscle Glycogen." *DVM Magazine* (September 1989), pp. 12, 14.

Kronfeld, D.S. and S. Donoghue. "Metabolic Convergence in Developmental Orthopedic Disease." *Proceedings of the American Association of Equine Practitioners* (1988), pp. 195 – 202.

Kurcz, E.V., L.M. Lawrence, K.W. Kelley, and P.A. Miller. "The Effect of Intense Exercise on the Cell-Mediated Immune Response of Horses." *Equine Veterinary Science*, Vol. 8, No. 3 (1988), pp. 237 – 239.

Laegreid, W.W., L.J. Huston, R.J. Basaraba, and M.V. Crisman. "The Effects of Stress on Alveolar Macrophage Function in the Horse: An Overview." *Equine Practice*, Vol. 10, No. 9 (1988), pp. 9 – 16.

Landeau, L.J., D.J. Barrett, and S.C. Batterman. "Mechanical Properties of Equine Hooves." *American Journal of Veterinary Research*, 44 (January

1983), p. 100.

Lawrence, L.M., K.D. Bump, and D.G. McLaren. "Aerial Ammonia Levels in Horse Stalls." *Equine Practice*, Vol. 10, No. 10 (November/December 1988), pp. 20 – 23.

Leadon, D.P., C. Frank, and W. Backhouse. "A Preliminary Report on Studies on Equine Transit Stress." *Equine Veterinary Science*, Vol. 9, No. 4 (1989), pp. 200 – 201.

Leadon, D.P. "A Summary of a Preliminary Report of an Investigation of Transit Stress in the Horse." *AESM Quarterly*, Vol. 3, No. 2 (1988), pp. 19 – 20.

Leadon, D.P., et al. "Environmental, Hematological and Blood Biochemical Changes in Equine Transit Stress." *Proceedings of the American Association of Equine Practitioners* (1990), pp. 485 – 490.

Lee, A.H., and S.F. Swaim. "Granulation Tissue: How to Take Advantage of It in Management of Open Wounds." *Compendium on Continuing Education*, Vol. 10, No. 2 (February 1988), pp. 163 – 170.

Lee, A.H., S.F. Swaim, et al. "Effects of Nonadherent Dressing Materials on the Healing of Open Wounds in Dogs." *Journal of the American Veterinary Medical Association*, Vol. 190, No. 4 (February 1987), pp. 416 – 422.

Lee, S. and C.L. Davidson. "The Role of Collagen in the Elastic Properties of Calcified Tissues." *Journal of Biomechanics*, Vol. 10 (1977), pp. 473 – 486.

Lees, M.J., P.B. Fretz, and K.A. Jacobs. "Factors Influencing Wound Healing: Lessons From Military Wound Management." *Compendium on Continuing Education*, Vol. 11, No. 7 (July 1989), pp. 850 – 855.

Lees, M.J., P.B. Fretz, J.V. Bailey, and K.A. Jacobs. "Second Intention Wound Healing." *Compendium on Continuing Education*, Vol. 11, No. 7 (July 1989), pp. 857 – 864.

Liu, I.K.M. "Update on Respiratory Vaccines in the Horse." *Proceedings of the American Association of Equine Practitioners* (1986), pp. 277 – 282.

Lopez-Rivero, J.L., et al. "Comparative Study of Muscle Fiber Type Composition in the Middle Gluteal Muscle of Andalusian, Thoroughbred, and Arabian Horses." *Equine Sportsmedicine* (November/December 1989), pp. 337 – 340.

Lopez-Rivero, J.L., A.M. Diz, E. Aguera, and A.L. Serrano. "Endurance Training in Andalusian and Arabian Horses." *Equine Practice*, Vol. 15, No. 4 (April 1993), pp. 13 – 19.

Lopez-Rivero, J.L., et al. "Muscle Fiber Size in Horses." *The Equine Athlete*, Vol. 3, No. 2 (March/April 1990), pp. 1 – 11.

Lopez-Rivero, J.L., et al. "Muscle Fiber Type Composition in Untrained and Endurance-Trained Andalusian and Arab Horses." *Equine Veterinary Journal*, Vol. 23, No. 2 (1991), pp. 91 – 93.

MacFadden, K.E. and L.W. Pace. "Clinical Manifestations of Squamous Cell Carcinoma in Horses." *Compendium on Continuing Education*, Vol. 13, No. 4 (April 1991), pp. 669 – 676.

MacNamara, B., S. Bauer, and J. Lafe. "Endoscopic Evaluation of Exercise-Induced Pulmonary Hemorrhage and Chronic Obstructive Pulmonary Disease in Association With Poor Performance in Racing Standardbreds." *Journal of the American Veterinary Medical Association*, Vol. 196, No. 3 (February 1990), pp. 443 – 445.

Mal, M.E., T.H. Friend, D.C. Lay, S.G. Vogelsang, and O.C. Jenkins. "Physiological Responses of Mares to Short Term Confinement and Social Isolation." *Equine Veterinary Science*, Vol. 11, No. 2 (1991), pp. 96 – 102.

Manning, T. and C. Sweeney. "Immune-Mediated Equine Skin Diseases." *Compendium on Continuing Education*, Vol. 8, No. 12 (December 1986), pp. 979 – 986.

Martin, R.K., J.P. Albright, W.R. Clarke, and J.A. Niffenegger. "Load Carrying Effects on the Adult Beagle Tibia." *Medicine and Science in Sports and Exercise*, Vol. 13 (1981), pp. 343 – 349.

McCarthy, R.N. "The Effects of Exercise and Training on Bone." *Trail Blazer Magazine* (August/September 1991), pp. 16 – 17.

McIlwraith, C.W., ed. *AQHA Developmental Orthopedic Disease Symposium* (1986), Amarillo, Texas.

McMiken, D. "Muscle Fiber Types and Horse Performance." *Equine Practice*, Vol. 8, No. 3 (March 1986), pp. 6 – 14.

Melick, R.A. and D.R. Miller. "Variations of Tensile Strength in Human Cortical Bone With Age." *Clinical Science*, Vol. 30 (1966), pp. 243 – 248.

Meschter, C.L., et al. "The Effects of Phenylbutazone on the Intestinal Mucosa of the Horse: A Morphological, Ultrastructural, and Biochemical Study." *Equine Veterinary Journal*, Vol. 22, No. 4 (1990), pp. 255 – 263.

Meyers, M.C., G.D. Potter, et al. "Physiologic and Metabolic Response of Exercising Horses to Added Dietary Fat." *Equine Veterinary Science*, Vol. 9, No. 4 (1989), pp. 218 – 223.

Moore, J.N. and D.D. Morris. "Endotoxemia and Septicemia in Horses: Experimental and Clinical Correlates." *Journal of the American Veterinary Medical Association*, Vol. 200, No. 12 (June 1992), pp. 1903 – 1914.

Morris, E.A. and H.J. Seeherman. "Clinical Evaluation of Poor Performance in the Racehorse: The Results of 275 Evaluations." *Equine Veterinary Journal*, Vol. 23, No. 3 (1991), pp. 169 – 174.

Morris, E.A., et al. "Scintigraphic Identification of Skeletal Muscle Damage in Horses 24 Hours After Strenuous Exercise." *Equine Veterinary Journal*, Vol. 23, No. 5 (1991), pp. 347 – 352.

Morris, E.A. and H.J. Seeherman. "Equisport: A Comprehensive Program for Clinical Evaluation of Poor Racing Performance." *Proceedings of the American Association of Equine Practitioners* (1989), pp. 385 – 397.

Morris, E.A. and H.J. Seeherman. "Evaluation of Upper Respiratory Tract Function During Strenuous Exercise in Racehorses." *Journal of the American Veterinary Medical Association*, Vol. 196, No. 3 (February 1990), pp. 431 – 438.

Morris, E.A. and H.J. Seeherman. "The Dynamic Evaluation of Upper Respiratory Function in the Exercising Horse." *Proceedings of the American Association of Equine Practitioners* (1988), pp. 159 – 165.

Mullowney, P.C. "Dermatologic Diseases of Horses, Part IV: Environmental, Congenital, and Neoplastic Diseases." *Compendium on Continuing Education*, Vol. 7, No. 1 (January 1985), pp. 22 – 32.

Mullowney, P.C. "Dermatologic Diseases of Horses, Part V: Allergic, Immune-Mediated, and Miscellaneous Skin Diseases." *Compendium on Continuing Education*, Vol. 7, No. 4 (April 1985), pp. 217 – 228.

Munroe, G.A. "Cryosurgery in the Horse." *Equine Veterinary Journal*, Vol. 18, No. 1 (1986), pp. 14 – 17.

Murray, M.J. "Phenylbutazone Toxicity in a Horse." *Compendium on Continuing Education*, Vol. 7, No. 7 (July 1985), pp. 389 – 394.

Naylor, J.M., et al. "Familial Incidence of Hyperkalemic Periodic Paralysis in Quarter Horses." *Journal of the American Veterinary Medical Association*, Vol. 200, No. 3 (February 1992), pp. 340 – 343.

Neely, D.P., I.K.M. Liu, and R.B. Hillman. *Equine Reproduction*. Hoffman-La Roche, Inc., 1983.

Nilsson, B.E. and N.E. Westlin. "Bone Density in Athletes." *Clinical Orthopedics*, Vol. 77 (1971), pp. 179 – 182.

Ogbourne, C.P. *Pathogenesis of Cyanthostome (Trichonema) Infections in the Horse*. Commonwealth Agricultural Bureaux, Slough, (1978).

Ogbourne, C.P. and J.L. Duncan *Strongylus vulgaris in the Horse: Its Biology and Veterinary Importance*. Commonwealth Agricultural Bureaux, Slough, (1977).

Oldham, S.L., G.D. Potter, et al. "Storage and Mobilization of Muscle Glycogen in Exercising Horses Fed a Fat-Supplemented Diet." *Equine Veterinary Science*, Vol. 10, No. 5 (1990), pp. 353 – 359.

Pascoe, J.R. "Exercise-Induced Pulmonary Hemorrhage." *Equine Veterinary Science*, Vol. 9, No. 4 (1989), pp. 198 – 200.

Peyton, L.C. "Wound Healing in the Horse Part 2: Approach to the Treatment of Traumatic Wounds." *Compendium on Continuing Education*, Vol. 9, No. 2 (February 1987), pp. 191 – 200.

Peyton, L.C. "Wound Healing: The Management of Wounds and Blemishes in the Horse—Part 1." *Compendium on Continuing Education*, Vol. 6, No. 2 (February 1984), pp. 111 – 117.

Piotrowski, G., M. Sullivan, and P.T. Colahan. "Geometric Properties of Equine Metacarpi." *Journal of Biomechanics*, Vol. 16 (1983), pp. 129 – 139.

Pollit, C. "Monitoring the Heart Rate of Endurance Horses." *Trail Blazer Magazine* (May 1992), pp. 16 – 17.

Pollit, C. "Monitoring the Heart Rate of Endurance Horses, Part 2." *Trail Blazer Magazine* (July/August 1992), pp. 8 – 11.

Pollit, C. "The Role of Arteriovenous Anastomoses in the Pathophysiology of Equine Laminitis." *Proceedings of the American Association of Equine Practitioners* (1991), pp. 711 – 719.

Pool, R.R. "Adaptations of Bones, Joints, and Attachments of the Limbs of the Horse in Response to Developmental and Infectious Diseases and to Biomechanical Forces Encountered in Athletic Performance." *Proceedings from the Denver Area Veterinary Medical Association Seminar* (January 1991).

Pool, R.R. "Developmental Orthopedic Disease in the Horse: Normal and Abnormal Bone Formation." *Proceedings of the American Association of Equine Practitioners* (1988), pp. 143 – 158.

Pool, R.R. "Pathophysiology of Athletic Injuries of the Horse: Bones, Joints, and Tendons." *AESM Quarterly*, Vol. 3, No. 2 (1988), pp. 23 – 29.

Pool, R.R. "Pathogenesis of Navicular Disease." *Proceedings of the American Association of Equine Practitioners* (1991), p. 709.

Porter, Mimi. "Physical Therapy for Equine Athletes." *AESM Quarterly*, Vol. 3, No. 3 (1988), pp. 40 – 43.

Porter, Mimi. "Techniques of Treatment." *Equine Veterinary Science* (March/April 1991), pp. 191 – 194.

Porter, Mimi. "Therapeutic Electricity." *Equine Veterinary Science* (January / February 1991), pp. 59 – 64.

Porter, Mimi. "Therapeutic Electricity: Physiological Effects." *Equine Veterinary Science* (March/April 1991), pp. 133 – 140.

Porter, Mimi. "Therapeutic Ultrasound." *Equine Veterinary Science* (July/August 1991), pp. 243 – 245.

Porter, Mimi. "Therapeutic Ultrasound." *Equine Veterinary Science* (September/October 1991), pp. 294 – 299.

Poulos, P.W., and M.F. Smith. "The Nature of Enlarged 'Vascular Channels' in the Navicular Bone of the Horse." *Veterinary Radiology* (1988), Vol. 29, pp. 60 – 64.

Powell, D., et al. "Rhinopneumonitis Roundtable Discussion." *Equine Practice*, Vol. 14, No. 4 (April 1992), pp. 8 – 12. *Equine Practice*, Vol. 14, No. 5 (May 1992), pp. 30 – 36. *Equine Practice*, Vol. 14, No. 6 (June 1992), pp. 17 – 20.

Pratt, G.W. "An In Vivo Method of Ultrasonically Evaluating Bone Strength." *Proceedings of the American Association of Equine Practitioners* (1980), pp. 295 – 306.

Pratt, G.W. "The Response of Highly Stressed Bone in the Race Horse." *Proceedings of the American Association of Equine Practitioners* (1982), pp. 31 – 37.

Pugh, D.G. and J.T. Thompson. "Impaction Colics Attributed to Decreased Water Intake and Feeding Coastal Bermuda Grass Hay in a Boarding Stable." *Equine Practice*, Vol. 14, No. 1 (January 1992), pp. 9 – 14.

Rabin, D.S., N.W. Rantanen, et al. "The Clinical Use of Bone Strength Assessment in the Thoroughbred Race Horse." *Proceedings of the American Association of Equine Practitioners* (1983), pp. 343 – 351.

Ralston, S.L. and K. Larson. "The Effect of Oral Electrolyte Supplementation During a 96 Kilometer Endurance Race for Horses." *Equine Veterinary Science*, Vol. 9, No. 1, pp. 13 – 19.

Ralston, S.L. "Common Behavioral Problems of Horses." *Compendium on Continuing Education*, Vol. 4, No. 4 (April 1982), pp. 152 – 159.

Ralston, S.L. "Nutritional Management of Horses Competing in 160 Kilometer Races." *Cornell Vet*, Vol. 78, No. 1 (1988), pp. 53 – 61.

Ralston, S.L. "Patterns and Control of Food Intake in Domestic Animals." *Compendium on Continuing Education*, Vol. 6, No. 11 (1984), pp. 628 – 634.

Reef, V.B., B.B. Martin, and A. Elser. "Types of Tendon and Ligament Injuries Detected With Diagnostic Ultrasound: Description and Follow-up." *Proceedings of the American Association of Equine Practitioners* (1988), pp. 245 – 248.

Reef, V.B., B.B. Martin, and K. Stebbins. "Comparison of Ultrasonographic, Gross, and Histologic Appearance of Tendon Injuries in Performance Horses." *Proceedings of the American Association of Equine Practitioners* (1989), p. 279.

Reilly, D.T. and A.H. Burstein. "The Mechanical Properties of Cortical Bone." *Journal of Bone and Joint Surgery*, Vol. 56A (1974), pp. 1001 – 1022.

Reinemeyer, C.R. "Anthelmintic Resistance in Horses." *Equine Veterinary Science*, Vol. 7, No. 6, pp. 390 – 391.

Reinemeyer, C.R., S.A. Smith, A.A. Gabel, and R.P. Herd. "Observations on the Population Dynamics of Five Cyathostome Nematode Species of Horses in Northern USA." *Equine Veterinary Journal*, Vol. 18, No. 2 (1986), pp. 121 – 124.

Reinemeyer, C.R. and J.E. Henton. "Observations on Equine Strongyle Control in Southern Temperate USA." *Equine Veterinary Journal*, Vol. 19, No. 6 (1987), pp. 505 – 508.

Richardson, D.W. "Pathophysiology of Degenerative Joint Disease." *Equine Veterinary Science*, Vol. 11, No. 3 (1990), pp. 156 – 157.

Ridgway, K.J. "Cardiac Recovery Index: Avoiding Inappropriate Utilization." *AERC Endurance News* (October 1991), pp. 5 – 7.

Ridgway, K.J. "Respiration as an Evaluation Parameter for Distance Riding." *AERC Endurance News* (October 1990), pp. 4 – 5.

Ridgway, K.J. "Exertional Myopathies." *Proceedings of the American Association of Equine Practitioners* (1991), pp. 839 – 843.

Robb, E.J. and D.S. Kronfeld. "Dietary Sodium Bicarbonate as a Treatment for Exertional Rhabdomyolysis in a Horse." *Journal of the American Veterinary Medical Association*, Vol. 188, No. 6 (March 1986), pp. 602 – 607.

Robinson, N.E. *Current Therapy in Equine Medicine 2*, WB Saunders Company, 1987.

Robinson, N.E. and R. Wilson. "Airway Obstruction in the Horse." *Equine Veterinary Science*, Vol. 9, No. 3 (1989), pp. 155 – 160.

Robinson, N.E., et al. "Physiology of the Equine Respiratory Tract and Changes in Disease: The Role of Granulocytes." *Proceedings of the American Association of Equine Practitioners* (1984), pp. 253 – 261.

Roche, J.F., L. Keenan, and D. Forde. "Some Factors Affecting Fertility of the Mare." *Equine Practice*, Vol. 9, No. 1 (January 1987), pp. 8 – 13.

Romeiser, K. "Tying-Up: Old Problem, New Twist." *Equus* 126, pp. 60 – 64, 128 – 129.

Rooney, J. "Passive Function of the Extensor Tendons of the Fore and Rear Limbs of the Horse." *Equine Veterinary Science*, Vol. 7, No. 1 (1987), pp. 29 – 30.

Rose, R. and Hodgson, D.R. *Manual of Equine Practice*, W.B Saunders Company, New York, (1993).

Rose, R.J. and D.R. Lloyd. "Sodium Bicarbonate: More Than Just a 'Milkshake'?" *Equine Veterinary Journal*, Vol. 24, No. 2 (1992), pp. 75 – 76.

Rubin, S.I. "Non-Steroidal Anti-Inflammatory Drugs, Prostaglandins, and the Kidney." *Journal of the American Veterinary Medical Association*, Vol. 188, No. 9 (May 1986), pp. 1065 – 1068.

Rude, T.A. "Vaccines, Bacterins, Toxoids Can Cause Allergic Reactions." *DVM Magazine* (May 1989), pp. 42 – 44.

Ruff, C.B. and W.C. Hayes. "Bone Mineral Content in the Lower Limb." *Journal of Bone and Joint Surgery*, Vol. 66A (1984), pp. 1024 – 1031.

Ruggles, A.J. and M.W. Ross. "Medical and Surgical Management of Small-Colon Impaction in Horses: 28 Cases (1984 – 1989)." *Journal of the American Veterinary Medical Association*, Vol. 199, No. 12 (December 1991), pp. 1762 – 1766.

Ruth, D.T. and B.J. Swites. "Comparison of the Effectiveness of Intra-Articular Hyaluronic Acid and Conventional Therapy for the Treatment of Naturally Occurring Arthritic Conditions in Horses." *Equine Practice*, Vol. 7, No. 9 (October 1985), pp. 25 – 29.

Schott II, H.C., D.R. Hodgson, J.R. Naylor, and W.M. Bayly. "Thermoregulation and Heat Exhaustion in the Exercising Horse." *Proceedings of the American Association of Equine Practitioners* (1990), pp. 505 – 513.

Schott II, H.C. "Aspects of Heat Production, Dissipation, and Exhaustion in the Exercising Horse." *AERC Endurance News* (November 1991), pp. 5 – 6.

Scott, B.D., G.D. Potter, et al. "Growth and Feed Utilization by Yearling Horses Fed Added Dietary Fat." *Equine Veterinary Science*, Vol. 9, No. 4 (1989), pp. 210 – 214.

Scraba, S.T. and O.J. Ginther. "Effects of Lighting Programs on Onset of the Ovulatory Season in Mares." *Theriogenology*, Vol. 24 (1985), pp. 667 – 679.

Shabpareh, V., E.L. Squires, V.M. Cook, and R. Cole. "An Alternative Artificial Lighting Regime to Hasten Onset of the Breeding Season in Mares." *Equine*

Practice, Vol. 14, No. 2 (February 1992), pp. 24 – 27.

Shaw, K., et al. *Strongid® C: A Roundtable Discussion*. Pfizer, Inc., 1990.

Shively, M.J. "Equine-English Dictionary: Part 1—Standing Conformation." *Equine Practice*, Vol. 4, No. 5 (May 1982), pp. 10 – 20, 25 – 27.

Smith, C.A. "Electrolyte Imbalances and Metabolic Disturbances in Endurance Horses." *Compendium on Continuing Education*, Vol. 7, No. 10 (October 1985), pp. 575 – 584.

Smith, J.D., et al. "Exercise-Induced Pulmonary Hemorrhage Findings, A Workshop." *Equine Practice*, Vol. 14, No. 1 (January 1992), pp. 19 – 25. *Equine Practice*, Vol. 14, No. 2 (February 1992), pp. 9 – 15. *Equine Practice*, Vol. 14, No. 3 (March 1992), pp. 28 – 32.

Smith, M.J. "Electrical Stimulation for Relief of Musculoskeletal Pain." *The Physician and Sportsmedicine*, Vol. 11, No. 5 (May 1983), pp. 47 – 55.

Snow, D.H. "Sweating and Anhidrosis." *Equine Sportmedicine*, Vol. 5, No. 2 (1986), pp. 4 – 5, 8.

Snow, V.E. and D.P. Birdsall. "Specific Parameters Used to Evaluate Hoof Balance and Support." *Proceedings of the American Association of Equine Practitioners* (1990), pp. 299 – 312.

Specht, T.E. and P.T. Colahan. "Surgical Treatment of Sand Colic in Equids: 48 Cases (1978 – 1985)." *Journal of the American Veterinary Medical Association*, Vol. 193, No. 12 (December 1988), pp. 1560 – 1563.

Spier, S.J. "Current Facts About Hyperkalemic Periodic Paralysis (HYPP) Disease." *The Quarter Racing Journal* (April 1993), pp. 44 – 47.

Spier, S.J. "Use of Hyperimmune Plasma Containing Antibody to Gram-negative Core Antigens." *Proceedings of the American Association of Equine Practitioners* (1989), pp. 91 – 94.

Spier, S.J. and G.P. Carlson. "Hyperkalemic Periodic Paralysis in Certain Registered Quarter Horses." *The Quarter Horse Journal* (September 1992), pp. 68 – 69, 120.

Spier, S.J., G.P. Carlson, et al. "Genetic Study of Hyperkalemic Periodic Paralysis in Horses." *Journal of the American Veterinary Medical Association*, Vol. 202, No. 6 (March 1993), pp. 933 – 937.

Spier, S.J., G.P. Carlson, et al. "Hyperkalemic Periodic Paralysis in Horses." *Journal of the American Veterinary Medical Association*, Vol. 197, No. 8 (October 1990), pp. 1009 – 1016.

Stabenfeldt, G.H. and J.P. Hughes. "Clinical Aspects of Reproductive Endocrinology in the Horse." *Compendium on Continuing Education*, Vol. 9, No. 6 (June 1987), pp. 678 – 684.

Stashak, Ted S. *Adams' Lameness in Horses*. Fourth Edition. Lea and Febiger, Philadelphia, 1987.

Stull, C. "Muscles for Motion." *Equine Practice*, Vol. 8, No. 4 (April 1986), pp. 17 – 20.

Subcommittee on Horse Nutrition, Committee on Animal Nutrition, Board of Agriculture, National Research Council, *Nutrient Requirements of Horses*. Fifth Revised Edition. National Academy Press, Washington DC, 1989.

Sullins, K.E., S.M. Roberts, J.D. Lavach, G.A. Severin, and D. Lueker. "Equine Sarcoid." *Equine Practice*, Vol. 8, No. 4 (April 1986), pp. 21 – 27.

Swaim, S.F. and A.H. Lee. "Topical Wound Medications: A Review." *Journal of the American Veterinary Medical Association*, Vol. 190, No. 12 (June 1987), pp. 1588 – 1592.

Swaim, S.F. and D. Wilhalf. "The Physics, Physiology, and Chemistry of Bandaging Open Wounds." *Compendium on Continuing Education*, Vol. 7,

No. 2 (February 1985), pp. 146 – 155.

Swann, P. *Racehorse Training and Feeding.* Racehorse Sportsmedicine and Scientific Conditioning, Australia, 1985.

Swann, P. *Racehorse Training and Sports Medicine.* Racehorse Sportsmedicine and Scientific Conditioning, Australia, 1988.

Sweeney, C.R., C.E. Benson, et al. "Description of an Epizootic and Persistence of *Streptococcus equi* Infections in Horses." *Journal of the American Veterinary Medical Association,* Vol. 194, No. 9 (1989), pp. 1281 – 1285.

Sweeney, C.R., C.E. Benson, et al. "*Streptococcus equi* Infection in Horses — Part 1." *Compendium on Continuing Education,* Vol. 9, No. 6 (June 1987), pp. 689 – 693.

Sweeney, C.R., C.E. Benson, et al. "*Streptococcus equi* Infection in Horses — Part 2." *Compendium on Continuing Education,* Vol. 9, No. 8 (August 1987), pp. 845 – 851.

Sweeney, C.R., et al. "Equine Roundtable Discussion: Respiration." *Equine Practice* (May 1989), pp. 16 – 24. *Equine Practice* (June 1989), pp. 10 – 16. *Equine Practice* (July/August 1989), pp. 29 – 40.

Swenson, M.J., ed. *Dukes' Physiology of Domestic Animals.* Ninth Edition. Cornell University Press, 1977.

Tarwid, J.N., P.B. Fretz, and E.G. Clark. "Equine Sarcoids: A Study With Emphasis on Pathologic Diagnosis." *Compendium on Continuing Education,* Vol. 7, No. 5 (May 1985), pp. 293 – 300.

Templeton, J.W., R. Smith III, and L.G. Adams. "Natural Disease Resistance in Domestic Animals." *Journal of the American Veterinary Medical Association,* Vol. 192, No. 9 (May 1988), pp. 1306 – 1315.

Texas Veterinary Medical Association Annual Meeting. "Hyaluronic Acid Use in the Horse: A Roundtable Discussion." Schering Animal Health, February 1988.

Thomas, H.S. "Using A Twitch." *American Farriers Journal* (July/August 1989), pp. 28 – 30.

Thompson, K.N., J.P. Baker, and S.G. Jackson. "The Influence of High Dietary Intakes of Energy and Protein on Third Metacarpal Characteristics of Weanling Ponies." *Equine Veterinary Science,* Vol. 8, No. 5 (1988), pp. 391 – 394.

Thomson, J.R. and E.A. McPherson. "Chronic Obstructive Pulmonary Disease in the Horse." *Equine Practice,* Vol. 10, No. 7 (July/August 1988), pp. 31 – 36.

Todhunter, R.J. and G. Lust. "Pathophysiology of Synovitis: Clinical Signs and Examination in Horses." *Compendium on Continuing Education,* Vol. 12, No. 7 (July 1990), pp. 980 – 991.

Traub-Dargatz, J.L., J.J. Bertone, et al. "Chronic Flunixin Meglumine Therapy in Foals." *American Journal of Veterinary Research,* Vol. 49, No. 1 (January 1988), pp. 7 – 12.

Traub-Dargatz, J.L. "Non-Steroidal Anti-Inflammatory Drug-induced Ulcers." *Proceedings of the American Association of Equine Practitioners* (1988), pp. 129 – 132.

Turner, A.S. "Local and Systemic Factors Affecting Wound Healing." *Proceedings of the American Association of Equine Practitioners* (1978), pp. 355 – 362.

Turner, A.S. and Tucker, C.M. "The Evaluation of Isoxsuprine Hydrochloride for the Treatment of Navicular Disease: A Double Blind Study." *Equine Veterinary Journal,* Vol. 21, No. 5 (1989), pp. 338 – 341.

Turner, T.A. "Hindlimb Muscle Strain as a Cause of Lameness in Horses." *Proceedings of the American Association of Equine Practitioners* (1989), pp. 281 – 290.

Turner, T.A. "Navicular Disease Management: Shoeing Principles." *Proceedings of the American Association of Equine Practitioners* (1986), pp. 625 – 633.

Turner, T.A. "Shoeing Principles for the Management of Navicular Disease in the Horse." *Journal of the American Veterinary Medical Association,* Vol. 189 (1986), pp. 298 – 301.

Turner, T.A., S.K. Kneller, R.R. Badertscher II, and J.L. Stowater. "Radiographic Changes in the Navicular Bones of Normal Horses." *Proceedings of the American Association of Equine Practitioners* (1986), pp. 309 – 314.

Turner, T.A., R.C. Purohit, and J.F. Fessler. "Thermography: A Review in Equine Medicine." *Compendium on Continuing Education,* Vol. 8, No. 11 (1986), pp. 855 – 861.

Turner, T.A., K. Wolfsdorf, and J. Jourdenais. "Effects of Heat, Cold, Biomagnets, and Ultrasound on Skin Circulation in the Horse." *Proceedings of the American Association of Equine Practitioners* (1991), pp. 249 – 257.

Turrel, J.M., S.M. Stover, and J. Gyorgyfalvy. "Iridium-192 Interstitial Brachytherapy of Equine Sarcoid." *Veterinary Radiology,* Vol. 26, No. 1 (1985), pp. 20 – 24.

Uhlinger, C.A. and M. Kristula. "Effects of Alternation of Drug Classes on the Development of Oxibendazole Resistance in a Herd of Horses." *Journal of the American Veterinary Medical Association,* Vol. 201, No. 1 (July 1992), pp. 51 – 55.

Uhlinger, C.A. "Equine Small Strongyles: Epidemiology, Pathology, and Control." *Compendium on Continuing Education,* Vol. 13, No. 5 (May 1991), pp. 863 – 868.

Valberg, S. "Metabolic Response to Racing and Fiber Properties of Skeletal Muscle in Standardbred and Thoroughbred Horses." *Equine Veterinary Science,* Vol. 7, No. 1 (1987), pp. 6 – 12.

Valberg, S. "Tying-Up Syndrome in Horses." *Hoof Print* (September/October 1991), pp. 35 – 36.

Van Den Hoven, R. "Mind Over Muscle." *Equine Veterinary Journal,* Vol. 23, No. 2 (1991), pp. 73 – 74.

Vanselow, B.A., I. Abetz, and A.R.B. Jackson. "BCG Emulsion Immunotherapy of Equine Sarcoid." *Equine Veterinary Journal,* Vol. 20, No. 6 (1988), pp. 444 – 447.

Veterinary Clinics of North America, Equine Practice, *Exercise Physiology,* December 1985, Vol. 1, No. 3.

Veterinary Clinics of North America, Equine Practice, *Parasitology,* August 1986, Vol. 2, No. 2.

Veterinary Clinics of North America, Equine Practice, *Behavior,* December 1986, Vol. 2, No. 3.

Veterinary Clinics of North America, Equine Practice, *Clinical Pharmacology,* April 1987, Vol. 3, No. 1.

Veterinary Clinics of North America, Equine Practice, *Management of Colic,* April 1988, Vol. 4, No. 1.

Veterinary Clinics of North America, Equine Practice, *Reproduction,* August 1988, Vol. 4, No. 2.

Veterinary Clinics of North America, Equine Practice, *The Equine Foot,* April 1989, pp. 109 – 128.

Veterinary Clinics of North America, Equine Practice, *Wound Management,* December 1989, Vol. 5, No. 3.

Veterinary Clinics of North America, Equine Practice, *Racetrack Practice,* April 1990, Vol. 6, No. 1.

Veterinary Clinics of North America, Equine Practice, *Clinical Nutrition,* August 1990, Vol. 6, No. 2, pp. 281 – 293, 355 – 371, 393 – 418.

Veterinary Clinics of North America, Equine Practice, *Respiratory Diseases,* April 1991, Vol. 7, No. 1.

Veterinary Clinics of North America, Equine Practice, *Advanced Diagnostic Methods,* August 1991, Vol. 7, No. 2.

Veterinary Clinics of North America, Equine Practice, *Stallion Management,* April 1992, Vol. 8, No. 1.

Veterinary Clinics of North America, Equine Practice, *Examination for Purchase,* August 1992, Vol. 8, No. 2.

Veterinary Clinics of North America, Equine Practice, *Tendon and Ligament Injuries,* August 1994, Vol. 10, No. 2.

Veterinary Clinics of North America, Equine Practice, *Emergency Treatment in Adult Horses,* December 1994, Vol. 10, No. 30.

Voges, F., E. Kienzle, and H. Meyer. "Investigations on the Composition of Horse Bones." *Equine Veterinary Science,* Vol. 10, No. 3 (1990), pp. 208 – 213.

Wagoner, D.M., ed. *Feeding To Win II.* Equine Research Publications, 1992.

Wagoner, D.M., ed. *The Illustrated Veterinary Encyclopedia for Horsemen.* Equine Research Publications, 1977.

Wagoner, D.M., ed. *Veterinary Treatments and Medications for Horsemen.* Equine Research Publications, 1977.

Wagoner, D.M., ed. *Breeding Management and Foal Development.* Equine Research Publications, 1982.

Waldsmith, Jim. The Equine Center. San Luis Obispo, California, personal communication.

Wanless, M. *The Natural Rider.* Summit Books, New York, New York, 1987.

Webb, S.P., G.D. Potter, et al. "Physiological Responses of Cutting Horses to Exercise Testing and to Training." *Equine Veterinary Science,* Vol. 8, No. 3 (1988), pp. 261 – 265.

Webbon, P.M. "Preliminary Study of Tendon Biopsy in the Horse." *Equine Veterinary Journal,* Vol. 18, No. 5, pp. 383 – 387.

White, G.W. "Adequan: A Review for the Practicing Veterinarian." *Equine Veterinary Science,* Vol. 8, No. 6 (1988), pp. 463 – 467.

White, N.A. "Thromboembolic Colic in Horses." *Compendium on Continuing Education,* Vol. 7, No. 3 (March 1985), pp. 156 – 162.

Wilson, G.L. and M. Mueller. *The Equine Athlete.* Veterinary Learning Systems Co., Inc., New Jersey, 1982.

Wilson, W.D. "*Streptococcus equi* Infections (Strangles) in Horses." *Equine Practice,* Vol. 10, No. 7 (July/August 1988), pp. 12 – 25.

Wood, C.H., T.T. Ross, et al. "Variations in Muscle Fiber Composition Between Successfully and Unsuccessfully Raced Quarter Horses." *Equine Veterinary Science,* Vol. 8, No. 3 (1988), pp. 217 – 220.

Woolen, N., R.M. DeBowes, H.W. Leipold, and L.A. Schneider. "A Comparison of Four Types of Therapy for the Treatment of Full-Thickness Skin Wounds of the Horse." *Proceedings of the American Association of Equine Practitioners* (1988), pp. 569 – 576.

Wynn-Jones, G. *Equine Lameness,* Blackwell Science, Oxford, 1982.

Yelle, M.T. "Clinical Aspects of *Streptococcus equi* Infection." *Equine Veteri-nary Journal*, Vol. 19, No. 2 (1987), pp. 158 – 162.

Yovich, J.V., G.W. Trotter, C.W. McIlwraith, and R.W. Norrdin. "Effects of Polysulfated Glycosaminoglycan on Chemical and Physical Defects in Equine Articular Cartilage." *American Journal of Veterinary Research*, Vol. 48, No. 9 (September 1987), pp. 1407 – 1413.

Figure Credits

Figure 1.1. Don Shugart.
Figure 1.6. Don Shugart.
Figure 1.7. Cappy Jackson.
Figure 1.13. Courtesy of *The Quarter Horse Journal.*
Figure 1.17. Courtesy of *The Blood-Horse.*
Figure 1.20. Equine Sports Graphics, Inc.
Figure 1.27. Courtesy of the International Arabian Horse Association.
Figure 1.29. Courtesy of the United States Trotting Association.
Figure 1.34. Courtesy of Don Stevenson.
Figure 2.1. J. Noye.
Figure 2.4. Courtesy of *The Blood-Horse.*
Figure 2.6. J. Noye.
Figure 3.4. Courtesy of the United States Trotting Association.
Figure 3.8. Courtesy of *The Blood-Horse.*
Figure 3.10. Cappy Jackson.
Figure 3.12. Cappy Jackson.
Figure 3.13. Cappy Jackson.
Figure 3.16. Courtesy of *The Blood-Horse.*
Figure 4.9. Courtesy of *The Blood-Horse.*
Figure 5.1. J. Noye.
Figure 5.6. Cappy Jackson.
Figure 6.1. Courtesy of the United States Trotting Association. Photo by George
    Smallsreed, Jr.
Figure 6.9. Courtesy of *The Blood-Horse.*
Figure 6.19. Courtesy of Dr Jim Schumacher, Texas A&M University.
Figure 6.20. Cappy Jackson.
Figure 6.21. Courtesy of Nancy Zidonis, Equine Acupressure, Inc.
Figure 6.30. J. Noye.
Figure 7.1. Courtesy of *The Blood-Horse.*
Figure 7.8. Courtesy of *The Horsemen's Journal.* Photo by Bill Witkop.
Figure 8.1. Courtesy of *The Blood-Horse.*
Figure 8.8. Cappy Jackson.
Figure 10.1. J. Noye.
Figure 10.5. Dudley Barker.
Figure 10.14. Courtesy of Mimi Porter, Equine Therapy.
Figure 10.15. Courtesy of Dr Dave Schmitz, Texas A&M University.
Figure 10.16. Courtesy of Dr Dave Schmitz, Texas A&M University.
Figure 11.1. Courtesy of Dr Ducharme, Cornell University.
Figure 11.4. Courtesy of Mimi Porter, Equine Therapy.
Figure 11.5. Courtesy of Mimi Porter, Equine Therapy.
Figure 11.6. Courtesy of Mimi Porter, Equine Therapy.
Figure 11.7. Courtesy of Mimi Porter, Equine Therapy.
Figure 11.8. Courtesy of Mimi Porter, Equine Therapy.
Figure 11.9. Courtesy of Mimi Porter, Equine Therapy.
Figure 11.10. Courtesy of Mimi Porter, Equine Therapy.
Figure 11.11. Courtesy of Mimi Porter, Equine Therapy.
Figure 11.13. Courtesy of Mimi Porter, Equine Therapy.
Figure 12.11. Courtesy of Nancy Zidonis, Equine Acupressure, Inc.
Figure 13.3. J. Noye
Figure 13.5. Courtesy of David Varra, DVM, MS
Figure 13.14. Courtesy of David Varra, DVM, MS
Figure 14.5. Courtesy of David Varra, DVM, MS

Figure 14.7. Courtesy of David Varra, DVM, MS
Figure 14.14. J. Noye.
Figure 15.30. Courtesy of David Varra, DVM, MS
Figure 16.11. Courtesy of David Varra, DVM, MS
Figure 17.10. Cappy Jackson.
Figure 19.1. Equine Sports Graphics, Inc.
Figure 19.3. Courtesy of the American Quarter Horse Association.
Figure 20.3. Barbara Ann Giove.
Figure 21.1. Courtesy of the American Quarter Horse Association.
Figure 22.1. Courtesy of Al Dunning Training Stables, Inc. Photo by Patty McClure-Hosmer.
Figure 22.2. J. Noye.
Figure 22.3. Courtesy of *The Blood-Horse.*
Figure 22.4. Courtesy of *The Blood-Horse.* Photo by Anne Eberhardt.
Figure 23.1. J. Noye.
Figure 23.9. Equine Sports Graphics, Inc.
Figure 23.12. Cappy Jackson.

Appendix
Count Fleet Courtesy of *The Blood-Horse.*

Glossary

abdomen, the cavity that lies between the diaphragm and the pelvis; contains the digestive organs, the liver, pancreas, kidneys and spleen

abdominocentesis, withdrawal of fluid through a needle inserted into the abdominal cavity

abort, to expel a foetus before it is able to live outside the uterus

abrasion, a wound caused by the wearing away of the top layer of skin and hair by friction

abscess, a localized collection of pus in a cavity formed by the disintegration of tissues

acetylcholine, a chemical neuro-transmitter, which enables a neuron to fire

acrosome, the 'cap' of the sperm cell which contains the enzymes necessary to penetrate the egg

actin filament, one of two types of filaments that make up a muscle fibre

acupressure, a form of acupuncture which seeks to stimulate specific nerve tracts and meridians without penetrating the skin

acupuncture, an ancient Oriental art which seeks to stimulate specific nerve tracts and meridians by needle penetration

acute, having short and relatively sudden course; not chronic

adenoma, a benign epithelial tumour in which the cells are derived from glandular epithelium or form glandular structures

adenosine diphosphate (ADP), product of the decomposition of the energy reserve of the muscles

adenosine triphosphate (ATP), represents the energy reserve of the muscles

adhesion, abnormal, firm, fibrous attachment between two structures, often formed as a result of inflammation

adjuvant, the liquid carrier which improves the efficiency of the vaccine

adrenaline, a powerful vasopressor that increases blood pressure and stimulates the heart muscle; also called epinephrine

aerobe, a microorganism that can live and grow in the presence of oxygen

aerobic, growing or taking place in the presence of oxygen

aerobic capacity, the ability to exercise without using anaerobic metabolism; increases with aerobic conditioning

agglutinate, clumping or massing together of cells or bacteria

agonist, a muscle opposed by another muscle, the antagonist

alcopecia, a loss of hair

alkalosis, increased alkalinity of blood and tissues; increased blood bicarbonate

allergen, a substance capable of causing allergy or hypersensitivity

allergy, a hypersensitive state acquired through exposure to a particular allergen; reexposure results in an altered capacity to react to the substance

alveolar macrophage, an immune cell which binds, internalizes, and inactivates microorganisms in the lungs

alveoli, a small cavity or pit, as in the air saccules of the lungs

amino acids, a class of organic compounds containing nitrogen; they form the building blocks of proteins

anabolic steroid, a chemical substance derived from testosterone; encourages protein-building

anaemia, a condition in which the number or volume of red blood cells, haemoglobin, and packed red blood cells is below normal

anaerobe, a microorganism that can only live and grow in the complete or almost complete absence of oxygen

anaerobic, growing or taking place in an environment lacking in oxygen

anaerobic threshold, the point at which lactic acid begins to accumulate in the muscles and bloodstream

anaesthetic, a drug or agent that is used to abolish the sensation of pain

anaesthetize, to abolish the sensation of pain with or without a loss of consciousness

analgesia, pain relief

anamnestic response, a state where the immune system 'remembers' a foreign protein and responds quickly to further insult

anaphylactic shock, anaphylaxis, an unusually severe, life-threatening allergic reaction to a foreign protein or drug

angioedema, a profound hypersensitivity reaction characterized by sudden swelling of the respiratory tract

angle of the bar, the bottom of the foot where the hoof wall meets the sole; also called angle of the sole

angle of the wall, the bottom of the foot where the hoof wall meets the heel

angular limb deformity, abnormality in the growth plate of the limb; examples include toed-out, pigeon-toed, knock-knee, and bowlegged conformational faults

anhydrosis, an abnormal deficiency of sweat

anoestrus, a period of sexual quiescence during which there is an absence of observable oestrus

antagonist, a muscle that counteracts another muscle, the agonist

anterior uveitis, inflammation of structures in the eye; characterized by pain, conjunctivitis, eye spasms and tearing

antibacterial, able to kill or inhibit the growth of bacteria

antibiotic, a chemical produced by a microorganism that can destroy or inhibit the growth of other microorganisms

antibody, a complex protein molecule which combines with molecules of antigen; antibodies participate in the immune response which protects against disease

antigen, a substance which the immune system recognizes as foreign and causes formation of antibodies

antigenic drift, a minor change in the structure or makeup of a virus; this process is called mutation

anti-inflammatory, an agent which counteracts or suppresses fever and the inflammatory response

antimicrobial, able to inhibit the growth and development of microorganisms

antiseptic, an agent which prevents the decomposition of tissue by inhibiting the growth and development of microorganisms

antitoxin, an antibody to the toxin of a microorganism that combines with the toxin, neutralizing it

anus, the exterior opening of the rectum

arrhythmia, any variation from the normal heartbeat

arteritis, inflammation of an artery

artery, vessel through which oxygen-enriched blood passes away from the heart towards the various parts of the body

arthritis, inflammation of a joint

arthrodesis, surgical fusion of a joint

articular, pertaining to a joint

arytenoid cartilages, paired cartilages in the larynx, collapse of one or both is involved in roaring

arytenoid chondrosis, abnormal calcification and abscesses of the cartilage in the larynx; leads to exercise intolerance and respiratory noise

ascarid, intestinal roundworm, a parasite particularly of young horses

asphyxiation, suffocation

aspiration pneumonia, an infection caused by inhaling contaminated food or other substance into the lungs

astringent, a drying agent that causes contraction and shrinking of tissues, and stops the flow of discharge from a wound

asymptomatic, without symptoms

ataxia, the inability to coordinate voluntary muscle movements

atlanto-axial joint, see no joint

atlanto-occipital joint, see yes joint

atlas vertebra, the first cervical vertebra after the skull

atrophy, decrease in size or wasting away of a body part or tissue

axial compression, a force directly down the limb which squeezes the bones and joints together

axial tension, forces which pull apart

axis vertebra, the second vertebra after the skull

bactericide, an agent that destroys bacteria

bacterium, any microorganism in the class *Schizomycetes;* (plural: bacteria)

bar shoe, a therapeutic shoe in which the heels are joined by a bar, creating a larger base of support for the foot

bars, structures on the bottom of the foot formed by the hoof wall as it turns forwards and inwards at the heels; they run on each side of the frog and converge on each other

bascule, the rounding of the neck and back as a horse jumps an obstacle

base-narrow, a conformational fault where the distance between the centre lines of the limbs at their origin is greater than the centre lines of the feet on the ground

bastard strangles, the strangles bacteria spread to the lymph nodes of the intestinal tract, abdominal organs, or brain

bench knee, a conformational fault where the cannon bone is offset to the outside of the knee

bevelled shoe, see slippered shoe

bicarbonate, basic component of some salts; sharp increase may cause elevation of blood pH

biomechanical stress, all the forces applied to a bone during weight-bearing

biopsy, the process of removing tissue from living patients for diagnostic examination; a sample obtained by biopsy

blackflies, ear midges which feed on blood in the ear pinnae; genus *Simulium*

bleeders, horses that bleed from the nose during a race due to exercise-induced pulmonary haemorrhage (EIPH)

bog spavin, excess joint fluid in the hock

bolus, a rounded mass of food or medicine which is given orally

bone marrow, the soft material filling the cavities of the bones; produces red and white blood cells

bone mineral content, the amount of minerals in a bone; a parameter of bone strength

bone spavin, a lameness originating in the hock which is characterized by either exostosis or cartilage destruction, particularly occurring on the inner surface of the hock

bots, the larvae of bot flies, which are parasitic in the stomach; *Gastrophilus* sp.

bowed tendon, damage to a tendon that results in inflammation and scarring

bowlegged, a conformational fault where the knees deviate away from each other; also called carpus varus

bradykinin, a strong vasodilator that increases the permeability of capillaries and constricts smooth muscle

breakover, the act of rolling the hoof forwards, lifting the foot from the ground heel first, as the horse moves forwards

broad spectrum, a wide range of activity, as in the variety of bacteria affected by a broad spectrum antibiotic

bronchioles, the successively smaller airways in the lungs into which the bronchi divide

bronchitis, inflammation of one or more bronchi, often marked by fever, coughing, and difficulty breathing

bronchoconstriction, reduced diameter of a bronchiole

bronchopneumonia, inflammation of the lungs that begins in the bronchioles, which become clogged with mucopurulent exudate

bronchi, any of the larger airways, including the two main branches of the trachea, one going to each lung, also including the large airways inside the lungs

bucked knees, see over at the knee

bucked shins, microfractures on the front and inside surfaces of the cannon bone, usually occurring on the forelegs of young horses that are strenuously exercised

bursa, a sac or sac-like cavity filled with fluid and situated beneath tendons where friction would otherwise develop

bursitis, inflammation of the bursa

caecum, the intestinal pouch between the large and small intestines; important for cellulose digestion

calf knee, a conformational fault where the knee is set too far back

camped out, a conformational fault where the hind legs are too far out behind

canker, chronic hypertrophy of the horn-producing tissues of the foot, beginning at the frog and extending to the sole and wall; characterized by foul-smelling, caseous, white discharge

capillaries, minute vessels that connect to the arterioles and venules, forming a network in nearly all parts of the body; their walls act as semipermeable membranes for the exchange of various substances between the blood and tissue fluid

capillary refill time, the time required for normal blood flow and colour to return to an area of the gum pressed by a fingertip

capped hock, inflammation of the bursa over the point of the hock caused by trauma

carbohydrates, organic compounds containing carbon, hydrogen, and oxygen; the chief source of energy; including starches, sugars and cellulose

carcinoma, a malignant new growth made of epithelium cells; a form of cancer

cardiac, pertaining to the heart

cardiac recovery index (CRI), a method of checking the heart rate recovery; the horse is trotted out 250 feet and the heart rate is counted after 1 minute from the start of the trot to determine if it has returned to the resting heart rate

cardiovascular system, the system formed by the heart, arteries, and veins; the circulatory system

carotid artery, the main artery of the neck, conducting blood to the brain

carpal, pertaining to the 'knee' of the front leg

carpitis, inflammation of the synovial membranes of the bones of the knees, causing swelling, pain and lameness

carpus, the 'knee' of the front leg

carpus valgus, see knock-knee

carpus varus, see bowlegged

carrier, an animal that carries a recessive gene or the organisms of a disease without showing signs of the condition; the animal may transmit the gene to its offspring or the organism to another animal; see also adjuvant

cartilage, a specialized type of connective tissue found in the joints, ears, nose, throat, and ribs; may be a precursor to bone

caseous, resembling cheese or curd; cheesy

Caslick's surgery, a process of stitching a section of the labia together to prevent air and contaminants from entering the reproductive tract; also called episioplasty

catalytic enzymes, enzymes that trigger reactions within the body

cataract, a condition where the lens of the eye becomes opaque

catheter, a flexible tubular instrument for withdrawing fluids from or introducing fluids into the body, e.g. urinary catheter, indwelling intravenous catheter, etc.

caustic, burning, corrosive, and destructive to living tissue

cell, the structural unit that is the living basis of all plant and animal life

cellular fluid, body fluid, composed mostly of water, which is both inside and outside of cells, and is constantly moving into and out of cells

cellulitis, inflammation and swelling of the subcutaneous tissue and muscle due to infection or trauma

cellulose, a carbohydrate that appears only in plants and is digested in the large intestine of horses by intestinal microorganisms; also called fibre

central core lesion, a common tendon injury which is associated with severe fibre disruption and haemorrhage, appearing as a black dot on an ultrasound image

central nervous system, the brain, spinal cord, cranial nerves, and spinal nerves; carries messages to and from the brain

cervical, pertaining to the neck, or to the neck of any organ or structure, such as the cervix of the uterus

cervical spine, the skeleton of the neck, made of seven vertebrae

cervicitis, inflammation of the cervix

cervix, the muscular, neck-like structure which separates the vagina from the uterus

check apparatus, the network of muscles, tendons, and ligaments, which allows the horse to stand with little or no muscle effort, and to sleep standing up

chemotherapy, the treatment of disease by chemical agents

choke, a partial or complete oesophageal obstruction created by swallowing too large a bolus of food or a foreign body

chorioptic mange, a skin disease caused by mite infection of the legs, frequently resulting in secondary infection and grease

chronic, a condition which persists for a long time with little change or progression; opposite of acute

chronic obstructive pulmonary disease (COPD), see heaves

cilia, minute finger-like projections whose whipping actions help maintain fluid transport over certain membranes

circulating antibodies, immune cells circulating in the blood and lymph

circumflex artery, the artery that runs around the bottom of the coffin bone

clinical diagnosis, diagnosis based on signs exhibited by the horse coupled with a physical exam

clot, a semi-solidified mass of blood

club foot, a foot configuration that may result in a high, upright heel and short toe; usually the result of a contracted tendon or nutritional deficiency in a foal

coagulate, to cause to clot, forming an insoluble fibrin clot

coffin bone, pedal bone surrounded by the hoof; also called P3, third phalanx

Coggins test, a test used to detect equine infectious anaemia antibodies in a blood sample

colic, acute abdominal pain due to a gastrointestinal disturbance

collagen, the predominant protein of the fibres of connective tissue, bone, and cartilage

collateral cartilages, the two cartilages on either side of the coffin bone

colon, the part of the large intestine extending from the caecum to the rectum; its length is about 10 – 12 feet

colony forming units (cfu), a bacterial colony created by rapid multiplication of a bacterium inoculated onto a nutrient medium

colostrum, the first milk after birth; important to the newborn foal's immune response

combined immunodeficiency disease (CID), a fatal disease; caused by a lack of an immune response in foals

common digital extensor tendon, a tendon located in front of the cannon bone

concentrate, high-energy feed, such as grains and pellets

concentric contraction, a muscle contraction where the muscle thickens as it shortens

conception, the combination of the genetic material of the sperm and ovum

concussion, a violent jar or shock

congenital, existing at, and usually before, birth

conjunctivitis, inflammation of the delicate membrane that lines the eyelid

connective tissue, fibrous tissue that binds and supports various body structures

contagious, able to be spread from one animal to another

contagious equine metritis (CEM), a highly contagious disease which causes inflammation of uterine, cervical, and vaginal membranes; caused by *Taylorella equigenitalis*

contracted heels, a condition in which the foot is contracted and narrowed, caused by a lack of frog pressure and moisture

contracted tendon, a condition where movement of the affected limb is limited and the limb is not fully extended at rest; the horse stands on its toe or buckles at the fetlock

contraction, the reduction in size of a wound; also muscle movement

contrast radiography, injecting a radio-opaque dye into a part and taking an X-ray

contusion, an injury incurred without breaking the skin

convection, natural air circulation due to hot air rising and exiting out the top and cool air entering from the bottom

COPD, chronic obstructive pulmonary disease, see heaves

coprophagy, manure ingestion

corium, modified vascular tissue inside the horn of the hoof which produces the horn: perioplic corium, coronary corium, laminar corium, sole corium and frog corium

corneal ulcers, a defect in the epithelium of the cornea

coronary, encircling like a crown, as applied to blood vessels, ligaments, or nerves; the coronary band encircles the hoof

coronary band, where the hoof horn meets the skin of the leg

coronary corium, a dense bed of connective tissue with an elaborate blood and nerve supply underneath the coronary band; responsible for new hoof horn growth

corpus luteum, the mass of endocrine cells formed in the ovary at the site of a ruptured ovarian follicle

corrective shoeing, the practice of trimming and shoeing so as to correct a defect in the way of travelling or to reduce pain

cortex, cortical walls, the outer layers of bones

corticosteroids, hormones of the adrenal cortex or any other natural or synthetic compounds having a similar activity; they have a systemic and metabolic effect; inhibit the inflammatory process

cortisol, a natural steroid hormone secreted by the body in times of stress which suppresses the immune system

coupling, how the hindquarter muscles connect to the back at the lumbosacral joint

cowhocks, a conformational fault where the hocks are pointed inwards when viewed from behind; the hocks are set closer in than the fetlocks

cracked heels, dermatitis found (usually) on the back of the pastern which may have numerous causes; also called grease heel, mud fever, scratches *Dermatophilus* bacteria often involved

cranial mesenteric artery, provides the main blood supply to the intestinal tract

crepitation, a sound like that of rubbing the hair between the fingers; caused by crackling from gas bubbles trapped under bruised or infected skin

cribbing, a vice of some horses in which it grasps the manger or other object with the incisor teeth, arches the neck, makes peculiar movements with the head, and sometimes swallows quantities of air

cross-protective antibodies, antibodies which will respond to variations of a virus strain, rather than only one strain

crude protein, percentage of protein contained in a feed

cryosurgery, the destruction of tissue by applying extreme cold; used to treat sarcoids

cryptorchidism, a condition in which one or both testicles are retained in the body cavity

Culicoides hypersensitivity, an allergic reaction to the bite of the *Culicoides* midge; characterized by intense itching

culture, a growth of microorganisms or living tissue cells

curb, strain of the plantar ligament on the back of the hock, causes inflammation and lameness

cutaneous habronemiasis, see summer sores

cutting, separating out cattle

cyst, any closed cavity or sac, lined by epithelium, particularly one that contains a liquid or semi-solid substance or parasite

cytology, examination of cells

debride, to remove dead and dying tissue with scissors or a scalpel

deep digital flexor tendon, one of two tendons located at the back of the cannon bone

degenerative joint disease (DJD), arthritis

degenerative myocardial disease, progressive disease of the heart muscle

dehydration, condition resulting from excessive loss of body water

demineralize, to eliminate mineral or inorganic salts from tissues, especially bone

demodectic mange, a skin disease caused by demodectic mites living in hair follicles and sebaceous glands, causing tissue damage through the production of toxins

dens, part of the axis vertebra that hooks under the atlas vertebra

denude, to make bare by removing the epithelial covering

deoxyribonucleic acid (DNA), the genetic code present in every cell of the body

dermatitis, inflammation of the skin

desmitis, inflammation of a ligament

desmotomy, the cutting or division of ligaments

developmental orthopaedic diseases (DOD), diseases of the bone in growing horses, including epiphysitis, osteochondrosis, osteochondritis dissecans

dew poisoning, see rain scald

dewormer, any of the many commercial products containing medications which destroy internal parasites; administered by stomach tube, oral syringe or through feed

diagnosis, distinguishing one disease from another, or identifying a disease from its characteristics and/or causative agent

diagnostic ultrasound, see ultrasound

diaphragm, the muscle membrane separating the abdominal and chest cavities, lying behind and beneath the lungs

diarrhoea, abnormal frequency and liquidity of faecal discharges

differentiation, process by which general cells develop into specialized structures during embryonic development

digestible energy, the portion of the gross energy in a feedstuff that the animal is able to digest and absorb

digestive tract, see gastrointestinal tract

digital cushion, a fibroelastic fatty pad forming the heel bulbs

dihydrostreptomycin, an antibiotic for infections in cattle

dilation, stretching or expanding

dimethyl sulphoxide (DMSO), an effective anti-inflammatory agent

disinfectant, chemical or physical agent used to kill bacteria on inanimate objects; too toxic for use on animals

dislocation, the displacement of any part, usually a bone

distal, furthest from the trunk

distal radius, the long bone above the carpus, or knee

distemper, see strangles

distension, being swollen or stretched from internal pressure

diuretic, agent that causes the secretion of urine

DL-methionine, a sulphur-containing amino acid

dorsal displacement of the soft palate, a condition where the soft palate rises upwards above the epiglottis and partially obstructs normal breathing

dorsal laminar arteries, branches of the circumflex artery that feed the front of the hoof

dorsiflexion, an unnatural limb configuration where the fetlock sinks towards the ground due to fatigued musculotendinous attachments; results in overstretched flexor tendons

drench, dose of medicine given to a horse by pouring it into the horse's mouth

droplet nuclei, droplets of water in the air which contain bacteria or viruses

duct, passage with definite walls

dystocia, abnormal or difficult birth

ear plaques, small grey or white spots found on the inner surface of the pinna

early embryonic death (EED), death of the embryo before day 30 of gestation

Eastern equine encephalitis, see encephalitis

easy twitch, a plier-like clamp that puts pressure on the horse's nose; a form of restraint

eccentric contraction, a muscle contraction where the muscle gets thinner as it lengthens

echogenicity, the amount of grey in the projection on an ultra-sound screen; indication of tissue density

efficacy, the effectiveness of a medication or treatment

egg-bar shoe, an oval-shaped shoe which helps correct for navicular disease

egg count, the number of parasite eggs per gram of faeces

ejaculation, emission of seminal fluid

elasticity, the ability of a bone to return to its original shape after being deformed by a stress

electrical muscle stimulation (EMS), high voltage electrical impulses which passively produce muscle contractions

electroanalgesia, electrically stimulating muscles to provide pain relief

electrolytes, salts in body fluids which are involved in various body functions, such as nerve impulses, oxygen and carbon dioxide transport, and muscle contractions

embolism, the sudden blocking of an artery by a clot or foreign material in the blood

embryo, in the horse, the unborn foal up to approximately 30 or 40 days of gestation

embryo transfer, a developing embryo is removed from its natural mother and implanted in the uterus of a host mother for the remainder of gestation

encephalitis, inflammation of the brain caused by an acute viral disease; three strains affect the horse: *Eastern equine e., Western equine e.,* and *Venezuelan equine e.;* also called sleeping sickness

encephalomyelitis, inflammation of the brain and spinal cord

endocrine, secreting internally; applied to various organs and structures which secrete hormones into the blood or lymph and have an effect on other parts of the body

endometrial cups, ulcer-like structures formed by the foetus in the endometrium of a pregnant mare; they secrete hormones necessary to maintain pregnancy

endometritis, inflammation of the endometrium

endometrium, the lining of the uterus

endorphin, a chemical released by the central nervous system to reduce and suppress the perception of pain

endoscope, an instrument for the visual examination of the interior of an organ such as the throat, trachea or stomach

endotoxic shock, shock caused by large amounts of endotoxin in the bloodstream

endotoxin, a toxin that is present as a component of the cell walls of Gram-negative bacteria

energy molecules, ATP; the product of metabolism

engagement, the use of the hindquarters to allow the horse to achieve self-carriage, or to use them under the body for braking and thrust for sliding stops or quick turns

enkephalin, a chemical released by the central nervous system to reduce and suppress the perception of pain

enteric, pertaining to the intestines

enteritis, inflammation of the intestine, usually the small intestine

enterolith, a stone that develops in the intestine, formed by salt deposits around a hard object

enzyme, a protein that acts as a catalyst to produce or accelerate change in a substance, as in digestion of food

epidermis, the outermost layer of the skin

epiglottic entrapment, a condition where the epiglottis is trapped in the arytenoepiglottic fold, causing exercise intolerance, noisy breathing and coughing

epiglottis, the thin plate of cartilage at the entrance to the larynx that prevents food from entering the larynx and trachea while swallowing

epinephrine, see adrenaline

epiphysis, a piece of bone that is separated by cartilage from the long bone in early life, but later becomes a part of the larger bone; it is at the cartilage growth plate that growth of the long bone occurs

epiphysitis, inflammation of the end of a long bone or of the cartilage that separates it from the long bone; more correctly called physitis

episioplasty, see Caslick's surgery

epistaxis, haemorrhage from the nose; nosebleed

epithelial, pertaining to epithelium

epithelialization, growth of new epithelium

epithelium, layer of cells of which skin and mucous membranes are formed

equine coital exanthema, a venereal disease caused by equine Herpes virus-3

equine distemper, see strangles

equine Herpes virus (EHV), a respiratory virus with two subtypes, EHV-1 and EHV-4; causes rhinopneumonitis

equine tumour necrosis factor (TNF), a by-product of the inflammation caused by endotoxins

equine viral arteritis (EVA), an infectious viral disease characterized by fever, depression, limb oedema or abortion

erectile tissue, tissue containing vascular spaces that become filled with blood

erection, the state of erectile tissue when filled with blood; particularly of the penis

erythema, redness of the skin

erythema multiforme, 'target' lesions caused by *Ehrlichia equi;* a form of hives

erythropoietin, a hormone which stimulates production of red blood cells in the bone marrow

eschar, a coagulated crust of skin debris which forms over the top of a rope burn

evaporation, transfer of water from a surface to the air

evaporative cooling, water vapour on the skin which is produced from the sweat glands pulls heat from the blood vessels, and the warmed water is then transferred to the air; a method of dissipating internal body heat

ewe-neck, a conformational fault where the topline of the neck appears to be put on upside down; instead of a crest, the neck has a dip in the neck along the topline

excretion, the act of eliminating the body's waste materials

exercise-induced pulmonary haemorrhage (EIPH), rupture of the capillaries in the lungs due to either previous lung infection or to obstruction of the upper airway; causes bleeding in the lungs, and sometimes from the nose

exostosis, an abnormal, benign growth projecting from a bone surface, usually capped by cartilage

exotoxin, a poison produced by a living organism

extender, formula used for semen dilution and preservation

extension, a movement that brings a limb forwards and into a straight line

extensor, any muscle that extends a joint

extensor process, a bony protrusion at the top of the coffin bone to which the extensor tendon attaches

exudate, fluid or cells that have escaped from vessels into tissues or onto tissue surfaces, usually a result of inflammation

faecal, relating to the bodily waste discharged from the intestines, consisting of bacteria, cells from the intestines, secretions (mainly of the liver), and food residue

fartleks, continuous exercise over long distances but periodically changing speed

fascia, supportive sheets of fibrous tissue located between muscles or beneath the skin

fast twitch high oxidative (FTa), a muscle fibre type that burns glycogen in the absence of oxygen

fast twitch low oxidative (FTb), a muscle fibre type which cannot use oxygen to burn glycogen for energy production

fatigue state, the point at which a bone begins to lose its elasticity after being deformed by loading and unloading cycles

fatty acids, key components of fats; an important muscle fuel for aerobic metabolism

feathering, long hair on the back of the fetlocks of cold-blooded horses

fermentation, bacterial or enzymatic decomposition

fertile, able to produce offspring

fertilization, the union of the sperm cell and the ovum

fetlock, the area or joint of the lower leg above the pastern and below the cannon

fetlock valgus, see toed-out; also called splayfooted

fetlock varus, see pigeon-toed; also called toed-in

fibrin, elastic protein released during blood coagulation

fibroblast, cell which produces fibrin, or collagen

fibroblastic sarcoid, a sarcoid which often develops after a wound and resembles proud flesh

fibroma, benign tumour of fibrous tissue

fibrosis, an abnormal increase in the amount of fibrous connective tissue in an organ, part, or tissue; scarring

fibrotic myopathy, adhesions which form between muscle masses of the thigh, sometimes after an episode of myositis

fibrous connective tissue, tissue consisting of elongated cells, fibroblasts, and collagen

fibrovascular callus, a structure composed of fibrin; a scaffold for granulation tissue and more fibrin to repair an injury

field fitness test, a test to determine a horse's aerobic capacity by measuring V_{200}, which is the horse's velocity at a heart rate of 200 beats per minute

fistula, an abnormal passage between two organs or from an internal organ to the surface of the body

fistulogram, the X-ray film taken of an area which was injected with a radio-opaque dye

flat feet, when the sole is not concave, which forces the horse to walk on the sole instead of the hoof wall, resulting in sole bruises

flexion, bending movement

flexion test, a diagnostic test for lameness where a specific joint is tightly flexed for 1 – 2 minutes, and the horse is trotted off

flexural deformities, a condition where the joint remains in flexion, for example, contracted tendons or club feet

float, to file down (rasp) the teeth, removing the sharp edges

flora, various microorganisms inhabiting an individual

flushing, a weight-gain programme instituted before breeding

focal ventral midline dermatitis, dermatitis on the abdominal midline caused by the horn fly, *Haematobia*

foetus, the unborn foal from approximately day 40 of gestation to birth

follicle, a small sac or cavity, such as in the skin from which a hair grows

follicle stimulating hormone (FSH), a hormone secreted by the anterior pituitary gland; stimulates follicular growth and controls oestrogen secretion by the ovary; in the stallion, FSH stimulates sperm production

founder, see laminitis

founder ring, see laminitic rings

fracture, the breaking of a part, especially a bone

frog, wedge-shaped mass of tissue; lies between the bars of the horse's foot; absorbs shock upon the hoof's impact with the ground

full-thickness, a wound or burn which penetrates through the skin

fungus, plantlike organism that feeds on organic matter; responsible for the mycotic diseases, e.g. ringworm

gangrene, death of tissue, usually due to loss of blood supply

gaseous colic, colic caused by the build-up of gas in the intestines

gaskin, the area between the thigh and the hock

gastric, pertaining to the stomach

gastric ulcers, ulcers of the inner wall of the stomach

gastrointestinal tract, digestive tract through which food passes where nutrients are absorbed; consists of mouth, pharynx, oesophagus, stomach, small intestine, caecum, large colon, small colon, rectum

gelding, a castrated male horse

gene, the functional unit of heredity carried by the chromosomes

genetic pool, all of the genes in a population

genital tract, reproductive tract; general term referring to the reproductive passageway and all of its associated organs

gestation, pregnancy

girth itch, see ringworm

gland, a secreting organ

glaucoma, eye disease marked by an increase in the intraocular pressure which causes changes in the optic disk

glucose, a simple sugar molecule derived from carbohydrates which is a principle source of energy

gluteal muscles, the muscle group over the croup and pelvis

glycine, an amino acid which functions as an inhibitory neurotransmitter, preventing the next neuron from firing

glycogen, a chain of glucose sugar molecules which may be stored in the liver and skeletal muscles and/or used as muscle fuel

gonitis, inflammation of the stifle

Gram-negative bacteria, the type of bacteria that, during Gram's staining process, lose crystal violet stain when rinsed with alcohol; unlike the Gram-positive bacteria, which retain crystal violet stain because their cell walls are composed differently

granulation tissue, the formation in wounds of small rounded masses of tissue, composed of capillaries and connective tissue cells which grow outwards to fill the wound defect; see second intention healing

granules, small particles or grains

grease heel, see cracked heels

gut sounds, sounds heard with a stethoscope in the horse's abdomen; indicates intestinal activity and level of dehydration

haemagglutinin (HA) spikes, a specific sequence of amino acids on the surface of viral particles; the part of the virus that is recognized as foreign by the immune system

haematoma, a blood pocket due to a ruptured blood vessel

haemoglobin, oxygen-carrying red pigment of the red blood cells

haemoglobinuria, the presence of free haemoglobin in the urine

haemolysis, the destruction or breakdown of red blood cells

haemorrhage, the leaking of blood from a ruptured blood vessel

haemospermia, the presence of blood in the semen

harvest mites, mites which cause trombiculiasis, characterized by small, crusty lesions

heart rate, the number of times the heart beats in 1 minute

heart rate recovery, the time required for the heart rate to return to the resting rate after exercise; depends on fitness, weather, and level of exertion

heat increment, heat generated by digestion and metabolism of food

heat index, a combination of the environmental temperature and the humidity

heat stress, occurs when body temperature climbs above 105° F and the body cannot efficiently cool itself

heave line, a line between the flank and the thorax created by overdevelopment of abdominal muscles; caused by heaves

heaves, respiratory disturbance characterized by forced expiration of breath; caused by allergies and dust; also called chronic obstructive pulmonary disease (COPD)

heel fly, see warbles

hepatic, pertaining to the liver

hepatitis, inflammation of the liver

heritable, capable of being genetically inherited

hernia, a condition where an organ protrudes through the structure which normally contains it

high-frequency electroanalgesia (HFEA), a type of electroanalgesia which provides pain relief faster but for shorter periods than low-frequency electroanalgesia

hindgut, portion of the digestive tract, including the caecum and large intestine

hirsute, abnormal hairiness related to an endocrine disorder

histamine, a chemical compound which dilates capillaries, constricts the smooth muscle of the lungs, and increases secretion of the stomach

hives, small, flat-topped bumps which may coalesce into larger bumps, usually found on the neck and shoulders, caused by an allergic reaction; also called urticaria

hobbles, a restraining device which restricts leg movement

hoof tester, pincer-type instrument used to gently pinch the hoof to find any inflamed and sore area

hormone, a chemical substance produced in the body by a gland or body organ which travels in the blood or lymphatic system to a distant specific organ, to regulate the activity of that organ

horn fly, *Haematobia,* a midge which causes dermatitis on the abdominal midline

horn tubules, hollow tubes of the hoof wall composed of keratin; running parallel and vertical as they grow down from the coronary band

host, an organism that harbours or nourishes another organism

humerus, arm bone, extending from the shoulder to the elbow

hyaluronic acid (HA), thick lubricating fluid in the joints

hydrotherapy, the application of water in any form, internally or externally, in treating disease or illness

hygroma, a sac distended with fluid

hymen, a fold of mucous membrane which partially or completely covers the opening of the vagina

hyoid apparatus, the bones which attach the larynx to the base of the skull

hyperirritability, pathological responsiveness to slight stimuli

hyperkalaemia, abnormally high potassium content of the blood

hyperkalaemic periodic paralysis (HYPP), skeletal muscle weakness associated with hyperkalaemia

hyperlipaemia, high levels of circulating fatty acids

hyperplasia, an increase in the number of cells in a tissue or organs, excluding tumour formation

hypersensitivity, a state of altered activity in which the body reacts with an exaggerated response to a foreign agent

hyperthermia, a method of therapy which uses a radio-frequency current to heat and destroy sarcoid tissue

hypertrophy, overgrowth, general increase in bulk of a part or organ not due to tumour formation; use of the term may be restricted to denote greater bulk through increase in size, but not in number, of the individual tissue elements

hypothalamus, the part of the brain which regulates part of the nervous system, hormone activity, and many body functions

hypoxia, lack of oxygen

icterus, see jaundice

ileus, a condition where intestinal movement has stopped

immune system, the organs and cells in the body which protect it from foreign bodies such as bacteria and viruses

immunity, the power to resist infection

immunodeficiency, a deficiency in antibody response, leaving the animal susceptible to infection

immunoglobulins, group of proteins, including antibodies

immunotherapy, introducing a foreign protein into an area to draw the immune system's attention to another problem in the area

impaction, the condition of being firmly lodged or wedged

implantation, attachment of the placenta to the uterine endometrium between days 45 and 150 of gestation

impulsion, the energy and thrust exhibited by the horse in motion

in utero, in the uterus, before birth

inactivated vaccine, a vaccine where the virus particles are treated so they are unable to damage the tissues

incubation, period between acquiring an infectious disease and its clinical manifestation

indwelling catheter, see catheter

infection, abnormal multiplication of microorganisms in the body

inflammation, the response of tissue to injury or abnormal stimulation, usually involving a reaction which leads to healing

influenza, an acute viral infection involving the respiratory tract; characterized by inflammation of the nasal mucosa, pharynx, and conjuctiva

infrared thermography, non-invasive method of identifying areas of inflammation by 'mapping' temperature differences in the tissues as related to increased or decreased blood flow and cellular activity

ingesta, consumed feed and fluids

inhalation, drawing air (or other substances) into the lungs

injection, forcing a liquid into a part, as into subcutaneous tissue, blood vessel, or muscle; a substance so forced

innervation, the distribution or supply of nerves or nerve stimulus to a part

insulin, a hormone produced by the pancreas; secreted into the blood to regulate sugar and fat metabolism

interactive system, a system in which all parts depend on the others for function

intercostal, between ribs

interference, striking of the inside of one leg with the inside of the hoof or shoe of the opposite leg; impact point may be from the coronary band up to the knee or hock

interval training, repeated sets of speed work and partial heart rate recovery periods; promotes lactic acid tolerance and increases speed

intestinal, pertaining to the intestines

intestinal flora, bacteria normally present within the intestine

intestinal threadworms, an internal parasite of foals caused by *Strongyloides westeri*; may cause foal diarrhoea and scours

intestinal tract, the small and large intestines

intestinal torsion, twisting of the intestines

intra-articular, within a joint

intradermal (ID), within the skin

intramuscular (IM), within a muscle

intravenous (IV), within a vein

intussusception, the prolapse of one part of the intestine into the lumen of an immediately adjoining part causing blockage

inversion, the respiratory rate remains faster than the heart rate after exercise; an inverted horse appears to pant

irritant, an agent that produces irritation

isometric contraction, a muscle contraction where the muscle stays the same length

isoxsuprine hydrochloride, a peripheral vasodilatory drug which improves the blood flow to the foot of navicular horses

jaundice, yellowish discoloration of the mucous membranes of the body; also called icterus

joint, an articulation; the place of union or junction between two or more bones of the skeleton

joint ill, see navel ill

jugular furrow, the groove on each side of the neck in which the jugular vein is located; also called jugular groove

jugular pulse, the rhythmic expansion of the jugular vein in the neck that may be felt with the finger

keloid, a sharply elevated, irregularly-shaped, enlarging scar

keratin, an insoluble protein which is the principal constituent of epidermis, hair, horny tissues, and the enamel of teeth

killed vaccine, a vaccine where the viral particles are dead and are therefore incapable of damaging the tissues

knock-knee, a growth plate abnormality in the distal radius that results in the limb deviating outwards from the knee down; may result from dietary deficiency; also called carpus valgus

labia, the vulval lips arranged vertically on either side of the vaginal opening

laceration, a torn, ragged wound

lactation, secretion of milk from the mammary glands

lactic acid, a toxic by-product of anaerobic muscle metabolism; causes muscle fatigue and soreness

Lactobacillus, bacteria in the gut that produce very large amounts of lactic acid from fermentable carbohydrates

laminae, thin plates or layers; a latticework of tissue and blood vessels

laminitic rings, rings around the hoof that result from altered keratin production in an attack of laminitis; also called founder rings

laminitis, inflammation of the laminae within the foot; also called founder

larva, an early developmental stage, usually the feeding form of an animal such as an insect or worm

laryngeal hemiplegia, when one or both arytenoid cartilages of the larynx collapse into the airway due to nerve damage; causes exercise intolerance and perhaps a roaring noise; also called roaring

laryngo-palatal dislocation, separation of the larynx from the ostium of the soft palate; results in reduced airway efficiency

larynx, a structure composed of nine cartilages located at the top of the trachea; contains the vocal cords

laser, an acronym for Light Amplification by Stimulated Emission of Radiation; generated by electromagnetic waves of the same wavelength that are aligned in both time and space, and travel in nearly the same direction

lateral, on the side; the outside

lavage, washing out a cavity or wound with a stream of fluid

lesion, abnormal change in structure due to injury or disease

lice, host-specific skin parasites that inhabit the topline; this infestation is called pediculosis

ligament, band of fibrous tissue which connects bones and cartilage, and supports the joints

lime, calcium oxide, used as a disinfectant

liniment, an oily, soapy, or alcoholic liquid preparation used on the skin and applied with friction

lip chain, a chain which is passed under the upper lip and over the gum as a method of restraint

lipoma, a benign fatty tumour

live foal guarantee (LFG), breeding contract provision which guarantees the mare owner a live foal as a result of the purchased breeding; usually gives the mare owner the right to rebreed the next season to the same stallion if the pregnancy fails

lockjaw, see tetanus

long-toe – low-heel (LTLH), a long-toe – low-heel foot configuration where the hoof–pastern angle is broken; leads to many lameness problems

low-frequency electroanalgesia (LFEA), a type of electroanalgesia which provides pain relief for 1 – 3 days

lumbar, pertaining to the loins, the part of the back between the thorax and pelvis

lumbosacral (L-S) joint, at the top of the croup; pivots and rotates the hindquarters and pelvis forwards under the body

lumen, cavity or channel within a tube or tubular organ

lymph, a transparent yellowish liquid containing mostly water and white blood cells, and derived from tissue fluids

lymphatic system, a system similar to the circulatory system which carries lymph from the tissues to the bloodstream

lysine, an essential amino acid for the growing horse

macrophage, an immune cell which binds, internalizes, and inactivates invading microorganisms in tissues

maiden mare, a mare that has not been bred

malabsorption, impaired intestinal absorption of nutrients

malignant, resistant to treatment; occurring in severe form, and frequently fatal; tending to become worse; in the case of a neoplasm, having the property of uncontrollable growth and/or recurrence after removal

malignant oedema, a disease caused by *Clostridium septicum,* characterized by the formation of large amounts of gas in the muscles, creating a crackling feel beneath the skin

malnourished, suffering from imbalanced or insufficient nutrient intake

malnutrition, a nutrition disorder caused by either an imbalanced or insufficient diet, or due to poor absorption and utilization of nutrients

mammary gland, the udder; a collection of highly modified oil glands in the mare's inguinal region that collect nutrients and synthesize and secrete milk

mandibles, jaws

mange, a contagious skin disease caused by various types of mites

mast cells, cells which release chemicals such as histamine

mastitis, inflammation of the mammary gland

meconium, the first intestinal discharge of the newborn

meconium impaction, an impaction colic which occurs if the first faecal balls are not passed soon after birth

melanin, dark pigment of the body; protects the skin from sunburn from UV rays

melanoblasts, immature melanocytes; germinal cells

melanocytes, the cells responsible for producing melanin

melanoma, a neoplasm derived from melanoblasts; may occur in the skin of any part of the body, in the eye, or in the mucous membranes of the genitalia, anus, oral cavity, or other sites

membrane, a thin layer of tissue which covers a surface, lines a cavity, or divides a space or organ

meninges, the three membranes that envelop the brain and spinal cord

meningitis, inflammation of the meninges, usually a complication of a pre-existing disease; generally characterized by incoordination, compulsive movement, convulsions, and a high but fluctuating body temperature

mesentery, tissue that supports an organ, such as that which supports the small intestine

metabolic, pertaining to metabolism

metabolic alkalosis, a condition where the bloodstream is excessively alkalinized due to bicarbonate retention by the kidneys

metabolism, chemical changes in a cell which provide energy for vital bodily processes and activities

metastasis, the spread of neoplasms from the primary site to other parts of the body

metritis, inflammation of the uterus

microbes, see microorganisms

microfilaria, minute, prelarval stage of some parasites

microflora, see flora

micronutrient, any substance that plays a nutritional role in the body and is required only in minute quantities in the diet

microorganisms, microscopic organisms such as bacteria, viruses, moulds, yeasts and protozoa

milkshake, a sodium bicarbonate drench; may buffer the effects of lactic acid in the bloodstream

mineralization, deposition of minerals (such as calcium and phosphorus), into a bone or damaged soft tissue

mitochondria, 'factories' within cells, which use oxygen to break down fuel into energy

mixed sarcoid, a sarcoid that has both verrucous and fibroblastic sarcoid characteristics

modified live virus, a virus that has been raised in a laboratory under somewhat unnatural conditions and therefore does not have the disease-causing abilities of a virus in the natural state, but still stimulates production of antibodies

moonblindness, see periodic ophthalmia

morphology, in semen evaluation, the examination of semen samples for normal sperm cell structure

motility, the ability to move; peristalsis when referring to the intestines; the ability of a sperm cell to move in a normal, forward manner; the percentage of sperm in a sample that are able to move normally

mucociliary apparatus (MCA), a one-way flow of mucus on top of the epithelial cells which line the airways; an airway clearance mechanism

mucopurulent, containing both mucus and pus

mucosa, mucous membrane

mucous, relating to mucus or a mucous membrane

mucous membrane, membrane that lines the hollow organs, air passages, digestive tract, urinary passages, and genital passages

mucus, clear, viscous secretion of the mucous membranes, consisting of mucin, epithelial cells, immune cells, and various inorganic salts suspended in water

mud fever, see cracked heels

murmur, a periodic sound of short duration of cardiac or vascular origin

muscle, an organ which contracts to produce movement

muscle relaxant, an agent that aids in reducing muscle tension

muscle tremor, an involuntary trembling or quivering of a muscle

musculotendinous, a muscle and its complementary tendon

mutation, the process by which the genetic code is altered

myalgia, aching muscles

myofibroblasts, fibroblasts that act like muscle cells; they pull the full-thickness skin at the wound margins in, reducing wound size

myoglobin, a molecule contributing to the colour of muscle and acting as a store of oxygen

myopathy, any disease of a muscle

myosin filament, one of two types of filaments that make up a muscle fibre

myositis, muscular inflammation; a common term to indicate disease of horses marked by a sudden attack of perspiration and cramping of the hindquarters, with the potential of passing light red to dark brown urine; occurs in horses that after engaging in continuous work are rested, well-fed and then returned to work; also called tying-up

nasopharynx, the part of the pharynx above the soft palate

navel ill, in foals, an infection within the joints that entered through the umbilical cord and spread through the bloodstream; also called joint ill

navicular, a small bone in the foot of a horse; common term for disease of the navicular apparatus

navicular apparatus, collectively, the navicular bone, navicular bursa, and deep digital flexor tendon

navicular disease, chronic inflammation of one or more of the structures of the navicular apparatus

necrobiosis, cell death and scar tissue build-up

necropsy, post mortem examination

necrosis, the pathologic death of one or more cells, or of part of a tissue or organ; characterized by atrophy of the affected area

necrotic, pertaining to or affected by necrosis

neoplasm, tumour; an abnormal tissue that grows by cellular proliferation more rapidly than normal and continues to grow after the stimuli that initiated the new growth ceases

nerve, cord-like structure, visible to the naked eye, comprising a collection of nerve fibres which convey impulses between a part of the central nervous system and some other region of the body

nerve block, a diagnostic test; local anaesthetic is injected into a nerve; if a lameness improves, the source of pain is identified

neurectomy, cutting a nerve, especially the palmar digital nerves as a treatment for navicular disease

neuroma, a painful lump of nerve tissue that sometimes forms after a neurectomy

neuromuscular irritability, the ability of a muscle to respond to nerve impulses

neutralize, to make a substance neither acid nor base

neutrophil, a white blood cell readily stainable by neutral dyes

nits, the eggs of lice

no joint, the joint between the first and second cervical vertebrae; moves the head side-to-side; also called atlanto-axial joint

nociceptor, see pain receptor

nodule, small node or knot which is solid and can be detected by touch

non-steroidal anti-inflammatory drugs (NSAIDs), drugs which limit inflammation, oedema, swelling, and pain

nuchal ligament, a fan-like structure forming the crest of the neck; extends from the base of the skull to the withers

nuclear scintigraphy, method of imaging an inflammatory condition by injecting a radioactive tracer material into the bloodstream; then a gamma camera 'images' areas of injured bone or soft tissue which has a greater uptake of the tracer

nutrient medium, gel-like substance containing nutrients which grow and sustain microorganisms for laboratory identification

occipitus, the base of the skull

occult sarcoid, a flat sarcoid, having thick, rough skin

oedema, accumulation of abnormally large amounts of fluid between the cells in the tissues

oesophagus, canal extending from the pharynx to the stomach

oestrogen, general term for any substance that exerts an oestrogenic effect; formed naturally by the ovary, placenta, and testicles

oestrous, pertaining to oestrus

oestrous cycle, the cyclic series of periods consisting of oestrus, metoestrus, dioestrus, and pro-oestrus

oestrus, period of sexual receptivity in the female; heat

onchocerciasis, a skin disorder which involves the larvae of *Onchocerca*, a parasitic worm; characterized by scaly, hairless lesions on the face, neck, or belly

ophthalmic, optic, pertaining to the eye

ophthalmoscope, instrument containing a perforated mirror and lenses used to examine the interior of the eye

opportunistic pathogen, an organism which does not usually cause illness until the immune system is depressed by another illness

organ, part of the body that performs a special function or functions

organization, replacement of blood clots by fibrous tissue

organophosphate, one of the phosphorus-containing chemicals which are used as drugs or pesticides

osmosis, diffusion through a semipermeable membrane that tends to equalize concentrations

ossify, to change or develop into bone

osteitis, inflammation of a bone

osteoblasts, cells that form new bone

osteochondrosis, a metabolic bone disease; incomplete maturation of growing cartilage in a joint, leading to cysts, fissures, or cartilage flaps

osteoclasts, cells that remove bone

ostium, a hole in the back of the soft palate through which a cartilage of the larynx fits during respiration

ovarian, pertaining to the ovaries or activity of the ovaries

ovary, one of the paired gonads in the female which contain ova (eggs)

over at the knee, a conformational fault where the knee is set too far forward; caused by excessive curvature of the radius; also called bucked knees

overtraining, exercising the horse too hard, too often without an adequate recovery period; characterized by weight loss or failure to gain weight, depression, exercise intolerance

ovulation, the release of an ovum from a mature follicle of the ovary

packed cell volume (PCV), the percentage of red blood cells in the blood

paddling, a gait defect in which the front foot is thrown outwards during flight; common in horses that are pigeon-toed

pain receptor, sensory nerve terminal which responds to stimuli of various kinds; also called nociceptors

palmar digital nerves, nerves on either side of the pastern innervating the back third of the foot

palpation, feeling or perceiving by the sense of touch

papule, small, circumscribed, solid elevation on the skin

paralysis, loss or impairment of motor function in a part

parasite, plant or animal which lives upon or within another living organism at whose expense it obtains some advantage

parathyroid gland, small bodies in the neck or near the thyroid gland in the neck which secrete hormones

parotid, situated near the ear

parrot mouth, a congenital defect in which the lower jaw is too short or the upper jaw is too long

partial-thickness, a wound or burn which does not penetrate through the skin

particulate, composed of separate particles

passive immunity, disease resistance acquired though the transfer of antibodies from another individual

pastern, the area between the fetlock joint and the coronary band

pathogen, any microorganism or other substance that causes a disease

pathogenic, disease-causing

pathological, pertaining to pathology

pathology, the study of the nature of disease; the causes, development, and results of disease processes

pectoral, pertaining to the chest

pedal osteitis, coffin bone inflammation

pediculosis, infestation with lice

pelvic brim, the most anterior portion of the floor of the pelvis

pelvic flexure, narrowing segment of the large intestine situated on the left side of the abdomen

pelvis, the ring of bone, along with its ligaments, formed by the os coxae (the pubic bone, ilium, ischium), sacrum, and coccyx

penis, the male organ of copulation; composed of veins and arteries, spongy erectile tissue, and a urethra

perineal, pertaining to the pelvic floor and the structures of the pelvic outlet

perineum, the area between the thighs, originating at the anus; in the male it ends at the scrotum; in the female at the mammary glands

periodic ophthalmia, recurrent episodes of anterior uveitis, the most common cause of blindness in the horse; also called moonblindness

periople, a very thin layer of cells forming the protective, waxy covering of the hoof

peristalsis, worm-like movement by which the digestive tract propels ingesta

peristaltic action, pertaining to peristalsis

peritendinous, pertaining to the tissues surrounding a tendon

peritoneal lining, peritoneum, membrane lining the abdominal cavity

peritonitis, inflammation of the peritoneum

pH, symbol for measuring alkalinity and acidity; pH 7 is neutral, greater than 7 is alkaline, less than 7 is acid

pharyngeal lymphoid hyperplasia, inflammation and enlargement of lymphoid tissue of the nasopharynx and epiglottis; similar to tonsillitis in humans

pharynx, the cavity which joins the mouth and nasal passages to the oesophagus and larynx

phonophoresis, using ultrasound over topical medication to encourage it to penetrate deep tissues

phosphocreatine, a compound of creatine and phosphoric acid; stored in and used by muscle cells as fuel for high-energy anaerobic muscle metabolism

photoaggravated vasculitis, inflammation of vessels made worse by sunlight

photophobia, abnormal aversion to light

photosensitization, excessive reaction of the skin to sunlight, resulting in swelling and inflammation

phrenic nerve, a nerve which passes directly across the heart muscle to the diaphragm; involved in thumps

phylloerythrin, a chemical which is a breakdown product of chlorophyll; accumulation in the skin causes photosensitization

physitis, inflammation of the end of a long bone or of the cartilage that separates it from the long bone; commonly called epiphysitis

pigeon-breasted, a conformational fault where the front legs are too far under the body; caused by a horizontal humerus

pigeon-toed, conformational fault where the feet point in because the forelegs are turned inwards; also called toed-in, fetlock varus

pigment, any colouring matter of the body

pineal gland, a gland in the brain behind the hypothalamus; may communicate with the photoreceptors in the eyes to determine the onset of oestrus

pinnae, the parts of the ears which project from the head

pinworms, an internal parasite, *Oxyuris equi,* which causes itching and rubbing of the tailhead

piroplasmosis, blood-borne protozoal disease transmitted by ticks; characterized by fever, depression, anaemia, and limb and abdominal oedema

pitting oedema, a swelling which, when pressed with a fingertip, retains an impression of a pit

pituitary adenoma, a tumour on the pituitary gland

pituitary gland, an organ at the base of the brain which secretes and stores hormones that regulate most basic body functions

placenta, a vascular organ that surrounds the foetus during gestation; connected to the foetus by the umbilical cord and is the structure through which the foetus receives nourishment from, and eliminates waste matter into, the mare's circulatory system

plaiting, a gait defect where one foot crosses over the other, resulting in interference

plaque, any patch or flat area; a horny, dry growth

plasma, liquid portion of the blood in which blood cells and proteins are suspended

platelets, disk-shaped structures found in the blood of all mammals and chiefly known for their role in blood clotting

pleura, the membrane enclosing the lungs and lining the thoracic cavity

pleurisy, pleuritis, inflammation of the pleura with exudation into its cavity and upon its surface

pleuropneumonia, pneumonia accompanied by pleurisy

pneumovagina, the presence of air in the vagina; a common cause of infertility in mares; also called windsucking

pododermatitis, see thrush

polyp, protruding growth from mucous membrane

polypeptides, a compound of two or more amino acids

post-legged, a conformational fault where the hind legs are too straight

poultice, soft, moist, mass of the consistency of cooked cereal, spread between layers of muslin, linen, gauze, or towels, and applied to an area to create moist local heat or to counter irritation

precipitate, a solid separated from a solution or suspension

prepatent period, the period from ingestion of infective larvae to egg-producing adults

prepuce, the fold of skin that covers the glans penis

primary immunization, the initial vaccine which primes the cells that produce antibodies

process, a projection, as of bone

progesterone, hormone produced by the corpus luteum which quiets uterine muscle contractions

prognosis, the prospect of recovery from a disease or injury

progressive motility, the ability of a sperm cell to move in a normal, forward manner

prophylactic, prevention; an agent that tends to prevent disease

prostaglandin, stimulant to intestinal and uterine muscle, and mediator of the inflammatory cycle

protein, any of a group of complex compounds which contain nitrogen and are composed of amino acids

proteinaceous, pertaining to or of the nature of protein

protozoa, primitive organisms which have only a single cell

proud flesh, exuberant granulation tissue

pruritus, itching

psoroptic mange, mange caused by a mite of the genus *Psoroptes;* occurs mainly on sheltered parts of the body, as on areas covered with long hair; also called scabies

psyllium hydrophilia mucilloid, a laxative which stimulates bowel movement and pulls fluids into the intestine; commonly known as Metamucil®

pulmonary, pertaining to the lungs

pulse, rhythmic throbbing of a vessel which may be felt with the finger; caused by blood forced through the vessel by contractions of the heart

pulsing electromagnetic fields (PEMF), two electromagnetic coils placed on opposite sides of the injured area to align the electro-magnetic field between them; allegedly promotes healing by improving oxygen supply

puncture, a wound that is deeper than it is wide

purpura haemorrhagica, a disease characterized by extensive collections of fluid and blood in tissues beneath the skin, occurring primarily on the head and legs; caused by an unusual allergic reaction to the bacteria responsible for strangles, *Streptococcus equi*

purulent, consisting of or containing pus; associated with the formation of, or caused by pus

pus, a liquid inflammatory product made up of immune cells and a thin fluid called liquor puris

pustules, visible collections of pus within or beneath the skin

pyloric sphincter, pylorus, tight band of muscle that regulates the juncture of the stomach with the small intestine

pyrogen, a fever-producing substance

quadriceps, the group of muscles covering the side of the thigh bone

quarantine, complete isolation from other horses

Quarter Horse, a small powerful breed originally bred for sprinting in quarter-mile races in Virginia in the late eighteenth century

rabies, an acute infectious disease of the central nervous system, usually fatal in mammals

radiographs, X-ray films

radio-opaque, opaque to X-rays; shows white on a radiograph

radius, forearm bone

rain scald, see cracked heels

rectal examination, examination of organs or structures adjacent to the rectum by feeling for size, texture, and other characteristics through the rectal wall; also called rectal palpation

rectum, the terminal part of the digestive tract

recurrent, returning after intermissions

red blood cells, haemoglobin-carrying cells in the blood that transport oxygen

regeneration, natural renewal of a tissue or part

remodelling, addition of new bone in response to stress, or removal of bone in an area that is not undergoing stress

renal, pertaining to the kidney

renal papillary necrosis, death of kidney tissue due to the antiprostaglandin effects of NSAIDs combined with dehydration

replication, reproducing or duplicating, as of a virus

resorption, the removal of an exudate, blood clot, pus, bone cells, etc., by absorption

respiration, the act of inhaling and exhaling air to exchange oxygen and carbon dioxide between the atmosphere and the cells of the body

retained placenta, placenta which is not expelled within 6 hours after foaling

retention, holding onto a fluid or secretion which is normally excreted from the body

retropharyngeal lymph nodes, lymph nodes under the throatlatch

rhabditic dermatitis, itchy, painful dermatitis caused by *Pelodera strongyloides* larvae

rhinitis, inflammation of the mucous membrane of the nose

rhinopneumonitis, inflammation of the nasal and pulmonary mucous membranes; an infectious disease caused by an equine herpes virus (EHV) subtype

rhinovirus (ERV), a respiratory virus for which there is no vaccine; symptoms include fever, swollen lymph nodes, and inflammation of the trachea and lower airways

rim pads, a pad between the hoof wall and the shoe

ringbone, bony enlargements and areas of new bone growth in the pastern or coffin joints due to degenerative joint disease

ringworm, a fungal disease causing circular patches of hair loss with scabby, flaking skin beneath; also called girth itch

roaring, see laryngeal hemiplegia

roping, catching cattle with a lasso

roughage, hay or pasture which provides fibre essential to intestinal function

ruminant, an animal which has a stomach with four complete cavities through which food passes during digestion; includes oxen, sheep, goats, deer, antelope

rupture, breaking or tearing of tissue

saccule, small bag or sac

saddle sore, an inflammation of hair follicles and skin caused by friction between the horse and the saddle

saline, relating to, of the nature of, or containing salt; physiological saline is a 0.9% sodium chloride solution

saliva, clear, alkaline, somewhat sticky secretion from various glands of the mouth; moistens and softens food for digestion

salve, a thick ointment

sarcoid, a benign tumour composed mainly of connective tissue which appears on the skin; the most common skin tumour of the horse

sarcoma, an often highly malignant tumour made up of a substance similar to embryonic connective tissue

sarcoptic mange, the most serious type of mange usually affecting areas where the hair is thin (head, neck, and shoulders)

scabies, see psoroptic mange

scale, a thin layer of cornified epithelial cells on the skin

scalenus muscles, muscles connecting the last four vertebrae to the first rib; they raise the base of the neck

scapula, shoulder blade

scapulo-humeral angle, the angle between the shoulder blade and the arm bone, which should be at least 90°

scar tissue, tissue remaining after the healing of a wound or other healing process

scope, the degree of freedom (extension and flexion) of the limbs and body while the horse is in motion

scratches, see cracked heels

scrotum, the pouch which contains the testicles

scurfing, the process of forming thin, dry scales on the skin

seasonally polyoestrous, having more than one oestrous cycle per breeding season

second intention healing, healing by granulation, without sutures; scar tissue will form

secondary condition, a condition caused by or consequent to a primary condition

secrete, to produce and give off cell products

secretory antibodies, immune cells found in body secretions, such as respiratory secretions in the nasal passages

sedative, a drug that reduces and controls excitement by its effect on the central nervous system

selenium, a trace mineral; toxicity causes tail and mane hair loss and, eventually, hoof sloughing

semen, fluid comprised of sperm cells and secretions of the testicles, seminal vesicles, prostate, and bulbourethral glands

semen evaluation, examination of semen for characteristics which indicate its fertility

semen extender, a formula used for semen dilution and preservation

semipermeable, permitting the passage of certain molecules and hindering the passage of others

septic shock, septicaemia, a systemic disease caused by pathogenic microorganisms and their toxic products in the blood

sequestrum, a piece of dead bone that has been broken off or become separated from the sound bone

scrotonin, a chemical released by the central nervous system which blocks pain impulses and reception by the brain

serous, pertaining to or resembling serum

serum, the clear liquid portion of the blood or any body fluid separated from its more solid elements; blood plasma with the fibrinogen removed

sesamoid, a small nodular bone embedded in a tendon or joint capsule

sesamoiditis, inflammation of the fetlock sesamoid bones usually involving both osteitis and periostitis

sheared heels, a syndrome where one heel bulb is higher than the other; results from improper trimming

sheath, a tubular structure surrounding an organ or part

shipping fever, disease related to stress of transport; symptoms include weakness, nasal discharge, discharge from the eyes, distressed breathing and coughing

shock, a condition of acute circulatory failure due to loss of circulating blood volume; caused by septicaemia, endotoxins, blood loss, colic, allergic reactions, or heart failure

shoe caulks, short protrusions from the underside of each heel of a horseshoe; used on racing shoes to provide better traction

sickle hocked, a conformational fault where the hind legs are angled beneath the horse

sign, evidence of a disease, as observed by someone other than the patient

silent heat, the mare does not display behavioural signs of oestrus, but she is ovulating

sleeping sickness, see encephalitis

slippered shoe, a shoe where the inside rim of the heel is thicker than the outside; also called bevelled

slough, dead tissue in the process of separating from the body

slow twitch (ST), a muscle fibre type which uses oxygen to burn glycogen and fatty acids to produce energy

sodium bicarbonate, may reduce effects of acidic environment in the exercising muscle; baking soda

sodium chloride, table salt; an essential electrolyte

soft laser treatment (SLT), laser therapy which uses a broad laser beam to stimulate wound healing and provide pain relief

soft palate, a sheet of tissue arising from the bottom of the hard palate and extending back and up across the nasopharynx towards the epiglottis

solution, the homogeneous mixture of one or more substances dispersed in a sufficient quantity of dissolving medium

somatomedin, a hormone which regulates growth

spasm, a sudden, involuntary contraction of a muscle or constriction of a passage

spasticity, increase in the normal tone of a muscle

spavin, an exostosis, usually medial, of the tarsus of equids due to degenerative joint disease

spavin test, a test in which the affected leg is held acutely flexed for about 2 minutes, then released immediately before the horse is trotted; considered positive for bone spavin or stifle problems if lameness is markedly increased for more than the first few steps

speculum, an instrument for enlarging the opening of a canal or cavity to permit examination; for vaginal examination, a hollow tube, usually about 16 inches long and 1½ inches in diameter, used to examine the vagina and cervix

spermicidal, destructive to sperm

sphincter muscle, circular muscle fibres or specially arranged oblique fibres which partially or totally reduce the opening of a tube or the interior of an organ

spinous processes, upward projections of the vertebrae

splayfooted, see toed-out; also called fetlock valgus

splint, inflammation of one of the two small metacarpal bones that run along the side of the cannon bone

spores, the reproductive elements of protozoa, fungi, algae, etc.

sprain, an injury in which some of the fibres of a ligament are stretched or ruptured

squamous, scaly or plate-like

squamous cell carcinoma, a malignant skin tumour derived from epithelial tissue; commonly called squames

Standardbred, a US and Canadian breed of trotting and pacing horse, used especially for harness racing

sterile, infertile or barren; or, having no infectious microorganisms on its surface

sterility, the inability to produce progeny

sternothyrohyoideus, the strap muscle which runs from the hyoid apparatus, down the underside of the neck, and connects to the sternum; helps keep the larynx and trachea open during athletic demand

sternum, the bone connecting the cartilages of the ribs; the breastbone

steroid, any member of the class of compounds that includes sterols, bile acids, and sex hormones

stethoscope, an instrument for hearing sounds made by the heart, lungs, and other internal organs

stiffness, the ability of a bone to resist being deformed by a stress

stimulus, an agent or action which produces a reaction

'stock up', swelling of the lower legs; caused by poor circulation due to pregnancy or restricted exercise

stomach worm, the internal parasites, *Habronema* sp. and *Trichostrongylus axei*; abnormal migration of *Habronema* larvae causes summer sores, or cutaneous habronemiasis

strain, an overstretching or overexertion of some part of a muscle or tendon; the degree to which a bone deforms to a stress

strangles, an infectious disease of horses caused by *Streptococcus equi* bacteria which invade the upper respiratory tract; characterized by enlarged lymph nodes under the jaw and throatlatch, and mucopurulent inflammation of the respiratory mucous membrane; also called distemper

strangulate, overloaded with blood due to constriction

straw itch mite, a mite whose bite causes small weals on the skin; commonly found in alfalfa hay or straw

streptolysin O, a toxin which remains in the bloodstream after a *Streptococcus equi* infection (strangles); allergic response to this toxin causes purpura haemorrhagica

stress tetany, a visible form of hyperirritability; signs include muscle twitching or spasms, the limbs stiffen, and the horse is nervous or jumpy

strongyles, various parasitic roundworms (family Strongylidae) commonly called bloodworms

stud chain, a chain which is passed over the nose as a method of restraint

subchondral bone, bone which lies underneath joint cartilage and supports it

subclinical infection, an infection which has no clinical symptoms, but can be spread to others

subcutaneous, beneath the skin

submandibular lymph nodes, lymph nodes under the jaw

subsolar corium, specialized skin tissue under the coffin bone which produces the sole and attaches it to the foot

sulci, the crevices of the frog

summer sores, sites of external inflammation caused by abnormal migration of *Habronema* larvae; also called cutaneous habronemiasis

superficial, near the surface; opposite of deep

superficial digital flexor muscle, the muscle attached to the superficial digital flexor tendon

superficial digital flexor tendon, one of two flexor tendons located along the back of the cannon bone

supportive treatment, that which is mainly directed at sustaining the strength of the patient

suppressor T-cells, cells of the immune system which suppress the action of other immune cells after the invader has been defeated

supraspinous, above a spine or spinous process

suspensory, a ligament, bone, muscle, sling, or bandage which holds up a part

suspensory desmitis, inflammation of the suspensory ligaments

swayback, a back deformity where the spine is concave when viewed from the side; common in older horses

sweat glands, glands near the skin surface which secrete sweat, which is composed of water, protein, and electrolytes

sweet feed, a concentrate grain mixture of corn, oats, barley, and molasses

symptom, evidence of a disease, as perceived and described by the patient; by definition, symptoms of a disease can truly only be found in humans

symptomatic, pertaining to or of the nature of a symptom

synchronous diaphragmatic flutter (SDF), see thumps

syndrome, a set of symptoms which occur together usually indicating a particular type of disease process

synovial capsule, the cavity containing synovia, or lubricating fluid, found in limb joints or bursae

synovial fluid, a viscous, transparent fluid, resembling the white of an egg, containing mucin and salts secreted by the synovial membrane and contained in joint cavities, bursae, and tendon sheaths for lubrication; reduces friction in the movement of joints, muscles, or tendons

synovial membrane, lining of a joint

systemic, relating to the entire organism as distinguished from any of its individual parts; pertaining to or affecting the whole body

teasing, showing a stallion to a mare to test her for sexual receptivity; especially useful when the mare exhibits no visible signs of oestrus

tendinitis, inflammation of tendons and musculotendinous attachments

tendons, bands of strong fibrous tissue that connect muscles to bones

tenosynovitis, inflammation of the tendon sheath

tension, see axial tension

testicles, the male gonads inside the scrotum which produce sperm cells and testosterone

testosterone, the male hormone produced in the testicles and responsible for the development and maintenance of secondary sex characteristics

tetanus, an infectious disease in which tonic muscle spasm and hyperreflexia result in lockjaw and generalized muscle spasm; caused by toxin of anaerobic *Clostridium tetani* bacteria

tetany, localized spasmodic contractions of muscles; may cause twitching or convulsions; caused by subnormal levels of blood calcium

therapeutic, relating to the treatment of disease; curative

therapeutic index, in drug use, the margin between the safe dose of a drug that will effect a cure, and the toxic dose that will kill the patient

therapy, the treatment of disease

thermoregulation, temperature control

thermoregulatory centre, that part of the brain which regulates internal body temperature within a very narrow range

third degree recto-vestibular laceration, occurs when a foal is delivered with a poorly aligned leg and the perineum is torn

thoracic, thorax, the chest; the part of the body between the neck and the diaphragm, encased by the ribs

thoroughpin, windgall of the Achilles tendon behind the hock

thromboembolic colic, colic due to obstruction of an intestinal blood vessel

thrombophlebitis, inflammation of a vein

thrombus, a clot in a blood vessel or in one of the cavities of the heart; caused by coagulation of blood in the area of damage

thrush, a degenerative condition of the frog; results from moist and unhygienic conditions; also called pododermatitis

thumps, repeated contraction of the diaphragm in rhythm with the heartbeat; caused by low blood levels of calcium, potassium, and magnesium; also called synchronous diaphragmatic flutter (SDF)

thyroid gland, an organ that secretes the hormone thyroxine, which increases the rate of metabolism

thyroxine, a hormone which acts as a catalyst and has wide-reaching effects on metabolism, growth, and immunity

tied in, a conformational fault where the measurement at the top of the cannon bone is less than the measurement at the bottom

tilted vagina, a conformational fault where the labia sit high above the pelvic brim, the anus is pulled forwards, and the vulva tilts horizontally; this often allows urine pooling on the vaginal floor

tipped vulva, a conformational fault where the vulva tilts forwards horizontally, allowing faeces to fall on the labia

tissue, an aggregation of similarly specialized cells united in the performance of a particular function

toed-in, see pigeon-toed; also called fetlock varus

toed-out, a conformational fault where the fetlock joint or carpus is rotated outwards; also called splayfooted, fetlock valgus, carpus valgus

topical, pertaining to a particular surface area, as in a topical ointment

torsion, twisting forces; twisting of the intestines in colic

toxaemia, a general intoxication or poisoning sometimes due to the absorption of toxins formed at a local source of infection

toxicity, quality of being poisonous

toxin, a poison produced by a living organism (endotoxin) or that is an integral component of a microorganism (exotoxin)

toxoid, a toxin which has been treated to inactivate its toxic properties but can still stimulate an immune response

trace minerals, mineral micronutrients required by the body in small amounts, for example, copper, manganese, and zinc

trachea, the windpipe, descending from the larynx to the bronchi

tracheobronchitis, inflammation of the trachea and bronchi

tranquillizer, an agent that produces a quieting or calming effect, without changing the level of consciousness

transcutaneous electrical nerve stimulation (TENS), a method of electrically stimulating acupuncture points to provide pain relief

transfusion, the introduction of whole blood or blood component directly into the bloodstream

transition zone, the areas just above and below a healing tendon injury

transitional period, the period which occurs at the beginning and end of the breeding season, marked by erratic oestrous cycles

transmission, a transfer of a disease, nerve impulse, or inheritable characteristic

trauma, a wound or injury

triglycerides, fat, composed of three fatty acids and one glycerol molecule

trombiculiasis, chigger bites

tubule, a small tube

tumour, a mass of new tissue which persists and grows independently of surrounding structures and has no useful function

turbulence, departure in a fluid or gas from a smooth flow

twitch, a device used to restrain a horse by placing pressure on the upper lip; also the contraction and relaxation of a muscle fibre

tying-up, see myositis

udder, see mammary gland

ulcer, a hollowed-out space on the surface of an organ or tissue due to the sloughing of dead tissue

ulcerated, affected with or of the condition of an ulcer

ultrasound, use of reflecting sound waves as a diagnostic tool to 'image' body parts or as a therapeutic tool to warm tissues

ultraviolet (UV) rays, light rays beyond the violet end of the light spectrum

upward fixation of the patella, when the ligament of the stifle is locked over the kneecap

urethra, the membranous canal for conveying urine from the bladder to the exterior of the body; also carries semen in the male

urethral extension surgery, surgery to 'build' a urethral tunnel so urine is voided clear of the mare's reproductive tract

urinalysis, a physical, chemical, or microscopic analysis or examination of urine

urine, the fluid excreted by the kidneys, passed through the ureters, stored in the bladder, and discharged through the urethra; healthy horse urine has a pale and cloudy yellow colour

urine pooling, collecting of urine on the vaginal floor; also called vesiculo-vaginal reflux (VVR)

urticaria, see hives

uterine biopsy, taking a tissue sample from the lining of the uterus to test for infection and abnormalities

uterus, the hollow, muscular organ, consisting of cervix, uterine body, and uterine horns

vaccine, a suspension of attenuated or killed microorganisms administered for the prevention or treatment of infectious diseases

vagina, the genital passageway that extends from the cervix to the vulva

vaginal speculum examination, examining the vagina and cervix using a hollow tube, usually about 16 inches long and 1½ inches in diameter

vaginitis, inflammation of the vagina

vagus nerve, the two recurrent laryngeal nerve branches which control the muscles controlling the arytenoid cartilages of the larynx; paralysis of the left branch is involved in roaring

vascular, pertaining to vessels

vasculitis, inflammation of vessels

vasoconstriction, diminution of blood vessels; leads to decreased blood flow to a specific area

vasodilator, causing enlargement of blood vessels

vector, an animal or insect that transmits a disease-producing organism

vein, a vessel through which the blood passes from various organs or parts back to the heart

Venezuelan equine encephalitis, see encephalitis

verrucous sarcoid, dry, wart-like, horny sarcoids which may resemble a cauliflower

vertebrae, the bone components of the spinal column

vesicular stomatitis, a localized inflammation of the soft tissues of the mouth, containing blisters or other lesions

vesiculo-vaginal reflux (VVR), see urine pooling

vessel, any channel for carrying a fluid

vestibular seal, a barrier to uterine infection created by the back of the vagina, the hymen, and the pelvic floor

vestibule, the vaginal area posterior to the hymen

villi, hair-like projections on certain mucous membranes

viral shift, the appearance of an entirely new strain of a virus due to the combination of two different strains

virulent, exceedingly pathogenic or noxious

virus, a microscopic agent of infectious disease which lacks metabolism and can reproduce only in living tissue or a culture medium

volar annular ligament, a non-elastic band of connective tissue running horizontally across the back of the fetlock

volatile fatty acids, an immediate aerobic energy source; produced from roughage fermentation in the large intestine

vulva, the external genitalia of the female, comprised of the labia, the clitoris, the vestibule of the vagina and its glands, and the opening of the urethra and of the vagina

wall, a layer enclosing a space (such as the chest, abdomen, or hollow organ) or mass of material (such as the hoof wall)

warbles, a genus of insects called *Hypoderma* whose larvae migrate through the skin to the back and are seen as a nodule with a breathing pore; *Hypoderma* adults are also called heel flies

warts, skin tumours caused by a papilloma virus

water-soluble, able to be broken down by water

wave mouth, a condition of uneven teeth wear found mainly in older horses

weals, smooth, slightly raised areas of the skin surface which are redder or paler than the surrounding areas

weaving, a nervous condition or habit affecting horses suffering from boredom; the horse continually shifts its weight from one leg to another and sways the upper torso

wedge pad, a pad that is thicker at the heel than at the toe

weight-bearing, applying normal body weight to a limb

white blood cells, immune cells responsible for protecting the body from microorganisms

white line, margin of horn between the sole and the hoof wall; acts as soft cementing material between the wall and sole; line through which nails should be driven when shoeing

white pastern disease, dermatitis caused by a staphylococcal bacterium

windgalls, inflammation of a joint and/or tendon sheaths

windsucking, see pneumovagina

winging, a gait defect in which the front feet are thrown outwards from the knee; common in base-narrow, toed-out horses

winking, protrusion of the clitoris between the labia, frequently observed in mares in oestrus

wobbler's syndrome, a disease that effects the cervical spinal cord and vertebrae of young horses; marked by incoordination

wolf teeth, small teeth that erupt in upper jaw, usually in front of the molars; vestigial premolar

X-rays, roentgen rays, electromagnetic vibrations of short wavelength that penetrate most substances to some degree, used to take radiographs of the body, thus locating fractures, etc.

yes joint, the joint between the atlas vertebra and the skull which moves the head up and down; also called atlanto-occipital joint

Index

gaskin, 20
gastric ulcers, 169, 289
girth sleeve, 364
glucose, 40
glycerol, 40
glycogen, 40, 41, 50–1
grain
  alternative to, 193
  barley, 184
  maize, 184
  oats, 184, 185
  overconsumption, treatment, 94–5
  proportions, 198
granulation tissue, 252, 371
gut sounds, 219

haemagglutinin, 119, 144
harvest mites (chiggers), 335
hay, 180, 182–3
  alfalfa, 185
  calcium to phosphorus ratio, 182
  grass, 182
  legume, 182
  moisture content, 183
  nutritional value, 182
  wetting, 128
head bumper, 449
head size, 3
heart murmurs, 168
heart rate, 144–8
  high altitudes, 233
  increase
    persistent, 217
    sign of discomfort, 441
  monitoring for stress, 145–8
  recovery, 145, 217–18
  see also inversion
heat increment (HI), 198–201
  grains versus roughage, 198–9
heat stress
  determining, 224–6
  prevention, 141, 197, 225
heat therapy, 240–2
heaves *see* COPD
heels
  cracked, 343–5
  expansion, 82

sheared, 83–4
herd instinct, 430
high altitudes, 233
  heart rate, 233
hill work, 55–6
hind legs, 22–4
hindquarters, 19–24
hives, 348–52, 403
hobble *see* restraint
hocks, 23–4
hoof
  alignment, 82
  balanced, 84
  biomechanics, 80
  care, 81
  colour, 68–9
  cracks, 77–9
  dressings, 71–3
  exercise, 73–4
  growth, 69, 72
  horn tubule
    abnormal growth, 73, 93
    growth, 70
  long-toe– low-heel (LTLH), 162
  size, 69
  strength, 70, 71–2
  toughening of, 71
  unbalanced, 162
  wall, 70
    elastic properties, 82–3
    growth rates, 69–70
    loss of flexibility, 82
    rings, 76, 88
  see also feet
hoof tester, 101
hoof–pastern axis angle, broken, 249
hormonal imbalance, 211–12
horn fly, 332
horse flies, 327
horseshoe *see* shoeing
hot climates, diet and feeding, 197–203
hyaluronic acid (HA), 218
hydrogen peroxide, 380
hydrotherapy, 242
hyoid, 110
hyperlipidaemia, 213

CONTENTS

POSSESSED
P.C. CAST

This one is for my man, the Rose. Thank you for reminding me about hope. I love you.

ACKNOWLEDGEMENTS

I want to send hugs and kisses to Gena Showalter! It is beyond awesome to be able to work on cool projects with my girlfriend. Ms Snowwater, I totally heart you!

A big thank you to my wonderful, long-time editor Mary-Theresa Hussey. It is *soooo* nice to be working with you again!

Katie Rowland—
THANK YOU FOR THE TU DETAILS.
Now go get ready for finals. Seriously.

As always, I appreciate, respect and adore my agent, Meredith Bernstein.

1

The bully's dad caused Raef to discover his Gift. It happened twenty-five years ago, but to Raef the memory was as fresh as this morning's coffee. You just don't forget your first time. Not your first orgasm, your first drunk, your first kill and, not for damn sure, your first experience of being able to Track violent emotions.

The bully's name was Brandon. He'd been a big kid; at thirteen he'd looked thirty-five—and a rough thirty-five at that. At least, that's what he'd looked like through nine-year-old Raef's eyes. Not that Brandon picked on Raef. He hadn't—not especially. Brandon mostly liked to pick on girls. He didn't hit 'em. What he did was worse. He found out what scared them, and then he tortured them with fear.

Raef discovered why the day Brandon went after Christina Kambic with the dead bird. Christina wasn't hot. Christina wasn't ugly. She was just a girl who had seemed like every other teenage girl to young Raef: she had boobs and she talked a lot, two things that, even at nine, Raef had understood were part of the pleasure and the pain of females.

Brandon didn't target Christina because of her boobs or her mouth.

He targeted her because somehow he had found out she was utterly, completely terrified of birds.

The part of the day that was burned into Raef's memory began after school. Brandon had been walking home on the opposite side of the street from Raef and his best friend, Kevin. On Brandon's side of the street was a group of girls. They were giggling and talking at about a zillion miles per hour. Brandon was ahead of them and, as usual, by himself. Brandon didn't really have any friends. Raef had barely noticed him and only kinda remembered that he'd been kicking around something near the curb.

Raef and Kevin had been talking about baseball tryouts. He'd wanted to be shortstop. Kev had wanted to be the pitcher. Raef had been saying, "Yeah, you got a better arm than Tommy. No way would Coach pick—"

That's when Christina's bawling had started.

"No, please no, stop!" She was pleading while she cried. Two of her friends had screamed and run off down the street. Two more had stayed and were yelling at Brandon to stop.

Brandon ignored all of them. He'd backed Christina against the fence to Mr. Fulton's front yard, taken the smashed body of what was obviously a road-killed crow and was holding it up, real close to Christina, and making stupid cawing noises while he laughed.

"Please!" Christina sobbed, her face in her hands, pressing herself against the wooden fence so hard that Raef had thought she might smash through it. "I can't stand it! Please stop!"

Raef had thought about how big Brandon was, and how much older Brandon was, and he'd stood there across the street, ignoring Kevin and doing nothing. Then Brandon pushed the dead bird into Christina's hair and the girl started screaming like she was being murdered.

"Hey, this isn't your business," Kevin had said when Raef sighed heavily and started crossing the street.

"Doesn't have to be my business. It just has to be mean," Raef had shot back over his shoulder at his friend.

"Bein' a hero's gonna get you in a lot of trouble someday," Kevin had said.

Raef remembered silently agreeing with him. But still he kept crossing the street. He got to Brandon from behind. Quickly, like he was fielding a ball, he snatched the bird out of Christina's hair, and threw it down the street. Way down the street.

"What the fuck is your problem, asshole?" Brandon shouted, looming over Raef like a crappy version of the Incredible Hulk.

"Nothin'. I just think making a girl cry is stupid." Raef had looked around Brandon's beefy body at Christina. Her feet musta been frozen because she was still standing there, bawling and shaking, and hugging herself like she was trying to keep from falling apart. "Go on home, Christina," Raef urged. "He ain't gonna bother you anymore."

It was about two point five seconds later that Brandon's fist slammed into Raef's face, breaking his nose and knocking him right on his butt.

Raef remembered he was holding his bleeding nose and looking up at the big kid through tears of pain and he'd thought, Why the hell are you so mean?

That's when it happened. The instant Raef had wondered about Brandon, a weird ropelike thing had appeared around the boy. It was smoky and dark, and Raef had thought it looked like it must stink. It was snaking from Brandon up, into the air.

It fascinated Raef.

He stared at it, forgetting about his nose. Forgetting about Christina and Kevin, and even Brandon. All he wanted was to know what the smoky rope was.

"Fucking look at me when I'm talking to you! It's sickening how easy it is to kick your ass!" Brandon's anger and disgust fed the rope. It pulsed and darkened, and with a whoosh! it exploded down and *into Raef. Suddenly Raef could feel Brandon's anger. He could feel his disgust.*

Completely freaked out, Raef had closed his eyes and yelled, not at Brandon, at the creepy rope, "Go away!" Then the most bizarre thing happened. The rope-thing had gone away, but in Raef's mind he went with it. It was like the thing had turned into a telescope and all of a sudden Raef saw Brandon's home—inside it. Brandon was there. So were his dad and mom. His dad, an older, fatter version of Brandon, was towering over his mom, who was curled up on the couch, holding herself while she cried and shook like Christina had just been doing. Brandon's dad was yelling at his mom, calling her an ugly, stupid bitch. Brandon watched. He looked disgusted, but not at his dad. His look was focused on his mom. And he was pissed. Really, really pissed.

It made Raef want to puke. The instant he felt sick, actually felt his own feelings again, it was like turning off a light switch. The rope disappeared, along with the telescope and the vision of Brandon's house, leaving Raef back in the very painful, very embarrassing present.

Raef opened his eyes and said the first thing that popped into his head. "How can you blame your mom for your dad being so mean?"

Brandon's body got real still. It was like he quit breathing. Then his face turned beet-red and he shouted down at Raef, spit raining from his mouth. "What did you just say about my mom?"

Raef often wondered why the hell he hadn't just shut up. Got up. And run away. Instead, like a moron, he'd said, "Your dad picks on your mom like you pick on girls. I know 'cause I just saw it. Inside my head. Somehow. I don't know how, though." Raef had paused, thought for a second and then added, trying to figure it out aloud, "Your dad was calling your mom an ugly, stupid bitch last night. You watched him."

Then the weird got, like, weird squared because Brandon reacted as if Raef had all of a sudden grown two feet, gained a hundred pounds and punched him in the gut. The big kid looked sick, scared even, and started backing away, but before he turned and sprinted down the street, he yelled the words that would cling to Raef for the rest of his life. "I know what you are! You're worse than a nigger, worse than a creeper. You're a Psy—a fucking freak. Stay the hell away from me!"

Oh, shit. It was true. No way…no way…

Raef had sat there, bloody, confused and—embarrassingly enough—bawling, while his best friend called his name over and over, trying to get him to snap out of it. "Raef! Raef! Raef…"

"Mr. Raef? Raef? Are you there, sir?"

Coming back to the present, Raef shook himself, mentally and physically, and picked up the phone, punching the intercom button off. "Yeah, Preston, what is it?"

"Mr. Raef, your zero-nine-hundred appointment is here, thirty minutes early."

Raef cleared his throat and said, "You know, Preston, it's a damn shame my Gift doesn't include predicting the future, or I'd have known that and been ready for her."

"Yes, sir, but then I would probably be out of a job," Preston retorted with his usual dry humor.

Raef chuckled. "Nah, there'd still be all that filing to do."

"It's what I live for, sir."

"Glad to hear it. Okay, give me five and send her in."

"Of course, Mr. Raef. Then I'll get back to my filing."

Raef blew out a breath, grabbed his half-empty coffee mug and stalked over to the long credenza that sat against the far wall of his spacious office. He topped off the coffee and then stood there, unmoving, staring out the window. Not that he was actually seeing the excellent view of Tulsa's skyline on this crisp fall day. Kent Raef was trying to scratch the weird itch that had been tickling his mind all morning.

What the hell was wrong with him? Why the walk down

memory lane this morning? God, he hated the thought of that day—hated remembering that scared, crying kid he'd been. He'd just wanted to be shortstop for his team, and try to fit in with everyone else. Instead, he'd been a psychic. The only one in his class. Norms didn't react so well to a Psy—especially not a nine-year-old Psy that could Track violent emotions, no matter how supportive his parents had been—no matter how cool it had been when the USAF Special Forces had recruited him. Raef hated remembering those years and the pain in the ass it had been learning to deal with his Gift and the way asshole Norms reacted to it.

It made him feel like shit to go back there—to revisit those memories. Today it also made him feel kinda shaky, kinda strange. If he didn't know better he'd think he was picking up emotions from someone—soft emotions, like yearning and desire, overshadowed by a deep melancholy.

"Shit, Raef, get it together," he grunted to himself. He did know better. Soft emotions? He snorted. *His* psychic powers didn't work that way—didn't ever work that way. A pissed-off jerk who took out his problems by kicking his dog was the softest Psy Tracking he'd ever picked up. "I need to get a life," he muttered as he returned to his desk and sat down, just in time for the single knock on the door. "Yeah, come in," he snapped.

The door opened, and his secretary, Preston, announced, "Mrs. Wilcox to see you, Mr. Raef."

Raef automatically stood as the tall blonde entered his office. He held out his hand to her, and ignored the fact that she hesitated well into the realm of rudeness before she shook it. A lot of Norms didn't like to be touched by his kind, but *she* had come to *him,* not the other way around, and so she was going to have to play by his rules. On his team, a handshake was nonnegotiable.

Of course, her hesitation might be due to the fact that his skin was too brown for her liking—she did have the look of one of those fiftysomething, old-oil-money cougars who were convinced that their shit didn't stink, and that the only reason God made anyone with skin a darker shade than lily-white was because of the unfortunate but unavoidable need for menial laborers.

"Constance Wilcox," she said, finally taking his hand in a grip that was surprisingly firm. He recognized the name as belonging to one of Tulsa society's elite, though he definitely didn't move in those circles.

"Kent Raef. Coffee, Mrs. Wilcox?"

She shook her head with a curt motion. "No, thank you, Mr. Raef."

"All right. Please have a seat." Raef waited for her to settle into one of the straight-backed leather chairs in front of his wide desk before he sat. He didn't particularly like the fact that he'd had old-world gentleman programmed into his genes, but some habits were just not worth the effort it took to break them.

"What can I do for you, Mrs. Wilcox?"

"Don't you already know that?"

He tried not to let his annoyance show. "Mrs. Wilcox, I'm sure my secretary explained that I wouldn't be Reading you. That's now how my Gift works. So, relax. There's no reason for you to be nervous around me."

"If you can't read my mind, how do you know that I need to relax and that I'm nervous?"

"Mrs. Wilcox, you're sitting ramrod straight and you've got your hands so tightly laced together that your fingers are white. It doesn't take a psychic to tell that you're tense and that your nerves are on edge. Anyone with half a brain and moderate powers of observation could deduce that. Besides that, my Gift deals with the darker side of the paranormal. People don't come to me to find lost puppies or communicate with the ghost of Elvis. People come to me because bad things have happened to them or around them, and bad things happening in a person's life tend to make him or her—" he tipped his head to her in a slight nod "—nervous and tense."

She glanced down at her clasped hands and made a visible effort to relax them. Then she looked back at him. "I'm sorry. It's just that I'm not comfortable with this."

"This?" No, hell, no. He wasn't going to make it any easier for her. Not this morning. Not when it felt like something was trying to crawl under his skin. He was fucking sick and tired of dealing with people who hired psychics from After Moonrise, but acted as if they'd find it more desirable to work side by side with someone who was unclogging their backed-up septic tank—by hand.

"Death." She said the word so softly Raef almost didn't hear her.

He blinked in surprise. So, it wasn't the psychic part that had her acting like an ice queen—it was the dead part. That was easier for him to understand. Death, specifically murder, was his job. But that didn't mean he liked it, either.

"Death is rarely a comfortable subject." He paused and, realizing there was a distinct possibility he had come off like a prick, attempted to look understanding. "All right, Mrs. Wilcox, how about we start over. You do your best to relax, and I'll do my best to help you."

Her smile was tight-lipped, but at least it was a smile. "That sounds reasonable, Mr. Raef."

"So, you're here because of a death."

"Yes. I am also here because I don't have anywhere else left to go," she said.

He'd definitely heard that before, and it didn't make him feel all warm and cuddly and saviorlike, as it would have made some of After Moonrise's other psychics like Claire or Ami or even Stephen feel. Which made sense. They could sometimes save people. Raef only dealt with the aftermath of violence and murder. There was no damn salvation there.

"Then let's get to it, Mrs. Wilcox." He knew he sounded gruff, intimidating even. He meant to. It usually made things move faster.

"My daughter Lauren needs your help. She's why I'm here."

"Lauren was murdered?" Raef dropped the gruffness from his voice. Now he simply sounded clinical and detached, as if he was a lab technician discussing ways to deal with a diagnosis of terminal cancer. He picked up his pen, wrote and underlined *Lauren* at the top of a fresh legal pad, and then glanced back at Mrs. Wilcox, waiting semipatiently for the rest of the story.

She pressed her lips together into a tight line, clearly trying to hold in words too painful to speak. Then she drew a deep breath. "No, Lauren was not murdered. She is alive, but she's not whole anymore. She's only partially here. I need your help to restore her spirit."

"Mrs. Wilcox, I think there has been a mistake made in scheduling. It sounds to me like you need to meet with another member of the After Moonrise team—one of our shamans who specialize in shattered souls. My powers only manifest if there is a murder involved." He started to lift the phone to buzz Preston, but her next words made him hesitate.

"My daughter *was* murdered."

"Mrs. Wilcox, you just said that Lauren is alive."

"Lauren is alive. It's her twin, Aubrey, who was murdered."

Raef put down the phone. "One twin was murdered, and the other's alive?"

"If you can call it that." Her face was pale, her expression strained, but she was keeping herself from crying.

Despite his bad mood his interest stirred. A living twin and a murdered twin? He'd never encountered a murder case like that before.

"Mr. Raef, the situation is that one of my daughters was murdered three months ago. Since then my other daughter has become only a shell of herself. Lauren is haunted by Aubrey."

Raef nodded. "It happens fairly often. When two people are very close—siblings, husband and wife, parent and child—and one of them dies or is murdered, the deceased's spirit lingers."

"Yes, I know," she said impatiently. "Especially when the murder is unsolved."

Raef sat up straighter. This was more like it. "Then you *have* come to the right psychic. I'll need to be taken to the murder scene, and will also need to speak with Lauren. If her twin is haunting her, then I can probably make direct contact with Aubrey through Lauren and piece together what happened. Once the murder is solved, Aubrey should be able to rest peacefully." He rubbed his forehead, wishing the uncomfortable feeling of yearning would get the hell out from under his skin. He was *not* that nine-year-old kid anymore. He was tough, competent, and he knew how to handle his shit.

"Yes, peace. That's what I'm here to find. For both of my girls."

"I'm going to try to help you, Mrs. Wilcox. You said Aubrey was killed three months ago? And the murder hasn't been solved yet? It's unusual that the forensic psychic wasn't able to close this file."

Her blue eyes iced over and the sadness that had been shadowing them was frozen out. "Is solving my daughter's murder what you mean by closing this file?"

Damn! He'd actually said that aloud. What the hell was wrong with him? He might not have the graveside manner of someone like touchy-feely Stephen, but Raef usually showed more tact than offhandedly insulting an already upset client.

"Yes, ma'am. I'm sorry that my wording seemed callous. I assure you that I am cognizant of, and sorry for, your loss."

She continued as if he hadn't spoken. "The reason Aubrey's file wasn't closed is because the police psychic couldn't communicate with my daughter about the murder. Either one of them."

Raef frowned. "That's highly unusual, Mrs. Wilcox. Did you give legal permission for your daughter's spirit to be questioned?"

"Of course," she snapped. "But it's not that simple with Aubrey and Lauren. It never has been."

"I'm sorry, ma'am. I don't understand what—"

Her imperiously raised hand cut him off. "Perhaps it would be easier if I showed you." Without waiting for Raef's response or permission, she stood and walked quickly to the office door. Opening it she said, "You can come in now, Lauren."

The woman who entered his office looked like a younger version of her mother—a leggy, twentysomething blonde with waves of platinum hair so light it was almost white. Her body was lusher than her mother's, who had the appearance of too many carb-free years and maintenance liposuction. Lauren, on the other hand, looked like she might enjoy a burger and a beer once in a while. Scratch that—the expensive silk knit sweater and the designer slacks and shoes said she might enjoy a fillet, a fancied-up potato and some expensive red wine once in a while.

His gaze traveled from her curvy body to her gray-blue eyes, and he felt his own narrow in response to what he saw—emptiness. Her smoky eyes were as expressionless as her face.

Lauren stopped in front of his desk and stared blankly over his shoulder. Then there was a shimmering in the air around her, and a transparent duplicate of her materialized.

It was as Raef got to his feet to face this new apparition that it hit him like a punch in the gut. The ghost radiated waves of emotion—yearning, desire, loneliness, longing—emotions Raef had never picked up from another human being, dead or alive, since his psychic talent first manifested that day so many years ago.

He tried to throw up his mental barriers, the ones he used at murder scenes to successfully block out the lingering spirits and their terror and pain and anger, the only emotions he had, until now, ever been able to Read. But his barriers weren't working. All he could do was stand there and be battered by the desire and longing that emanated from the ghost.

"Kent Raef?" The spirit's voice drifted through his mind.

He cleared his throat before he answered, but his voice still sounded scratchy. "Yes. I'm Kent Raef."

The spirit sighed with relief. *"Finally!"* She glanced at her twin. Lauren blinked, as if coming awake after a long sleep, and the ghost and the girl exchanged smiles. *"Good job, sis."*

"You knew I'd figure it out eventually," Lauren said.

"And you know it bothers me terribly when you speak to the air like that," said Mrs. Wilcox.

"I can tell that corncob is still firmly inserted up your butt, Mother," said the ghost.

Lauren coughed to cover a giggle, which was echoed by the ghost, who laughed out loud.

The laughter in the room raced across his body like static electricity, tingling and bringing all the nerve endings in his skin alive, totally disconcerting him.

Raef pulled his thoughts together. *Ignore the emotions. You can figure out what the hell is going on with that later.* Right now he just needed to do his job—solve the murder, put the spirit to rest, close the case file.

"Aubrey, why don't you tell me about your death and from there I can "

Raef was interrupted by a shriek that moved across his skin with the force of a blow. Aubrey's mouth was wrenched open as she screamed in agony, a sound that was echoed eerily by her living sister, then her spirit wavered, like heat waves off a furnace, and she disappeared.

2

"So you saw, or at least heard something?" Mrs. Wilcox's words were clipped, and in the silence that followed Aubrey's disappearance her voice sounded unnaturally loud.

"Aubrey manifested and spoke to me. Briefly." Raef answered her, although he didn't look at the older woman. Instead, he was watching Lauren carefully, noting that her empty expression hadn't returned, and even though her face couldn't be called animated, she at least didn't look zombielike anymore. And also noting that the torrent of emotions that had poured from Aubrey had been abruptly cut off. He cleared his throat, wishing like hell his coffee had a shot of Jack in it. "Please have a seat, Miss Wilcox. There are several things I need to go over with both you and your—"

"Why don't you go home, Mother?" Lauren surprised him by interrupting in a brisk, no-nonsense voice as she sat in the chair beside her mother's. "It would probably be better if I answered his questions alone."

"What if it returns, Lauren?"

"Mother, I've told you before that I see Aubrey a lot. She's dead. That doesn't make her an it. She's still Aubrey."

"I wasn't speaking of your sister's ghost," Mrs. Wilcox said coolly. "I'm referring to the horrid fugue state that sometimes comes over you."

"Mother, I've tried to explain this to you before, too. It doesn't just 'come over' me. There's a reason for it." Mrs. Wilcox's face remained implacable and Lauren sighed. "I'm not going to be driving. If I zone out again I'm sure Mr. Raef can babysit me long enough to get me home."

"Lauren, I…" her mother began, and then seemed to check herself. She stood and inclined her head formally to Raef. "I assume you will be certain my daughter returns home safely?"

"I will," Raef said, not liking the family drama he'd stepped into.

"Then I will speak to you later, Lauren. It was a pleasure to meet you, Mr. Raef."

After the door closed behind her mother, Lauren sat and met Raef's gaze. "She's not as cold and uncaring as she comes off as being. But all of this is just too much for her."

"Define *this*," he said.

"*This* would be my sister's death and the fact the police have been unable to solve it. Add a dash of Aubrey haunting me with a sprinkle of possession and stir in a big blob of my soul being drained and you get a recipe that would freak out anyone's mom." Lauren's voice was calm, her body appeared relaxed. It was only in her blue eyes that her desperation showed.

Raef got up and walked to the credenza. He topped off his coffee and then poured a generous cup for Lauren. "Cream or sugar, Miss Wilcox?" he asked over his shoulder.

"Both, and if we're going to work together I wish you'd call me Lauren."

He fixed the coffee and then handed it to her. "Lauren it is. My friends call me Raef." He resumed his seat and gave her a brief smile. "Actually, my enemies call me Raef, too."

"Do you have many enemies, Raef?"

"Some," he said. "Do you?"

She shook her head. "No."

"How about your sister?"

"No. That's just one of the reasons this whole thing is so awful. None of it makes sense."

"Tell me what you know about your sister's death, and I'll see if I can begin making some sense out of it."

"I don't know where to start." Lauren's impassive expression tensed and when she sipped her coffee Raef noticed her hands were trembling.

"Start at the beginning. When was she killed?"

"July 15. She was alone, even though she shouldn't have been. I'm almost always with her on jobs—" She paused, flinched in obvious pain. "I mean, I *used to* almost always be with her." Lauren corrected herself and regained her composure, then continued in a steadier voice. "July is in the middle of our busy season for maintenance, so we often had to split up to finish jobs on time."

"Maintenance? What type of work did you and your sister do?"

"Landscaping. July can be a rough month on plants if we don't get enough rain and the Oklahoma heat turns up early, like it did this past July. Plants burn up if they're not maintained properly through the heat. Aub and I own Two Sisters Landscaping. Or at least we did." She faltered again, and took another sip of her coffee. "I'm sole owner now."

"Of the company? As in you are the biggest stockholder?"

"Own the company as in Aubrey and I started it, ran it

and were its first two employees." She met his eyes. "Yes, we actually got our hands dirty. A lot." She held up one hand and Raef's brows lifted in surprise when he saw that instead of being well manicured and delicately white, Lauren had short, bluntly clipped nails and obvious calluses on her work-hardened palm. He would have never guessed that the daughters of a rich Tulsa socialite would be into something as blue-collar as landscaping.

"I would have thought a psychic would be better at hiding his thoughts," Lauren said.

Raef looked from her hand to her eyes. Then, much to his own surprise, he heard himself admitting, "I usually am."

"Dirt-digging girls from rich families must seem pretty unusual to you," Lauren said.

Raef gave her a lopsided smile. "Sounds like it's a reaction you're used to."

"Let's just say our family wasn't thrilled when Aubrey and I opened the business six years ago. We were lucky they couldn't stop us."

"Explain that," Raef said. He didn't feel the prickle of foreboding he usually did when he stumbled on what would eventually become a lead for solving a murder, so he really didn't need to question Lauren about her family's attitude about her business, but he realized he *wanted* to question her—wanted to know more.

And that was odd as hell.

"Aubrey and I received an inheritance from our grandfather when we turned twenty-one. It was ours to do whatever we wanted with—so we started our own business, but instead of buying a chic little boutique in Utica Square someone else could run, or following family tradition and investing in real estate, we bought plants and dirt. At least, that's how our mother put it. Our decision wasn't popular, but it was ours to make."

"So, how was business?"

"Excellent. It still is. We have five employees and have had to actually turn away jobs. That's why Aubrey was alone that day—we'd overextended and she was the expert in aquatic plants. So she went by herself to Swan Lake."

Raef felt a shock of recognition, and couldn't believe he hadn't put two and two together before then. "Aubrey Wilcox, middle of July, electrocuted to death while she was working with the water plants on the Swan Lake island." Then he realized why he hadn't recognized the name on his appointment book. It wasn't a murder investigation. The death had been ruled accidental. What the hell?

"It wasn't an accident," Lauren said firmly, as if she was the mind reader.

"But if I pulled the police report it would say your sister's death was accidental, wouldn't it?"

"Yes. Does that mean you won't take the case?"

"No, I'll take the case." Which was nothing unusual. Sometimes families needed his services for closure. Hell, not just *his* services, but psychics in general. The police could tell the bereaved over and over that it was suicide, or an accident, and they would still hold on to the hope that there was a bad guy, a reason, a focus for their rage and despair. That's where a Psy came in—and it was one of the reasons they'd become big business, even in a world that was mostly filled with Norms who were uncomfortable with psychic Gifts. By communicating with the spirit of the dead person directly, a psychic could help families come to terms with the truth, move on, find closure. Of course, Raef personally usually preferred a good, old-fashioned murder case—hatred and anger he could deal with. Despair was another story.

"Aubrey told me she was killed."

Raef shook himself mentally. "I thought your sister's spirit was having a hard time communicating about her death." He'd witnessed that. He'd asked her about her murder and she definitely *hadn't* communicated with him.

"She *is* having a hard time communicating. When I say she *told me* I don't mean that she actually said, 'Hey, sis, I was murdered.' I mean she told me in here." Lauren closed her fist over her heart. "There are things she's not allowed to put into words, but I can *feel* them. She and I have always been two halves of the same whole. I don't know how else to explain it because if you're not us, it might be impossible to comprehend. Add to the whole confusing mix that whatever is going on after Aub's death is affecting me, and you have some serious weirdness. Raef, the truth is, even I don't understand what's really happening. I was hoping you could help me—help us. Please help us, Raef."

Raef paused, studied Lauren and collected his thoughts. When he finally spoke it was slowly, as if he was processing information aloud. "The police ruled her death an accident, but your twin has made it clear to you, and only you, that she was murdered. Is that correct?"

"Yes."

"And even though she manifests to you, which I've witnessed, there still seems to be some barrier between the two of you, as if she's being blocked or controlled by another force?"

"Yes, especially when she tries to communicate with me directly about her murder." She sounded incredibly relieved. "You can't know what a relief it is to talk to someone who doesn't call me a freak and who will actually listen to me!"

His smile was authentic, but grim. "Try being a nine-year-old who can Track negative emotions, and only negative emotions. I understand what it's like to be discounted and called a freak."

Lauren expelled a long breath in a relieved sigh. Her shoulders relaxed and she finally took a sip of her coffee. "Good. Then we talk the same language."

"So your sister is actually possessing you," he said, looking up from the notes he was taking. That was unusual. Possession by a spirit wasn't unheard of, of course, but spirits didn't usually possess family members. He couldn't remember ever hearing of one twin possessing another.

"Well, I don't know if you'd call it real possession. She manifests, like she did earlier, and we can talk." She paused, blinking hard as if trying to keep herself from crying. "I miss her. A lot. I don't feel normal without her." Lauren shook her head and wiped at her eyes. "But that's not what's important. What's important is that when she does try to communicate with me about her death, she gets ripped away from here and I can feel what's happening to her, and it's like…" Lauren's words trailed off. She shuddered. "It's like I'm being killed, too."

"Hang on. Your sister's already dead. Maybe what you're feeling is her struggle to stay attached to you while her spirit is being drawn to the Otherworld. Lauren, the truth is that for most spirits it is difficult for them to remain on this plane of existence. They should be moving on." He tried to speak soothingly, but he wasn't good at the touchy-feely stuff. Plus, it was looking more and more as if he should just refer Lauren and her family, dead and alive, to the After Moonrise medium.

"You're not getting it," Lauren said, looking more and more

animated. "Aubrey isn't moving on. She can't. He's not done killing her."

"Come again?"

Lauren sighed. "This is what Aubrey has been able to tell me: her killer has bound her spirit. He's bound all of their spirits. Physical death was just the beginning of their murders. He doesn't stop until he drains their souls of life, too. You have to find him. He's not done killing."

3

"And you know that this psychic serial killer is draining spirits because your sister told you in there." Raef pointed to where Lauren still clenched her fist over her heart.

Her spine stiffened and her chin went up. "Don't patronize me, Raef. I know it the same way you know you're talking to ghosts of the dead instead of your own overactive imagination, even though no one else can see and feel what you do."

"All right." He nodded his head slowly. "You got me there." He stood up and took his keys from his desk drawer. "Then let's go."

"Go?"

"To the scene of Aubrey's accident."

"You mean to the place she was murdered," Lauren said firmly.

"Either way, I need to check it out." He raised a dark brow at her when she didn't move. "You did know that it is my standard procedure to go to the site of the death, didn't you?"

"Yes—yes, I knew," she stuttered. "It's just that, well, I haven't been back there since."

"Not once? Not even when your sister has been manifesting to you?"

Lauren shook her head. "No." The word was a whisper.

"I can take you home first," he said, walking around his desk to her. "We can talk afterward and—"

"Would it be better if I come with you?" she interrupted, her voice sounding firmer. "I mean, for you and the investigation."

"It probably would be, especially because your situation is so unique."

Lauren stood. "Then I'll go."

THE TRIP FROM THE After Moonrise downtown offices to Midtown's Swan Lake was short and silent. Not that Raef minded. He was naturally quiet and never had understood the need most people felt to chatter uncomfortably to fill a peaceful lull. He also had to ready himself for what would happen when he visited the site of a death and opened himself to the psychic images left there. Accident or murder, it wasn't exactly a walk in the damn park, and it was always better to take a quiet moment to center himself first.

As he drove down Utica Street, he glanced at Lauren. Her face was pale and set. She was staring straight ahead. He thought she looked like a marble sculpture of herself.

"It's not going to be that bad," he said, turning right at the entrance to the lake and parking his car along the curb that ringed the area. "I'm the psychic, remember?" Raef tried to add some lightness to the moment.

She turned cold blue eyes on him. "She was my sister. My

twin. We've been together since we were conceived. Psychic or not, going to the place where she was killed scares me."

Before he could even try to come up with something comforting to say, her gaze moved from his to Swan Lake. She shook her head and gave a little humorless laugh, saying, "It's stupid to call this place a lake. It's tiny. Except for having water, there's nothing 'lake' about it."

"They call it Swan Lake because Swan Pond doesn't sound right," he said.

She looked back at him. "I hate this place."

He nodded. "That's a normal reaction, Lauren. Your sister died here—of course you have a strong negative reaction to it."

"There's more to it than that."

He wanted to tell her that the relatives of the dead always felt like there was more to it than simple death, even if it took their loved one peacefully, in the middle of the night, during the winter of life. Instead, he swallowed back the condescension and said, "Are you ready? You can wait here if you need to."

"I'm ready, and I'm going with you."

She sounded one hundred percent sure, but her face was still unnaturally pale as they walked slowly to the sidewalk that circled the oblong-shaped body of water. Raef thought that Lauren had been right—the place was no damn lake, even if it was pretty and well tended. The sidewalk had only a fourth of a mile circumference, or at least that's what the helpful signpost said. It was the same signpost that talked about the different types of waterfowl that could be found in the area, in particular noting the mated pair of swans for which the lake had been named.

The sign also asked visitors not to feed the fowl, including the swans. And it insisted everyone except "authorized personnel" remain outside the fence that ringed the area.

"The entrance to the dock that takes you to the island is over there." Lauren pointed down the sidewalk to their right.

Raef nodded and they continued walking. He glanced around them. The October morning hadn't turned cold and cloudy yet, as Channel Six weather had predicted. Big surprise that they got it wrong. So it was a gorgeous morning, but an off hour, only just before 10:00 a.m. Too late for morning walkers and bird-watchers, and too early for those who liked to eat their lunch at the park. There was only a retired couple sitting on a bench on the opposite side of the lake, reading a paper together. *Good. Less gawkers,* he thought, while he followed the line of the sturdy green fence that ensured park visitors didn't disturb the waterfowl. A flurry of honking and splashing pulled his gaze to the lake. One of the swans was bullying a group of ducks that must have drifted too close to his personal space.

"They're mean," Lauren said. "Doesn't matter how pretty they are—they're mean and dirty. And the biggest reason my company has to come out here so often."

"You still have the contract to maintain the plants here?"

Lauren nodded, but she looked uncomfortable. "Aubrey wants it that way. She doesn't like to let a little thing like her death get in the way of good business."

"But you said you hadn't been here since her death."

"I haven't. I have five employees, remember?"

Then Lauren's use of the present tense about her sister's wishes caught up to his thoughts. "So she communicates with you about your business?"

"She communicates with me about lots of things, just not about her murder. Actually, I don't feel right unless she and I

are talking. I don't feel whole without her...." Lauren's words
trailed off as she came to an awkward silence. As if just realizing what she'd said, she shook her head and attempted a
smile. "I'm repeating myself, but it's hard not to. My life isn't
the same without her."

Raef started to comment, but Lauren's humorless laugh
silenced him. "Yeah, I know. It's normal for me to feel her
loss. Normal for things to be different. Normal to grieve."
She shook her head, looking out at the small lake. "I've heard
it all. Not one single person really gets it."

There didn't seem to be anything Raef could say to her
that hadn't been said, obviously to no effect, by others. Plus,
maybe Lauren was right. He'd never heard of a twin manifestation and possession before. Maybe there were unusual forces
at work in this death. Who was he to scoff at the abnormal?
Hell, he lived in Abnormalville; even the other psychics at
After Moonrise kept him at a distance. You don't have to be
a Greek god to know that if you invite Discord to a party, all
hell is gonna break loose.

Shit, his life sucked.

They'd come to a locked gate in the fence, and Lauren
stopped. Just inside the gate there was a small wooden dock
and a slim, slatted walkway that led from it to the island of
craggy stone, foliage and a waterfall-like fountain cascading
down one side of it that sat in the middle of this end of the
lake. "There." Lauren's voice was pitched low. "It's out there
that it happened." The eyes she turned to him were haunted
with sadness. "You'll need to go out there, won't you?"

"Yes."

She drew a deep breath. "Then let's go." Lauren flipped
open the metal cap that held an elaborate keypad for the locking mechanism on the gate. Her hands shook only a little as she

pressed the series of buttons that made the gate whir and click, and finally open. Without waiting for him, she strode through it and onto the dock. It was only then that she stopped, hands fisted at her sides, eyes looking at her feet, at the water, at the shore. Everywhere except out at the island.

"I'll be right behind you," Raef said.

"Okay. Yes. Okay. I can do this."

Lauren stepped onto the walkway. Raef stayed close to her, worried that she might pass out and fall into the damn water. That was something neither of them needed. They were halfway to the island when Raef steeled himself and then dropped the barriers he usually kept firmly locked around his mind.

Death, he whispered to himself, *come to me.*

He braced himself for the influx of terror and anger and hurt and pain that always flooded him so near the site of a death.

And there was nothing. Absolutely nothing.

The only thing he felt was the brush of the unseasonably warm October breeze and his own confusion.

"Here." Lauren had reached the island. Raef realized he'd stopped and quickly closed the distance between them. "This is where it happened." She pointed a shaky hand at the base of the rocky island where it met the water. There were several floating plants that looked to Raef like lily pads, along with some bushy clumps of underwater grasses. "Aubrey was replacing the water lilies, trimming the black bamboo and cleaning the algae from the spirogyra. She stepped down there—" Lauren motioned to a ledgelike edge of the island "—and was working with the plants, half in and half out of the water. The mechanism that powers the pump to the waterfall is under that ledge. The police say she cut the electrical line while she was working with the plants. The pump shorted out, sending an electrical current through the water and killing Aubrey. Technically, that's what happened. But it was no accident."

"Are you sure?"

Lauren's pale cheeks flushed. "I already told you. I am absolutely certain my sister was killed!"

"That's not what I'm asking. I want to know are you sure that this is where she died."

"Of course I am."

"Her death happened here and not at St. John's?" Raef made an impatient jerk of his chin at the hospital that was directly across the street from Swan Lake.

"Yes. She was dead when the joggers found her. They even came to her funeral. I talked to one of them myself. She was floating facedown in the water right there, tangled in the spirogyra grass." Lauren's hand was still a little shaky when she pointed to the spot below them where her sister's body had been discovered. "There—right there is where they pulled her from the pond."

Raef didn't say anything else. He just continued to stare at the water and the odd, curling grass that floated like Medusa's hair just beneath the surface.

Nothing. He felt nothing.

"Raef, what is it? What's happening?"

"Your sister couldn't have died here."

Lauren frowned at him. "Of course she did. That's the one part of the police report that was completely accurate."

"How about the coroner's report? Are you sure it concurred?"

"Yes. The coroner listed her time of death as more than an hour before the joggers called 9-1-1."

"You've read it? You've seen the report?"

"Yes and yes. I've scoured over it. I practically have it memorized, much to the TPD's irritation. Raef, what is it?"

"There's nothing here. No psychic Tracing of a death at all. And that is impossible."

Lauren opened her mouth, but instead of speaking, a strangled gasp wrenched from her. She swayed, her eyes fluttering, and Raef moved quickly to her side, steadying her by grasping her arm.

"Easy there. I'll figure this out and—" His words broke off abruptly as emotions rippled through him. But they weren't death scene emotions, familiar if numbing in their violence. Instead, joy and warmth and a poignant sense of longing filled him. He tried to throw up his mental barriers, but his traitorous Gift ignored it, leaving him naked and defenseless to the onslaught. Then the air beside Lauren rippled and her twin's ethereal body manifested.

"I knew you'd come. I knew you wouldn't let us down. I remembered you from that article in Oklahoma Today *magazine last year."* She grinned impishly. *"It said you were the best psychic detective in Oklahoma—that you were like an Old West sheriff. You always got your man."*

Raef swallowed hard, trying to pull himself together. *I can feel her joy!* Never before. Never during the twenty-five years his Gift had manifested had he ever felt a positive emotion from any spirit.

Aubrey laughed and the sound washed through his body like magic, sensitizing his nerves and his skin so that the fine dark hair on his forearms prickled as if she had just run a teasing, caressing hand over them.

"Ah, come on, Kent, relax. You look like you've seen a ghost," she said, still smiling joyously.

"Raef." He ground the word out automatically, the usual

gruffness of his voice intensified by the force of the emotions filling him. "People call me Raef."

"I'm not going to," Aubrey said. *"I like Kent better. Plus, you can't really call me a person anymore, can you?"*

Raef just stared at her. Had a spirit ever called him anything? No, hell, no, none of them had. He usually just Tracked the negative emotions left by the bad guys. He followed violence and hatred and fear until it led him to a living murderer. Ghosts didn't have shit to do with him.

Until *this* ghost.

Aubrey's gaze went from him to sweep around Swan Lake. *"It's beautiful here, don't you think? The trees are particularly lovely. So wise and strong, like soldiers standing guard."* She turned shimmering blue eyes back to him. *"They must take a lot of care."*

As soon as she'd spoken the words Raef felt it. The slicing pain hit him as Aubrey's semitransparent body doubled over. Lauren moaned, and her arm trembled violently under his grasp.

"Kent!" Aubrey gasped. *"Help us!"*

She disappeared as Lauren collapsed into his arms.

4

"Oh, God," Lauren groaned. "I think I'm going to be sick."

"No. Not here." Raef slid an arm around her waist and half carried, half dragged her from the dock and through the gate. He'd retraced their path and was almost to the car when Lauren spoke again.

"Wh-where are we going?"

"Don't know. Right now I'm just getting us the hell outta here," he said, wrenching open the door to the car and guiding her semicarefully into the passenger seat. He hesitated, watching her closely as she sat, face in hands, and trembled. "You still gonna be sick?"

"Maybe," she muttered into her hands.

Yeah, well, me, too, he thought, but instead said, "Try not to be," then closed her door and hurried around the car, putting it in gear and getting the hell outta there. Silent and on autopilot he drove, turned left on Lewis and was halfway to Fifteenth Street before he realized he was heading for his house. *What the fuck is wrong with me? I'm taking a client home?* Raef glanced at Lauren. She'd taken her face from her hands. Her arms were wrapped around her, as if she was literally trying to hold herself together. Her face had gone from dead pale to splotchy pink. She was still trembling.

Suddenly she reminded him of Christina Kambic all those years ago, and he had a terrifying urge to protect her. *Shit! Shit! Shit! What's wrong with me?*

"I'm not going to be sick. At least, not right now," Lauren said stiffly, definitely misunderstanding his sideways glances.

"Want me to take you home?" he asked inanely.

"No." Lauren made two quick shakes of her head.

"Your mother's place?"

"Hell, no." She looked straight at him then. "Anywhere but there."

He only met her blue-gray eyes for a moment before making his decision. Raef grunted and turned right on Fifteenth, catching the green light and taking a quick left on Columbia, entering the quaint little neighborhood that was hidden between busy Fifteenth Street and kinda dicey Eleventh Street. He drove down a couple side streets, took another left and then pulled into the cobblestone driveway of the 1920s-era brick house he called home.

Raef turned off the car and looked at Lauren, who was gazing at him, an obvious question mark on her flushed face. He blew out a long, frustrated breath, got out of the car and opened her door for her. "It's my place," he explained. "I don't take clients here."

"Yet here I am," she said as he closed the car door behind her.

"Yeah, well, that's just part of a list of *don'ts* that I've broken today." As they walked together up the curving sidewalk that led to his spacious front porch, he held up his hand and ticked off fingers like an umpire keeping count of strikes. "First, I *don't* usually feel as fucking bizarre as I did right before I met you." He paused when they were standing on the porch and added, "And your dead sister." Another finger went up. "Then I *don't* go to a murder scene—a documented scene of a death—and not pick up death emotions."

"Death emotions?" she interrupted.

He bit back his annoyance and answered her with a sharp nod and a sharper tone of voice while he dug in his pocket for his house key. "Yeah, death emotions. Bad ones. Like fear and panic and agony and hatred. Being able to Track negative emotions is my Gift."

"That sucks," she said.

He shrugged. "It's the way it is—the way it's been since I was nine."

"Yeah, don't take this the wrong way, but a Psy Gift is really pretty weird. I mean, it's not like anyone can predict it."

"You're telling me?" He snorted, and then opened the door for Lauren and motioned for her to go inside, following her closely, still explaining but also watching how her eyes opened in surprise as she took in the sheen of the hardwoods and his antiques that were comfortable as well as expensive and tasteful. "Which leads to don't number three." He put up the last finger. "I *don't* feel what I felt when your twin manifested— joy." Raef paused again and shook his head, remembering. "I even felt her laughter. *Her laughter.*"

Lauren's brow furrowed. "But you're a psychic. Feeling emotions is what you guys do."

"It's not that simple. No one just gets a blanket ESP stamp, like, *Hey, here ya go, buddy, now you're a psychic so you can read everyone's minds,*" he said sarcastically.

"Look, you don't have to sound like that. I don't know

about this psychic stuff. No one really does—or at least I don't think anyone really does." She put her hands on her hips. "It's not like your people are superopen with how the Gift works."

"It's not like *your* people really give a shit," he countered.

"Well, I give a shit now!" Lauren shouted, surprising both of them. She sighed and ran her fingers through her hair. "Sorry. I'm not usually such a bitch."

He chuckled. "Yeah, well, I'm usually such a bastard."

The air around them shimmered, and then, in the middle of Raef's living room, Aubrey manifested, saying, *"No wonder you don't bring women home."*

This time her emotions were muted. Her sparkle wasn't totally gone, but it had definitely dimmed. Still, she smiled at him, and as she did Raef felt a flutter of pleasure wash against his skin as, once again, he picked up her emotions. *She's pleased to see me,* Raef realized. *That's what I'm feeling.*

"He didn't say he didn't bring *women* home." Lauren broke into his internal dialogue. She shook her head at her twin, speaking to her in a totally normal, if tired, voice. "He said he didn't bring *clients* home. I've been telling you for years, if you're gonna eavesdrop, get it right."

"Touché," Aubrey said, grinning at her sister.

Raef frowned at both women. "It's not just about me not bringing clients here. I also don't bring work home. Period."

"You mean this cool old house is a no-ghost zone?" Aubrey said impishly.

Raef didn't say anything because he was feeling her playful sense of humor, and that feeling had his voice lodged somewhere in his gut.

"I have to sit down," Lauren said, glancing at him and then the wide leather couch. "Do you mind?"

"Yeah, I mean, no. Hell, I mean, yes, you may sit," Raef stuttered like an idiot.

Aubrey giggled, obviously getting some of her sparkle back.

"You're freaking him out," Lauren said as she sat heavily. "And you're exhausting me."

Aubrey's sparkled dimmed. "Sorry, sis," she said. She didn't move to sit beside her sister, whose face was back in her hands, but Raef watched her lift a semitransparent hand toward her, like she wanted to touch her. He felt her sadness then, and realized he hated it and had a ridiculous urge to do something, anything, to erase her sadness and bring back her joy—her joy he could feel.

And that was just fucking not normal.

"Okay, that's enough," he said gruffly. Both women, alive and dead, turned their pretty faces to him. "I need to know what the hell is going on here." He pointed at the ghost. "Were you murdered or not?" Raef watched the twins exchange a look.

Lauren spoke first. "Tell him. He'll see, and it'll make the explanation easier."

"It'll hurt," Aubrey said.

"I know. Just do it fast and get it over with. I'll see you again soon," Lauren said.

Aubrey nodded and then faced him. She met his gaze for a long time—long enough for Raef to be struck by her beauty. Yeah, she looked a whole lot like her twin, that figured. But she was softer, curvier, shorter—and her hair was longer. Just then it was lifting around her in response to a nonexistent wind.

"I know you can help us. I believe in you, Kent."

He knew she was telling the truth. He could feel her belief. It was warm and strong and very, very disconcerting—which left him utterly unprepared for her next words, and the flood of agony that followed them.

"My body was murdered by a man who has trapped my soul and the souls of a lot of other people. He's feeding off our pain. His name is—" Aubrey's words were sliced off as her ghost was ripped in half and Lauren shrieked with her twin in agony—an agony Raef felt all too well, an agony so great that it had his vision narrowing and his heart racing. The torn pieces of Aubrey's ghost were burned away like morning mist before sunlight and she was gone. Again.

Raef realized he had staggered to the couch and was clutching the back of it to keep himself upright. He raised a shaking hand and wiped sweat from his brow. The sound of a body dropping to the floor had him struggling to refocus in time to see that Lauren had slumped, unconscious, from the couch.

"Shit!" Raef hurried to her, carefully lifting her back on the couch, laying her down and checking for a pulse. "Strong and steady," he muttered. "Good—good. Hey, come on. Wake up. You're fine. Everything's fine," he said, more for himself than for her.

Lauren's eyelids fluttered and then opened. He started to breathe a long, relieved sigh, but then he realized how vacant those blue-gray eyes looked. Not only was the light not on, but nofuckingbody was home.

And that scared the shit out of him, so much so that he automatically fell back into what he knew best about dealing with while scared. His voice deepened, hardened, and MSgt Raef barked at her like the Special Forces NCOIC he'd once been. "Lauren! Get your ass back here on the fucking double! You haven't been given permission to go any damn where!"

Lauren blinked, shook her head as if she'd just come in

from the rain, and then her eyes animated and she focused on his face. "Raef."

Even though the name wasn't a question, he nodded. "You're back. Good."

"Feel bad, though," she said weakly.

He grunted and nodded. "Bet you do. Your soul's attached to Aubrey's, isn't it?"

"Yes. Always." The two words were whispers.

"All right. Well, that explains a lot about this cluster fuck." He stood.

"Are you leaving?"

"Sadly, no. You're in my house, remember?"

Lauren looked around, as if she hadn't remembered until then. "Oh, yeah, that's right. You don't bring clients here."

"I don't brew strong tea with honey for them, either. Which is what I'm going to do for you. Sit. Don't move. Don't faint. And don't fucking disappear on me again."

"Yes, sir," she said with what he already understood was uncharacteristic meekness.

He stopped halfway to the kitchen. "And for Christ's sake, don't call me sir. I was an NCO. I used to work for a living, unlike a fucking officer."

He didn't need to be psychic to feel Lauren's confusion all the way from the living room. "Civilians..." he grumbled as he clattered through his orderly cupboards and flipped on the electric kettle, tossing a bag of English breakfast tea, a dollop of local honey, a squeeze of fresh lemon *and* a healthy slosh of single-malt Scotch into each of the large mugs.

When he brought the brewed and spiked tea to the living room he was relieved to see that Lauren was sitting up and studying the art on his fireplace mantel. She turned and raised a brow at him. "Erté?"

"Yep," he said, handing her the mug of tea. She took the couch and he sat in a leather chair across from it.

"Your wife likes Erté?"

"Not married. Anymore. And no, she did not. I like Erté."

"Erté was gay."

"Yes, I'm aware of that."

She raised a brow at him. "You were military, weren't you?"

"Air force—OSI, that's Office of Special Investigations to civilians. Ten years—been out for almost five now," he said, sipped his tea and then added, "FYI—most military men don't give a shit whether the guy beside him is gay. They care more that the guy will stay beside him and cover his back. You shouldn't stereotype, Miss Wilcox, since you don't appreciate it when people assume you're just some stuck-up rich bitch who doesn't work for a living."

Her other brow raised at the word *bitch,* but she just sipped her tea, nodded and said, "Scotch and lemon and honey is my sister's favorite kind of tea."

"Was," Raef corrected her. "She's dead. Let's start right now with dealing with that, even though you can still see her and talk to her. That might help you start separating yourself from what's happening to her—at least long enough for me to try to figure out how to catch the guy who's doing it to her."

"She's not going to be able to help you do that."

"Because he's keeping her from helping me," Raef said.

"He's keeping her from helping anyone—even me. Any time Aubrey tries to talk about her murder, even tries to hint about it, it's like he has some kind of electric line into her soul." Lauren shook her head and Raef could see she was fighting back tears. "How the hell can he keep causing her such pain even after her body is dead?"

Raef didn't have one damn clue about how to answer that

question, so he countered with one of his own. "It's not just Aubrey who feels pain caused by him. It's you, too."

"Yes, it's me, too. And that's not all. She's getting weaker. He's draining her, and the weaker she gets—the more she's drained—the weaker I get. Somehow he can use her, and apparently several other people, even though they are all dead." Lauren stared into his eyes. "How? How is he doing it?"

"I'm going to be straight with you, Lauren. I've never heard of anything like this. Even when I was in the air force and Tracked terrorists. I experienced some really bad stuff, and some really bizarre stuff, but nothing that was leeching a ghost's soul *and* the ghost's living twin. Sorry, but I just don't have the answers for you."

"So, basically, you don't know what you're doing."

"Basically, you're correct. With your case I do not."

"Well, then, what am I going to do? Just fade away with Aubrey where we'll exist forever somewhere between agony and darkness?" This time a tear escaped Lauren's eye and rolled down her smooth cheek.

"Not if I can help it," Raef heard himself say.

Lauren threw up her hands and repeated, "How?"

"By doing something I hate like hell. I'm going to call in the cavalry and ask for help, even though it's a damn annoying cavalry and she's going to be obnoxiously pleased that she's going to have to bail me out."

5

"She's way too small to be the cavalry," Lauren whispered from beside Raef.

They were sitting at his huge old desk peering into the big-screen Mac as the redhead answered the video call. She raised a scarlet brow and turned clear green eyes on Lauren, saying, "I don't know what you mean by cavalry, but *she's* not deaf."

"Hey, I'm sorry," Lauren began. "I didn't mean to—"

"Yeah, yeah, stand down, tough girl," Raef interrupted. "Milana Buineviciute, this is Lauren Wilcox. She's a client of mine and *I* called you the cavalry, she didn't." Raef moved his gaze from the quick-tempered little redhead to Lauren. "Lana is the head medium for our Oklahoma City branch of After Moonrise. She's a pain in the ass, and even though she claims to be Lithuanian I suspect her of being a Russian spy, *but* she knows more shit about ghosts than anyone I've ever met. Not that that's a compliment."

"Atsiknisk," Lana told Raef blandly. "Which means 'fuck

off"—in Lithuanian, *not* Russian. Try moving into the twenty-first century, Raef. The Cold War has been over for longer than I've been alive." She looked at Lauren. "Good to meet you, Lauren." Lana glanced back at Raef. "Hey, *sudzius,* she's not a ghost."

"I've worked with you long enough to know you're calling me a shithead, and I know Lauren isn't a ghost, Nazi. It's her twin sister who is dead."

"Nazis were German, not Russian or Lithuanian," Lana told Raef smoothly before turning her attention back to Lauren. "A twin's death is always difficult. Her ghost, she is with you?"

Lauren nodded. "Yes, quite often, actually."

"What you are doing with this girl?" Lana snapped the question to Raef, her accent suddenly becoming more pronounced with her annoyance. "She should be working with a medium. If Vivian Peterson isn't the right choice there in Tulsa, bring her here to me."

"Her sister was murdered—that's why she's here with me, not because I'm into overtime or trying to poach someone's clients. You should know that," Raef said, not caring that he sounded as pissed as he felt.

Lana's expression softened and she brushed back a strand of bright red hair from her forehead. "Sorry, Raef. You are right. I've been going through my own *sudas* lately."

"Which makes you the shithead?" he said with a quick smile.

"*Taip.* Definitely. And now that we've established that, I am ready to listen." Lana picked up a legal pad and a pen. "Tell me what has happened."

Raef quickly recapped Aubrey's death and the events that had followed, reluctantly admitting everything, even the fact that he could feel her softer emotions, and ending with her latest manifestation in his living room. While he talked, Lana took notes, asked just a few pointed questions and looked grimmer and grimmer. When he was done she sighed and ran her hand through her fiery hair again.

"Do you know what he is? This murderer who steals souls?" Lauren asked into the silence.

"I do, but only through rumor and what amounts to fairy tales used to frighten children."

Lauren looked confused and Lana smiled. "I should clarify and say fairy tales used to frighten *psychic* children."

Raef felt a sliver of shock and sat up straighter. "The murderer is a psychic."

"Taip," Lana agreed. "But more specifically, the murderer is a psychic whose Gift has to be much like yours."

"Mine?" Raef shook his head. "What are you talking about?"

"You said you felt her emotions, and they were all softer, positive emotions. That's not the norm for you, Raef."

"To say the least," he snapped.

"And this ghost, she seems to be filled with positive emotions?" Lana said.

Lauren nodded. "Aubrey was full of joy and positive energy in life—she still is in death."

"When Aubrey tries to talk about her murder, when she gets anywhere close to darker, more negative emotions, like the fear and pain and even anger or hatred that remembering what happened to her evokes, that's when she dissipates, correct?" Lana asked.

"Yeah, it's like he has a hook into her that he can reel back whenever he wants," Raef said.

"Not *whenever.*" Lana continued, "Lauren, if Aubrey manifests and says nothing about her murder, if she simply visits you, does the killer pull her back to him?"

"No, but we always end up trying to talk about her murder. She's being drained. Even when we don't say anything about her death at all. She's still being drained," Lauren said.

"Because he's feeding off her emotions—the negative ones—fear, pain, panic, hatred. He can't tap into the softer emotions. My guess is he can't even Trace her spirit when she's feeling them." Lana met Raef's gaze. "He's a psychic like you gone bad."

"Shit. I knew this was a cluster fuck of massive proportions," Raef said.

"Why? If he's like you, then it should be easier for you to find him," Lauren said. "Can't you use your—" she paused and made a vague gesture with her hand "—your Gift or whatever and Track him down?"

Raef jerked his chin at Lana. "Ask the cavalry. She's the ghost expert."

Lana's green eyes sparkled and her smile reminded Raef of a ginger cat who had just lapped a bowl of cream. "Oh, Raef can find him, but he cannot use his Gift like he usually does. The murderer has that way blocked. You already told me what happens whenever your sister tries to speak of her death."

"He knows it. He stops her," Lana said. "And he hurts her more."

"Which proves Aubrey does know who killed her and could lead us to him—if he let her," Raef said. "Damn! It's frustrating as hell!"

"Aubrey can still lead you to her killer, she just has to do so through positive emotions. Use them to Track him."

"Positive emotions?" Raef snorted. "How the hell do I

learn about Tracking with those? Joy isn't gonna lead me to a murder site and a serial killer."

"You don't have to learn about positive emotions, *sudzius*. I have told you before, if you let go of your attachment to negative emotions, your soul will naturally reset itself and begin to accept and understand their opposites."

"And I've told *you* before—I'm not like the rest of your touchy-feely gang," Raef said.

"Great, you mean *he* has to get happy to find my sister's killer?" Lauren said.

"What the fuck is this, a motivational speech? I don't have any attachments to negative emotions. Negative emotions are my damn job. I don't need to get happy. I just need to find a murderer," Raef told the two women.

Both women smiled knowingly back at him.

He considered pouring more Scotch into his tea. Instead, he faced Lana. "So, that's the bottom line? I have to move through positive emotions to find this killer?"

"That's the bottom line," Lana agreed. "Like you, the guy is a fish out of water when he's not attached to hate and fear and pain. Let Aubrey show you how to flank him through joy and love and happiness."

"Flank him, huh? I knew you were a Russian spy," Raef muttered.

Lana grinned. "Here's the good news. All human soul are designed to accept love and happiness and joy, or at least they are if they can let go of their attachments to hate and fear and pain. And you're human, even though you are a man. Good luck. You'll need it." Lana waved a goodbye to Lauren and then disconnected the Skype call.

Raef and Lauren sat in silence, watching the screen saver come on—a series of pictures of a North Side beach house in

Grand Cayman where he vacationed every year. At that moment Raef wished desperately he had his ass in the sand and a cold beer in his hand.

"Do you think that's true?"

Lauren's question seemed loud and out of place, but weirdly enough Raef thought he knew exactly what she was asking.

"You mean the part about all human souls being designed to accept love and happiness and joy?"

"Yes, that's what I mean," she said.

"No," he said. "I don't."

"I don't think I do, either, but I can promise you Aubrey would think it's true—even now. Even dead."

He looked at her and saw how tired she was and how dark and sunken her blue eyes were. "I guess it's a good thing Aubrey's leading this hunt, then."

"She won't be doing anything for a while. When he jerks her back like that, so hard and so painful, it takes a lot out of her and she doesn't manifest for hours, sometimes a whole day."

"It takes a lot out of you, too," Raef said.

Lauren shrugged. "I'm still alive."

"You need to rest. Let me take you home, or to your mom's. Whichever you'd rather," he said, disconcerted by how hollow the thought of Lauren being *not* alive made him feel.

"Thanks. You're right. I'm exhausted. You can take me to my home. Not my mother's. Never my mother's, no matter how out of it I am."

"You're not out of it. Actually, I think you're doing pretty damn well for someone who's being soul sucked by a serial killer."

Lauren smiled as they walked back to the car. "That shouldn't make me feel better, but it kinda does."

"Hey, that's me. Mr. Warm and Fuzzy."

Lauren laughed then, and Raef was taken aback by how much she suddenly reminded him of Aubrey—so taken aback that he didn't have much to say as he drove the short way to Lauren's house, which was in the Brookside area of Midtown Tulsa, just a few miles away.

When he pulled up in front of the neat little bungalow, Lauren said, "Thanks, Raef. I guess I'll see you soon."

"I'll call you tomorrow. Let me do some digging about this soul-sucking crap and then you and I will take another whack at working with Aubrey."

"Sounds like a good plan."

Raef went around and opened her car door for her, and when she hesitated, obviously gathering her energy to get out of the car, Raef took her arm and guided her to her feet.

"Thanks," she said. "I'll be fine from here."

"I'm going to make sure you stay that way," he said.

Lauren looked up at him, and as their eyes met and held, Raef felt a sensation deep inside him—one he hadn't felt in a very, very long time.

"I believe in you," Lauren said, eerily echoing her twin. Then she went up on her tiptoes and kissed his cheek softly before turning away from him and going into her dark house and leaving Raef to drive away rubbing his cheek and muttering, "Cluster fuck…a total goat-herding, cat-roping cluster fuck…"

6

Raef didn't go home. Instead, still muttering to himself about *un*natural disasters, he stopped by his After Moonrise office and grabbed some Psy books from a very surprised Vivian Peterson, who was their resident expert on ghosts.

Raef didn't like her. Never had. She was just too damn ooie-ooie. Her hair was green, for God's sake.

On the way back to the house he stopped for take-out pizza at the Pie Hole and a six-pack of Blue Moon beer—both the liquor store and the pizza place were within walking distance of his house.

"Which is just one of reasons this place is so perfect for me." Raef sighed with contentment as he chugged the first bottle of beer between bites of the Everything Pie Hole Special. He didn't open the first research book until he'd worked his way through half of the pie *and* half of the six-pack. *Then* he started reading.

Within fifteen minutes he was shaking his head and opening another beer. He flipped through the chapters of the first

book, *The Spirit Hunter's Guide,* reading quickly. "'Possession, succubus infestation, poltergeists, noxious aroma inva-
sions…'" Raef read aloud. "This ghost stuff is some seriously
not right shit." He swigged another beer and tossed that book
aside, picking up a slimmer volume titled *Shamanic Retrieval.*
Paging through it Raef found essays sectioned off with the
titles "Soul Theft and Loss," "Souls Lost to Love" and finally
"Retrieving a Stolen Soul."

"About damn time," he said under his breath and began
to read.

Retrieving a stolen soul must be done with skill and care.
Remember, we must act in harmony with the universe—
harming others, even others who have stolen souls, puts
us out of harmony.

Raef snorted. "Like I give a fuck?" He kept reading.

Soul thieves usually take spirits because they believe
they need the power to live. This is rarely true. Only one
psychic in thousands can actually feed from the energy
of another's soul. The problem is some less than scru-
pulous psychics can convince themselves that they can
use the power of another—therein you find a soul thief.

"The problem is the asshole I'm dealing with *can* feed from
souls." Raef continued.

Because of the power attachment to the stolen soul, it
is complicated to convince the thief to release it. There
are two basic ways to attempt, with responsibility to universal order, to retrieve a stolen soul.

Then in bold writing Raef read:

1) Offer the thief a gift to replace the soul. Sometimes an animal spirit can be traded for the human soul.

"That sucks for the poor dog," Raef said.

2) Trick the thief by distracting him or her, and then pull the soul away yourself. Of course, this takes the well-honed skills of a shaman or a medium, and should not be attempted by a psychic with a different Gift. To do so may cause harm to the thief and, possibly, the stolen soul, as well as the inexperienced psychic.

Raef sat back, sipping his beer and thinking. Should he bring in another psychic like Lana? He didn't give a shit about the thief's safety—the guy was a killer. Even though he'd rather not get his own ass in a bind, he wasn't particularly worried about himself. Raef had been handling his own shit for decades. He did care about Aubrey, as well as her sister— which was almost as irritating as it was unusual.

It just wasn't normal for him to care.

"Hell, this isn't a normal case," he reasoned aloud. "And this isn't a normal soul stealing, either," Raef rationalized aloud. "It's a murder. The soul part is only secondary. So, the ooie-ooie crap needs to take second place to the murder. And I'm the right man to take care of the murder part." He reread number two. "'Trick the thief by distracting him or her, and then pull the soul away yourself.' How 'bout I do the distracting, like get this guy arrested and put away for life, and Aubrey just runs like hell—so to speak."

Nodding to himself, Raef paged through, skipping the sections on "Restoring a Soul's Light" and "Finding Shattered Souls," but stopping at the heading "Retrieving Souls from the Land of the Dead."

The Land of the Dead is not the equivalent of a Christian heaven or hell. It is not one of the three layers of the Otherworld. It is a place for lost and broken souls— be they dead or alive. It is a dangerous place, even for a trained shaman or medium. It's filled with hopelessness. Sometimes shattered souls can be found there. Sometimes soul thieves choose the Land of the Dead as a holding place for their victims. Whether you are healing a shattered soul or retrieving a stolen one, enter the Land of the Dead without protection and experience, and you risk becoming lost, too.

"Jackpot!" Raef said. "Definitely sounds like the place I need to go." He skipped the rest of the warnings and went straight to the heading titled "Entering the Land of the Dead."

Begin by lighting a candle. You are seeking shadow and smoke, death and darkness, you will need to keep a light close to you, both figuratively and literally.

Reluctantly, Raef got up and went to his bedroom where he always kept a vanilla candle ready to burn. He used to like the way the candlelight flickered off his wife's smooth skin. Kathy had been lush and sexy, and the warm light of a flame used to make her look like a love goddess come to earth. Of course, he hadn't actually burned the damn candle in years, not since his wife had decided she couldn't live with his job— or in her words, *I can't stand what your job does to you, Raef. It makes you sad, and nothing I do ever changes that.*

Raef paused halfway back to the living room, candle in hand. "Why the fuck am I thinking about that? Kathy's been gone five years. The candle only stayed because I like the way it smells." Raef stifled a sigh of annoyance. So, yeah, it would be nice to see another naked woman in candlelight, but that hadn't happened in a long time. "Too long," he said as he lit the vanilla candle and picked up the book and the beer again. "All right, what next?"

Shamanic battles of life and death can happen in the Land of the Dead. If you attempt to go there you must be skilled and courageous and well protected.

"Yeah, yeah, get to it," he mumbled.

The Land of the Dead can be found past the Other-world boundary. Think of the Otherworld as if it were an ancient map when man believed the world was flat, and if you went too far you fell off into nothingness. That nothingness is the Land of the Dead.

To find it, keep the light of your candle strong in your mind's eye. Then begin to meditate upon the reason for your quest. A shaman or medium can Track a soul with the help of his or her Gift.

"Huh." Raef snorted. "I'm not an ooie-ooie shaman or a medium, but I can Track things. Usually murderers, but what-ever. Nothing is normal about this case. Maybe I can Track more than I thought I could, or at least when it comes to Aubrey and Lauren maybe I can." He kept reading.

> Know that once you have Tracked the soul to the
> Land of the Dead, your psychic Gift will cease to work.
> You must use mortal guile and your own wisdom to re-
> trieve the lost one.

"First good news I've heard yet," he said, chuckling softly.

Raef closed the book and looked at the candle. He stared at the flame until it seemed as if the light was burned into his mind.

Then he began thinking of Aubrey.

She made him feel joy.

She laughed. She laughed a lot, especially for a dead girl.

She was blonde and beautiful and had a sparkle that even death couldn't dim.

She called him Kent. No one called him Kent.

Raef closed his eyes, held the light in his mind and Aubrey in his heart and, just as he did at a murder scene, began to feel around with his Gift...seeking...questing...searching.... Only this time he wasn't trying to Track rage and fear and pain. This time he was questing after a sparkling blonde whose laughter reminded him of champagne.

When he actually found her it jolted him with surprise. Murder victims he'd Tracked before had led him to their killers with dark, smoking trails—or rivers of pain and hatred like oil slicks. Aubrey's trail was a shimmering thread of joy that flickered bright and then dim. *Why?* he wondered. *What's going on with her?* Then he recognized the dimming— he'd seen it before; it was worry. Raef reached with his Gift to grab on and Track the illusive, glittering thread, but instead of Tracking he felt an already familiar sensation pass over his skin, and her voice, somewhere between annoyed and surprised, sounded in the air around him.

"Kent, what are you doing?"

He opened his eyes. Aubrey had materialized in front of him, between the couch and the old steamer trunk he used as a coffee table. It had gotten dark while he'd been reading, and the living room was dim —the only real light cast by the vanilla candle. The lack of light agreed with Aubrey. She looked almost substantial, and Raef noticed she was wearing only a slip of a dress, one of those silk things that laced up the front and hugged women's curves so well. And Aubrey had some serious curves to hug.

The joy that had been dimmed by worry sparkled alight as Aubrey cocked her head to the side, studied him and then began to laugh. Her laughter skittered across his skin, raising the hair on his forearms, and calling alive sensations that had been dead within him a lot longer than Aubrey had been.

"What?" he said, scrubbing a hand roughly across a forearm. "Why are you laughing?"

"'Cause I just realized what you're doing."

She grinned, but didn't continue until he prodded, "And what do you think I'm doing?"

"It's not think, Kent. It's know. I know you're checking me out."

Raef frowned, trying to ignore the crackle of humor that lifted around her and washed against him. "That's not what I was doing before you showed up, and why does that make you laugh?"

"Because it means your love life is even deader than me." She giggled.

"That's not funny," Raef said. "And before you showed up I was trying to Tr—"

"No!" For a moment she sounded frantic, and the humor that had been bubbling around him faded. Then, she reached up and took hold of one of the diaphanous laces that held the front of her dress together. Aubrey smiled teasingly at him. *"No, let's not go there. If we go there, then I'll have to leave, and neither of us wants that. How about we go here instead."* With one deft pull, she undid the tie and the lacing fell open, exposing her naked flesh.

"You're naked!" Raef blurted, and then mentally smacked himself. *Were boobs all it really took to make me forget she's dead?*

"No, I'm naked under this." Aubrey slowly ran her hands down the front of the silk dress, lingering over her breasts until her nipples began to harden. She gasped in pleasure. *"Wow—"* her voice was a breathy whisper *"—I feel amazing."* Still touching herself, Aubrey half walked, half floated closer to him. *"You can feel me, Kent. I know you can."*

She was only an arm's length from him, and she was so fucking sexy there in the candlelight, all skin and lush curves and nipples that were tight and ripe and ready for his tongue. Raef reached for her, and felt a shock and a chill when his hand met with nothing but air.

Her laugher bubbled around them. *"Not like that, silly! Feel me in there."* Aubrey took one hand from her body, leaned forward and pressed her hand against his chest, over his heart.

He didn't feel the pressure from her hand. He didn't feel anything except her laughter and his raging hard-on. "I don't feel shit! You're a ghost. I don't know what the fuck I'm doing."

"I've made you feel before. I can do it again, and it's important that you do. It's the only way we can move forward. The only way we can fix what's wrong." She was standing right before him. Her hands went to one of the loosened laces of her dress. She tugged again, this time harder, and the silk slid through, open-

ing the dress completely. With a teasing smile she shrugged her shoulders and it slid from her body to pool in a semi-substantial puddle at her feet.

"Oh, God. You are so damn beautiful," Raef couldn't stop himself from saying.

"Then feel me, Kent. Let go of all of that baggage you have because of the past, and allow yourself to feel pleasure again." Aubrey caressed her breasts. Then slowly, she moved one hand down her body, over the curve of her belly, and slid her fingers under the triangle of blond curls between her legs.

Raef couldn't take his gaze from her. His body was aching in hot, hard response. Automatically, he rubbed his hand over his jeans and down the long length of his swollen cock.

"Yes! Let me see you. Let me watch you."

"Then let me feel you!"

"Kent, baby, you can do that yourself. Just let it happen. Let go of the past and be willing to feel pleasure in the present."

"Yeah, okay. Anything," he said. "I let go of all that crap."

"Why? Tell me why," Aubrey whispered.

"Because I want to feel pleasure. With you!" He almost shouted the words.

As soon as he'd spoken it hit him—her emotions. He'd felt her laughter before. He'd even felt her joy. But what he was feeling now sliced through him like a sword: joy, laughter, lust, desire, pleasure, all wrapped together. The emotions entwined and implanted within him. Raef ripped open the front of his jeans and took his cock in his hand, stroking himself as he watched her blue eyes widen.

"You are incredible!" Aubrey said. *"And you do feel me."*

"I do feel you," he gasped. "I feel what you do to yourself. I feel what you do to me."

"Then feel this...." Aubrey's gaze never left his as her fin-

gers moved more quickly over herself. Raef was staring into her eyes as they both came to orgasm—he was still staring at her when she whispered, *"This makes you closer to me, and the closer to me you get, the closer you'll be to finding him. But you can't do it through negative emotions. You have to Track him through the opposite—joy and pleasure, happiness and hope. He can't fight that, and he won't be able to stop you from—"*

This time the soul thief didn't rip Aubrey in half when he jerked her back to him. This time he made her explode into little pieces, so that her scream was cut off like a snuffed candle, leaving Raef drained, confused and alone in the darkness without her.

7

"I just jerked off with a ghost. I am seriously fucked up."

Raef stared at the ceiling, lifted the bottle of single-malt Scotch he'd retrieved from the kitchen and took several long drinks. He meant to go back to reading the soul-retrieval stuff. Instead, he stared at nothing and thought about Aubrey. "She staged the whole thing," he mused aloud between gulps of Scotch. "She has to be guiding me. She's probably getting info from her connection with Lauren. And hell, she's the one trapped. She's gotta have something figured out about what would get her free. She obviously knows I can't Track this guy through negative emotions. He has them blocked. But he's not gonna pay attention to positive emotions because guys like him—and me—aren't good at the softer side of emotions. We're not used to 'em."

He blew out a long breath. How long had it been since he'd had sex, anyway? "More than a year since my *relationship* with Raven had crashed and burned. Christ, her name had been *Raven*. What the fuck had I expected?" He shook his head at his own stupidity, and at online dating in general, and realized the room was spinning a little around him.

Raef snorted and took another drink of Scotch. By now he hardly felt the burn. "Aubrey's good at positive emotions. Hell, Aubrey's good at a lot of things." He stared at the ceiling until his eyes blurred, blinked and finally closed.

Later he would remember that his last thought that night wasn't about Aubrey's hair or her boobs or how hard she'd made him or the way she touched herself—his last thoughts had been about her laughter and how the sound and feel of it had been better than all of the sex stuff...and the sex stuff had been really good.

THE BANGING ON RAEF'S front door woke him. It was loud and jarring, and only slightly less obnoxious than the pounding pain in his head. "Yeah, Jesus, yeah, I'm coming." He glanced at the clock before wrenching open the door— 8:30 a.m.? Damn, he was going to be late for work. Which meant he should have opened the door with a thank-you-for-being-my-alarm-clock instead of a snarl, but life just wasn't fair. "What the hell do you—" His words broke off when he saw Lauren's raised brows.

"I'm a morning person. I figured you'd be on your way out the door for work. The cab dropped me off 'cause I thought I'd go with you," she said unapologetically, though she did raise her hands, which were holding two tall cups of QT coffee. "I come bearing offerings."

He opened the door, took one of the coffees, stepped back and, with a grunt, gestured for her to come in.

She walked past, giving him a Look. "You're not ready to go to work."

"No kidding." His voice sounded like there was gravel in his throat.

"You look bad. Real bad," she said.

"Scotch. A lot of it," he said.

She shuddered. "I did that once. Never again."

"I'm a slow learner," he said. "I got some Merritt's dough-nuts in the kitchen. They're only two days old so they're not too much like bricks. Make yourself at home while I'm in the shower." He disappeared into the bathroom, closed the door, and as memories of the night before flooded his mind, Raef thought seriously about using the razor to slit his wrists. "Why can't I be one of those drunks who don't remember anything?" Raef asked his rough-looking reflection in the vanity mirror. He shook his head. Slightly. It still hurt like hell. "You had sex with a ghost, and that ghost's twin sister is in your kitchen." He sighed and started to lather up his face, muttering, "Might as well be a freshly shaven, clean perv."

When he got out of the shower and opened the door to the hall, Raef was confronted by two things—the smell of bacon and eggs, and Lauren. She had *Shamanic Retrieval* open in her hand and was carrying it back to the kitchen. Looking up from its pages she stopped to stare at him.

Color bloomed in her cheeks.

Raef tightened the towel that was around his waist, feeling even more naked than he was—and he was pretty damn naked.

"I made breakfast," she said, before turning away and hurrying the rest of the way to the kitchen.

"I'm hungover," he called, hurrying the rest of the way to the bedroom.

"I know. It's good for you, though. Trust me. I was a biology major in college," she called in return.

Raef pulled on jeans and an old air-force sweatshirt. As he walked into the kitchen he told his phone, "Call work." Feeling oddly like an obedient child, he sat at the breakfast-nook table, where Lauren had already placed a full plate of eggs, bacon and toast—along with a cup of fresh coffee and a shot of what smelled and looked suspiciously like single-malt Scotch. He raised a brow at her as he spoke. "Preston, reschedule my appointments for today. I'm still on the case I took yesterday and I'll be working in the field. Thank you." Raef hit the end-call button, forked up some eggs and bacon, and said to Lauren, "What does being a biology major in college have to do with hangovers?"

She sat across from him with her own plate of breakfast. "Simple. Hangovers are biological. Food helps. So does hair of the dog. Actually, I'm not sure if the hair-of-the-dog part is biological or psychological, but it works."

"Yeah, this isn't my first rodeo. I'm just surprised there was any Scotch left in that bottle." He gulped the shot and grimaced, reaching for the coffee.

"Well, there was barely a whole shot left. I'm assuming the bottle was mostly full when you started?"

"Yep," he said through bites of eggs and bacon that were really tasting damn good.

"Rough night?"

He swallowed and avoided her eyes. "Yeah."

"Okay, well, sorry about your rough night, and like I said yesterday, I'm not usually this bitchy, but hungover or not we have work to do. Aubrey should be able to manifest again by now, so as soon as we're done eating I'll focus my thoughts and she should—"

"Oh, go ahead and eat. I don't mind watching. I'm finding out that I kinda like it."

Aubrey's giggle washed around them as she materialized and Raef almost choked on a mouthful of eggs.

"Good morning, sis. Morning, Kent."

"Hey, Aub, you look good. All bright and happy," Lauren said.

"I had a verrrry interesting night."

The smile she sent Raef was brilliant and sparkling, and seemed to catch him in a spotlight. He felt it. He actually *felt* her happiness. It was like an endless Saturday, or having box seats at the World Series, or knowing you're going to have lots of sex. Lots of really good sex.

"Oh. My. God. You two did it. I don't know how it's possible, but you two *did it* last night," Lauren said, glaring from Raef to her sister.

"How the hell could you know that? You're a Norm! You're not psychic." Raef threw up his hands in exasperation.

Aubrey giggled some more, causing Raef's skin to prickle. *"She knows because Lauren and I have always been connected. I think you'd call it our own interpersonal psychic link, which means you really do have to stop lumping us with the Norms."*

"Which also means you two did do it last night."

"What we did was create pleasure, and pleasure is definitely a positive emotion. Right, Kent?" She grinned at Kent.

"Doesn't feel like it right now," he mumbled.

"Cheer up. It's not like she got you pregnant," Lauren said. Then raised her brow and, sounding so much like her mother that Raef even recognized it, announced, "You didn't masturbate, did you, Aubrey Lynn Wilcox? You know what I told you about that." And then Lauren Wilcox dissolved into giggles that included a very unladylike snort.

Aubrey laughed with her sister, full-throated, filling the breakfast nook with joy that washed through Raef. He couldn't help it. He couldn't stop it. Raef threw back his head and laughed along with the ghost and her twin sister. *Happy,* he thought. *I'm happy around her—around them. And I haven't been happy in a very long time.*

"*That's right, Kent. Feel it. Feel it with me. Pleasure and humor, joy and happiness. Feel them and keep them close to you, like shields. Because when you stop looking at the forest and find the tree, you'll only get one piece of the puzzle. He has the rest of the pieces hidden where only you can find them when you follow me. You won't be able to use your Gift there, but you can use—*"

"No, Aubrey! Don't!" Raef shouted, and came to his feet so fast the chair toppled over behind him. But he was too late. Aubrey's semitransparent body had already been ripped away.

"Oh, no!" Lauren gagged. Holding her hand over her mouth she staggered to the kitchen sink and puked up eggs and bacon and coffee.

"Here." Raef handed her a paper towel. "Just breathe."

She took the paper towel with a hand that trembled and wiped her mouth. Raef went to the fridge and grabbed a can of Sprite, popped the top and held it out for her. "This'll help. Rinse your mouth and then sip it."

Lauren didn't take the can. She just stood at the sink, wiping her mouth over and over again, staring blankly out the kitchen window to Raef's backyard.

"Lauren?"

She didn't even blink. He jerked the paper towel from her hands, threw it into the sink and then took her shoulders into his hands, turning her to face him.

"All right. That's enough. Come back now."

She stared straight ahead at his collarbone. He hadn't realized until then how short she was—petite, really. And those sharp blue-gray eyes of hers were still vacant and glazed. Raef gave her shoulders a shake. Not too rough, but hard enough it should bring her attention back to her body. He deepened his voice and took all the emotion out of it. "I said that's enough. Get back here, Lauren!"

Like throwing a switch, the light came into her eyes. Lauren blinked and looked up at him. "Raef? What—" Her whole body started to tremble and, feeling totally in over his head, he did the only thing he could think to do—he pulled her into a hug.

She buried her head in his chest and shook.

"Hey, it's okay. You're back. You're fine," he said inanely, thinking how small she was—God, would she even weigh a hundred pounds soaking wet?

"It's getting worse," she said against his chest.

"Where were you? Where do you go when that happens?" he asked.

She stepped back out of his arms and looked at him in surprise. "Ohmygod, Raef! I never even thought about where I go, just how I feel." She shook her head and went back to the breakfast table, pushed aside her half-eaten plate and sat heavily. Lauren wrapped her hands around her mug of coffee and took a sip. Raef righted his chair and did the same.

"So, describe it to me," he said.

She looked over her mug at him. "It's foggy there. And cold. Ugh, and it's wet, too."

"Wet? It's raining?"

Lauren shook her head. "I don't think so. Maybe it's not really wet, but that place makes me feel like I'm drowning," she said.

"Could be part of the spiritual draining. That must be how your body and mind are interpreting it."

"It's so hard to tell you anything for sure because everything is in black and white, but foggy or blurred, like one of those old silent movies." Her eyes narrowed contemplatively. "Actually, it's a lot like a silent movie. Things skip around, like movie frames freezing."

"Is anyone else there?"

"Yes," she said without hesitation, and then added more slowly, "Aubrey is there, and there are other people, too. But they're hard to see. They fade in and out. They're only vague images. I do know they're in pain. They're all in pain." She shook her head again. "I've known it all along and just refused to think about it because it's so, so terrible there. But it has to be where the murderer is keeping his victims' souls."

"The Land of the Dead," Raef said.

"What?"

He snagged the slim book from where Lauren had left it on the kitchen counter. "It's in here. It's also what Aubrey's talking about when she gets ripped back there by him."

"Bread crumbs. She's trying to lead us to her with bread crumbs, but they keep getting eaten," Lauren said.

"Maybe not totally eaten." He got up, refilled their coffee and brought a legal pad and a pencil back to the table. "So, whenever Aubrey's emotions change—whenever she tries to talk about her death or her killer—he can sense it and he rips her away from here. Correct?"

"Correct. But it happens so fast that she never really gets to tell us anything."

"But she tries," Raef said. "Maybe we should listen better."

"Okay, well, I'm not going to be very good at that because I feel her pain and I get ripped away with her. Or at least part of me does—that part that's attached to Aub."

"I get that. So let me help, or at least help with what I've witnessed. The first time Aubrey disappeared was in my office when you hired me and I asked her to tell me about her murder."

Lauren nodded. "I hired you because she told me to, and that took her a while because she kept getting ripped away. She finally just described you and then said 'KooKoo Kitty.' I figured it out from there."

"KooKoo Kitty? How the hell did you find me from that?"

Lauren smiled. "It's twin speak. We had a cat when we were twelve. Someone had dumped her on our grandparents' ranch by one of our guest cabins. She was, of course, pregnant. She was a sweet, friendly little thing, so Mother let us keep her as one of the barn cats, but said we'd have to give away the kittens and get her spayed. We called her Cabin Kitty. Well, she had her kittens and then promptly lost her mind protecting them. She attacked every cat, dog, chicken and even horse at the ranch. We renamed her KooKoo Kitty."

"Nice story. Still don't know why the hell that led you to me."

"Oh, that's easy. After Moonrise and the whole Psy thing is seriously cuckoo, and you're the only tall, dark and handsome working there."

"Thank you. I think." Then he tried not to dwell on the fact that Aubrey described him as handsome. "So, that was time number one."

"Obviously the murderer doesn't want you involved in his case."

"Yeah, well, too late. Second time was at Swan Lake." Raef thought back, frowning. "I don't remember her saying anything even vaguely pertaining to her death, do you?"

"Actually, I do remember what she was saying because it seemed harmless." She moved her shoulders. "Sometimes I can tell she's getting ready to get ripped back. I mean, I know that she's trying to tell me something."

"Like today."

"Exactly. But yesterday she was totally happy. All she was doing was talking about the trees. She called them soldiers, wise and strong, and said they must need a lot of care. And that was it. He took her away."

Raef's eyes widened. "I'm an idiot. She wasn't talking about trees—at least, not just about them. She had to have been giving us a clue about the murderer for him to have jerked her away." He sat up straighter. "Ah, shit. She did it again today. She said when I stop looking at the forest and find the tree I'll get a piece of the puzzle."

"Raef! Whoever killed her must have been working on the trees at Swan Lake," Lauren said.

"Puzzle piece found," Raef said grimly. "And that tree-loving bastard better watch the hell out."

8

"So what you're saying is on July 15 there were no city tree trimmers at or around the area of Swan Lake?" Raef was talking into his cell as he paced across his home office.

"That's correct, Mr. Raef, I see no record of having sent our tree trimmers out to Midtown at all that day." The city worker's voice sounded like she was talking to him through a tin can. Hell, with the City of Tulsa Works Department and their crappy budget, that might be true. He glanced at Lauren where she sat at his computer. She looked up at him. He shook his head, and she went back to concentrating on the computer. "Could you double-check your records, ma'am?"

"Certainly. Hold please," she said.

"I'm on hold. Again." Raef growled and continued prowling around his office. Finally the tin-can voice returned.

"Sir, I have checked and rechecked our records for that day and the day before. All of our tree-trimming teams were in the Reservoir Hill neighborhood on the fourteenth and the fifteenth of July. I am sorry I couldn't be of more help."

"Yeah, me, too, but thanks," Raef said, disconnecting. "Struck out," he told Lauren.

"Well, I think I just hit a home run," she said, excitement raising her voice.

"How so?" He went to look over her shoulder at the Swan Lake website she had up. She'd clicked into several of the pictures and was studying them intently.

"First, I've quit thinking like a grieving sister and started thinking like a landscaper. Those are elms." Lauren pointed at the picture. "Actually, almost all the larger trees lining the pond are elms."

"Okay, why is that important?"

"Because of our weather patterns elms are especially susceptible to Dutch elm disease. It can be devastating to them."

"And?" Raef prompted.

"And the pretty neighborhood around Swan Lake wouldn't stay pretty if its biggest shade trees withered and died from a nasty, highly contagious fungus. These trees are healthy—strong and soldierlike, as my sister would say. That tells me Midtown has an arborist."

"A what?"

"Tree doctor. This many elms, old and young, tell me they've been well cared for. Hang on, if I remember correctly…" Her fingers flew across the keyboard as she searched and clicked. "And I do! There's an innovative preventative treatment for Dutch elm disease that needs to be applied in the spring and early summer." She looked at him. "Mid-July would have been a perfect second-application time."

"I was calling the right department, but asking the wrong question," Raef said, but before he punched the city number again, Lauren's words had him pausing. "He has more souls trapped than just Aubrey's. I can feel them."

"He's a serial killer," Raef said grimly. "I wonder how many more *accidents* have happened to people in Tulsa in the past year or so, and how many of them were close to other well-tended groves of trees." Raef hit the number to the After Moonrise office. "Preston, I need you to get into the database and do a search for me. Deaths ruled as accidental in the past year. I'll need specifics on the death sites. Pay special attention to details about the trees in the area—like, did the accident happen in Mohawk Park or did someone fall down the stairs at the BOK Arena. I'm interested in the trees, not the structures. Our killer has a connection to trees, might even be a tree doctor. Got it?...Good. Call me back ASAP." He disconnected and glanced at Lauren.

Even though she was completely focused on the computer she must have felt his look because Lauren said, "I'm already checking arborists in the area. Call the city back."

Raef did as he was told.

"So, the city uses three arborists. Chris Melnore, out of Hardscape in Bixbie, Steve Elwood, who has his own tree-trimming business in Broken Arrow, and Dr. Raymond Braggs, who is a professor at TU." Raef read from the list the public-works director had given him. "All three have serviced Midtown. Murphy's Law is working well, which means the city had a major computer crash last week, so they don't have a record of which one of the three might have been to Swan Lake in July. They're gonna check and see if anyone kept any physical notes, but it's doubtful that they'll find anything. It was back in July and this is October."

"Can't we just call the three men and ask if he was at Swan Lake that day? We could pretend like we're calling from the city for, uh, tax records or something like that," Lauren said.

"We could, but you see how jumpy the guy is already. He jerks Aubrey outta here if she so much as mentions a damn tree. I don't want him going rabbit on me."

"Then how do we figure out which one he is?" Lauren rubbed a hand over her face and brushed back a strand of long blond hair.

She looks tired, he thought. *Again. I have to remember that this is draining her along with Aubrey.*

"Well, we can't do much until we get the list of accidental deaths from my office. Then we'll check out the death scene and see if there is any link to a tree doc, and go from there."

"Or we could print off pictures of each of the three guys and when Aubrey manifests next see if she can point us to one of them."

"You mean before she screams and gets torn into pieces and part of you gets sucked away with her? No. How 'bout I try some old-fashioned detective work instead."

"Aubrey and I can handle it. We've been doing this for months."

"How much longer do you think you two have?" he asked bluntly, his voice a lot colder than he meant it to be.

Her face lost the little color it had had. "I don't know," she said listlessly. "I can't tell because I don't feel right—don't feel whole—without Aubrey. So a piece of me is missing whether I'm being drained by a serial killer or not."

"All right, then, let's not push it." He gentled his voice. "You're tired."

"I'm always tired."

"I'll take you home. You can rest and I'll call you as soon as I have something."

"Do you have to?"

Raef raised a brow at her. She looked away and he saw some

color in her cheeks. Before he could say anything she seemed to collect herself and turned her eyes back to his. Their gazes met and held.

"I know you have a thing for Aubrey. That's fine." Lauren looked away.

"That's weird," he said, wishing she'd meet his gaze again. "She's dead."

"That's fine," she repeated as if he hadn't spoken. "I don't want to stay because I want to have sex with you or anything like that." When he just stared at her, she added, "Not that you're not an attractive man. You are. Really. Obviously my sister thinks so, and she and I have similar tastes in men." She pushed a thick strand of blond hair from her face, looked up at him. This time her cheeks were bright pink.

She was beautiful.

His throat felt dry. He cleared it. When she didn't continue speaking he prompted, "You and Aubrey liked the same guys?" Then he realized what he'd said and he hastily added, "Not that I'm into twin sex fantasies or anything too weird."

"Define *too weird*." Her eyes found his again.

And damned if *his* cheeks didn't suddenly feel hot. "Well, after what happened last night between your sister and me, I think my definition of *too weird* is changing."

Lauren's smile was warm—so warm it made his skin tingle. She gave a little laugh. "Okay, before this gets too crazy, let me start over. Raef, I'd really appreciate it if you'd let me stay here until we find my sister's killer. I mean, if you don't mind too much."

"That might be days or weeks," Raef said.

"It can't be," she said, no longer smiling or blushing. "There's no way Aubrey and I have that long." She drew a long breath. "The truth is that every time Aubrey gets ripped out of here and takes part of me with her, I'm afraid I may never come back. For some reason you are able to get me back. I don't think you always will be able to, but for right now being around you makes me feel as safe as I'm able to feel."

Ah, shit, no! he thought. What he heard himself say was, "Fine. You can stay. But you get the couch."

"That's perfect. I like to go to sleep watching TV."

"That shows a lack in your upbringing," he said.

"To say the least."

"What, rough time with nannies?" he asked sarcastically.

"Mother doesn't believe in nannies. She didn't have any. Mother also doesn't believe in children, especially not girl children. Sadly, she had two of them. And our father never paid any attention because we weren't a son. Here's a news flash— you don't have to live in a trailer to be abused as a child."

"Hey, sorry. That was out of line of me," he said, feeling like a douche bag.

"Don't worry about it. Almost everyone assumes Aub and I are spoiled rich girls." She shook her head wearily. "*Were,* I mean. She's dead. I have to start remembering that."

"All right, that's enough. Let's go." Raef gestured for her to come out from behind his desk.

"Are you making me leave?"

He hated the soft, scared tone of her voice. "No, I said you could stay. I may be an ass, but I don't break my word. What I'm making you do is take a nap."

She stopped halfway down the hall. "Seriously?"

"Naps are healthy. Again, this shows another lack in your upbringing."

"I can assure you that's only the second of many," she said, following him to the wide leather couch that was already loaded with soft pillows and a faux-fur throw. She plumped a pillow, kicked off her shoes and curled up on her side, pull-ing the throw up to her neck. "You know, it really does look like a girl lives here."

"I didn't realize pillows, a blanket and a few antiques and art were gender specific."

"Your pillows are baby-blue and cream, your throw is faux leopard and your art is Erté. I have two words for you, and they're hyphenated—girl-like."

She was looking at him through big blue eyes that were ringed with shadow, her hair was already rumpled and she was all curled up in a ball that he thought was so little he could almost pick her up and toss her into the other room—but she had an impish smile and a lifted chin that said she'd dare him to try.

Raef liked her. Really liked her.

He leaned down, clicked on the universal remote and handed it to her. "Girl-like or not, I also have all the cable channels—in HD."

"That's not girl-like. That's civilized."

He chuckled all the way back to his office.

RAEF TRIED TO WORK, but it was an exercise in frustration. He searched the internet for everything he could find about the three tree doctors, and then stared at their websites. Nothing stood out and screamed *psychic serial killer* about any of them. Melnore, a white guy in his mid-thirties, was divorced and had a part-time kid, or at least that's what his Facebook page said. Elwood, another white guy, didn't have a Facebook page. His website had a fish with a cross in it and by his Photoshopped picture he looked to be late thirties to early forties and in de-nial about balding. "Great, a church boy. He's gonna be fun to research." According to the TU faculty website, Braggs completed the white, middle-aged trifecta. He was single and newly tenured at the university. His faculty picture was standard conservative suit and tie. He looked professorially boring. His bio didn't mention any family. He needed a haircut, but besides that looked as harmless as the other two. "Could be any or all of them."

Raef pushed his chair back from his desk and rolled his shoulders. He felt like shit. Not hungover anymore, but tired and woolly-headed. He glanced at the computer clock—just after noon. Preston would be at lunch. He wouldn't call for at least the next hour or so.

"Combat nap time," he told the air around him, then he padded quietly down the hallway and stole a peek at Lauren. The TV was on, but turned way down. The day had become overcast, and the room was dim, but he could see by the light from the TV that her eyes were closed. *Good. We'll both be better off after forty winks.* Raef reclined onto his wide bed, fully clothed, put his phone on Vibrate, slid it into his jeans pocket and closed his eyes. Sleep came to him like it had since his days in the military—fast and easy.

Which was exactly how he came awake, too, when the feeling intruded on an excellent dream he was having about playing shortstop during the World Series.

Hope! I know it's ridiculous, impossible, but I can feel hope. Raef lay there for a moment, just soaking in the emotion. God, it felt good. Better than pleasure. Better than joy.

And then he realized why he was feeling it.

Aubrey had to be here.

Quickly, quietly, he padded on sock feet to where he could look into the living room. He'd been right. She was there, sitting on the couch beside Lauren, who was awake. They were talking in low voices, their heads tilted toward each other, and

Raef was struck by how alike they were. It wasn't just how they looked. It was the way they moved—the way they both talked with their hands. As he watched, Aubrey swept back a strand of diaphanous blond hair that had floated over her face, just like Lauren had been doing all morning. She said something Raef couldn't hear, but it had Lauren giggling and then pressing a hand over her mouth, as if she'd just laughed at something mischievous—*or raunchy,* Raef thought as he watched Lauren fan herself like her face was suddenly hot.

He didn't think he'd made a noise, though he was smiling, but Aubrey chose then to look around her sister and straight at him.

"Come on in, Kent. We have a proposition for you," she said, sounding both mischievous and raunchy.

9

"What's the proposition?" he asked, wondering why even though he sounded reluctant his feet were propelling him quickly to join the two women.

"Aubrey wants to give you something," Lauren said, still looking flushed-cheeked and sounding a little breathless.

"*But I need Lauren's help.*" Aubrey grinned at her twin. "*And she's agreed. Happily.*"

Raef was almost as suspicious as he was curious. Almost. "All right, what do you want to give me?"

"*We'll tell you—or rather, we'll show you—but first I want you to promise me you'll open your mind and your heart and be willing to just go with it.*"

A red flag went up for Raef, but it was hard to assess the warning when Aubrey and Lauren were both beaming full-wattage smiles at him. "I need to know what it is I'm being open about before I make that promise." Even he could hear the bullshit in his voice. Hell, he'd agree to be open to sprouting wings and jumping off the fucking garage if those two kept smiling at him like that.

"It's part of being open, Raef. You don't get to know what you're promising—you get to be *open* to all sorts of possibilities." Then Lauren giggled, and her cheeks got even pinker.

Raef went from being curious to intrigued, and that trumped suspicious. "All right. I promise. Now, what are you two cooking up?"

Aubrey stood. *"Just a little hope, and that plus pleasure and joy makes for a feast."* The ghost lifted her hand and Lauren stood beside her. The women smiled at each other. *"Are you ready?"* Aubrey asked her.

"As I'll ever be," Lauren said. Raef thought she sounded nervous.

"It'll be fine. I'll drive," Aubrey said teasingly.

"You always were better at *driving* than me," Lauren said. She shook back her hair and laughed. "Just do it. I'm ready to take one for the team."

Aubrey looked from her twin to Raef. She *really* looked at Raef—moving her gaze from his feet, all the way up, slowly, to meet his eyes. Raef felt himself start to harden. *What the hell? Just her look does that to me?*

Then Aubrey turned her gaze back to Lauren. *"Oh, please, sis! Take one for the team? This is going to be better than buttered popcorn and Raisinets!"*

Raef thought he heard Lauren whisper something that sounded like "Nothing's better than popcorn and Raisinets…" but he couldn't be sure, and what Aubrey did next blew his mind so totally and completely that he forgot everything except what was happening right before him.

Aubrey and Lauren were facing each other. Lauren opened her arms and Aubrey stepped into them, as if they were going to embrace. But their joining didn't end with a hug. Aubrey seemed to melt into Lauren. Slowly and without any of the ripping or tearing or shattering that had come before, Aubrey disappeared.

Lauren was silent and still for several moments. Then she lifted her right hand. Staring at it, she traced the fingers of her left hand down her palm, wrist and forearm. "Wow, I'd forgotten."

"Lauren?" Raef asked, even though his gut told him her answer before she did.

She turned blue eyes to him. Her smile widened. "No, Kent, not Lauren. Or at least not *just* Lauren."

"Aubrey!"

She closed the few feet between them. "Yes, it's me." She lifted her right hand again, cupping his cheek. "You shaved just this morning, but you're already stubbly. All that dark, manly stubble. I like it. It's going to feel wonderful against Lauren's soft skin."

"Possession—it's, uh, dangerous." He sounded like an idiot, but her touch had his pulse jumping and his dick hardening.

Her hand went from his cheek to his neck. Her fingers were soft and delicate and so, so warm. They slid from there down the front of his sweatshirt, pausing over his nipple, where she used her nails, lightly, to caress him.

He inhaled sharply.

She smiled.

"For most people it is dangerous, but we're twins. We shared the same womb. It's different for us." As she spoke, Aubrey moved her hand to the waist of his jeans. There she paused again, and slipped her hand up under the edge of his sweatshirt, until her fingers touched the skin just beneath his belly button. There she used her fingernails again. Lightly she stroked naked flesh, following the waistline of his jeans.

"It's still not healthy. Not right." Raef was breathing so hard he sounded like he was running a damn marathon.

"This is where the part about promising to be open comes in." Her fingertips moved down until they found his erection, and then she traced the long, hard line of his cock—slowly—up and down. "Kent, you strike me as a man who keeps his promises," she whispered as she leaned into him. "Am I wrong?"

"No!" The word came out with a moan of desire. "But you're not alive. And you're not Lauren."

"Kent, just open yourself to me and let yourself feel it." She lifted her other hand and curled it around his broad shoulder.

"Feel what? All I can feel is you, and I'm fucking sure that's not right!"

She smiled. "Yes, feel me, but also let yourself feel hope—the hope that there is more to this life than what you've known, or even what you've believed yourself capable of." Then, before he could say anything, or move away, or second-guess what was happening, Aubrey kissed him.

She was sweet and soft, and so damn warm. Her mouth was open and inviting, and he could not say no. His arms went around her and his tongue met hers, touching, tasting, desiring, and as he moaned again and lost himself in the taste of her, he *felt* it —hope. It filled him to overflowing. He'd been right in the bedroom. It was better than pleasure and joy. It was a rare and wonderful thing that lit him from within.

Raef stopped kissing her long enough to look down at her flushed, smiling face. "I don't care that you're dead. I don't care that this is Lauren's body. Right now—for this moment—I'm going to hope that somehow this is all going to turn out right. And I gotta have you, Aub. I gotta."

"Then I'm yours—for this moment." She gave him a little

push and he sat back on the couch. Lauren had been wearing a pullover sweater the color of her eyes, and a pair of ass-hugging jeans. Still smiling at him, Aubrey pulled off the sweater and unzipped, then stepped out of, the jeans. She paused for a moment, looked down at herself and laughed softly. "French lace from Muse at Utica Square. Sis, I knew I could count on you for the sexy specialty lingerie." Her eyes found Raef again. "Do you like it?" Aubrey touched her nipple through the pink lace.

How the hell could pink lace be so damn sexy?

Raef nodded and swallowed. His mouth felt dry. "Yeah," he said gruffly. "I like it. A lot."

"And this?" Her hand moved caressingly down her softly rounded, womanly belly to the tiny triangle of pink lace that was the matching thong panty.

Raef thought his dick was going to explode. He nodded again. "Yeah, and that." Then he had her gasping as he moved quickly, reaching around her to cup her curvy ass in his hands, and pulling her forward so that he could press his lips against the blond triangle of curls he could see through the lace.

With a laugh that was definitely more breathless than she'd been before, Aubrey stepped back, just out of his reach. "Now it's your turn." She gestured at his clothes. "I want to look, too."

Raef didn't have to be asked twice. He peeled his sweatshirt off and tossed it across the couch and, with a quick motion, stripped off his jeans and kicked them away.

Aubrey widened Lauren's eyes. "Commando? Always?"

"Always," he said. "Your turn." His eyes went from her bra to her panties.

"Well, it only seems fair," she said teasingly, reaching around to unhook the bra, and shimmying out of it. She took off the panties more slowly, letting him watch her glide them down her thighs and lift her gorgeous little feet up, one at a time, and step delicately from them.

"Will you come to me now?" Raef opened his arms to her. "Please."

"Yes, Kent. Yes, I will."

The wide leather couch became an erotic playground as Raef explored her body. Her nipples were tight under his tongue, and he loved how they filled his hands, but he stopped only briefly there—he had to taste her, he had to feel her against his mouth. He moved down to the damp blond curls between her legs. She opened her legs for him and he pressed his lips against her mound. Then his tongue found her clit, and she moaned his name as he teased it—back and forth. His mouth moved down, to the very center of her, and he guided her hand so that her fingers took the place of his tongue. He looked up at her and met her gaze. "Will you touch yourself for me like you did last night?"

"Yes," she whispered.

And then her whisper turned to gasps and moans as her slim fingers stroked herself, and his tongue teased and caressed along with it until he felt her thighs tense and her body tremble. She called his name out as she came and he pressed his mouth to her, tasting the waves of pleasure that washed through her body.

Aubrey surprised him then, by reaching down and pulling him up to her. She was laughing and flushed, and her hair was wild all around her shoulders. "Your turn. Again." She shifted her body so that she was on top of him, and then, with a mischievous grin, began moving down his body.

He didn't have to tell her. She already seemed to know his hot spots—those two places on his body that drove him mad. Her tongue found the first—his nipples—and he couldn't hold back the moan of pleasure. She glanced up. "Yeah, that's what I thought." Then she dipped her head and her tongue went back to work on his nipple, lightly and quickly, teasing him while she flicked the other one gently until it, too, was taut and ready for her tongue.

When she took his cock in her hand he had to grind his teeth together and try like hell to think of taxes so he didn't come. Her hand was as warm and teasing as her tongue, and she worked both of them together. Just when he knew he was going to explode, she stopped, pressed her breasts against his chest, and kissed him deeply, playing the same game with his tongue that she had with his nipples. In one motion, she shifted again, and straddled him. Tossing back her hair, she sank onto him, consuming him with her wet heat. While their gazes met and held she began moving up and down, sliding the length of him.

"Do you feel it? Do you feel me?" she asked him breathlessly.

"Yes, oh, God, yes." He did. He felt the heat of her body and the pleasure it was giving him, and he also felt her emotions—joy and pleasure and hope, most of all hope. His hands found her waist and he guided their tempo so that his reality narrowed to only her. He was looking in her eyes as his orgasm took him, an earthquake of feeling that shook the very foundations of his world. He cried her name, too—the name of a ghost, the name of a woman he couldn't hope to really have, but who had somehow breathed life into his battered soul.

When she collapsed on his chest he held her tightly, feeling her heartbeat against his, feeling the slickness of their sweat between them. She nuzzled his neck and kissed him and murmured something sleepily. He stroked her hair, loving the silky feel of it. She sighed then, and lifted herself just enough to look into his eyes.

"I have to go now," Aubrey said softly.

There was a terrible tightness in Raef's chest. "I know."

"Even though we're twins, this is hard for Lauren."

Raef started to draw away from her, trying to gently slide her aside. "I hope she isn't—"

Aubrey pressed her fingers against his lips. "Shhh, don't say it. Lauren isn't sorry. Lauren isn't upset. She's been here the whole time." Aubrey took his hand and put it over her heart. "She's just letting me drive, that's all."

"This isn't easy for me," Raef admitted, his voice hesitant.

"Me, either. But we're going to make it through to a happily ever after," Aubrey said.

"God, I hope so," he said.

She smiled. "Hope—I like that. Hold on to it, Kent."

Then Aubrey closed Lauren's eyes. Her body went limp in his arms. Raef felt a chill pass over him. He didn't look. He didn't need to. He knew Aubrey was gone.

In his arms Lauren stirred and looked up at him, blinking groggily.

"Hi," he said, not sure what the hell to do and wishing Aubrey had at least waited to get dressed before she'd unpossessed her sister.

"Hi," she said.

Lauren didn't move out of his arms, but he could feel the tension in her body—her very naked body—because it was pressed against his very naked body.

"So," she said, "how do we make this not awkward?"

"I have no idea," he said honestly.

At that moment his cell phone, which was still in the front pocket of his discarded jeans, had the good sense to start vibrating.

10

"Might be the office," he said, carefully pulling away from her, grabbing his jeans and the phone in one quick motion. The number was from After Moonrise, and, grateful for the reprieve, he punched the accept-call button. "Yeah, Preston, what do you have for me?" Raef spoke into the phone, keeping his back to Lauren while he pulled on his jeans.

"Got the results of the accidental-death search," Preston said.

"Hang on, I'm gonna put you on Speaker." Raef turned around to find Lauren in the process of pulling on his USAF sweatshirt.

"Let me get some paper first," she said when her head popped into view. She hurried back to his office and he numbly muttered something to Preston about waiting a second.

Actually, he didn't remember much of what he'd said to Preston. Raef was too busy staring at Lauren going and coming. His sweatshirt was huge on her, coming almost to mid shapely thigh, but somehow it was even sexier than the damn pink lace.

She sat on the couch, crossed her legs demurely, brushed back her hair and held the pencil expectantly. "Okay, I'm ready," she said.

He pressed the speaker button, thinking that he'd never look at that old sweatshirt the same way ever again.

"Let's hear it, Preston."

"So, I think there are two cases over the past twelve months that you'll be interested in." Preston's voice was as business-like and efficient as he was. "One happened last January. Remember that bad snowstorm just before the long weekend?"

"Yeah, I do," Raef said. Lauren nodded agreement.

"On January 20, some local teenager, Charlie Padgett, took his daddy's Camaro for a joyride to Mohawk Park, along with a case of beer. The storm dumped six inches of snow in an hour. Police report said the kid got drunk and then stuck in the snow. He tried to walk out of the park and fell down and froze to death instead. It was ruled an accident."

"I'm hoping the tree connection is more than just the fact that Mohawk Park has trees," Raef said.

"Definitely. The kid's body was discovered by a tree-trimming team," Preston said.

"Is there anything in the report besides the tree trimmers being there for regular maintenance?" Lauren asked. "Were they there for a more specific reason?"

Into Preston's stunned silence Raef explained, "That's Lauren Wilcox. She's working her sister's case with me."

Preston cleared his throat. "Oh, well, okay. Yes, Miss Wilcox, the police report was thorough. TPD questioned the trimmers extensively. Apparently they were under the direction of a consulting arborist who was overseeing the cleanup after the storm."

"Did they list the tree doc's name?" Raef asked.

"Let me check." Preston paused while Raef heard the tapping sounds of a keyboard. "No, the report just says that they were under the direction of a city-hired arborist."

"What about the other death?" Raef asked while Lauren took notes.

"The other was in April. Caused by a frat-boy binge, complete with the kid choking on his own vomit, even though he was described by all of his friends as a nondrinking nerd. There's no direct arborist connection listed, just a coincidental tree connection. The body was found by the campus landscapers behind a very expensive pallet of saplings the university had spent lots of alumni money on to replace the trees that didn't make it through the last ice storm in February. I figured no one would spend so much money on a bunch of trees without consulting an arborist, so I thought you might be interested."

"Please tell me the university you're talking about is TU and not OSU-Tulsa or TCC," Raef said.

"As a matter of fact, it is," he said.

"Preston, you might have just served our killer to me on a silver platter. Take the rest of the day off."

"You know it's already an hour past quitting time, don't you?" Preston said.

Lauren hid her giggle with a cough.

"Right. I've been, uh, busy." Raef didn't meet Lauren's gaze. "So, what I meant to say was for you to take the morning off. Tomorrow. And good job."

"Thanks, boss," Preston said, with only a hint of sarcasm before disconnecting.

"It's Braggs," Lauren said.

"Good possibility it is," he agreed.

She tapped the paper she'd been taking notes on, frowning. "January, April, July." Lauren looked up at him. "If this is him, he's killing in three-month cycles. Raef, it's October."

"He's due," Raef said.

"So we're going to go apprehend him, right?" Lauren was already getting up and heading toward the pool of pink lace that was very near his feet. "I mean, we'll question him and see if he squirms?"

He sighed and grabbed her by his sweatshirt, lifting her up so that she wasn't bending over and showing way too much of her pretty little ass. "*We're* not. *I* am."

She frowned up at him. "I'm going with you."

"To confront the serial killer who murdered your twin sister, still has her soul trapped and is ready to murder again? No, you're not."

Instead of pulling away from him, Lauren pressed her hand against his chest. "I have to. It's logical."

"Putting you in danger isn't logical." Her touch was doing weird things to him, and he had to keep reminding himself that she was not Aubrey. *But, damn! She felt like her and looked like her and even if she wasn't Aubrey he really liked her and--* Raef shook his head, trying to clear his thoughts. "I'll check him out and tell you everything. You'll be in on all of it, but from a safe distance."

"There is no safe distance for me, Raef! I'm being drained just like Aubrey is being drained. We don't have time to mess around with this. The bottom line is that it's logical that I come with you because you'll know as soon as he sees me if he's the killer."

Raef stared down at her. She was right. If Braggs was the killer the sight of Lauren, looking so much like one of his murder victims, would evoke strong, negative emotions from him—emotions Raef's Gift would definitely be able to pick up.

He blew out a long breath of frustration. "You can come, but it has to be on my terms."

"Anything," she said, hugging him hard.

Raef let himself hold her and breathe in her scent. "Stay close to me. Stay quiet. And if bad shit starts going down you run like hell and call 9-1-1. Promise me."

"I promise," she said, and squeezed him tightly before letting him go.

"And I want my sweatshirt back, too," he said.

She had bent over to pick up her panties. She paused, straightened, and with a smile that had his heartbeat speeding up, Lauren pulled his sweatshirt over her head and tossed it at him. Then, very slowly, she said, "Be careful what you ask for, Raef."

He swallowed, muttered, "Thanks," and retreated into his bedroom as fast as his rubber legs could carry him.

THERE'D BEEN A MAJOR redo to the University of Tulsa's campus over the past couple of years. What had once been a nondescript entrance to a cluster of light-colored stone buildings mixed with modern stuff stuck in a kinda dicey part of town at Eleventh and Harvard had turned into a real university campus—complete with a swanky stone-and-wrought-iron perimeter fence and excellent landscaping.

Hell, they even had a fountain.

Raef was an ex-TU student. He hadn't graduated, but he liked to think that the several thousand dollars he'd paid in tuition during his three long years there had bought at least a few yards of the new fencing. Or maybe a portion of the fountain. Whatever. He still knew enough about the campus to pull into the main entrance at Tucker Drive and take a right to snake around to the bio building, Oliphant Hall. He parked in the west lot, shut off the car and turned to face Lauren.

"Okay, here's why we're here. We need Dr. Braggs's advice on how to save the big old elm in my front yard because we heard he's an expert on curing Dutch elm disease."

"There is no real cure for Dutch elm disease," she said.

He sighed. "Look at me. Do you think he'd think I know that?"

She raised her brows, and even though her eyes were tired and shaded, they sparkled at him. "Probably not."

"Exactly. So, if this is our guy you need to understand that his first sight of you will elicit some strong negative emotions. He'll be in turmoil, even if he looks totally calm to you. I'm going to ask for his business card—so I can reach him later about my elm, because right now we're in a hurry to get to a dinner date. You stay behind me. I'll be between you and him. You'll be near the door. We'll get in, and get out, and if I pick up negative emotions from him I will make a call to TPD. They'll take it from there."

"And I'm supposed to?"

"Play blonde. You can do that, right?"

Instead of getting pissed and narrowing her eyes at him, she blinked guilelessly and fell into a very good Okie accent. "Why, what do ya mean, sir? I'm simply standin' by my man like any well-trained woman would. Could ya please help him so that he's in a real good mood when he lets me fry him up some dinner while he 'reads'—" she air quoted "—the *Sports Illustrated* swimsuit issue?"

"Stop scaring me," he said, trying—unsuccessfully—to hide his smile.

"You lead and I'll follow," she said, obviously not trying to hide her smile.

"Hey," he said before she could get out of the car. "Remember that this isn't a game. If Braggs is our guy he's a killer."

Her blue eyes met his steadily. "I'll never forget that. Don't worry about me. Do your part. I'll be the silent bait and then I'll stay out of your way."

He started to tell her that she wasn't the damn bait, but she was already out of the car and standing on the sidewalk that led to the front entrance of Oliphant Hall.

Raef, you have lost your fucking mind, he told himself.

Lauren didn't stay on the sidewalk long. When he joined her she was crouched over some short greenish bushes inspecting their leaves.

"Azaleas," she said, before he could ask the question. "Sleeping ones, actually, which is what they're supposed to be doing this time of year. They're well tended—definitely in good shape. The groundskeepers know their business here."

"Ted Bundy had a girlfriend who said he was a good guy—and all the while he was slaughtering young coeds."

"Who?"

"How old are you?"

"Twenty-seven. What does that have to do with—"

"Never mind," he interrupted, feeling old and worried and insane, all at the same time. "Just keep in mind not everything is how it looks. And do exactly what I tell you to do."

"Okay, I got it." Then she touched his arm. "If it's Braggs and he's arrested, what happens then?"

"Well, I'll let the police know about the psychic entrapment, and that we believe he's taken his victims' souls to the Land of the Dead. They'll bring in a shaman who specializes in soul retrieval."

"Right away?"

He hated that she sounded so scared. "Yeah, I'll make sure of it." *And if they don't move fast enough, I'll Track the bastard to the Land of the Dead and kick his ass myself,* Raef added silently.

"Then Aub will go free?"

"That's the plan," Raef said, his stomach suddenly feeling not so good.

Lauren looked out across the campus, shivered and whispered, "Yes, that's what has to happen, no matter what it does to me."

"Lauren," he said, sounding sharper than he'd meant to because of the worry for her that spiked in his twisting gut. "You won't be drained anymore. You'll be able to—"

"I know," she interrupted him, back to her steady, no-nonsense self. "It'll be okay. Aub and I will be okay." Lauren took her hand from his arm and started walking briskly down the sidewalk.

He didn't have a clue what the hell to say to her. All he could do was try to wade through the conflicting emotions this damn case was making him feel while he caught up with her as Lauren followed the sidewalk around the light sandstone building. Together, they turned to their left to walk beneath white pylons that gave way to a very ordinary-looking glass door.

Raef had taken classes in Oliphant Hall—more than a decade ago, but the smell had stayed the same. "Books and formaldehyde mixed with testosterone and stress. I'll never forget that smell," he said.

"It was the same at OU. I think it's a common higher-education smell. Well, minus the formaldehyde."

A petite girl with big blue eyes and straight, well-maintained blond hair was coming toward them. She had a ridiculously thick anatomy-and-physiology tome clutched against her chest and an it's-midterm-and–I-gotta-study frown creasing her otherwise lineless forehead.

"Excuse me." Raef smiled at her. "Do you know where we can find Dr. Braggs?"

The girl blinked as if coming up through layers of essay test hell, and pointed at the ceiling. "He's probably still in the dissection lab on the third floor—room 303."

"Do you know if he has a class right now?" Lauren asked.

"No," said the college coed. "Lab is done for the day."

"Thank you," Lauren said.

The girl smiled, nodded vaguely and hurried on her way from the building.

Raef called on the recesses of his college experience and accessed a few brain bytes that he hadn't killed with alcohol poisoning. "Over here." He led Lauren a little way down the wide hallway to an industrial-looking metal door that had been painted the same unpleasant yellow as the rest of the first floor. "It's the stairwell that leads up to the third floor. If I remember correctly, and don't quote me because halfway through my freshman year I changed my major from Environmental Science to Beerology, this is how we get up to the third-floor classrooms."

"You went here?" Lauren asked as they climbed the stairs.

"For almost three years this is where I matriculated."

"Which means you didn't graduate," she said.

"Not even close," he agreed. "College and I didn't agree."

"Makes sense to me. OU and I had a fundamental disagreement, as well."

"Which was?" he asked, realizing he was actually interested in her answer.

"Well, they thought their students needed to attend class.

Even if said students could *not* attend class and just show up for tests and still make decent grades." Lauren shrugged. "OU and I agreed to disagree."

"You agreed to leave and they agreed to let you?"

Her smile was sly. "No, I agreed to let Mother endow a chair in the botany department, and OU agreed to give me a BS." Her smile turned into a giggle. "A BS! It still makes me laugh. That's exactly what it was—bullshit."

"What about Aubrey?" He couldn't seem to stop himself from asking.

Her gaze met his. He tried to read her eyes and found all he could decipher was weariness and a healthy dose of cynicism.

"Aub graduated with honors—*without* Mother bribing anyone. She has always been the smart one."

"And which one are you?"

"I'm the pragmatic one. Which one are you?" she fired back at him.

"I don't have a twin."

"Let's pretend like you do."

"All right. I'd be the grumpy one," he said.

As he grabbed the metal handle of the door to the third-floor hallway, she said, "Really? My guess is you'd be the lonely one."

11

The smell hit him right away. It had been bad enough on the ground floor. Up here in the dimmer, cooler third-floor hallway it was downright disgusting.

Lauren wrinkled her nose. "Eesh, what is that?"

He glanced at her. "You were a botany major but you didn't take any labs?"

She rolled her eyes at him. "I told you—I *took* a bunch of classes. I just didn't *attend* many of them. So, what's the smell?"

"Death," he said. "Formaldehyde only preserves bodies for so long. It never completely covers the scent of decay."

Lauren looked horrified. "There are dead bodies up here?"

"Yep. Humans, animals and probably a bunch of bugs, too."

She shuddered. "No wonder I never went to class."

"Stay close," he said.

"Don't worry about that. I'm not going anywhere." She wrapped her arm through his.

Raef moved forward with Lauren practically stuck to his

side, trying not to think about how good she felt and how badly he wanted to keep her safe.

The classrooms were clearly labeled and in numerical order, with odd numbers to the left and even on their right. Room 303 was only a few yards from the stairwell exit.

"Ready?" he asked her.

She unwrapped her arm from around his and lifted her chin. "Ready."

Speaking quietly, he said, "This isn't going to take long. Remember, let him see you, but then I'll move between the two of you. Stay behind me."

"And close to the door," she whispered back. "I remember. Let's just get this over with."

He nodded tightly, and pulled the door open by the cold, metallic handle. Only half of the fluorescent bulbs in the classroom were on and very little light managed its way through the high, rectangular windows. Black lab tables were clustered in pods. The smell was bad, but the tables and the aluminum lab chairs—which looked ironically like bar stools—were spotless. The wall closest to them was decorated with large feline physiology posters that were almost as gruesome as the stuff that was floating in huge jars on the shelves that lined two of the other walls. The place was so dim and creepy that at first Raef didn't think anyone was in the room. Then, from the head of the classroom, a man cleared his throat and said, "May I be of some assistance to you?"

"Dr. Braggs?" Raef asked in his best nice-guy voice.

The professor pulled off his glasses and rubbed the bridge of his nose with the back of his hand, which was covered in a latex glove.

"Yes, I am Dr. Braggs. How may I help you?"

"Well, if ya have a sec I'd like to ask you 'bout a tree,"

Raef said, adding a healthy dose of Okie and country-ing up his words.

Braggs blew out a little sigh. "I'm a bit busy setting up tomorrow's lab. But I can talk while I work."

"Hey, great! That'd be great," Raef said, and started moving toward the front of the room, staying ahead of Lauren.

"All right, then. Ask away." Braggs put his glasses back on and bent over the large metal tray that was mounded with something Raef couldn't quite make out. He studied Braggs as he approached him.

Had Raef not been so accustomed to the many faces of evil, he would have automatically discounted Braggs. The guy was absolutely average. His height was average—his balding was average—even the slight paunch he was working on was completely average. He appeared as harmless as Raef's dorky tenth-grade math teacher.

But Raef had spent ten years with the OSI in the air force, and he'd been involved in the apprehension of men who looked like Mr. Rogers, even after they'd strapped explosives to women and babies and intimidated them into going into restaurants to blow themselves up, along with innocent civilians, just to make a pseudo-religious point. It'd been tough to learn to separate the seen from the unseen, but he'd damn well figured it out—lives had depended on him. He'd been good at his OSI job then, and that military experience had helped him become one of the best psychic murder investigators in the U.S. of A.

So, Raef looked past what his eyes could see, reached out and tested the invisible energy around him. Nothing. He felt nothing. Not even the slight hum of irritation Braggs should have been feeling at being interrupted.

"I'm Buddy Chapman," Raef began when they were within handshaking distance of Braggs, "and this is my wife—"

But Raef didn't get a chance to finish his introduction. Lauren, who had been following just a little behind him, had stopped like she'd run into a glass wall. Her eyes were wide, staring at the tray Braggs was working on, and her voice was unusually loud. "You're cutting up a cat!"

Braggs looked up, pulled off his glasses again, his average brown eyes blinking like he was having trouble focusing on Lauren. "Young woman, I am dissecting the internal organs of a feline specimen for tomorrow's nursing students to identify in their anatomy and physiology midterm," he said patronizingly. "I realize this might appear unsavory to an outsider, but I hope you will try to realize that this creature died for the greater good of science." He hesitated and blinked again. Then, as if his vision had finally cleared, his eyes widened. He smiled at Lauren. "You look familiar. Are you a graduate of TU?"

It was when Braggs smiled that the bedlam of emotions hit Raef. Braggs's expression never changed—never wavered from the benign dismissiveness and slight curiosity he was showing Lauren—but inside the *real* Braggs was a seething cesspool of hatred and rage, lust and fear, all mixed with the most disturbing wash of greed and violence Raef had ever felt.

"Graduate of TU? My wife?" Even though Raef was being battered by emotions, Raef forced himself to keep his tone normal, his voice jovial and as mildly patronizing as Braggs's charade. "No, sir. My little woman here married me right outta high school. She went straight to the college of havin' babies, if you know what I mean." As Raef spoke he kept his eyes on Braggs, moving one more step forward, and positioning himself directly in front of the professor, who was on the opposite side of the dissection table, and between him and Lauren. "Hey, I gotta apologize. We shouldn't have barged in here on ya. I just got a question about the big elm in my front yard. It's lookin' sickly and I hear you're a damn good tree doctor."

"Well, thank you," Braggs said, sounding calm and cordial, even though Raef could feel that he roiled with hatred and a deep, desperate need for violence. "I truly do not mind that you and your lovely wife have sought me out."

"Yeah, but you got your work to do, and the wife, she's a little squeamish." Raef tried to chuckle, but only managed to clear his throat. "How 'bout you give me your card and I call and set up an appointment proper?"

"Whatever you wish, Mr. Chapman. I have cards here in my desk, and I do see that your wife is looking rather faint."

Braggs opened the top drawer of the dissection table, and Raef took the opportunity to glance back at Lauren saying, "Honey, you go on back to the car and the kids. I'll get Dr. Braggs's info and meet you—"

"Raef! Watch out!" Lauren screamed, eyes wide and terrified.

Raef lunged to the side, reaching for the concealed Glock he kept in his side holster, but Braggs was already over the table and on him, striking with superhuman speed at his arm with a dissection blade that was so sharp it slit through Raef's sweater and sliced a long, deep path down his arm from bicep to wrist, causing him to drop the gun. It skittered across the slick floor as if it had been paved with ice.

"Lauren, go! Now!" Raef couldn't even look at her. All of his attention was focused on Braggs, who had suddenly morphed from average Joe Blow to a slashing, cutting machine.

Raef grunted with effort as he dodged the guy's blows. His body was taking too damn long to respond. *No, it's not me.*

It's Braggs. He's abnormally fast—abnormally strong. Braggs struck again. Raef couldn't be quick enough. This time the blade sliced a red line across his chest, but Raef's adrenaline was pumping so hard he only felt the warm wetness of his blood. The pain would come later—if he lived until later. *Gotta buy Lauren time to get out of here—to get help.*

Braggs slashed again, ripping a line of blooming scarlet down the inside of Raef's thigh. As Raef staggered, Braggs rushed around him.

"No!" Raef snarled, reaching out and catching the edge of his lab coat and pulling him back. "You're not getting her unless you go through me."

Braggs laughed. Raef thought it was the most terrible sound he'd ever heard. "She's as dead as you are." His words were filled with venom. His face was twisted with anger. "I won't go after her until you bleed out. She can run as far as she wants. I'll find her. I'll kill her. I'll drain her. Just like I did her sister."

Raef didn't see her coming. Neither did Braggs. But suddenly Lauren was there, behind the professor. She swung the long metal pipe she was holding in both hands like a baseball bat, connecting with the back of Braggs's head as she yelled, "Like hell you will!"

Braggs dropped to the floor where he lay utterly motionless.

Lauren was actually descending on him, pipe raised, to hit him again when Raef caught her in his arms. "Stop—he's unconscious. We got him. We got him."

Lauren hugged him hard and then abruptly pushed away from him, her trembling hands hovering over his bleeding knife wounds. "He cut you. Oh, God, Raef. You're bleeding so much."

"I'm gonna be okay." He wanted to touch her face—to hold and reassure her—but she was right. He was bleeding. A lot.

"Lauren, I'm going to cuff Braggs. You call 9-1-1." Stifling a painful groan, Raef crouched over Braggs and took out his handcuffs.

"I can't. I tried, but there's no reception up here. At all." Lauren's breath caught on a sob. "Raef, God, the blood!"

"I'm okay," Raef repeated, trying to sound calm even though he could already feel that he was getting light-headed. He managed to roll Braggs over and cuff him. "Here's what you need to do. Go outside. Call 9-1-1. Get help." He staggered over to where his Glock had slid to a stop against the classroom wall. When he bent to retrieve it his legs gave way so he sat beside the gun, and started to unbuckle the belt to his jeans.

"I'm not going without you." Lauren rushed to his side and was trying to take his hand, obviously thinking she could tug him to his feet.

"Lauren," he said, speaking as quickly and clearly as possible as he cinched the belt around his thigh. "I'm six foot four. I weigh two hundred and thirty-five pounds. You can't even drag me out of here. I've got a tourniquet on this leg wound. The rest will wait. If you get your very shapely little butt outside and call 9-1-1. Understand?"

"Yes. Sorry." She wiped tears from her face, leaving bloody smears across her cheeks. "I'm going right now." She hesitated only long enough to lean down and kiss his forehead. "Don't you dare die on me."

"Not planning on it," he muttered as she turned and started to hurry away.

It was then that Braggs sat up.

His entire face had changed. His eyes were larger, darker and sunken into his head. Blood flowed freely from the cut in the back of his scalp—it ran down his neck and seemed to cloak him in crimson. Raef had no idea how it could be, but the professor looked as if he'd lost half his body weight in a matter of minutes. He'd become almost skeletal and looked more reptilian than human.

"You have both been very inconvenient. I will take particular pleasure in draining you." Braggs drew a deep breath, and with that inhalation Raef could feel the surge of siphoned violence and hatred that filled him, and as it did Lauren dropped to her knees with a terrible moan of agony.

"Lauren!" Raef shouted.

Lauren's gaze met Raef's. "He's draining Aubrey now!" she gasped.

"I've never had twins before," Braggs said. "It's like a two-for-one special." He lifted his arms and snapped the handcuffs as if they were a child's plastic toy, spread his arms and embraced the flood of terror and pain that cascaded into him.

The raw sound of agony that escaped from Lauren sliced through Raef. "He's killing us," she sobbed.

"No, he fucking is not." Raef lifted his Glock and, in one smooth, quick movement, shot Braggs between his eyes, blowing away the entire top of his head.

Even though the world was going oddly gray around the edges, Raef could hear Lauren whimpering not far away from him. "Hey, it's okay. The bastard's dead. It's over. Just don't look at him—it's not a pretty sight."

When Lauren didn't respond, Raef dragged himself over to her, thinking she must be in shock. "Lauren, honey, you gotta pull it together and get me some help. I know I look indestructible, but—" His words cut off as he reached her. She was in a fetal position, her arms wrapped around herself. Her face was absolutely colorless, her eyes blank, open and staring. "Lauren!" With a trembling hand he felt for a pulse. It was weak, but there. "Lauren, damn it! Don't do this! He's dead. He can't hurt you or Aubrey anymore."

The air above Lauren shimmered as Aubrey tried to materialize. Raef could only catch fleeting glimpses of her silhouette.

"Aubrey, what's happening? I got the guy—I killed him!"

Like her spirit, her voice was a weak, whispering shadow of itself, and all Raef heard before Aubrey faded away was, *"You killed his body. It's his soul that's draining us. Save us, Kent...."*

12

"Fuck! I'm a moron!" He closed his eyes against the pounding in his head. "Okay, yeah, I can do this. I Track murderers. Just because the asshole's dead doesn't mean I can't Track him." Raef drew a deep breath and reached out with his Gift.

Nothing.

The only negative emotions left in the room were his own. There was no murder trail. The murderer was dead.

"Save us, Kent..." seemed to hover in the blood-scented air around him.

"How?" Raef shouted. "How the hell do I save you? I can't Track a dead guy!"

The realization hit him and Kent's eyes opened. "I can't Track a dead guy, but I have Tracked a dead girl. I found Aubrey before—I can find her again. And when I find her, I find the bastard that killed her."

Raef only had a moment to feel the relief of his discovery when the world pitched and rolled, and suddenly he was on his back lying beside Lauren's motionless body.

"Hang on, Lauren! I'm not going to die on you!" he tried to shout, but the words came out as barely a whisper. He was losing strength fast…fading fast….

Lauren was going to die. He was going to die. Aubrey was going to cease to exist—they all would. He was going to fail. He was going to die….

So this was it? Time to quit—to give up? He tried to sit, to do something, anything, but his body wasn't obeying him, wasn't working. He knew it because his fucking mind wasn't just working—it was working with bizarre clarity.

Raef might have smiled, but he couldn't be sure because his face had gone numb.

To hell with this Negative Nancy bullshit, Raef growled silently to himself. *If I have to go to the Land of the Dead, being almost dead has gotta be a plus. So all right. Let's really get this thing done.*

Raef closed his eyes and focused on his breathing while he tried to recall what he'd done the night he'd Tracked Aubrey— the night she'd materialized and *felt* with him. What had that damn book said about soul retrieval and the Land of the Dead?

As his body continued to get weaker, Raef's mind became sharper and sharper. Snippets of the book he'd breezed through that night came back to him.

…enter the Land of the Dead without protection and experience, and you risk becoming lost, too…

"Too late," Raef mumbled, and then he continued to recall.

Begin by lighting a candle.

Well, he didn't have a candle, but he did have the memory of a light that he'd never forget—Aubrey's shimmering thread of joy. What was next? What were the rest of those damn directions?

They came to him along with another surge of dizziness.

Once you have Tracked the soul to the Land of the Dead, your psychic Gift will cease to work. You must use mortal guile and your own wisdom to retrieve the lost one.

"That's right. That part seemed like good news then. Now I'm not so sure about my level of guile, let alone wisdom." Raef's voice sounded weird, like it wasn't really attached to his body. Hell, he felt weird, like *he* wasn't really attached to his body.

"Probably more good news for where I'm going." Then Raef shut his mouth and, after one last look at Lauren, closed his eyes.

He thought of Aubrey. Her laughter and her joy. The way she made him feel. No, not just hot and hard and sexy. Aubrey made him *feel*. Ironically, a dead girl had breathed life into a whole world of emotions he'd believed had been irrevocably lost to him because he'd spent most of a lifetime dealing with death and destruction.

And she called him Kent. No one but Aubrey had called him Kent since his Gift had been discovered.

Raef held the light of Aubrey in his mind and in his heart, and with every bit of his skill as a psychic, he reached with his Gift, seeking, searching....

He found her more easily than he'd expected to, even though Aubrey's light wasn't a glowing, ribbonlike trail anymore. All that was left of the shimmering thread of joy he'd glimpsed before was a single, thin beam of light the color of champagne gone flat. The dimness of Aubrey's light scared him so deeply that it severed the tie that remained with his body, and Raef felt his spirit shoot away from the cold classroom. He didn't waste time worrying about how the hell he was going to get back. He didn't hesitate. Instead, he rushed after Aubrey's fading light, Tracking her with a speed and ease he'd never before experienced, which was good and bad. It was good because it was like he'd been fired from a cannon straight and sure into the Land of the Dead. It was bad because it was like he'd been fired from a cannon straight and sure into the Land of the Dead—and had less than a heartbeat to prepare himself for the experience.

Though I don't know how the hell anyone could be prepared for this shit, Raef told himself as he drifted to a halt, watching Aubrey's fading light disappear into the seething caldron of misery below him.

The sound of it hit him first. Voices drifting up to him were an awful mixture of sobs and screams and pleadings. He tried to make out single words, but it was difficult. It was like he had landed in the middle of an amphitheater that was hosting a chaotic symphony of hopelessness. He stared, trying to find the source of the voices. It was tough to get a good look at what was below him because a thick fog drifted over everything. Raef made himself drop closer to the land, and pockets of fog parted to reveal a landscape of utter desolation. It was like the Mojave mixed with the Arctic mixed with a nuclear wasteland. Almost totally devoid of color, the land lacked anything that was growing or sheltering, and all over the place was littered with what Raef at first thought were bizarrely shaped stones, jutting up from the bleak, drought-cracked ground. It wasn't until one of the stones moved that he realized they weren't rocks at all—they were bodies that had become grotesquely fused to the land. A shoulder jutted, an eyeless head was frozen, faceup, an arm protruded.

And even more awful, Raef watched as one of the fused bodies opened its mouth and shrieked.

Raef shuddered with revulsion. The bodies still had life in them, even though they lacked color or animation or expression, and they had actually become part of the land.

Aubrey? Oh, God, is one of them Aubrey? And Lauren? Is that how Braggs has them trapped—not by his own force, but by the force of this terrible place?

Almost in a panic, Raef reached out again for her slim beam of light, but he found nothing—felt nothing. He couldn't Track her at all.

Then he remembered—the book had said when he reached the Land of the Dead his Gift wouldn't work, that he'd have to use his brains and his wits. *So think!* he ordered himself. He'd Tracked Aubrey here—it was just when he actually arrived that his Gift had gone.

He stared around him, trying to clear his thoughts. Okay, maybe he should just start going from body to body and calling her name.

No. That felt wrong, and he didn't have time to waste searching aimlessly. *Think! Use some of that fucking wisdom both girls believe you have!* He stared around him. What a colorless, hopeless place. There was not one green thing—not one bit of sunlight or blue sky or even the familiar brown of a winter-nude tree.

Wait, he thought. *I might have something. Aubrey has color! Her spirit, even though it's trapped here and being drained, has enough color left in it to leave a trail for me.*

He didn't need to search the pathetic, colorless people who

had utterly given up and had no more light about them at all. He just needed to search for light—any light.

Raef shifted his attention from the horrible, fused figures and began drifting. As he did he searched, sweeping his gaze back and forth, peering through fog and darkness, until off to his right a slight flicker of something like a candle caught in a great wind pulled at the edge of his sight. Raef redirected himself until he was hovering over the spot he was sure he'd seen the glimmer of color.

The damned fog was everywhere and he made himself drop down, closer to the ground itself. When he got lower the fog parted and the land beneath him fell away, leaving Raef staring down at a huge pit that was filled with a sewerlike, vitreous liquid that roiled and churned. With a shudder of disgust, Raef saw that people were bobbing around in the liquid, frantically trying to stay afloat. The people appeared to be as colorless as the bodies fused to the land, but as he watched, light fluttered across the face of one of the swimmers—right before she was engulfed in a wave and her head went under—only to reappear with a gasp and a terrible scream of agony a moment later.

It was the voice he recognized before he recognized her pale, terrified face.

"Lauren!" he shouted, commanding himself to go even lower—to go down to her.

"Raef! He's here! He—" Lauren's head went under again.

"Hang on! I'm coming!" Raef reached into the oil-slick water, feeling through the cold, dark liquid for her, but his search was suddenly stopped as something hard caught him in his gut and hurled him into the air and away from the pit.

He gasped with shock as pain lashed through him, blurring his vision. Raef blinked hard. When his focus finally came back he was looking down at a creature that was circling the top lip of the pit. Lizardlike, its body stretched all the way around the circumference of the pit. It had multiple tails that whipped in agitation at Raef. It opened its fang-lined maw to hiss at him—a sound that made the fluid in the pit churn even more crazily and had the swimmers, whose lights were now barely visible, crying out and struggling even harder to stay afloat.

"*Stop!*" Raef shouted at the creature. "*You'll drown them all!*"

The lizard thing opened its horrible mouth again and familiar laughter drifted across the liquid pit and up to Raef. "*Yessss,*" it hissed. "*I will drown them, but slowly, after I have bled everything I can from them. Are you here to join them? Your scarlet light will make a nice addition to my collection.*"

Raef met the creature's dark eyes—eyes Raef recognized as easily as he had the laughter and the voice.

Raef looked from the Braggs creature to the pit, and saw Lauren's head go under again. The sight worked like a goad on him and his answer rang clear and strong through the sounds of misery around him. "*I didn't come to join them, but I'll take their place. You can have me and my light, just let the twins go.*"

"*No, Raef!*" Lauren shouted. The Braggs creature reached into the pit and swirled the liquid with a claw, and Lauren's head was engulfed in another oily wave.

"*Look!*" Raef felt foolish, but he waved his arms like he was trying to flag the attention of a charging bull. "*You don't want her. She's almost used up. I'm not.*"

The Braggs creature paused, drawing his claw from the liquid. His dark eyes met Raef's gaze. *Hatred,* Raef thought. *I don't need my Gift to know that Braggs is hatred become tangible.*

Braggs's soulless laughter drifted around him again. "*No,*" he said. "*I will not trade with you. Between us there is that little matter of the fact that you killed my body. That will be inconvenient for me until I can find another to take its place."*

I need my fucking Glock right now, Raef thought.

"And if I remember correctly, back in the mortal realm your body is very busy dying. Soon you will be just another lost soul here. Who knows, you might accidentally stumble into my pit."

"Hey, it doesn't have to be like this. Maybe we can make a deal." Even though he felt like he was grasping at straws, Raef spoke quickly. At least while he talked Braggs was more focused on him than on pushing under the heads in the pit and slowly, slowly, while he spoke, Raef drifted closer and closer to Lauren. *"You say you need a new body. Take mine. I'll trade it for the twins."*

Braggs's laughter was a hiss. *"No, your body is dying."*

"I'm tougher than you think. Afghanistan couldn't kill me. I'll bet you didn't, either. That Glock makes one hell of a roar. Paramedics are probably on their way to TU right now."

"Perhaps. We could wait and see. If you drop to the land—you have died. If not—maybe you'll live. Maybe we'll trade then."

"No, Kent!" Aubrey's voice was weak. He could see that her mouth was barely above the churning liquid. *"You can't trade with him! He'll cheat you. You have to beat him. Remember what I taught you! That's all you need to—"*

Braggs snarled, and one of his tails snaked out and forced Aubrey's head under the liquid. Raef wanted to go to her—wanted to kick Braggs's ass and pull her and Lauren out of there—but Braggs was so fucking big that he covered the entire lip of the pit. Raef glanced down at himself, hoping for just an instant that he might have materialized in this realm as something other than his all too human, and all too vulnerable, body.

Sadly, he had not been turned into a knight in shining

armor. He was just himself, albeit a less substantial version of himself.

The creature of hatred continued to circle the pit, watching him warily, tails writhing, jaws snapping. *"Why not come even closer? Let's fight for the twins."*

Raef wanted to—he wanted to so damn bad! But he wasn't an utter moron. Until he'd brought out the Glock, Braggs had been beating him. Actually, Braggs had probably killed him.

"Fight for the twins? If I'm gonna come down there to kick your scaly ass, I want more than just two women if I win." Raef stalled as Braggs taunted him, hissing insults while his tentacled tail tortured the struggling souls in the pit.

Think! Raef ordered himself again. *Listen to Aubrey! Remember what she taught me.*

What the hell had she taught him? She'd made him feel. She'd taught him that instead of holding on to suspicion and negativity, he could feel joy and laughter. She'd reminded him that there was pleasure to be had in life.

She'd taught him to have hope.

Hope was exactly what was missing in the Land of the Dead!

As the understanding came to him, Raef felt the truth of it swell within him—and joy and laughter, happiness and pleasure and hope filled his floating spirit, warming him like a hearth fire.

"What are you doing?" Braggs snarled. He'd turned all of his attention from the pit to Raef.

Raef looked down at himself and blinked in amazement at what he saw. From the middle of his chest light glowed scarlet and orange, yellow and white, like an otherworldly flame. *"I—I don't know. My Gift's not supposed to work here."*

He hadn't realized he'd spoken aloud until Aubrey, obviously using the last reserves of her strength, shouted up at him. *"It's not your Gift—it's you. It's who you really are, so you brought it with you."*

"Silence, bitch! It is time for you to cease to exist!" Braggs pressed a clawed foot against Aubrey's head, holding her under the liquid.

"No, Braggs. It's time for you to cease to exist!" Acting on instinct Raef reached within himself and found the Gift that was truly his—the joy and pleasure and hope that Aubrey had awakened in his life. And, like he was the starting shortstop back in middle school—back when he'd been an unlikely hero for anyone who was weaker than himself—Raef threw the ball of luminous emotions directly into Braggs's face.

Blinded, the creature shrieked and began lunging and snapping and biting so violently that it attacked itself—tearing huge hunks from his own flesh, which seemed to goad him on, making Braggs writhe and shriek and bite himself even more desperately.

With no hesitation, Raef rushed down, slipping past the creature that, blinded by hope, was destroying itself. He found Lauren first and held out his hand to her. *"Grab my hand!"* he shouted over Braggs's panicked roars.

Lauren grasped his hand, but as he began pulling her up she shook her head and resisted. *"No, I won't go without Aubrey."*

"I'll come back for her. I'll come back for as many as I can," he said.

"No. I'm not leaving without her—not without the rest of them."

"Lauren, we don't have time for this. I don't know what the hell is happening back in Tulsa with my body. You're alive. You're the only one here who I am one hundred percent sure is alive."

"If you believe that, we're all doomed," Lauren said.

"Damn it! I'm just being logical. I can't pull you all out. No damn

way I'm strong enough. I'm gonna lose everyone that way. I have to—" His words cut off as Raef realized what he was doing. It wasn't force or logic that had blinded Braggs and caused the creature to turn on itself. It was hope and joy, pleasure and laughter. He met Lauren's eyes and smiled. *"You're right, girl. We're all going home today. Find her. I know you can do it, and I've got you until you do."*

Lauren's smile was almost as brilliant as the beam of light that shot through Raef's body, sizzling with heat and hope, speeding down into Lauren, lifting her as it lifted Raef. As Lauren's body slid from the slimy pit, the ray of light extended down and Raef watched as a hand reached from under the surface, grabbing on to it. Aubrey's head broke the surface. She gasped and coughed, but she held tight to the ribbon of light, which passed through her and snagged another fading swimmer—a teenager. Lifting, Raef saw another swimmer grab the life light, and another and another until he had all of them free of the pit and of the creature of hatred as it completely self-destructed.

Raef's ribbon of light whipped up and up, carrying a whole trail of spirits, bright and glistening, all with colors of their own. Laughter filled the air, along with luminous light as the spirits Raef had freed floated around him, causing the bleak sky over the Land of the Dead to shimmer and shine, rainbow-like. And then, with a bright flash, each of the spirits began spinning off, reminding Raef of shooting stars, until he was left there hovering with Lauren and Aubrey.

"You did it!" Lauren cried. She was still holding tight to his hand, which she lifted to her lips, kissing his palm softly. *"Thank you, Raef. Thank you so much."*

He started to respond. To tell Lauren that she'd had a whole hell of a lot to do with the saving part, but before he could speak her eyes widened in surprise, then she gasped and disappeared.

"*Lauren? What the hell?*"

"*She's not dead, Kent,*" Aubrey said, drifting to him. "*She went back to the mortal realm, back to her body.*" She smiled, and even though joy sparkled like champagne all around her, tears filled and then spilled over her eyes. "*You'll go back soon, too.*"

"*I don't want to go back.*" He reached for her. "*Not without you.*"

Aubrey wrapped her arms around him. "*I wish I'd met you before,*" she whispered to him.

"*I can feel you,*" he said, holding tightly to her.

"*It's our souls. They know each other. Maybe they always will.*" Aubrey kissed him then and Raef's spirit trembled at her touch. "*I never doubted that you would save us,*" Aubrey said against his lips. "*Never.*"

"*I didn't save you—you saved me. Because of you I learned to laugh again. To feel again. To hope again. Without you I wouldn't have been able to—*"

Raef didn't get to finish. He didn't even get to say goodbye. His words were cut off as pain sliced through him and his spirit was ripped from Aubrey's arms, returning to his body with a terrible jolt of agony.

"That's it! We got him back! Hang in there, man, we're almost at St. John's."

Raef blinked up at the EMT who was putting the paddles back in the slots on the crash cart. There were tubes in his nose and arms and he felt like his chest was on fire.

"Aubrey," Raef tried to shout, but the name was barely audible. The EMT bent over him, putting pressure on his chest wound, and Raef repeated weakly, "Aubrey."

"She's fine. Just shaken up and a little shocky. The cops are bringing her in behind us."

"No," Raef whispered. "She's dead." Then he closed his eyes and the world went black.

RAEF CAME TO SLOWLY. At first he didn't know where he was, and his immediate thought was that he was really going to have to lay off the single malt. He was getting too damn old for two hangovers in as many days. He felt like utter hell. Shit, his chest hurt! Not even eighteen-year-old Macallan was worth this. He must have had more to drink than he'd had that night he'd gotten so shitfaced that he'd forgotten Aubrey was dead and...

Aubrey. His eyes opened as his thoughts caught up to her name and he remembered. *I'm not dead, but she is.*

He must have made some kind of noise because Lauren lifted her head from where she'd been resting it on the side of his hospital bed. "You're awake! Finally," she said with relief.

He tried to smile. "Are you okay?" His voice sounded gruff and his throat hurt like hell, but at least he didn't sound all whispery and weak.

"Yeah, we are." Lauren was much more successful with her smile. She beamed joy at him, and Raef could almost see it glistening in the air around her.

Which was bullshit. Raef couldn't feel positive emotions, or at least he couldn't feel them anymore. That ability had died with a dead girl.

The thought of Aubrey, and all that he'd lost with her, made his heart hurt like hell. Raef turned his head. He couldn't look at Lauren just then. Honestly, he might not ever be able to look at her again.

"Hey," Lauren said softly, touching his cheek familiarly

and gently guiding his head toward her. "Kent, please don't turn away from me."

"Don't call me that." He didn't want to hurt her feelings. He really did like Lauren, really did care about her, but there was no damn way he was going to be able to handle her calling him Kent.

"Why not? I always have," she said.

"Bullshit—that was Aubrey. You've always called me Raef," he said, not sure if he wanted to cry or smash his fist into something.

"Yeah, well, we decided when we joined that we liked you as Kent best. So it's Kent you're going to be from now on," she said.

Raef blinked at her, utterly confused. "Pain meds. That has to be what's going on. You aren't making one damn bit of sense."

Lauren smiled into his eyes. "You are on pain meds, but that's not what's going on. What's going on is that we're both here—Lauren and Aubrey—together, forever."

Raef felt a rush of hope that he tried to squelch. "No, that's not possible. It can't be."

"Why not? We were never whole without each other. It only makes sense that we share one body since it seems like we share one soul."

"Aubrey?"

"Absolutely. And Lauren."

Raef looked into her shining blue eyes and saw her there—saw both of them there, and then he *felt*. An emotion flooded through his body that was so intense—so incredible—that he suddenly found it hard to catch his breath.

"What's wrong?" She was on her feet, reaching for the nurse's call button, when Raef intercepted her hand.

"It's not bad," he assured her. "It's just a feeling like nothing I've ever felt before."

His soul mate let out a long breath of relief and gently cupped his face in her hands. Before she kissed him she whispered, "That's the one last feeling I had to teach you, Kent—love...."

★ ★ ★ ★ ★

HAUNTED
GENA SHOWALTER

To she-just-gets-hotter P. C. Cast—
aka Miss P. C. Snowater-Cole—for the phone calls, the emails
and the laughs. I had so much fun playing in your sandbox!
And of course, I love you!

To my editor Margo Lipschultz for the keen insight
and kind assurance!

To my agent Deidre Knight, for always being in my corner!

To Jill Monroe, for bouncing ideas and making me laugh
with her stories of dog vomit. (But if you baby talk just
one more time…I'll still love you, *sigh*.)

prologue

The woman lay naked atop a cold slab of metal, her wrists cuffed above her head, her legs shackled apart. Frigid air that smelled of blood and disinfectant had turned her skin into a layer of ice over muscle too weak to even tremble. Determination to escape had drained out of her after the thousandth attempt, though the tears she'd shed forever ago were still crystallized on her cheeks.

This was it for her, she thought. The last day of her life. Sadly, there would be no changing course. The ship had already sailed and the storm had already begun.

She hadn't asked for this, certainly hadn't wanted it, but she'd gotten it. Now all she could do was fight. And she would. With every ounce of her strength, she would.

A muffled mewling sound echoed somewhere beyond her.

Though she was bound too tightly to twist and look, she knew her replacement had just woken up and realized she was locked inside a dog cage, only a metal slab and another female's shame visible. She knew—because she had once been locked inside that cage herself.

She had been forced to watch as the psycho who'd stunned her and stuffed her inside of his car had finished off the *other* woman who'd been on this slab. The one before her, now dead, killed in the most horrendous way.

"Do yourself a favor and shut up," she told the girl. Now wasn't a time for gentleness. "It's better to remain silent than to give him what he wants—and he wants you to cry. He wants you to scream and beg and tell him how badly it hurts."

The mewls increased in volume.

"Or continue doing that and make him the happiest murderer in the world," she added with a grumble.

The thump of booted footsteps suddenly filled the room. Her heartbeat spiked into a too hard, too fast beat. One second passed, two, before the hinges on the room's only door groaned. Sickness churned in her stomach.

He was here.

Was she really going to do this?

"Good morning, my lovelies." Such a smug tone, layered with threads of glee and malicious intent. "How are we feeling today?"

Yeah. She was.

Cries emerged from the cage as she said, "I'm feeling like it'd be fun to do a role reversal with you. What do you think? You on this bed, me with a low IQ, a tiny penis and—stop me if I'm wrong—big-time mommy issues."

A hiss of breath slithered in her direction. "You will never mention my mother again, do you hear me?" Anger had replaced the smugness, knives and other toys clanging together as he searched for the instrument he desired.

"If by 'never mention again' you mean 'never stop talking

about it,' then, yeah, I heard. So, why don't you pretend I'm your therapist and this is a free-of-charge session?"

"Enough!"

Hardly. "Tell me. Did Mommy Dearest not breast-feed you? Or did she breast-feed you far too long?"

A heavy silence crawled through the small enclosure.

Dig the knife deeper—he soon will. "Come on, you can trust me. I'll keep everything on the down low, and only bring up your deep, dark secrets on my blog. Well, and maybe my Twitter feed. Oh, and Facebook. Possibly a video diary on YouTube. Other than that, my lips are sealed."

The metal crashed together with more force. At last he found what he wanted—an eight-inch serrated blade. Holding it up so that the silver gleamed in the too bright overhead light, he turned to face her, a half grin, half scowl lifting the corners of his lips.

"Darling," he said to the other captive, pretending to ignore her. He couldn't hide the clenching of his teeth. "You'll want to pay special attention to what happens next because if you displease me, you'll experience it yourself."

The cries became muffled whimpers, the cage rattling as the female tried to slink through the bars.

Never again will I give him that kind of satisfaction. "Oh, goodness, oh, no," she said, mocking him. "The psycho killer has a knife. Someone cue the spooky music and my terrified screaming."

His narrowed gaze landed on her, and he waved the blade back and forth, back and forth. "Have you not yet realized the beast you provoke?"

"Uh, hello. Obviously I have. He's as tiny as the rest of you, which is why I'm grinning."

He popped his jaw. He wasn't an ugly man, was actually

quite beautiful, with golden curls, eyes of the sweetest honey and features as innocent and guileless as a child's.

Such a cruel, cruel mask.

When she'd first woken up in that cage she'd thought he was here to save her. A notion quickly disabused as he hauled her out, cut away her clothing and laughed with chilling delight.

"I can make this painless…or excruciatingly painful. Watch yourself," he snapped.

"Did I hurt your feelings?" she said. "Bad prisoner. Bad, bad, bad prisoner."

Steps slow and measured, he approached her. "Think you're so brave? Well, let's see what I can do to change your mind, shall we? I know you can't see her, but the girl in the cage is—drumroll, please—your only real friend. You remember her, don't you? Of course you do. She's the pretty one."

The first spark of heat ignited in her chest as she craned her neck to try to peer into the cage, but again, as tightly bound as she was, she was unable to contort herself as needed. She saw only the wall of pictures. Photos he'd taken of the other females he'd violated.

Tomorrow, her image would join them.

"You're lying, trying to hurt me because you're a miserable little runt whose heart has rotted and you can't find any other way to get to me."

Hatred flared in his eyes, creating deep, dark pits of evil. "You think so? Well, why don't you ask the girl and find out whether or not I spoke true."

Her fingers curled into fists. He wasn't lying. Was he? A liar would not appear so satisfied. Would he? "Say something," she commanded the girl.

Silence.

His smug chuckle resounded between them. "My deepest apologies, but she'll not be saying anything. She's mouthy, your friend. You know she is. I'm afraid I was forced to cut out her tongue."

Another spark of heat, this one containing fiery strands of rage. Growing...growing... Her friend *was* mouthy, and this man was vile enough to take her—and just cruel enough to stop her from ever speaking again. Anything to add to the torment he'd already unleashed.

How dare he abduct her friend! How dare he force such a precious girl to endure the horrors he'd visited upon her! Growing...growing...

"You sick, disgusting...argh!" she rasped, jerking at her cuffs. No description was foul enough. "I'll end you. You'll never be able to hurt her again. Just wait... I'll...end...you." *Don't cry. Don't you dare cry.* But she was having trouble catching her breath, forming words.

With his free hand, he stroked along her brow, his touch gentle, almost tender. "You've always thought yourself stronger than you really are. It's your biggest flaw. One I'll enjoy culling from you."

She tried to bite him.

He laughed. "I can't wait to show my newest plaything pictures of our time together. Think she'll be jealous?"

The rage spread through the rest of her, burning, blistering, causing any hint of tears to evaporate. "You can kill me, but I'm staying here, I promise you." There was her voice, stronger than before, dripping with determination.

He quirked an eyebrow in mock fear. "Oh, scary. And just how will you manage that, hmm?"

"I'll find a way. There's *always* a way, and good *always* overcomes evil."

"So certain," he said, and tsked under his tongue. "I've heard a strong spirit can prove victorious against anything, even death, but, darling, as I've tried and tried and tried to tell you, you aren't very strong."

"We'll find out." An accepted fact in their world: there was indeed an afterlife. Some people moved on to a better place. Some, to a worse place. But she wasn't going anywhere until her friend was safe.

"Well, I hope you're right. Just think, if you remain here on earth, we can be together again." He raised the blade, grinned—and plunged the metal deep.

1

Oklahoma City, Oklahoma

SIG-Sauer: eight hundred dollars.

Case of bullets: thirty dollars.

Shooting your neighbor in the face for going through your trash after you'd already warned him there would be consequences if he ever dared to do it again: priceless.

And I'll do it, too, Detective Levi Reid vowed as he polished the gun in question. *My stuff is my stuff. Even my trash!*

He'd moved into the King's Landing apartment complex three weeks ago, but he still wasn't sure why. Or how. Fine, he knew how. He didn't like it, and would never admit the truth to anyone but himself, but every day he experienced some sort of blackout. He would snap out of it missing anywhere from five minutes to five hours. Or, in the case of this apartment, seven days.

Honestly, here's what he knew about the events leading up to such a major loss: he'd followed a suspicious-looking guy to the building's back entrance. The end. He'd next woken up inside this very room, all of his things surrounding him. He had no idea when he'd packed his stuff, given his home of six years to a stranger or rented this spacious though run-down two-bedroom hellhole totally *not* suitable for a king.

His coworkers hadn't come looking for him because he was currently on a forced leave of absence. He didn't have a girlfriend and had already canceled all of his "mandatory" appointments with the shrink. So, he'd decided to stay put, just in case another blackout struck and he came to some-place worse.

First he'd fumed about his total lack of control—and there were holes in his walls to prove it. Then he'd sunk into a (manly) depression. Manly: no crying or whining, just star-ing stoically—if not sexily—into the darkness. Now he pon-dered. He should have manned up and moved somewhere better, but some part of him had actually grown to like it here, despite everything.

Situated at the edge of downtown Oklahoma City, his new home gave him an up close and personal view of the homeless who littered the streets, the prostitutes who constantly hunted prey and the dealers who made back-alley sales day and night. He'd come to this area countless times while on the job, and it had always given him the creeps. (Again, in a manly way.) And okay, okay. The building wasn't as bad as he remembered. Someone had fixed it up, made it habitable.

His neighbors weren't so bad, either, he supposed. They had their quirks, but who didn't?

The guy in 211 skulked around every corner as if a serial killer had his number—and that number was up. Any time Levi heard a suspicious noise and decided to check the halls, the guy glued himself to Levi's side, crying and begging Levi to help but refusing to answer any questions or share any details.

The girl in 123 liked to tiptoe up and down the halls at all hours of the day and night, stopping to attempt to X-ray vision her way past every door she encountered. Any time Levi walked past *her*, her attention would swing to him and she would say something spine-chilling like, "I miss my baby. Will you be my baby?" Or, his favorite, "What will you do when you're dead? Dead, dead, dead, you're so dead."

The guy in 409 was Mr. Dumpster Diver.

As of last week, a redheaded stunner and her pretty blonde roommate had moved in. They might be as weird as the rest of them, but he was thinking about asking the redhead out. He wasn't a fan of dating, but he sure did like getting laid.

Right now he sat at his kitchen table, his SIG in pieces and mixed with his cleaning supplies. He greased the gun's rails, put the slide on, removed the slide and wiped off the rails, each action automatic. He'd done this a thousand times before, and now found the act calming.

Calm, something he was supposed to maintain. Apparently, if you were on the job and attacked an alleged serial killer who liked to store body parts in his freezer, you'd be told you had "temper issues" and needed to take time to "think and rest."

What he really needed was a distraction. So, okay, fine. No more thinking about asking Red out. He'd just do it. Hopefully, she was into rough-looking homicide detectives who were possessive of their stuff but trying to learn to share. Also, Levi wasn't interested in one-night stands and actually expected commitment. And despite popular opinion, he did know how to smile.

A hard knock at his door brought his head snapping up.

Probably just another neighbor here to ask to hide from Johnny Law or to tell him the end was near. "Go away. No one's here."

Another knock, this one harder, more insistent. "I won't bite," she said. "At least, not more than a few times."

He liked her voice. Soft and sweet, yet determined. Still, an intelligent person didn't offer to nibble on strangers.

Motions swift, he put his gun back together and shoved it in the back of his running shorts. The weight created big-time sag, never a good thing but especially not when he was shirtless. His uninvited guest would probably get a peek at his goods, but by the time he finished with her that wouldn't be the worst of her worries. She needed to learn the consequences of this kind of behavior.

But...then he glanced through the peephole and spied the redhead's roommate, the pretty blonde. Teaching her a lesson took a backseat to getting rid of her. Last time he'd seen her, she'd made him feel a tide of guilt and shame. Why, he didn't know. Didn't care. He just didn't want to deal with her.

The moment he opened the door, however, urgency took a backseat to concern. She was highlighted by flickering overhead light, chewing on her nails and shifting nervously from one foot to the other. Crimson specks marred her cheeks and splattered her hands. Blood?

Frowning, he opened the door wider. "Are you okay, ma'am?"

Eyes of ocean-blue narrowed on him, her gaze becoming a laser that sliced through flesh. She stopped chewing and shifting at least, and no feelings of guilt or shame rose to the surface. "Ma'am? Did you just call me ma'am?"

"Yes, ma'am. Are you okay?"

"Wow, that hurts!" she said, ignoring his question a second time. "Just how old do you think I am?"

A minefield of a query, and one he was better off disregarding. He motioned to her stained hands with a tilt of his chin, even as he reached for the handle of his gun. "Let's try this again. Are you hurt?" He scanned the walkway. Empty. No suspicious shadows, marks or noises. "Is someone following you? Bothering you?"

"Why would you—" She glanced down, chuckled and wiggled her fingers at him. "This is paint. I'm a painter."

Paint. No mortal danger, then. His concern faded, and the surliness resurfaced. "Then what are you doing here?" Okay, so he probably should have pretended to be nice. She'd tell her friend he was a tool, and the friend would tell him she'd rather date a dishrag when he finally asked her out.

"As I was saying," she continued blithely. "My amazing art does not contain…" A shudder of revulsion shook her. "You know."

What? Blood? Probably. So many people had an aversion to the stuff, but he'd never had such qualms. "'You know'?" he parroted.

"Yeah. The elixir of life."

You're kidding me. "And the elixir of life is?" Levi was having what he suspected was fun for the first time since his suspension. The girl was brave enough to knock on a stranger's door and demand he open up, but she couldn't say a certain five-letter word? How cute was that?

She ran her tongue over her teeth and whispered, "Fine. I can do this. It's *B-L-O-O-D*." Another shudder shook her.

Would it be rude to laugh at her? She'd actually spelled the word rather than said it.

His stance softened, and he allowed his arm to fall to his side. "So you're an artist, huh?"

"An *amazing* artist."

"I don't know about amazing," he said, "but you're defi-

nitely modest." And she was more than cute, he realized. She
was short and curvy, her face something you might find on a
little girl's favorite doll, with big blue eyes, a button nose and
heart-shaped lips. She was utterly adorable.

"By the way," he added, "being called 'sir' would be a reason to have a hissy. Ma'am's all good. I say that to everyone
with—" his gaze automatically dropped to give her a once-
over, but he got caught on her breasts, which were straining
the fabric of her pajama top. He managed to jerk his attention
back up and choke out "—estrogen." Girl was *stacked*.

"Good point," she said, tossing that tumble of pale hair over
one shoulder, "but I assure you, I'm all woman."

Noticed. Believe me. Rather than voice the sentiment aloud—
and risk finding his testicles in his throat—he gave her a single
nod of affirmation. "No argument here."

A relieved breath left her. "Thank you for not telling me I
need to double-check my woman card."

"A double check isn't necessary." *Are you...flirting?*

"Well, isn't the big, strong he-man sweet?"

"Yes, ma'am, he is."

He wasn't the type to flirt, but yeah. Yeah, he was flirting,
and she was flirting back.

He'd planned to ask the redhead out, not really wanting
anything to do with the blonde and all that guilt and shame
she'd caused, but now, with the emotions out of the way, he
changed his mind. He wanted this one.

In female-speak, that meant he wanted to get to know her
better. In male-speak, he wanted her in his bed, like, now.

She was young, probably in her mid-twenties, with that cascade of wavy blond hair, blond brows and blond lashes, those
delicate doll features and the fair skin of someone who preferred to hiss at the sun rather than to bask in it. And she was—

Familiar. He knew her, he realized. Somehow, someway, he knew her. Finally, an explanation as to why he'd felt what he'd felt when she'd first moved in, and yet he had no idea when or where they would have met.

"You're staring," she said, chewing on her bottom lip.

A nervous habit, definitely. One that made him think she was slightly…broken.

A protective instinct he usually only experienced on the job sprang to life. Annnd, yes, there was the guilt and the shame again.

Why? Why would he feel this way about her?

Well, no matter the answer, Red was back in the running. Levi didn't date the broken. Ever. He protected, he avenged, but he didn't fix. How could he? He couldn't keep his own life on track. Besides that, he didn't like feeling this way.

"Seriously. What?" she demanded.

"Just wondering if we've met before." Even as he asked, his arms felt heavier, the muscles tense, as if memory had been stored there and he was now reliving his time with her. But…that would mean he'd held her. That wasn't something he would forget.

Her nose scrunched up endearingly. "Is that a line? Because that sounds like a line."

"Actually it's a question—" *can't date her, can't date her, really can't date her, even though you dig her straightforwardness* "—and an answer would be nice."

"Oh." Was that disappointment in her tone? "Well, the only answer I can give you is no. I would remember someone with your particular…attitude." Her gaze raked over him, and the little tease shuddered as if they were discussing *B-L-O-O-D*. "And for your information, I'm entirely lacking in modesty about my paintings because there's no need for it. I'm an in-credible artist. Incredible!"

Confidence was more of a turn-on than straightforward-ness, and she possessed more than most. There was no way she could be the broken girl he'd imagined her. Right? And guilt and shame weren't that bad. *Right?*

"Never said you weren't incredible. And what's wrong with my attitude?"

"It kind of sucks, but I'm sure you're told something similar all the time." Up her hand went, her nail back in her mouth, her teeth nibbling. "I, uh, smell coffee," she said, a sudden tremble in her voice, "and yes, I'd love some. Thanks."

She darted around him and breezed inside, a waft of cinna-mon and turpentine accompanying her. As he watched, mo-mentarily speechless, she stalked to his kitchen.

His brain eventually chugged out of the station. Who did she think she was? His home was his sanctuary and strangers were never allowed. Not even hot ones.

To be honest, this girl was the first person other than him-self to ever step inside the apartment. His partner was avoid-ing him, and his family was...well, he had no idea where. At eighteen, he'd left home and had never looked back. His par-ents had died when he was six, and none of his relatives had wanted him, so he'd hopped from one foster family to another until the age of thirteen, when a depressed housewife and her emotionally abusive husband had adopted him. Good times.

So, yeah, call him paranoid, call him domineering and self-ish and rude, but what was his was his, and he never shared.

But you're learning to share, remember?

Not anymore!

He would kick her out after scolding her for her daring—

and, as a courtesy, he wouldn't shoot her in her pretty face—and then they could discuss going to dinner, maybe a movie.

He would have the blonde or no one, he decided.

But he took one look at her and found himself rooted in place. Her motions were stiff, jerky, as she gathered the supplies she needed. A cup, the sugar, a spoon. As many interrogations as he'd conducted over the years, he knew when someone wanted to say something but hadn't yet worked up the courage. His new neighbor was desperate to confess a secret; she just needed a little push.

Take control of the situation. "Hey, lady. You need to get something straight."

"'Lady' is just as bad as 'ma'am.' I'm Harper," she called over her shoulder.

Harper. The name didn't quite fit her.

He closed the distance, checking the living room to make sure he'd cleaned up after himself. Besides the shirt and pants he'd draped over the side of his couch, he had, thankfully, done a little picking up. As for his furniture, the dark leather of his couch and love seat were scuffed but of high quality, his coffee table as polished as his gun, and his rug threadbare only where he liked to pace. The floorboards creaked with his every step, but then, creaks, groans and moans as wood settled and hinges dropped were the standard sound track, blending with chatter that could be heard through the ultrathin walls.

"Listen up," he said.

"Okay, I've waited long enough for you to offer," the woman—Harper—interjected. "What's your name?"

"Levi. Now why are you here?" He gripped the counter to stop himself from shaking her. Shaking was bad. Very, very bad. Or so his captain was always saying.

Clutching *his* cup, sipping *his* coffee, she turned to face him. Only, rather than spilling her reasons, she grimaced and gasped out, "What *is* this crap? Because honestly? It tastes like motor oil."

So he liked his joe strong. So what? "Maybe it *is* motor oil."

"Oh, well, in that case, it's actually pretty good." She took another sip, sighed as though content. "Definitely grade-A motor oil." Her gaze slipped past him. "You know, your place is so much bigger than mine, with much better lighting. Who'd you have to sleep with to get it?"

She's as weird as the rest of them. "Who says I had to go all the way?" *Apparently, I am, too.*

A laugh bubbled from her, and she choked on the coffee. "Dude. Do you know what you just implied?"

"Uh, yeah. That's why I said it." Now, then. He'd allowed her to dominate the conversation long enough. He needed to move this along before she gave another one of those laughs. *Gorgeous.*

He sidestepped the counter, moving closer to her, closer still, the fragrance of cinnamon thickening the air between them, the turpentine fading. He claimed the cup, set it aside and crowded her personal space, forcing her to back up until she ran into the cabinets.

She peered up at him, those ocean-water eyes haunted... and, oh, so haunting. Just then, she reminded him of a fairy with a broken wing.

Broken. There was that word again.

Muscles...tensing again...

In his experience, everyone had secrets. Clearly Harper was no exception. He recalled the day she moved in. She'd kept her eyes downcast, the long length of those pale lashes unable to mask the shadows underneath. There'd been a hollowness to her cheeks that had since filled out, and a stiffening of her spine every time someone had neared her. And wow, he'd noticed a lot considering he'd hadn't allowed himself to watch her.

"You have five seconds to start talking," he said more harshly than he'd intended. There was no reason to break her other wing, but dang, his instincts to protect those weaker than himself were taking over, every part of him rebelling at the thought that someone had hurt her. "Why. Are. You. Here?"

She gulped, and her trembling increased. "Can't a girl get to know a guy before she begs him for a favor?"

"No." Evasion never worked with him. "Are you in some kind of trouble?"

Color darkened her cheeks, even as the rest of her blanched to chalk-white. "Not exactly, no." Softer voice, danger hidden by silken threads of...fear? Yeah, definitely fear. No longer was her gaze able to meet his.

More gently he said, "Explain 'not exactly.'"

And there went her nails, smashing into her teeth. "Word on the street is, you're a detective with the OKCPD."

"I am." No reason to mention his forced leave of absence.

Those ocean-water blues finally returned to him, so lovely in their purity his breath actually snagged in his throat. "What kind of cop are you?"

"A detective, as we've already established."

"Like there's a difference. A badge is a badge, right? But I meant, are you the good kind or the bad kind? Do you care about justice, no matter the cost, or do you just like closing a case?"

He pressed his tongue into the roof of his mouth and reminded himself that he was a calm, rational being (with a gun) and she probably hadn't meant to insult him and his coworkers.

"Harper." A swift rebuke, her name uttered as though it was a curse. He should have called her "ma'am" again, but since he'd teased her about how he'd gotten the apartment, formalities were out. "You're seconds away from being arrested for public intoxication, because only a drunk person would say something like that."

A relieved sigh left her. "The good kind, then. Otherwise, you'd try and convince me of just how good you are, rather than taking offense."

"Harper."

She swallowed. "Okay, fine. I told you I'm a painter, right?"

"An *incredible* painter."

Her chin lifted, those haunting secrets in her eyes momentarily replaced by affront. "Well, I am," she said, having to speak around her fingers. "Anyway, I, uh, hmm. I knew this would be hard, but wow, this is worse than the time I had to tell Stacy DeMarko her butt did, in fact, look fat in those jeans."

I am not amused. He wrapped his fingers around her wrist and pulled her hand away from her mouth.

The contact jolted her, and she gasped. It jolted him, too. Her skin was unbelievably soft, decadently warm, something out of a fantasy. Her pulse hammered erratically, every pound caressing him. He let her go, stepped away.

"Last chance, Harper. Just say what you came to say. That's the only way to get what you need."

She rubbed at the elegant length of her neck, the picture of feminine delicacy, and whispered, "I'm painting something... from memory, I think, and...the problem is...I don't really remember, but it's there, in my head, the horrible image, I mean, and...and...I think I witnessed a murder."

2

Aurora Harper, named after Sleeping freaking Beauty—and if anyone dared call her by the awful name they'd soon get a personal introduction to the razor in her boot—sat "calmly" on her neighbor's couch. He was peering at her, silent, waiting for her to answer his latest question.

Her tongue felt thick and unruly, unusable, and there was a lump growing in her throat, making it difficult for her to swallow. She hated talking about this, hated *thinking* about it, and would have given anything to slink away unnoticed, soon forgotten.

Thing was, Levi would not be forgetting her. After her grim announcement, he'd gone stiff and jarringly quiet, then had ushered her into his living room, gently pushed her onto the couch cushions and pulled a chair directly in front of her. He'd spent the next half hour drilling her for information.

She'd had no idea what to expect from him, had known only that he was the most rugged-looking man she'd ever seen. Oh, yeah, and every time she'd glanced in his direction he'd made her heart pound with an urge to fight him or to jump into his arms and hold on forever—she wasn't yet sure which.

He had wide shoulders, muscled forearms and the hard, ridged stomach of an underwear model. Dressed as he was in black jogging shorts, she could see that he had scarred knees and calves. He was barefoot and his toes were strangely cute.

She forced her gaze up. Black hair shagged around a face honed in the violence of a boxing ring, or perhaps even the down-and-dirty streets, with still more scars crisscrossing on his forehead, his cheeks sharp and skirting the edge of lethal, and his nose slightly crooked from one too many breaks. A shadow of a beard covered his jaw.

He was just as bronzed up top as he was below, and she would guess his ancestry Egyptian. His eyes, though...they were the lightest green, emeralds plucked from a collector's greatest treasure. Long black lashes framed those jewels, almost feminine in their prettiness.

Not the only thing pretty about him, she thought then. His lips were lush and pink, the kind her best friend and roommate Lana would "kill to have...all over me."

And, okay, enough of *that.* Harper wasn't here for a date, wasn't sure she'd ever date again. The past few weeks, she could not tolerate even the thought of being touched. Maybe because every time she closed her eyes she felt phantom hands whisking over her, heard the laugh of a madman who enjoyed inflicting pain, and smelled the coppery tang of blood deep in her nostrils.

She could have written off the sensations as an overactive imagination, except...sometimes she fell asleep in one room and woke up in another. Sometimes she would be in her kitchen, or in her studio room painting, or anywhere, really, and would blink and find herself standing in a neighborhood she didn't recognize.

The blackouts freaked her out, filled her with soul-shuddering panic, and each time she realized she was someplace new, her mind would paint her surroundings with blood, fill her ears with screams...such pain-drenched screams.

The only explanation that fit was that she'd witnessed a murder, but had suppressed the details. Suppressed until she painted, that is, the blurred images of horrors no one should ever have to bear taking shape and emerging unbidden. Either that, or crazy had razed the edges of her brain and she needed to be locked away for her own safety.

"Honey, I asked you a question and you need to answer it."

The harshness of Levi's voice jerked her out of her mind. Guess he was done calling her by her name and even the old-lady "ma'am," and was now resorting to endearments that sounded more like curses.

"No," she said, just to pick at him. "Not 'honey.' I told you. I'm Harper."

One black brow arched into his hairline, and for a moment he appeared amused with her rather than accusatory. "Is that a first or last name?"

"Does it matter?"

"Yeah."

She popped her jaw, finding strength in the familiarity of an irritation she'd never been able to shake. Her mother had named her after a fairy-tale princess and had expected Harper to mimic her namesake. Years of training in manners and deportment, followed by years of competing in a pageant circuit she'd despised, had nearly drained the fighting spirit out of her. Nearly. "Well, I'm not telling you the rest of my name." He'd laugh; he'd tease her.

He shrugged those beautifully wide shoulders. "Easy enough to find out. A few calls, and boom." He paused, clearly waiting for her to jump in.

"I will never willingly volunteer it, so you'll just have to make those calls."

A gleam of challenge entered those green, green eyes. "So be it." He rested his elbows on his knees and leaned closer to her, the scents of minty toothpaste and pungent gun oil intensifying. Scents she really, really liked, if the flutter of her pulse points was any indication. "Let's backtrack a bit. Tell me again what you think you're painting."

This was the third time he'd demanded that information, and she'd watched enough cop shows to know he was testing her, looking for any mistakes between her first and subsequent telling. If he found them, he could write her off as a liar.

"Shouldn't you be taking notes?" she said, stalling.

"No."

"You'll forget—"

"I never forget."

"Anything?"

"Not anything like this."

How intriguing. "Really, because that's—"

"Talk," he barked.

His intensity gave her the strength to obey. "Okay." She closed her eyes and forced the painting to the front of her mind. "There's a cold metal slab, stainless steel, I think, and it's splattered with dried b-blood. There are shackles at the top and bottom, holding a woman's wrists and ankles, and those are also splattered. There are holes on the slab and floor... drains, I think, and they're splattered, as well. There's a man. He's clutching a knife over the woman's abdomen." Every word caused her heart rate to quicken and little beads of sweat to dot her skin. Sweat, yet her blood had thickened with ice.

"Describe the man."

"I can't." Her lashes fluttered open as a shudder rocked her. Nausea rolled through her stomach, a common occurrence these days. "I haven't yet painted his face." Wasn't sure she wanted to see it. Even the thought of him made her want to hide under her covers and cry.

"What *have* you painted of him?"

"His lower body. His arms. Some of his chest."

"And he's wearing...?"

Good question. She'd been so focused on what was happening in the picture that she hadn't paid any attention to the little details her mind had somehow caught. "A white button-up shirt and dark slacks."

"Possibly a businessman, then. Gloves?"

"No."

"Is he pale, tan, black, what?"

"Tan, though not as tan as you."

"Okay, now describe the woman."

"I can't," she repeated, a mere whisper. She flattened a hand over her stomach, hoping to ward off even a little of the sickness. "Not her face, I mean. She's naked, and her skin is pale."

"Does she have any birthmarks or scars?"

Harper licked her lips, pictured the female and shook her head. "If she does, I haven't added them yet."

His gaze sharpened on her, more intense than before and kind of, well, terrifying. This was not a guy to anger, or taunt, or even to play with. He would retaliate, no question. "How much of her have you painted?"

"All but the head."

"Is she a brunette, blonde or redhead?"

"How would I—"

His pointed gaze explained for him.

"Oh. Uh, I don't actually know. The bottom half of her is blocked by the man's torso."

"Is she alive or dead in the painting?"

"Dead, I think." And probably happy to have escaped the pain.

Silence once again permeated the room, thick and oppressive, reminding her of exactly why she hadn't wanted to come here. She'd known he would doubt her—as she sometimes doubted herself—or suspect her of playing a part in the murder.

Lana believed the woman was indeed real and Harper had stumbled upon the scene. As an employee of the Oklahoma City branch of After Moonrise, a company specializing in grisly murders and the spirits those murders sometimes left behind, she ought to know. But her belief stemmed not from the painting, but from the fact that there were two weeks neither Harper nor Lana could account for. Harper could have been trapped with the man and his victim, and somehow, miraculously, have managed to escape.

Her friend had showed the painting to her coworkers, but they hadn't taken the case. Lana had even begged—which, in her case, meant she'd cracked heads around—and they'd finally given in and said they would look into it, but so far, they'd discovered nothing. *If* they'd even tried. Lana was doing everything she could on her own, but as someone used to dealing with spirits rather than bodies, this wasn't her area of expertise.

So, when Lana heard a detective was living in their building, she had insisted Harper nut up and speak out.

This tormend you, she'd said in a Lithuanian accent that came and went with her moods. When she was happy, she sounded as American as Harper. When she was scared or angry, hello, the accent appeared, as thick as if she'd just stepped off the plane. So often now, she was sad, and at the time she'd been filled with so much sorrow over what Harper might have endured that her teeth had chattered. *Let man help you. That girl…she deserve peace, rest. Please.*

I can't. He'll suspect me of hurting her.

Maybe at first, but then he see the trut…. Please, do for her, for you, for…me.

Given the fact that Lana had spent every night of the past few weeks sobbing for the pain *Harper* suffered over the entire ordeal, well, Harper had been willing to do anything her friend asked, no matter the consequences to herself.

"Harper." The curt bark of Levi's voice jolted her out of her thoughts. "You with me?"

"Well, I am now," she grumbled. "Do you have an inside voice?"

His lips twitched at the corners, hinting at an amusement he'd so rarely shown. That humor transformed his entire face. Those emerald eyes twinkled, little lines forming at the corners. His mouth softened, and his skin seemed to glow.

"Have you ever painted anything like this before?" he asked.

"No. I love painting people, but not like this. Never like this. Why does that matter?"

"Once, and it's plausible you stumbled upon some kind of scene. Twice, and it's more plausible your mind manufactured everything."

Okay, that made sense. "Well, it was only once. And just so you know, I can't see the dead, so it wasn't a bunch of spirits putting on a show for me, either." She wasn't like Lana, who had always had the ability to see into that other realm.

"I'll need to view your new painting, as well as a sample of your usual work," Levi said.

"All right. The new one isn't done, though. Obviously."

His head tilted to the side, his study of her intensifying. "When did you begin painting it?"

"About two weeks ago." She tried not to squirm or wring her fingers under such a probing stare—until she realized that his probing stare was a good thing. Criminals would not stand a chance against this man's strength and ferocity. If her painting were a depiction of a real-life event, Levi would find out the identity of the man responsible and punish him. "Little by little, I've been filling in the details."

Another bout of silence before he sighed. "Let's switch gears for a minute. Forgetting the fact that you've never before painted anything like this, what makes you think this is a memory?"

Bottom line, she wasn't ready for a stranger to know about her blackouts and to, perhaps, use them against her, yet neither was she ready to lie to a man who could have kicked her out but hadn't. He'd listened to her, had asked her questions and truly seemed interested in helping her.

So, she said, "I'm struck by moments of absolute terror," and gazed down at her feet. Her pink snakeskin boots were one of her favorite possessions. She'd had to sell four paintings to buy them, as well as live off peanut butter and jelly for a month, but she'd never regretted the choice. So pretty. "Moments I can almost feel the shackles around *my* wrists and *my* ankles."

"Delusions hold that same power," he pointed out.

Don't act surprised, you knew it would come to this. And better this than the other avenue he could have taken: blame. "Well, I hope it *is* a delusion," she whispered.

"Me, too, Miss…Harper?"

"Just Harper." She would *not* be tricked into revealing her full name, thank you.

"Had to try," he said with a shrug. "What if you discover you were the one on that table, that you somehow escaped but repressed what happened?"

"Impossible. I was only gone——" She pressed her lips together, stopping her hasty confession before it could fully emerge. "I would have had bruises at some point, and I haven't."

He sat there a moment, silent again, before nodding as if he'd just made a decision. He pushed to his feet and stuck a finger in her face. "Stay there. Do not move. I'll get dressed and we'll walk to your apartment together. Nod if you understand."

"And there's that lovely attitude again," she muttered.

"Nod."

Oh, very well. She nodded.

"Good. Disobey, and I'll cuff you faster than you can say, 'I'm sorry, Levi, that was the dumbest thing I ever did.'" Without waiting for her reply—because he clearly didn't expect her to have one—he turned on his heel and headed for the hall.

"Uh, just thought you should know that your gun is showing," she called.

Just before he disappeared around a corner, she thought she heard him say, "Honey, you're lucky you're only seeing the butt of it."

She wasn't *that* bad. Was she?

Harper waited. The click of a closing door never sounded. Well, she wouldn't let that stop her; she stood with every intention of walking around his place and checking out his things.

Maybe she *was* that bad.

"I told you not to move," Levi called with more than a hint of annoyance.

He'd heard the quiet swish of her clothes? "Tell me you don't talk to your girlfriend with that tone." The moment her words registered in her head, she groaned. Basically, she'd just asked him to marry her and have a million babies.

"No girlfriend." A tension-ripened pause. "You?"

"Nope, no girlfriend, either." The jest served a dual purpose. One, lightening the mood, and two, discovering whether or not he cared to know her lack-of-boyfriend status. If he pushed for more info, he might just be as fascinated by her as she was by him.

And she was, wasn't she? Fascinated by this rough-and-gruff detective with the jewel-toned eyes. *Thought you weren't interested in dating anyone.* She wasn't. Right? She hadn't taken one look at a grumpy cop and changed her mind, *right?*

"Boyfriend?" Levi barked out, and she nearly grinned. *You're in trouble, girl.* "Nope, no boyfriend."

She scanned his walls. There were no photographs, no artwork, nothing hanging anywhere to inform her of his tastes so that she could peel back the curtain surrounding his life and reveal the man he was with others, when he was relaxed. Did he ever relax, though? Probably not. Judging by his permafrown, it would take a miracle.

"Your decorating...did you decide to go with Minimal Chic?"

Stomping footsteps echoed, and then he was there, in front of her again, tall and dark and ruggedly delicious, an erotic dream come to life in a black T and black slacks.

She'd bet his gun was still at his back. He was a warrior, a protector. A danger. Sweet heaven, but she had to paint him, she decided. He wasn't handsome in the classic sense, but, oh, he was so much *more*. He was interesting.

She'd always favored interesting.

"We're not discussing my decorating," he said.

"You mean your *lack* of decorating."

"Whatever. Lead the way."

"So you can stare at my butt?" Sometimes her tongue got the better of her, and now was definitely one of those times. There was no way he could respond to that without—

"Exactly."

—making her sigh dreamily.

She was in *big* trouble. "I'm not interested in dating anyone, just so we're clear."

He glared down at her. "Good, because I was thinking about asking out your friend."

Oh, ouch. Yet wasn't that always the case? Men slobbered all over Lana like babies who'd just found fuzzy candy on the floor.

"Good!" she said with a huff. "Rude isn't my type." She turned, giving him her back, and marched out.

"But then I met you and changed my mind," she thought she heard him grumble from behind her.

3

Harper was utterly baffled when Levi gave her painting a once-over, asked a single question, then turned and left her apartment. He did this *after* she'd overcome her urge to vomit and placed the wretched canvas—though perfectly painted—in the heart of her living room, just for his benefit. Sure he'd paused to eye Lana, as any man with a pulse would have done—and even some without, surely—but he hadn't so much as called out a token "Don't leave town." Or even a very necessary "I'm on the case, no worries."

The door slammed ominously behind him, echoing throughout the somewhat dilapidated two-bedroom apartment with plush furnishings Lana had restored with loving care, a hobby of hers. *Their* decorating style was Match Smatch. Every piece was an odd color and shape, and nothing harmonized.

Levi's question played through her mind. "You said there was blood. Where is it?"

The answer was simple. Seeing the blood on the canvas freaked her out, so every morning, after her subconscious mind forced her to add it back, she erased it, leaving the walls pristine and clean.

"That has to be a record for you," Lana said, her Lithuanian accent nonexistent because her darker emotions weren't yet engaged.

Harper purposely kept her back to the gruesome scene of torture and death she had created and kept her gaze on her friend. "I have no idea what you mean."

Had the painting disgusted Detective Snarls? Was he even then searching for his handcuffs, intending to take Harper into lockup? No. No way. He would have dragged her with him, not allowing her out of his sight. He wasn't the type to cross his fingers and hope she stayed put. Even when he'd left her alone in his living room, he'd kept his bedroom door open so that he could hear her movements.

"I've seen you scare off a man within an hour of meeting you, but five minutes? You must have done something *really* special to this one."

Harper snorted. "Wasn't like I asked him to meet my parents or anything." And, bonus, she never would. Three days after her fourteenth birthday, her dad had taken off and never looked back. After that, Mommy Manners had forced her to become even more involved in pageants, and Harper had eventually cracked, poisonous words she still regretted spilling out. Though she'd tried to make amends, her mother hadn't spoken to her in years. "But you know, he could have had the decency to invite himself to breakfast." They had details to hammer out, right? "I mean, he wants to ask you out. Shouldn't he try to butter me up or something, so I'll put in a good word for him?"

"Uh, no, no, he not be asking me out."

"He said he would."

"Well, he lied or changed his mind because that man has a jones for a hot blonde with a taste for destroying fairy-tale princess."

Hope fluttered through her, causing her heart to skip a beat. "First, the taste is justified. Sleeping Beauty sucks. Evil showed up and instead of fighting she took a nap."

"Is that reason enough for you to buy figurines of her likeness just to smash when you're angry?"

"Yeah. And second," she continued, "there's just no way you're right about the cop wanting me. But go ahead and tell me why you think so, beginning once again with how smoking hot you think I am and ending with how you think he's willing to drop to his knees and beg me to go out with him, and don't leave out a single detail."

Lana rolled her eyes. The bold shadow she wore gave those eyes an exotic, smoky look, extending all the way to her temples in glittery points. "You are hot. He will beg. You will say no—and don't try to deny it. I noticed your antiman campaign. I will call you stupid. You will paint a mustache on my face while I sleep. I will carve the legs out from under your bed. We will laugh. The end. Now, tell. Will he help you or not? Because I will hurt him if not."

Okay, so it wasn't the story she'd hoped for but it was true nonetheless. "I might have you hurt him, anyway. After I'm done with him, of course." He was surly with a capital S-U-R-L-Y, glaring at her when she'd entered his apartment after he'd clearly invited her in—with his eyes. "He needs someone to turn his frown upside down. By hanging him out of a window by his ankles."

"Just say a word, and it is done."

Oh, how she adored Lethal Lana.

They'd met in junior school, when Lana's family moved

to the States, and their instant connection had changed the very fabric of Harper's life. Harper, the "lady" of her mother's dreams, had been fascinated by Milana Buineviciute, the wild child of her mother's nightmares.

A (now reformed) smoker, drinker and full-time cusser who never backed down from a fight, Lana had taught Harper how to get down and dirty with brass knuckles and steel-toed boots. Harper had taught Lana to channel the jagged edges of her emotions into art, and the exchange had bonded them.

They balanced each other, even in looks. Lana's hair was naturally dark, almost jet, but she'd bleached the straight-as-a-board strands and then dyed them neon red, a color that complemented her cream-and-rose complexion perfectly. Her features were bold, aggressive, and yet her green eyes were always at half-mast, a sultry invitation to peel away her clothing and have your wicked way with her. Or so Harper had gathered from any man who'd ever looked at her.

Even as fatigued as Lana currently appeared, and had, for these past few weeks, with bruises marring the delicate tissue under her eyes, her lips chapped from constantly being chewed, and the weight she'd dropped from her already slender frame, the girl was a showstopper.

"Maybe we should move," Harper said. "We'll just pack my precious valuables and your crap and—"

"No!" Lana shouted, then repeated softly, "No. I stay here."

A relieved breath escaped her.

After Harper had snapped out of her first blackout and seen what she'd painted, she had walked the streets trying to reason things out. Lost in her thoughts, she'd unknowingly entered the worst part of town. She'd ended up in front of this building, and a desire to live here had instantly consumed her. She'd raced home to tell Lana, and Lana had paled, burst into tears for no reason. Well, there had been a reason, but she still refused to say.

Eventually Harper managed to talk her friend into subletting their place and moving here. But where Harper had thrived, Lana had declined all the more. And yet, she couldn't be dragged out with a tank.

Harper felt guilty about that, she did, but she had no idea what to do.

"By the way, we are not done talking about the cop," Lana said, calm now and rubbing her hands together with glee. "I saw the way you looked at him so I must ask. By 'done with him' did you mean you will hurt him when you jump into his arms and beg him to marry you?"

Harper rolled her eyes, and it was then that she noticed the black shadow creeping along the walls of the living room. Dread poured through her veins, hot and as slick as oil. She knew that shadow, had battled it each time a blackout descended, and knew it would crawl down the walls, consume the entire room and try to swallow her whole.

"I'm sorry, but I have to go," she muttered, grabbing her purse and stalking into the hallway outside their apartment, overly warm air enveloping her. The darkness would catch up to her, but that wouldn't stop her from running.

The floor whined with her every step, other apartment doors slammed closed and the overhead light flickered on and off, on and off. Creepy, yes, but it suited her new frame of mind.

Lana, in her long-sleeved top and pajama pants with a tool belt painted around the waist, stayed close at her heels. "You okay?"

"I will be." *I hope.* Only Harper was able to see the shadows, and she could guess why. Either she was halfway down the road to crazy or she was already standing at the edge, waving goodbye to the life she'd once lived.

She quickened her pace. As always, a pretty young girl stood in front of one of the doors, trying to peer inside an apartment that was not her own. Black hair fell in silky waves to her shoulders. Usually when Harper passed her, the girl remained quiet and unaware, her attention locked on whatever she saw through the obstruction. This time, her head whipped in Harper's direction and violet eyes more otherworldly than human pierced her to her soul.

"Such a naughty girl," said the teenager in a voice chilled by lack of emotion. "You should have known better."

Surprised, Harper stumbled over her own foot.

Lana flipped the girl off and said, *"Tu mane uzknisai."* She waited for Harper—who knew she'd just told the girl how ticked she was—to straighten up before hurrying on.

"What'd I do?" Harper demanded of the girl, looking over her shoulder. She hadn't had a serious boyfriend in over a year and hadn't been on a date in months, even before her whole "no touching" rule. There'd been no naughtiness in her life. None. Well, not until today, when she'd eaten Levi up with her eyes. "Were you listening through the cop's walls while I was with him, you little—"

"I never should teach you to fight." Lana motioned her forward. "She clearly out of mind. Pay no attention or she drag you into her insane."

Another full-on appearance of her accent, proving Lana was as affected by the girl's taunt as Harper. For that reason, she let the subject drop. Until Harper solved the painting mystery, Lana had enough to deal with—whatever "enough" entailed.

A few minutes later, they were outside, the pulsing heart of Oklahoma coming into view. Tall structures with chrome and glass on every floor knifed toward a baby-blue sky with no hint of clouds. Thick green trees with curling branches lined the river walk and overly crowded sidewalks. Sidewalks far more crowded than usual, in fact. On the streets, cars of every color whizzed past, the speed limit clearly a suggestion not to be heeded.

There was a deep chill in the November air, yet Harper remained unfazed. "So, anyway," she said, getting them back on track, "if you hate the apartment so much, why do you want to stay?" She asked even though the very idea of leaving made her quake. She asked even though she'd asked before and Lana had not answered.

"I don't hate the place. I belong there."

That was something, at least. "But—"

"Give me another but, and I smack yours!"

Harper laughed, she just couldn't help herself.

A man and woman walking toward them jumped, as though startled by the sound of her voice. The pair gave her a strange look before passing her. So she was in her winter pj's, like Lana. So the heck what!

"So where we go?" Lana asked.

After a moment's thought, a heavy sigh left her. "Let's go to the place that started us on this journey. Maybe if I figure out what happened to me, I'll stop hearing screams of pain in every single one of my dreams."

REMAINING IN THE SHADOWS, Levi kept pace behind the two females. What a striking pair they made. The tall redhead and the petite blonde, both feminine beyond imagining. Nearly every guy that passed them stared at the redhead, dismissing Harper as if she just couldn't compare.

Idiots, he thought. There was a delicacy to Harper, a fragility, yet when she opened her mouth you discovered just how much of a ballbuster she was. The contrast was exhilarating.

But those blue, blue eyes of hers—those haunted eyes with their secrets and pain and a thousand questions waiting to be answered—continued to, well, *haunt* him. As much as they would have turned him off any other woman, and should have turned him off her, he wanted her more with every second that passed. The shame and guilt were completely gone, and now, every time he caught sight of her, an urge to protect her rose up, one stronger than before, nearly overwhelming him.

A man had to touch a woman to protect her, and he really wanted to touch Harper again. That softness…that heat…

Figure out her mystery first.

He'd walked into her apartment, and for a second he'd seen crumbling walls, even a rat racing across his feet. But then in a snap, he'd seen freshly painted walls of bright yellow and blue, colorful furniture and every surface scrubbed clean. The momentary hallucination had freaked him out, but he'd said nothing. Then, after viewing her painting, a gruesome thing to be sure and exactly as she'd described it—a man standing over a bound, battered and naked female, a knife in his hand—he'd needed a moment to collect himself. Part of him had wanted to gather Harper close and make sure she was kept safe, even from the past. The other part of him had wanted to shake her for not coming to him sooner.

If what she'd painted hadn't sprung from an overactive imagination, the only way to have witnessed such a scene was to have been in the room with the killer. A room like that wouldn't have windows. So, discarding the overactive imagination argument for the time being—something he would do until proven otherwise—she had either aided and abetted the killer or had been captured herself and had somehow managed to escape. Levi doubted the first. Harper's aversion to blood was real; no one could fake the draining of color from their face. And that, of course, left the second option....

Actually, there was a third possibility, he realized. She could have been captured and killed.

Death wasn't the end of life. He knew that beyond any doubt. Knew spirits existed eternally. Only problem was, he'd never developed the ability to see the spirits in the unseen realm, and at thirty-four, he doubted he ever would.

He'd been told only specifically gifted people could see into the invisible world around them. He'd also heard that with specific exercises, the gift could be developed over time, but he'd never tried any of them. Now he kinda regretted that. Two of his coworkers possessed the ability and they always uncovered answers pertaining to the worst of cases, even those deemed unsolvable, when no one else could.

Levi could have used some of that uncovering now.

He'd get his answers soon enough, though. He always did. And yeah, he should be on the phone, finding out what he could about Harper and her past, as well as her roommate's past, but he'd heard the pair stomping and chattering down the hall and he'd decided to follow them instead. He was glad he had.

A few interesting tidbits he'd already picked up. They loved each other, were comfortable together. They talked and laughed, teased each other good-naturedly. Yet ninety percent of the people who passed them eyed them as if they were certifiable, even the males drooling over Lana. And as beautiful as the redhead was, and as fragile as Harper appeared, not a single male approached them.

Of the remaining ten percent, well, five percent eyed them with amusement, but the other five eyed them with fear. That same remaining five-and-five eyed *him* with sheer terror. He was used to people turning away from him, or outright running from him, as if he were a mass murderer with a blood vendetta or something. But usually those people were criminals, and he'd just caught them committing heinous crimes.

Finally the two women stopped in front of an art gallery, their happy moods draining and leaving only grim expectation. The place was small but open, with big glass windows staring into an elegant space with columns and hanging lights.

Harper flattened her hand on one of the panes. "I was here, I remember that much."

"Yes, and you sold bazillion paintings that night."

The accent...Czech, maybe.

"And you..."

"Left early on arm of some loser." Guilt saturated the redhead's tone.

"Yes, and I failed to come home."

Neither female knew he was here, listening. The fact that they were searching for answers ruled out the possibility of an overactive imagination entirely. Yeah, people could convince themselves of the strangest things and actually think they were real, but they usually couldn't get someone else to agree with them.

The hand on the pane, so delicate and tiny in comparison to his, fluttered to Harper's neck. She closed her eyes and breathed deeply, seeming to ponder the fate of the world before a slow smile curled her lips, lighting her expression with a mix of pride and sadness. "I was so happy by the end of the show, my nervousness gone. My first genuine presentation was a raging success, more so than I could ever have dreamed, even as amazingly talented as I am, and every painting sold."

Yeah, there was no way this woman could have aided a

murderer. He knew criminals, had dealt with them on a daily basis for years, and yeah, some of them were good actors, well able to mask the monster within, but that smile...that sadness...combined with her physical reactions, there was just no way this was an act.

If he was wrong, he'd shoot *himself* in the face.

He was going to find out the truth. He was going to help her.

"What next? You remember?"

He watched as a tremor rocked the curve of Harper's spine, spiraling into her limbs. Nearly knocked her off her feet. "I...I..." She wrapped her arms around her middle, skin turning a light shade of green.

"You do not do this now," the redhead rushed to add. "We come back later."

"No," Levi said, stepping from the shadows, "you won't. You do this now, Harper." As sick as she currently appeared, she might not work up the nerve to return.

In unison, both women spun to face him. Harper reacted first. With a face bathed in panic and a mouth hanging open to unleash a scream, she jacked up her knee—and nailed him in the balls.

4

Deserved this, Levi thought. He never should have snuck up on Harper. He'd known better. Women were more unstable than C-4.

What? They were.

Silence permeated the tension-filled space between Levi and Harper as he struggled to find his breath and forget the fact that his testicles would probably need to be surgically removed from his throat. Even the crickets were too uncomfortable to laugh about what had just happened.

Harper's eyes were wide, her hand now over her mouth, and the friend was—doubled over laughing, he realized as the haze of pain gradually faded. Okay, so *she* wasn't too uncomfortable. Suddenly he was glad he hadn't gotten around to asking her out. *So not my type.*

Harper, on the other hand... His fairy with the broken wing and secrets in her ocean eyes had a nasty flight-or-fight response. It wasn't such a wonderful thing when he was on the wrong end of her knee, sure, but it'd be white-hot sexy when he wasn't, he was certain.

Still. Lesson learned. Never again would he underestimate her. But next time—and considering the amount of time they would have to spend together, working this case, there would be a next time—if given a choice, he would much rather chase her. Then, at least, he'd get to tackle like the good ole days when he'd played for OU.

Finally oxygen passed through his nostrils, filled his lungs. He smelled car exhaust and sunshine and...cinnamon. Her. He liked the smell of her.

Her hand fell away from her mouth. "I'm not going to apologize," she said, chin lifting. With the morning sun stroking her exposed skin, flushing her cheeks to a deep rose, she practically sparkled with vitality. "You scared me, and I reacted. Deal with it."

"You don't need to apologize. I do." He rubbed the back of his neck, grunted out a quick "Sorry" and left it at that. It was more than he'd given anyone in years, and you know, it hadn't left the bleeding, gaping wound that he'd expected.

The stiffness drained from her, and she worked up a beautiful grin that lit her entire face. It was genuine, with no hint of sadness, and she looked as if she'd swallowed the sun. Her hand fluttered just over her heart as she said, "Wow. Never has a more poetic apology been spoken. I'm all warm and tingly inside."

His body reacted to her words—warm and tingly—heating, tensing. He really had to get this attraction thing under control. He didn't mind wanting her, liked it, in fact, but he did mind the growing intensity of that wanting. "So you disappeared from this place?"

"I think." The grin was the next to drain away, followed by that gorgeous light. "Maybe."

"Maybe?"

"I just remember bits and pieces."

He heard the frustration and anger in her tone and sympathized. Levi knew he'd attacked the serial killer, but didn't know what he'd done or what had provoked him. He had flashes of flying fists, could even hear grunts of pain, but that was it. And for a man who prized his memory, having never forgotten a locker combination or even a file number, that irked.

"Ever talked to the owner of the gallery, asked questions? Ever talked to anyone who was there the night you're speaking of and might know?"

"No, but—"

"I have," the redhead said.

He arched a brow at her, a silent demand for her to continue.

Harper waved a hand between them. "Levi, meet Lana. Lana, meet Levi."

"You are so pleased to meet me, I know. Now, no one knew or saw anything," Lana said, the accent vanishing with an obvious, concentrated effort. Her hand had fluttered to her neck, where her fingers tapped against her pulse, seeming to mimic the cadence of her voice.

"I need the names of the people you talked to, and anyone else you remember being there."

As she rattled off the names, he read the hours of operation listed on the gallery's window. It was eight in the morning, and the place wouldn't open for another hour. He checked the door. Locked. He knocked, just in case someone was in back doing inventory or something. No one answered.

"Shouldn't you be writing down these names and numbers?" Lana asked.

"No," he said without looking at her.

"Apparently, he remembers things," Harper said drily.

He rattled off every name, every number, and both women
gaped at him. With two fingers, he helped Harper close her
mouth. "Anything else either of you want to share before I
start looking into this?"

Harper gave a little gasp, as though surprised by his agreement to help—or by his touch—and shook her head, but
Lana shifted nervously from one foot to the other. Suddenly suspicious, he homed his gaze in on her. She licked
her lips, narrowed her eyes, shifted from one foot to the
other. He remained silent, waiting for her to crack. They
always cracked.

Determination filled those green eyes. "Nope, nothing,"
she said.

Oh, she knew something, and he *would* find out what it was.
But not here, and not now. He'd dig up some details about
her, Harper, the art gallery, the owner, the people who had
attended Harper's gala, and go from there. The more armed
he was with information, the better chance he'd have of intimidating Lana and forcing her to talk.

He only hoped Harper was safe with her.

Has been so far, he told himself. "I'll swing by this evening,"
he told Harper, crowding her backward and forcing her to
stop against the building. Their gazes were locked, the air
charged between them. For a moment, her breath hitched in
her throat.

He leaned down, careful not to touch her a second time—
would she gasp if he did?—and whispered straight into her

ear, "Consider this your first and only warning. Next time your knee goes near my balls, I'll retaliate. But don't worry... I think you'll like it."

WHEN THE ELEVATOR DINGED and opened up to the OKCPD bull pen, Levi tensed and he wasn't sure why. He recognized the sights: guys in button-ups and slacks, guys in uniforms, cubbies and desks, computers, criminals cuffed to chairs, papers all over the walls. He recognized the sounds: heavy footfalls, the clack of high heels and the stomp of boots, inane chatter, angry shouting, fingers tapping keyboards, phones ringing. And the smells: coffee, aftershave, soap, unwashed bodies, perfume, sugar.

He just wasn't sure he belonged here anymore. He felt disconnected, separated, and wasn't sure it had anything to do with his suspension. So...why?

Your neighbors' crazy is rubbing off on you, that's all.

Small comfort. He maneuvered around the cubbies, throngs of people headed in every direction, each too busy to pay him any attention. He reached his partner's office and rasped his knuckles against the already open door. Vince sat behind his desk, head bent over a file. His gaze flicked up, landed on him, but quickly returned to whatever he was reading. His features were pale, drawn, and lines of tension branched from his eyes. Though he was only thirty-four, he appeared fifty and unable to care for himself, his cheeks hollowed, his sandy hair disheveled and his white shirt coffee-stained.

"Ignoring me still?" Levi asked. Vince had yet to forgive him for attacking the suspect and placing himself in the line of fire.

A reel of memory suddenly played, startling him. He and Vince had stormed into a small basement room. The perp had raised his arms, seemingly accepting of his arrest, and smiled. Smiled, smug and proud of all he'd done to his victims—and silently promising to do it all over again if ever he was released.

Levi had worked too many gruesome crime scenes because of the man, the last one enough to turn even *his* iron stomach. A young female had been staged, her lifeless, bruised and battered body pinned to a billboard for all of Oklahoma's downtown commuters to see as they hurried to work.

That smile had razed the jagged edges of his already shaky composure, a desire to protect the rest of Oklahoma's females rising up inside him. A desire he hadn't been able to fight. He'd rushed forward, busted the guy around—and gotten busted around himself.

In the present, he experienced a pang in his side. His kidney must have taken a couple shots.

"Come on, Vince," he said, and was once again ignored.

Detective Charles Bright stalked down the hall, spotted him and did a double take. "Levi?" His gaze roved the area just over Levi's shoulder before returning. "What are you doing here?"

He watched as Vince finally glanced up. Jaw clenched tight, he gritted, "What do you think I'm doing here, Bright? Working. Maybe you should do the same."

Talking through him. "Real mature," Levi said, flipping him off.

Bright waved Vince off, then led Levi to the office at the end of the hall. He closed and locked the door, and motioned for Levi to sit as he claimed the chair behind a desk scattered with papers.

Levi had always liked Bright. Guy had dark skin and eyes and kept his head shaved to a glossy sheen. He was a laugher, truly cared about the victims he fought to protect and would work himself to death to solve a case.

"I can't believe Vince is so mad he refuses to speak to me."

A soft, sad smile greeted his words. "Had you put him in danger, he'd be over it and you'd be forgiven. But you put yourself in danger, and that's harder to forget. He loved— loves—you like a brother."

"He better still love me." Vince was all the family he had.

"He does. Give him time. He'll come around."

Levi understood the need for time, he did, but his balls were sore and he wasn't exactly in the best of moods, so he decided to forget Vince for now. "Listen, I'm not actually here to beg my partner's forgiveness. My neighbor thinks she witnessed a murder and I promised to help her find out the truth. I can't access any databases, so I need your help."

Bright frowned, instantly intrigued. "Your neighbor?"

"Yeah. I don't know if I told you but I moved into an apartment building downtown, close to Brick Town. She just moved in, too."

"Her name?"

"Harper."

"And the rest?"

"Just a minute." Levi shifted to dig in his back pocket. He withdrew the driver's license he'd slipped from her purse when he'd backed her into the building. After reading the text, a laugh bubbled from him. "Aurora Harper." How freaking adorable. Aurora fit her in a way Harper did not.

Fingers clicking on the keyboard, Bright was silent for a long while. He would stop and read, then type again, then stop and read again, then type again. With every pause, his frown deepened. The wait for answers nearly drove Levi to pace, punch a wall, *something*.

"Okay, here's what I know," Bright finally said, propping his elbows on his desk. "Your Aurora—"

"Harper. She prefers Harper, and she isn't mine." He paid no attention to the fact that having her referred to as "his" affected his body just as strongly as her nearness had. Heat and tingling and want...so much want.

The denial earned him a swift grin. "All right. Well, Ms. Harper is twenty-seven. Five foot two. One hundred and ten pounds. She's gotten three tickets for speeding, one for parking illegally, and was in a car accident two years ago, but it wasn't her fault and she walked away with only a few bruises."

Silence.

"That's it?" Levi demanded. "That's what had you frowning?"

Bright drew in a deep breath, slowly released it. He settled back in his chair and folded his arms over his middle. "Milana Buineviciute, her roommate, works for After Moonrise and has the ability to see and communicate with the dead. Ms. Buineviciute reported her missing five weeks ago."

Milana Bonnie Wee Cutie. Now there was a name. Five weeks ago. Early October. She'd been in the apartment for a week, so that left four weeks unaccounted for. And the After Moonrise thing wasn't a point in her favor.

A few times, an After Moonrise agent had helped the OKCPD with a case. And for each of those few times, Levi had had to deal with a wealth of irritation. A.M. came in with their fancy equipment and superior attitudes and simply took over, acting as if the detectives couldn't find their way out of a paper bag. But his favorite? They'd called him a "norm," as if it were a four-letter word.

Wait. It was. Whatever! It had ticked him off.

"Inquiries were made, and it was discovered that Harper was last seen at Carmel Art Gallery, on October fifth around midnight." Bright paused, flicked his tongue over an incisor.

"That gallery certainly has been popping up on our radar a lot lately. Seems your boy Cory Topper bought a few paintings there. Only came to light a few days ago, since the sales were made under the table. We didn't think to tell you because you're, uh, off the case."

His stomach clenched. Topper. The serial killer who'd kept pieces of his victims in his freezer. The lunatic who'd tortured women in his basement. The psychopath who'd left a dead body on a billboard. The smug little ant whom Levi was now suspended for brutalizing.

To find out there was a connection between Topper, a dirtbag scum with evil in his veins, and Harper, a delicate, fragile little thing with knees of iron...he didn't like that. At all. But to learn that she'd been missing, to now know beyond any doubt that something *had* happened to her, was even worse.

He brought her painting to the forefront of his mind. The male Harper was bringing to life certainly fit Topper's body type, he realized now. Average height, slim build, deceptively gentle-looking hands.

"Where was Harper found?" he rasped. "When? And where had she been?"

"Oh, hmm." Bright glanced at the screen. "She wasn't found. At least, nothing has been entered into the system."

"I don't understand. What do you mean?"

"The case is still open."

Irritation laced with anger flooded him, and he popped his jaw. Why hadn't Lana reported her as found? Why hadn't Harper come forward? Fear that Topper would find her again? But then, that would mean she remembered him, if he was truly the one responsible, and it was clear that she didn't.

Levi replayed his new memory of the night he'd come face-to-face with Topper. Topper had been standing beside...

what? All he could picture were rivers of blood. Lots and lots of blood, flowing this way and that way and all around. Had there been any secret rooms? Someplace Harper could have been stashed, bound and helpless, forced to watch? Someplace she could have accidently stumbled upon and hidden?

A cage flashed through his mind.

A cage?

"Was there a cage in Topper's home?" he asked. "Actually, don't tell me. Just give me the crime scene photos." He'd never seen them.

"You know I can't do that," Bright said sternly.

"All I want is a glance at them." He could compare them with Harper's painting.

A sigh met his words. "I've always been a sucker. I'll see what I can do."

"Thanks. So how's our man Topper doing?"

Bright rolled his shoulders, easing tension. "He recovered from the injuries you gave him and is now locked up without bail, awaiting trial. We managed to find evidence of his crimes *after* his arrest."

Meaning, everything they'd found the day they'd arrested him had been thrown out because of Levi and they'd needed something new. And thanks be to God, they'd gotten it. Levi had read what had been fed to the media and knew there was more, but he wasn't going to ask. Yet.

Don't make everything a battle, son, his dad told him once. He didn't remember this on his own. He'd seen a home video of the two of them together. *You do, and you'll never win 'em all.*

"You got anything else on Harper?" he asked.

"A bit." Bright gave the computer screen another read. "The night of her disappearance, the art showing had wound down and only the owner remained in the building when she left, but he claims he was counting receipts in the back room and heard nothing unusual."

"Any connection between Topper and the owner?"

"Not that we've found."

"Are there *any* suspects in Harper's case? An ex-boyfriend with an ax to grind? A neighbor with a record? A stepdad with a grudge?"

"Oh...no, but I'll be sure and...close things now, and I suppose there's no real reason to press charges for withholding information."

Why the hesitation?

Bright cleared his throat and said, "Why don't you bring your Harper in? To me, only to me," he added in a rush, "and *I'll* question her about what happened."

"What do you know?" Levi demanded.

"What do you mean?"

"You're acting weird, hesitating to say certain things."

The detective pinched the bridge of his nose. "I'm telling you everything I can, Levi. Given that you're on a leave of absence, in fact, I'm telling you more than I should, and could even lose my own job over this." Bright's scolding tone lacked anger but was filled with understanding. "Now, what about bringing her in? I'll make sure she's protected while she's here."

No one was better at interrogation than Bright, and he'd be as gentle as possible, but... "Questioning her right now won't do any good. She doesn't remember. Whatever happened—" and it had to be bad for her to have repressed it as deeply as she had "—she's painting the image of a murdered woman."

Another frown tugged at the corners of Bright's mouth. "A woman? Describe the woman you're talking about. Could she—" a pause, a shifting in his seat "—*be* Harper?"

"No. You know I can't see the dead." His stomach clenched

as he once again brought the painting front and center and saw the pale skin of the woman, the delicacy of her bone structure. "There are similarities, granted, but no. And I can't tell you much more because Harper hasn't yet painted the face."

Bright worried two fingers over his stubbled chin. "Bottom line, there's a chance she saw the guy torture someone else."

"Yeah."

There was a whoosh of air as Bright straightened in his seat. "I want to see the painting. If we are, in fact, dealing with Topper, I want every piece of evidence I can gather. Yeah, he's going away for life, will probably be put to death, but maybe this is the way we'll find the bodies of his other victims."

If there was anything left of them. Levi had no idea why Topper had deviated from his usual M.O. and bound that woman—with all her parts—to that billboard. He had no idea why he'd kept mementos of some but not others. But really, did Levi *want* to know the twisted reasons of a psycho? "I'll take a picture and email it to you."

"Good, for starters."

"And I'll want a copy of the missing-person's report."

"Fair is fair, but I'm only giving you a glimpse of it." A few clicks and the papers began printing. "You can't take it with you. And don't dare ask if I'll do the same with the crime scene photos. That's a bigger deal, and you know it."

Disappointment struck him, but he said, "All right. Understood."

Bright held out the paper, and Levi scanned the contents. He didn't try to sort things out; he simply memorized every detail for later. When he finished, he stood. "Thanks for everything. I appreciate it."

"Anytime. And keep me updated on what you learn about Harper, okay? I'll work a few angles from this end."

Meaning, legitimate ends. He nodded and trudged to his partner's office, only to find that Vince had left. Whatever. They'd talk eventually. Next time, he wouldn't let Vince ignore him.

Now to dig through the report, and question Lana. That guilt he'd glimpsed at the gallery...she knew something more. Had she helped the abductor? But why report Harper missing? To hide her own actions? And yet, he doubted that was her motive. Genuine affection existed between the pair. Although, a lot of people could be bought, whether they loved someone or not.

Great. He was talking himself into believing in Lana's culpability, then talking himself out of it. Well, he wasn't going to wait until Lana cracked. Tonight, he was going to crack her open...himself...and...darkness...so much darkness...closing in....

No, he nearly roared. Ice crystallized in his veins, while sweat beaded over his skin. Breath boiled in his lungs.

Right there in the bull pen of the OKCPD, a shroud of black fell over his mind, slowly at first, stealing his thoughts one by one. He tensed, hating this feeling, knowing what happened...next—how he would lose...hours...perhaps days—but what he didn't know was *why* this kept happening or what—

Black...

Nothingness...

Empty...

5

Not again, Harper thought, panic rising as she peered down at her paint-splattered hands. She clutched a paintbrush, the tip drip...drip...dripping crimson onto her bare feet. Sickness bloomed in the pit of her stomach like a poisonous flower, its pollen drifting through the rest of her, sticking and growing until her blood was ice and her skin fire, her breath jagged and burning as it rasped against her lungs.

Before she looked up and faced the reality of what she had created, she spun and checked her surroundings. She stood inside her apartment's studio. Her shoulders sagged with relief. Okay. She could deal with anything else. Right?

Her gaze took in other details. The clock on her wall flashed 12:01—no, 12:02. The dark of the night seeped through the five-inch crack in the red, orange and yellow curtains Lana had made, and the scent of rain saturated the air, a roll of thunder booming.

Once upon a time, she had loved storms. Had loved the smells and the drop in temperature, the feel of raindrops against her skin. But lately they reminded her too much of Lana's tears, and even the tears *she* sometimes wanted to shed. Now that love was dead. *As dead as the girl you're painting.*

Ugh. The sickness intensified. So...she must have blacked out. Last thing she remembered was sitting on the couch, talking to Lana, waiting for Levi to come over, praying he'd learned something, *fearing* he'd learned something. Then... nothing.

Lightning suddenly struck, blazing the sky with gold and—a scream lodged in her throat, her heart pounding uncontrollably. A girl stood on the balcony outside her window, staring in at her with violet eyes. Other details registered. A fall of black hair, the wistful features of a young woman ready to fall in love, happy with her life yet somehow miserable at the same time.

How long had she stood there, watching? Had she noticed the scene unfolding on the canvas? As the questions filled Harper's mind, anger filled her chest. The peeping had to stop. Now.

Harper dropped her brush, heard the plop of it against the plastic covering she kept over the floor and stomped to the window.

By the time she had the pane lifted, the girl was gone.

Cool, moist air wafted inside the room, carrying the scents of floral spices and freshly cut grass; both failed to calm her, only ratcheted her anger higher. Harper pressed her tongue against the roof of her mouth as she snapped the pane back in place and threw the lock. She closed the curtains, being sure to hook the edges and prevent even the smallest fissure from forming, then she stood there for several minutes, knowing she was stalling, knowing she needed to turn, to face the truth one more time. Maybe this time would be the last. Maybe this time she had finished the painting, and all the answers would slide into place.

Maybe.

But hopefully not.

As much as she wanted to know, she *didn't* want to know.

"I can do this," she muttered. Slowly, so slowly, she turned on her heel. Deep breath in, deep breath out, she lifted her gaze.

And there it was, her painting. The overhead light seemed to spotlight the entire canvas, and...oh, no, no, no! She hadn't finished it, hadn't given the man a face, but she *had* finished the woman.

Lana was the woman on that slab, a bloody blade poised over her heart.

Lana. *Her* Lana.

No, no. *No!* That wasn't possible. Couldn't be possible. Lana would have told her if she'd been in that nightmare situation and somehow managed to escape. Lana was alive, and like Harper, Lana had never come home with injuries.

How would you know? You black out, lose track of time. What if her injuries healed during one of those blackouts, huh? No, no, no, she thought again. Panic...rising...

Maybe she was mistaken. Maybe the woman only looked like Lana. But black hair bleached and colored red cascaded over slender shoulders—and how many women had hair like that? Long black lashes cast shadows over hollowed cheeks. A perfectly sloped nose, lips red and raw, chewed from worry.

Though Harper had painted over all the cuts and bruises, though the woman's skin was smooth and creamy, blood spilled from her neck, her wrists, her stomach, her legs, her feet. Blood splattered the walls, pooled on the floor.

Blood.

Lana's blood.

Lana's. Blood.

If this truly were Lana—no, no, no, it couldn't be...just couldn't—how could Harper have known what happened to her? Lana hadn't told her. Or...what if she *had* told her, but Harper had repressed the memory, as she'd first feared?

Harper raced to the bathroom and dry heaved, thoughts batting through her mind one after the other. Every time Lana viewed the painting, she paled and clutched her stomach. The first time, she had actually vomited. Could she have repressed the memories, too, after confessing? Could something inside her recognize the pain she had endured?

With shaky hands, Harper brushed her teeth, splashed water on her face. "You have to confront her," she told her reflection. "Have to learn the truth. For both of you."

Determined, she stalked down the hallway. She'd forgotten to turn off the hall lights again—either that, or she'd turned them on during her blackout.

She stood in front of Lana's bedroom door. Her hand shook with more intensity as she wrapped her fingers around the knob and twisted. As the hall light spilled across the bed and the woman lying in the center, enveloped by a familiar rainbow-colored comforter, her red hair tangled over her pillow, her eyes closed in the sweet retreat of slumber, relief filled Harper to the point of bursting.

Whatever happened, she survived.

Did she really want to awaken Lana to a nightmare?

Harper gulped, the heavy question weighing her down. No. No, she didn't. The truth could wait until morning.

As quietly as she was able, she closed the door, checked every other door and window in the apartment. Levi had said he would get in touch with her yesterday evening, but he hadn't and now she was done waiting for him. She'd waited all day, in fact, and hadn't even received a hastily scribbled "Can't make it" note under her door. Well, he would now have to deal with the consequences of breaking his word.

She stomped out of the apartment, locked up after herself, double-checked the lock, triple-checked the lock, then padded to Levi's and—dang it! She'd forgotten to pull on a pair of sneaks. Someone had spilled a soda, so the carpet was cold and wet. Shivers were soon raking the length of her spine, intensifying when a clap of thunder boomed.

A hard rap at his door, shifting from one increasingly irritated and sticky foot to the other while glancing around to make sure no one tried to sneak up on her. When she spotted the freaky girl with the violet eyes gliding toward her, *dry* black hair floating back in a breeze Harper couldn't feel, her own bare feet seeming to lift off the ground, panic threatened to engulf her. How had the girl gone from outside to in so quickly, without getting wet?

"Such a naughty girl." In a voice as eerie as the rest of her, the teenager added, "You should have been nicer to him. He loved you, loved you so much."

Could she be… Was she a spirit, maybe? Harper had never possessed the ability to see into that other realm, but this was just too weird to be natural.

And, to be honest, she wanted no part of it. "Levi." Another rap, this one harder, yet still Levi failed to respond. "Levi, it's Harper! Open up."

The girl was coming closer and closer…. Harper tried the knob. It twisted easily. She darted into the apartment, quickly barricading herself inside. One minute passed, two, but the girl never misted through the door as Harper had been half convinced she would, never so much as knocked.

Still trembling, she peeked through the peephole but found the hallway empty. As the panic left her, common sense piped up. Lana could see the dead. Lana had always been able to see the dead. She knew the difference between living and un-living at a single glance, and she would always tell Harper when she spotted a spirit. Not once since they'd moved into this building had she pointed one out.

Tomorrow, Harper was doing a little research of her own, and maybe she would try to speak to an expert on those who developed a latent ability to see into the spirit realm—and find out if it were possible for someone to *lose* the ability. She wouldn't speak with Lana's coworkers, though. If Lana was having trouble, she didn't want anyone else to know it. But then, who did that leave?

"Levi, it's Harper," she called. "Are you here?"

Silence.

No, not silence. Another crack of thunder boomed, practically splitting the air in half. She yelped, her heart hammering against her ribs.

"Levi!"

Again, silence.

Why would he leave his place unlocked? That wasn't very coplike. And why wasn't he here? He'd said he was girlfriend free. Unless…maybe, while looking into Harper's story, he'd met a woman and stayed the night at her place.

Why that thought irritated her so much, she wasn't sure. She liked the look of him, yeah, but her life was a mess and she was pretty sure she'd already decided not to pursue any-thing with him, so— *Oh, why are you trying to fight it? You like more than the look of him. You like his strength and his intensity and that take-charge attitude of his. He makes you feel safe—when he's not sneaking up on you—and that's something you don't get from anyone else. You'll never know if something more could grow between you unless you try.*

Well, well. An intelligent line of thought, bypassing her qualms. That's how badly she wanted him, she supposed.

And he wanted her, too, which was an unusual occurrence, really. Most guys went for Lana and never changed their minds. But would Levi be okay with dating Harper, considering the trouble she was bringing to his door?

"Levi," she called again. "This is your last chance to announce your presence before I start nosing around your place. If you shoot me after I've given you this warning, I'll be very upset."

Again, silence.

"All right, then." No way was she going back into that hall. Sighing, she flipped the light switch, chasing away the darkness and illuminating his living room.

She walked forward, intending to wash her feet in his bathroom—only to stop short.

He was here.

He was sitting on his couch.

And he was staring at the wall with a blank expression on his face.

Concerned, Harper approached him. "Levi?" She bent down and waved a hand in front of his face, but he gave no reaction.

He wore the same clothes he'd changed into the first time she'd been here. Black T-shirt, black slacks. A quick check of his pulse proved his heartbeat was strong and steady, but his skin was chilled. Alarmingly chilled. His pupils were unresponsive to the light, his ears somehow unaware of the now-constant roll of thunder.

Harper reached out, intending to pat his cheek to gauge

his responsiveness to a more direct touch. He reacted with reflexes as swift as the lightning outside, grabbing her by the wrist and stilling her.

He blinked. A moment later, his gaze locked with hers. Awareness hit her with the force of a jackhammer. He smoldered with rumpled sex appeal.

"Harper?" Her name was little more than a growl.

"Yes."

"What are you doing here?"

"I needed to talk—"

"Never mind. Talk later." He jerked, and she landed in his lap.

6

One moment Levi was trapped in a world of black and help-lessness, and the next Harper was spotlighted in front of him, all that he saw, all that he wanted to see. Like an angel, her pale hair had seemed to form a halo around her, her concerned gaze so gentle it caressed him. She had been his only anchor to the world, a tether that would not allow him to slip away.

He'd remembered going to the station, speaking to Bright. Remembered finding out Harper had been reported missing, and her roommate had failed to tell the police she'd returned home. He'd had every intention of interrogating Lana, but then the darkness had come for him, right there in the sta-tion. And now he was...somewhere else, and Harper was with him....

"Levi?" she said.

Had he called her and asked her to come over? Dragged her here? He *hated* not knowing.

Frowning, he glanced around. He was inside his apartment, the lights switched on, bright enough to make his eyes water, though he couldn't remember how he'd gotten here. He was sitting on his couch, and Harper was in his lap.

He liked that she was in his lap.

Was she truly here, though? Was she real? Was she healthy, whole, *alive?* Unharmed by a murderer? He had to know... and he had to taste her, he thought, the need consuming him in an instant. She would keep the darkness at bay. She would keep him in the here and now. And he would protect her, he vowed.

He pressed his lips into hers.

The moment of contact, she gasped, and the moment her mouth opened, he took full advantage, kissing her as if she possessed everything necessary for his survival.

Maybe she did.

No one would hurt this woman. Not ever again. He wouldn't allow it.

At first she was stiff, but as his tongue rolled against hers, she melted against him, her hands making their way into his hair. Nails dug into his scalp. Her legs straddled him, those lethal knees pushing into the back of the couch.

How sweet she tasted, like an aged wine, heady and something to savor. He forced himself to gentle, sipping from her for as long as his control would allow, then he drank deeply, already addicted and needing more. He wasn't sure he'd ever get enough, but, oh, he would try. He would take everything she had to give, and still demand more.

He didn't like the circumstances that had brought them together, but he was glad they *had* been brought together, that something good could come of something so ugly.

"Harper."

"Yes?"

He meant to say something, but once again he got caught

up in kissing her and couldn't remember what it was. Him, a man who could memorize any number at any time, now so forgetful. But what better thing to concentrate on? Her moans of approval blended with the rough rasp of his breaths; they strained against each other, his need for her deepening, spiraling, threatening to burst from his skin.

And she was with him all the way—until his hands began to roam down her back, circle around her hips and slip up… up…toward her breasts. She gave another gasp, this one laced with fear. She jerked away from him, stumbling into his coffee table, tripping to the side, falling, then crab-walking away from him until her back hit the far wall.

Fear…that fear permeated the cloud of desire in his mind. "Harper," he said in a voice still affected by smoky desire. "What's wrong?"

"I'm not ready," she said with a tremble in her voice. "I can't. I can't, and you can't make me. Please don't make me."

I'm not ready. The words echoed through his mind, and he froze. *I can't, and you can't make me. Please don't make me.* Had someone once forced her? His hands curled into fists. No. He didn't want to believe it, was sick at the thought. This had to be about the painting. A lone female, bound to a cold slab of metal, naked, tools of torture hanging on the walls.

"Harper," he said. She was breathing too heavily, would probably pass out if she failed to calm.

He'd once looked at her and thought her somehow broken. Now he knew beyond a doubt. She was—but she was so much more. She had stalked into the apartment of a man she'd never before met and asked for help. She'd had the strength to patch herself up, to hunt for answers.

"Harper," he repeated as he stood.

A little mewl left her.

One step, two, he approached her, his steps unhurried, as nonthreatening as possible. He held his hands in front of his body, palms out. "I'm not going to make you do anything, okay?"

Another mewl.

"You're here with me, with Levi, and you're safe." Before, he'd told himself he would leave her alone if she was broken in any way, that he was too weighed down with his own concerns to help someone else recover. Now he knew there was no way he could stay out of her life. Not just because he wanted more of her, more of everything she had to offer, but because he hated seeing her like this. He wanted his smiling, teasing Harper back.

When he reached her, he crouched down, careful not to touch her. "Harper, sweetheart. Can you hear me?"

A tear rolled down her cheek.

A sharp pang in his chest had him biting his tongue to stop a curse from forming. Slowly, so slowly, he extended his hand to brush the hair from her brow. He wasn't sure what he expected, but what he got wasn't it. She erupted into a blaze of motion and fury.

"No!" Her fist struck him in the eye.

A surprising amount of pain exploded through his head, considering her tiny size, but still he remained immobile. He'd been hit enough times in his life that being smacked with a semi probably wouldn't have fazed him. But she wasn't done, and next did her best to rain a world of hurt on him. He let her. By the fifth punch, his adrenaline was so high he hardly felt a thing, anyway. It was only when she began to kick and to twist, trying to claw her way out through the wall, that he reached out to stop her.

He caught himself just before contact. If he touched her too soon, her terror and desperation would only be driven higher and he'd have a whole new set of injuries to contend with. He would have to wait this out. Shouldn't be too much longer now. Her motions were slowing…slowing.…

Finally, the fight left her entirely. She collapsed on the floor, sobbing, breaking his heart into so many pieces he wasn't sure he'd ever be able to glue them back together.

He said gently, "Harper, sweetheart?"

"Levi?" she asked with a sniffle.

Thank God! Springing into motion, he scooped her up and cradled her against his chest. She allowed this, her head burrowing into the hollow of his neck. He could feel the wetness of her tears, and wanted to howl.

He carried her to the couch and eased himself down, still holding her close. Several minutes ticked by in silence. He'd dealt with victims of abuse before, but never this up close and personal. So, because he wasn't exactly sure of what to do, he went with his instincts and massaged the back of her neck, played with the ends of her hair, traced his fingers along the ridges of her spine.

"Tell me what happened," he said.

She drew in a deep, shuddering breath, released it. "I don't know. One minute I was kissing you, and the next I was on the floor, crying. That happens sometimes. Not that I've kissed a lot of guys," she babbled. "Even the most casual of touches can set me off. Lana and I don't even high-five anymore."

He frowned. "So…you have blackouts?"

A heavy pause. Then a whispered, "Yes."

That little ball of information did more than land in his yard. It shattered his window. She had blackouts, just like him. A strange coincidence. Far too strange. His Spidey senses were suddenly tingling.

"Did I do something to you?" she asked, hesitant. "Say something I shouldn't have?"

"We kissed, only kissed, and you jumped to the floor. That's all, I promise. I never even made it to second base," he said with as teasing a tone as he could muster. *But I will. I will help you, and we will do more, all.* "And just so you know, I have blackouts, too."

She jerked upright, twisting to fully meet his gaze. "What! Really? You're not just saying that to— Oh, my goodness! What happened to your face?" she ended, horrified.

He could only imagine what he looked like. The beginning of a black eye, surely, as well as a swollen cheek and busted lip. A lip that ached as it twitched at the corners. How could she amuse him in the worst of situations?

"What's wrong with it?" He placed his hands on the couch, off her body. Just in case. He didn't want a repeat of the Episode; he just wanted her, but he was willing to wait.

"Everything! You look hideous!"

Won't grin. But man, he liked her honesty. "You should see yourself."

Her eyes were red, swollen, and her skin spotted with pink. Strands of pale hair were stuck to her cheeks, saturated from her tears. "What's wrong with me?"

"Nothing." She was the most exquisite creature he'd ever beheld.

The thought made him cringe. He so was not a poet.

"You're *that* disgusted by me?" she squeaked.

He rolled his eyes. "You're hot. I'm hooked. And if what just happened didn't scare me away, nothing will."

Her features softened. "So what *did* just happen to you?"

"I got into a fight," he said, unwilling to say more if she couldn't remember.

"When? With who?"

He loved that, even though her hands were probably throbbing, she refused to consider herself.

"I promise you," she continued, "I'll *ruin* him. Me and Lana, we have a system."

He donned his best "I'm a cop and you're in trouble" expression. "What system?"

"Oh, uh. Hmm. Never mind about that."

As if he'd really arrest her for defending him. A body-cavity search, maybe. A stint with the cuffs, definitely. But anything behind bars? Probably not. "So how long have you been having those blackouts?"

"I don't want to talk about it," she muttered.

"Do it, anyway."

"No."

Stubborn. "Here's how this is gonna work. You're gonna show me yours, and I'm gonna show you mine."

A calculating gleam entered her eyes. "I do want to see yours, so...okay. Yes." She nodded. "They started just before I moved here."

His frown returned. "Same for me."

"So you really do have blackouts?"

"I do."

A thousand different emotions played over her features. "I can't believe... You're the first person... Levi, do you know what this means?" she asked, adjusting herself on his lap, once again straddling him.

"No." Only the memory of what had happened the last time they'd been in this position kept his hands at his sides.

"I'm not alone! Do you know how thrilling that is? I mean, no, not thrilling, that would be a terrible thing to feel." Her nose scrunched as she struggled to experience what she deemed appropriate. "I'm sorry you've had to deal with something like that. It's terrible. *But I'm not alone!*"

"Me, either." And he was as thrilled as she was, he realized. For the first time since his parents' death, there was someone who understood him.

"What do you think this means?"

"I don't know. Does Lana have them, too?"

"No. I asked."

But had the secret-keeping Miss Bonnie Wee Cutie told the truth? He *had* to interrogate that woman.

"That's what was wrong with you when I first got here, I bet," she suddenly exclaimed. "You were in the middle of a blackout, weren't you?"

"Yeah."

"Do you know what time or where you were when it began?"

"It hit a short while after I left you. I had just talked to my friend at the station, was walking to the elevator to leave, and that's the last thing I remember."

She toyed with his shirt, twisting the material. "I can fill in a bit of the missing time. I came over around midnight to speak with you, but you didn't answer. The door was unlocked, by the way. When I came in, you were sitting on your couch, staring into the darkness, unaware of anything around you."

Relief cascaded through him. He'd always wondered—fine, feared—what he'd done while lost to the darkness, and sitting on his couch hadn't made the list. "What did you want to speak with me about?"

Her hand flattened over his heart, her nails almost cutting past his shirt. "Well…the blackout here wasn't the only one I experienced today. One second I was waiting for you, the next I was in front of my painting. I'd filled in a few more details."

He was gripping her by the waist, holding on to her as if she would slip away at any moment, before he even realized he'd moved. "Tell me."

"I… The girl I'm painting…it's Lana."

Lana? Impossible. But…the secretiveness, the trepidation, the odd behavior, reporting her friend missing but never reporting her found…yeah, the pieces could fit. "Where's the painting now?"

"My apartment."

He would study it—in a bit. "So, you think she was abducted, tortured and somehow escaped," he said, a statement, not a question.

"Yes. I mean, I know I told you the girl in the painting was dead, but I had to be mistaken about that."

"And?"

"And I think I went looking for her…saw her trapped, hurt."

Poor darling. "Have you recalled anything from the scene itself?"

"No." The rapid puffs of her breath were the only sound in the room. "I'm stumbling on one fact, though. Like me, Lana wasn't ever found with injuries."

There was that, wasn't there. "Maybe she healed during one of your blackouts."

Her shoulders drooped. "Maybe."

"There's one way to find out what happened to her," he said.

She sighed. "I know. I don't like it, but I know."

7

Though Harper knew Levi expected to return to her apartment that very second, shake Lana awake and treat her to an intense interrogation, and though Harper needed to hug her friend and cry with her and promise to make everything better, her emotions were still raw, the fear of sinking into another black hole a living entity inside her. She wanted to stay here, inside Levi's apartment, safe from the sorrow that awaited her for just a little longer.

He just smelled so good, heat radiating off him in continuous waves, wrapping around her. One of his hands caressed her back, and the other stroked the side of her leg. Both soothed her, despite the fact that she usually hated being touched, and all too soon her eyelids grew heavy. She yawned.

"Can we postpone?" she asked. "Just until morning. Please."

"Begging doesn't work with me. This needs to be done, Harper."

"I know, but I'm not at my best and I want to be at my best when we do this. *Pleeease*."

A pause. A sigh. "Begging didn't used to work," he grumbled, and he stayed put.

A soft chuckle escaped her. "Don't beat yourself up. I'm irresistible."

He said something to her, but he sounded far away. She tried to respond, she really did, but...

...floated away...into another darkness, though this one offered comfort rather than terror. Maybe because she could still smell the musk of Levi's scent, could still feel the warm pulse of him, not just at her side but all over.

When the weight finally lifted from her eyelids, she blinked awake. A frown formed as she cataloged her surroundings. She was inside a strange apartment, stretched out on an unfamiliar couch. The overhead light was on, sunlight streaming through a dark curtain.

Morning had arrived, she realized. The last thing she remembered was talking to Levi, and agreeing to speak with Lana.

She sat up—or rather, tried to. Strong arms were banded around her, holding her in an intractable grip. Panic sparked to life while she attempted to orient herself. Warm breath trekked over her neck. A man's breath. A man who was aroused.

Had she blacked out, left Levi and gone home with a stranger? Bile burned a path up her throat as she struggled against that vise grip.

A growl rumbled from the man. "I've got you," a raspy voice said. "Be still."

A raspy voice she recognized.

Levi. Frowning, she glanced down, spied the bronze of his skin and the light dusting of dark hair. Drank in the strength of his fingers, and the thin scars that crisscrossed his wrists.

As quickly as it had formed, the panic left. Relief danced

through her. But...this made no sense. They weren't inside his apartment. The furnishings were different. Before, there'd been no artwork on the walls. Now portraits of animals playing poker...and golf...and baseball filled the walls. Walls that had gone from white to pale blue in a single night.

"Levi," she said.

"Harper," he replied, his tone letting her know her name was a curse.

"You awake?"

"I'm talking, aren't I?"

Growling, more like. "Not a morning person, huh?"

"Not a morning, afternoon or evening person. You'll just have to deal with it because, this time, you're to blame. You stood up three times, and once even made it to the hallway outside."

Sleepwalking. The number-one reason she'd become a fan of insomnia. "I don't remember any of that," she admitted.

His arms tightened around her for several seconds before he sat up, dragging her with him. Sadly, he severed contact and she found herself mourning the loss of his strength and his heat. How unlike her. But then, with his confession about his own blackouts, his determination to help her, Levi had busted through her instinctive safeguards, making her as comfortable with him as she was with herself.

"So where are we?" she asked, smoothing her hair from her cheeks.

"Where else? My apartment."

She blinked over at him, confused. "And you decided to do a little redecorating while I was sleeping?"

"What are you talking about?" Frowning, he stood and padded to the kitchen, where he stumbled around as he gathered supplies for coffee. His shirt and pants were wrinkled. Sometime during the night he'd removed his shoes and socks and now his feet were bare. "You fell asleep, I helped you get comfortable, got comfortable myself and was out soon afterward."

"But your walls." She waved her hand over the portraits.

He glanced over his shoulder to examine them. "Yeah. What about them?"

She looked at his face, intending to gauge his reaction to her next words, but she got caught on another thought trail. The swelling had gone down in his eye and cheek, and his skin was only slightly discolored. Last night, he'd been black-and-blue. The split in his lip had already scabbed over.

"You heal quickly," she announced.

"Harper," he said on a sigh. "The walls."

Right. The walls. "Yesterday they were naked."

He froze, his hand raised to pour in the grounds. Slowly he set everything down and turned toward her. "You're sure?"

"Yes. I always study a person's walls."

His brows knitted. Suddenly he looked as confused as she felt. "Why?"

"Art. Why else? You can learn so much about a person that way."

He shook his head, as if dislodging a pesky thought. "And mine were…naked, you said."

"Yes. And a different color!"

His gaze swept over each of the portraits a second time, lingering, taking in every detail. "I recognize every piece, recognize the color. That's how they've looked since I moved in."

Her stomach bottomed out, the implications almost too much to take in. "One of us is mistaken."

"Or both of us are right and something weird is going on." He rubbed the back of his neck. "Forget the coffee. Let's shower, and go chat with Lana."

"Shower…together?"

"Well, not now," he grumbled. "You can use the guest bathroom if you want."

"I do. Thank you." Though she was tempted…

As he stalked out of the kitchen and into his bedroom, Harper lumbered to her feet.

She found the guest bathroom easily enough, only to discover a still-packaged toothbrush, a fresh tube of toothpaste and every feminine product known to man. Or woman.

As hard and gruff a guy as Levi was, he sure was prepared for female guests—something Harper wasn't sure she appreciated. Was he a player?

It wasn't like Harper had any type of claim on him, especially considering she'd just denied him, but still. He'd held her all night long. Before that, he'd kissed her. So…*she had a claim on him.*

Yeah, she'd first thought to keep things purely professional between them. But guess what? She'd just changed her mind. For sure this time. If he'd wanted to enjoy his bachelorhood, he should not have invited her to happy shower time. He should have kept his lips and hands to himself. He should have refused to snuggle her and keep her safe.

When she stepped out of the stall, dripping wet and wishing she'd looked for a towel before making use of the water, she found a small pile of clothes resting beside the sink. A T-shirt and a pair of sweatpants—neither of which belonged to her.

That Levi, she thought, unsure whether she wanted to grin or slap him. She'd locked the door, but he'd come in, anyway. At least the clothes belonged to him rather than another woman.

By the time she finished rolling the soft material at her wrists, waist and ankles, he was in the living room, waiting for her. He eyed her up and down, nodded his approval despite the fact that her hair was wet and the bulk of the clothing made her look as if she'd gained twenty pounds since they'd last seen each other.

While her heart drummed erratically, she gave him the same perusal. He wore another black shirt and pair of black slacks, but he somehow looked more delicious than ever. So unfair.

As he ushered her into the hallway, she said, "So those tampons in your guest bathroom…"

"They aren't mine, that's for sure," he said, locking his door.

"I know that. Moron! So whose are they?"

"You're not gonna like the answer."

"Tell me, anyway."

"They belonged to my ex, and I failed to throw them out." He escorted Harper down the hall and up the stairs to her apartment.

"Why would that make me angry?"

"You might think I kept them because I still had feelings for her. I don't. You might think I meant to let your roommate use them, since I'd planned to date her. You might think I'm obsessive about keeping what's mine…and you'd be right, and the knowledge might scare you away."

She locked on to one thought. He'd first wanted Lana. "Why did you kiss me if you wanted to date my roommate?" she gritted out. Oh, he'd mentioned his desire to hook up with Lana before, but they'd just met and she'd just irritated him and that could have been a taunt. This wasn't.

"See?"

"Answer me."

"I didn't say I *still* wanted to date her."

"But she was your first choice."

"A choice made in a moment of insanity."

"So?"

"So, you're going to throw it in my face the whole time we're together, aren't you?"

The whole time we're together. That was relationship talk, and it was the only thing that mollified her. "Yeah," she said. "I am."

"I probably shouldn't admit this, either, but that's kinda hot."

And he was hooked on her, she remembered him saying. Well, okay, then. She wouldn't punish him *too* badly.

"Lana," she called when she was inside their place, hoping to give her friend time to wake up, dress or whatever she needed. "Lana!"

Silence.

"Wait here," she said, and went to Lana's bedroom. Inside, she flipped on the light. The bed was empty, the covers askew. The closet was empty, as well, no clothes remaining.

As she flattened her hands over her stomach to ward off an oncoming ache, she felt rather than saw Levi come up behind her.

"What's wrong?" he asked.

"She's gone." And she'd left in a hurry. Some of her things were on the floor—a shoe, a pair of panties and a brush—as if they had fallen out of a hastily thrown-together bag.

Levi brushed past her and searched every inch of the room. She stood there, numb, as she watched. Why had Lana left her? And she *had* left her.

"What are you doing?" she asked when Levi crouched on the floor and traced his fingertips over the carpet fibers.

"Checking for foul play." He went through the entire space from top to bottom before ushering her to the dresser and motioning to a wrinkled piece of paper. "Read it, but don't touch it, okay? I want it dusted for fingerprints. And tell me if it's her writing and if she sounds normal."

Harper's eyes watered as she glanced down. She had to wipe them three times before she could make out the words.

Please do not be mad, Harper. Your painting...I do not know why you paint me. I was not there, I swear to you. Nothing was done to me, and I witness nothing done to anyone else. I do not know what it means, but this has scared me. I will take off for a while. I must figure some things out. Don't worry about me, okay? I will be fine. And so will you. Your detective will take care of you now. I am sorry I couldn't. I love you more than anything on this earth and nothing will ever change that.

P.S. I know I told you the OKC branch of A.M. did not wish to take your case, but that was a lie. I do not want them involved in this, no matter what. Promise me. Instead, I want you to go to Tulsa and visit the A.M. offices there. I called, and they expect you. They will take you seriously. Go to them, please, you and your detective both. What if you've seen into future?

Harper could see the tearstains on the paper, knew Lana had cried while she'd written this. "She definitely wrote this, and not under duress, but I don't understand it," she whispered.

What if Lana was right and she had seen into the future? What if Lana would one day suffer atrocities at some madman's hands? What if—

"I can see where your thoughts derailed, and you need to get back on the right track. *What if* can be two of the cruelest words ever created if you let them."

True. They lit a fire under fear while proving nothing, stopping nothing. And they could be wrong, her worry pointless. "If the painting is a glimpse of the future, why am I missing so much of my life in the here and now? Why am I having blackouts, but Lana's not?"

"Maybe she is. Maybe she lied. Why would she not want you to visit After Moonrise here in Oklahoma City?"

Lied…lied… Lana could have lied to her. Always they'd shared everything. Money, clothes, cars, food, sorrows and pains, joys and rewards. Brutal Honesty had been their motto.

Do I look fat in these jeans?

As a rhino.

What if my date tries to kiss me?

He won't. Not with that garlic breath.

"Maybe she didn't want her coworkers involved in my potential crazy," Harper said. Maybe. So many maybes.

Levi's hands settled on her shoulders. "I'll ask one of my friends to track her, watch her, guard her. She'll be kept safe, I promise you."

He hadn't said "and question her" but she heard the words in his tone. No matter how much Harper hated the way things were playing out, an interrogation needed to happen now more than ever. "Thank you. She's my best friend. I love her no matter what, same way she loves me, and I want her safe."

"She will be."

Emotion clogged Harper's throat, and her chin trembled. "What are your plans today?" he asked.

"I want to paint the killer's face." She *had* to paint it. No longer would she resist.

Even thinking about him caused a flicker of rage to erupt inside her. If he had—or would—hurt the girl in the painting, then he had hurt other women, and would doubtless hurt many more. He had to be stopped.

"Okay. All right. I'll give you a few hours, but then we're taking Lana's advice and heading to Tulsa. We'll take your painting, whatever shape it's in, and let them have a look, tell them what's been going on. I want to hear what they have to say."

"O-okay." Maybe they could explain the blackouts, too. Because…no matter how wonderful it was to know she wasn't alone in her suffering, it was bizarre that both she and Levi were experiencing them, that they'd started at the same time. "You don't have to work?"

Guilt filled his eyes, quickly masked. "Not today. Why don't you get started? I'll make that call about Lana, gather a few things from my apartment and come back. I don't want you alone today."

"Okay," she repeated, peering down at the note. Why had Lana taken off without some kind of a confrontation? Running wasn't like her. In fact, Lana had never backed down from a challenge, any challenge. And where had she gone? Like Harper, she was without any family. They only had each other. Now she was out there, alone, scared.

Strong hands cupped her face. "Harper. Look at me."

A tear trekked down her cheek as she obeyed.

"Everything's going to be all right," he said gently. He wiped the tear away with the pad of his thumb.

"I don't like the uncertainty. I don't like that every time I get a question answered, a thousand more pop up. And I *hate* being afraid."

He kissed the tip of her nose. "I won't let anything happen to you, either. You have my word." He didn't wait for her reply, didn't ask permission, but lowered his head the rest of the way and claimed her mouth.

Without any hesitation, she wound her arms around him,

holding on tight, allowing him to consume her bit by bit. Glad for him, glad for this, shocked by her need to touch and be touched, but more so by her lack of panic. This was real, and this was necessary. This was everything she hadn't known she'd needed. If any man could protect a woman from harm—from unseen forces, even—it was this one. He knew his power, his authority, and he wasn't afraid to wield it.

When he pulled away, lines of tension branched from his eyes. He opened his mouth to say something, thought better of it and stomped out of the apartment. Through the wooden door she heard him growl, "Lock this."

On shaky legs she followed his trail. Even her fingers shook as she flipped the lock.

"Good girl," he said, his footsteps sounding a moment later.

She rested her forehead against the door. That man...oh, that man. The kiss hadn't panicked her, but now the thought of losing him did. In a very short time, she'd come to depend on him...to need him. And maybe he needed her, too. He could have washed his hands of her. After all, this wasn't his problem. But he hadn't. He'd immediately taken up the reins of control, arranging their next steps. A good thing. She wasn't sure she would have had the strength to visit After Moonrise without him.

You're wasting time. Buck up and get to work. For Lana. She had to save Lana—so that she could yell at her for daring to abandon her.

With a sigh, Harper marched into her bedroom.

8

Levi merged onto the highway. First he'd had Harper in his apartment, now his car. He'd allowed her to borrow his clothes—which she'd changed out of, and he kind of wished she hadn't. Letting someone else play with his toys should have put him on edge, but he was strangely settled. This felt right. He liked having her near, within reach, surrounded by his things.

"Did you reach your friend?" she asked. She chewed on her nail, watching as cars and buildings whizzed past. "Is he going to track down Lana?"

"Yep."

"You trust him? He's decent at what he does?"

"Yep."

"Well, that's good enough for me, I guess."

Her grumbling tone told him she reeeally wanted him to elaborate, but how could he elaborate, when the details were sparse? Why did he trust Bright? Instinct. How long had he known the guy? Years. What kind of cases had he solved? Complicated.

Half an hour of silence followed that little interaction before Levi could stand it no longer and asked, "Were you able to paint the guy's face?" He'd hoped she would open up on her own, and he wouldn't have to press. He wanted her to be comfortable with him, but he was also tired of waiting.

"No," she said, and he caught the taunt in her tone. He'd given little, so she would give even less.

This woman really cranked his chain. "Why not?"

"Blocked."

"Is there anything I can do to help?" He purposely didn't mention Topper because he didn't want to increase her worry for her friend. Not unless absolutely necessary.

"Yes," she said, and he could feel her gaze on him, as if she were judging his reaction. "You could pretend you know how to have a conversation and, I don't know, stop barking out one-word answers anytime I ask a question."

Won't grin. "Sure."

"Argh!" She leaned over and punched him in the arm. "You're a hard nut to crack, you know that?"

"Yes."

That earned him another punch. "Well, despite your sparkling wit, I'm going to let you stay with me tonight. I paint in my sleep, but fear somehow finds me and wakes me up, stopping me from finishing. If you're there, I'll feel safe and I'll continue painting until it's done. I know it."

Safe. Good. "Consider me there." Over the years, with as many victims as he'd dealt with, he'd learned a thing or two about fear. You absolutely could not meditate, or feed upon, thoughts that scared you. You had to cast them away, and force yourself to focus on something else. He would be her something else…his hands…his lips… He'd move slowly, take a little at a time, demand a little at a time, until she was ready.

Then he'd take all. Everything.

She must have sensed the direction of his thoughts because she said, "Now then, about the kiss."

"Yeah. What about it?" He wanted more, and if she expected him to enter some kind of friend zone, they'd have a problem.

"This is gonna tick you off."

"Say it, anyway."

"I know we've only kissed, like, once, but you're staying the night tonight, and…well…"

"And, well, you want me to keep my hands to myself." It was better than the total rejection he'd anticipated from her, and something he could work around.

"Not at all," she said, surprising him. "You can get handsy if you want…maybe…if you go slow. But I don't want you seeing another woman while we're…you know, involved."

Wait, wait, wait. She was demanding exclusivity from him? Giving him exactly what he wanted from her? He gave a mock sigh. "If you insist…"

"I do."

He liked knowing she was as possessive as he was. "Then I guess I can—"

"Oh, just forget it!" she huffed. "I'm not dog food, you know. I don't want a man who's this resistant. I don't have to throw myself at anyone, so you can just—"

"You're not throwing yourself at anyone. You're with me, and there will be no other men for you." Anger with himself—shouldn't have teased her over such an important subject—morphed into anger with any other man who'd try to hook up with her.

"You're sure?" she said in a snippy tone.

"Very. You?"

From the corner of his eye, he saw her flick her hair over one shoulder. "Kind of."

Really won't grin. She was sure all right, but her mean streak had kicked in.

Now to figure out what was happening to the world around them.

Finally they made it into Tulsa. Here, the trees were thicker and there were a few more hills. There were buildings of brownstone and stucco, brick and siding, some tall, some short, some thin, some wide. The sky created an eerie backdrop, a long expanse of dark gray layered with fat, rain-heavy clouds.

After Moonrise came into view. Eight stories high, with smoked-glass windows and a waterfall in front, it was one of the city's classier structures. The front doors were arched, all about the welcome.

He parked in one of the only empty slots, got out and moved to the other side of the car to help Harper. Clutching the sheet-covered painting in her hands, she gifted him with a soft smile of thanks. He couldn't stop himself from smoothing a strand of hair from her cameo face and luxuriating in the perfection of her silky skin.

She leaned into his touch, her eyelids dipping to half-mast—but not before he caught a glimpse of apprehension. Not directed at him, but at the coming meeting, he was sure. He knew she expected to be told she had predicted her best friend's death, knew part of her also expected to be told there would be nothing she could do to stop that death from occurring. He knew because he'd battled the same thoughts.

"Let me ask you a question," he said. "When you first came

to my apartment, what would you have done if I'd kicked you out without listening to you?"

Her brow furrowed as she gave serious consideration to her response. "I guess I would have annoyed you so badly you would have done anything to get rid of me. Even listen."

Exactly what he would have guessed. "How would you have annoyed me?"

A shrug of those delicate shoulders as she said, "By knocking incessantly on your door, following you around like a puppy and ultimately shoving the painting in your face."

"That would have taken balls of steel."

"And I polish mine every night. So what?"

Again, exactly what he would have guessed. "So," he said, trying not to grin, "I just wanted to remind you that you do, indeed, have them." He linked their fingers, confiscated the painting with his free hand and dragged her to the entrance.

As they strode across the pavement, he heard her praying under her breath. "Lord, give me the strength to hear what I need to hear and to do what I need to do. Thank You."

A bell rang as they stepped from outside to in. Soft music played in the background. The temperature rose considerably, from misty and cold to dry and bone-meltingly hot. Incense saturated the air, sweet and spicy at the same time, somehow pleasing and repugnant at once. His nostrils burned, but he endured the sensation as a necessary evil.

He scanned the area, taking in every detail at once. There was a reception desk, a long table with coffee and other refreshments, and a waiting room with big, comfortable-looking chairs.

Six people—four males and two females—reclined in those chairs, but only the little dark-haired girl perched on her mom's lap paid Harper and him any attention. She smiled and waved, and Levi waved back, charmed. The mom looked over at him, frowned and gently admonished the girl to behave and mind her own business.

The lady at the reception desk alternated between answering the phone and typing into her computer. In her mid-fifties, with hair dyed the darkest of jet, skin aged from sun exposure and features that were lovely nonetheless, she glanced up at his and Harper's approach—

—and screamed.

Her hand fluttered over her heart, and she jumped to her feet. "What are you doing here?"

He was used to alarming people with his gruff appearance and no-nonsense demeanor, but screams and accusations at minute one, when he wasn't waving a gun? Yeah, that was a first.

"It's okay, Mommy," he heard the little girl say. "He's not gonna hurt anyone. He just looks scary."

"My name is Detective Reid, OKCPD," he said loudly, hopefully calming the people in the waiting room who'd begun to mutter in distress. He lowered his voice and added, "Milana Bonnie Wee Cutie should have called to tell you we were coming. We have a few questions for whoever's in charge of…" Just how did you explain the weird things happening to Harper? And to him, for that matter.

"Lana works for the OKC branch," Harper blurted out. At least she kept her hands at her sides, opting not to chew on her nails.

The receptionist exhaled with relief and said, "Okay, yes. Yes. I—I remember getting her call. I just wasn't expecting—" she waved her hand up and down to encompass Levi's big body "—this."

This. "What's wrong with *this?*" he growled.

"You're not a little blonde with a Napoleon complex, are you?" she snapped. "I was told to expect a little blonde with a Napoleon complex."

"Okay, taking over now," Harper muttered. "Here's the deal. I might be painting the future, and Lana thought you could help me. And besides that, other things have us freaked out, like the fact that Levi's apartment changed its furnishings in a single night, but he didn't do the changing and it still looks the same to him. This agency specializes in the paranormal, right? Well, there's nothing normal about anything that's happened to us lately, and I want answers. Like, yesterday."

The lady glanced between them, her color high but gradually lightening. "Just...stay where you are." Never taking her gaze off them, she bent down and picked up the phone.

A whispered conversation took place, and Levi thought he heard "I don't know" about a thousand times. Finally, she replaced the phone in its cradle and said, "Agent Peterson will be right out."

A few seconds later, a big man with a big scowl stomped from the elevator. A smaller man holding a stack of files raced behind him, desperate to catch up.

"Headed out, Mr. Raef?" the receptionist called.

"Yeah." Mr. Raef stopped, gave Levi a once-over, and glared. The smaller man rammed into Mr. Raef's back, dropping his papers, but the guy hardly seemed to notice. "What are you doing here? What do you want?"

"He isn't as evil as he looks," the receptionist said.

"You're sure?" the man demanded, taking a menacing step in Levi's direction. "My woman is waiting for me, and even the thought of being late makes me killing mad, so if any killing needs to be done..."

Levi rolled his eyes and wished he still had his badge.

"Ms. Peterson is taking— Ah, there she is," the receptionist said with relief as a woman stalked out of a second elevator. She was of average height—meaning Levi towered over her and she towered over Harper—and average weight. Meaning Levi could snap her spine with a single twist of his giant man-hands.

Peterson had short hair dyed pink and lacquered into tiny spikes. Her eyes were brown and rimmed by eyelashes she'd also dyed pink. She wore a dog collar, had brass knuckles tattooed on her fingers and was clad in a plaid shirt with ruffles and baggy black pants tucked into combat boots. She stopped abruptly when she spotted them and flashed her teeth in a scowl.

"What are you doing here?" she demanded.

Seriously. Could no one treat him like a human being? "We're friends of Lana's."

"Lana?" Mr. Raef cursed under his breath. "They're all yours, Peterson," he said with a mean-sounding chuckle, and exited the building, the other man scurrying behind him.

Peterson ran her tongue over her teeth. "Lana didn't say you looked like...this."

"Hey! What's that supposed to mean?" Harper snapped.

Levi swallowed a laugh and put his hands on her shoulders, holding her in place. He had a feeling she was seconds away from leaping on Peterson like an injured wolverine interested in a last meal.

Peterson's gaze danced between them before she nodded. "All right, fine. I'm choosing to believe you are who you say you are. So don't just stand there. This way." She motioned to the elevator with a sweep of her hand. "Fifth floor."

On the walk to the office, he counted three gasps, two

weird looks and one murderous glare, but other than that, he was ignored.

"I'm telling you, I'll be fine," Peterson said as she closed the door, sealing herself inside with him and Harper. Levi had no idea who she'd been talking to, since everyone had beat feet out of the hallway, but whatever. He just wanted to get this over with.

They each took their seats, and he carefully leaned the painting against his leg.

The office itself was normal, with white walls, brown carpet, a desk, a computer, a phone system and papers scattered everywhere. Even the portrait hanging over the desk was something you'd find in any other establishment: pink rosebuds surrounded by green foliage.

Peterson leaned back in her swivel chair, crossed her arms over her middle and said, "All right. Why don't you tell me why you're here. That wasn't a question or a suggestion, by the way. Lana was vague, and I don't have a lot of time."

"Why don't you tell me your qualifications first," Levi replied, his voice wielding a sharp edge.

One of her brows shot into her hairline. "Qualifications for what?"

"For dealing with a situation like ours," Harper said. Her nerves must have kicked back into gear, because the tip of her nail found its way into her mouth. "Besides the obvious, of course."

Peterson drummed her fingers together, but replied, "Well, I can see into the spirit realm and I'm usually given the cases dealing with people no one else wants to deal with. It's my sparkling personality. I can put anyone at ease. What else, what else. I've solved murders gone cold, helped lost souls figure out why they're still here, and aided families who've just lost a loved one."

"Are you trying to tell me Lana is...dead?"

"Do you think she is?" Peterson countered. Great, they'd been stuck with the paranormal equivalent of a shrink.

"She isn't. And you're not the one we need," Levi said. "Let's go." He reached for Harper, intending to stand. "We'll knock on every door in the building until we find someone who can actually help us."

"What do you need, then?" Peterson asked, seemingly unconcerned by his threat. "Exactly. Lana mentioned a few details, but I want to hear everything from your point of view."

He relaxed, willing to take a moment to test her out, and nodded to Harper. "Tell her."

She explained about her blackouts, the changes in Levi's apartment, about the painting she usually only worked on while she was sleeping and the fact that she'd just filled in Lana's face. As she spoke, Peterson finally softened, her features radiating something akin to sympathy.

"Let me see the painting," she ordered.

"Can you help us?" Levi asked.

"Maybe."

For now, that was enough. Levi lifted the canvas from its perch on the floor, keeping the back to Harper despite the fact that a sheet draped the front. A long while passed in silence as Peterson studied the thing from top to bottom. She would stare, then write a note, stare, then write another note. Finally she returned to her reclined position and sighed.

"I've spoken to Lana hundreds of times, but I never pictured her like *that*."

"What do you want to know about the painting?" Harper asked as he re-covered the source of her nightmares and lowered it to the floor. Shifting nervously, Harper licked her lips. "Did I paint the future?"

A decisive "No" cut through the tension. "Definitely not."

"You're sure?" she asked, relief already dripping from her.

"Didn't you catch that 'definitely'?"

Defensive, Harper said, "But how could I not have painted the future when what you saw hasn't happened...to my knowledge?" she added reluctantly.

"Well, how do you know I'm actually sitting here in the room with you?"

Her brow furrowed in confusion. "Uh, I just do."

"Bingo. I just know, too. It's my job, and I'm very good at my job."

That time, Harper accepted what she'd been told and fell against the back of her chair. "Thank you. Thank you so much."

Though he hated to ruin that relief, Levi couldn't let the facts slide. "What else could it be? Like she said, what's in the painting hasn't happened yet. Lana claims she hasn't lost days of her life, not like we have, and Harper never saw any injuries on her. Are you saying the painting is a figment of Harper's imagination?" He knew it wasn't.

"No, that's not what I'm saying, but thank you for putting words in my mouth," Peterson retorted. She massaged the back of her neck, murmured something that sounded like, "I have my temper under control, I have my freaking temper under control," and said loudly, "Look. Did the two of you recently move into an apartment building near Oklahoma City's Brick Town?"

"Yes," he replied with a frown. "Both of us. How did you know that? Lana?"

"I told you. Lana was in a hurry and left out quite a few

details. But I want to look around both of your apartments before I tell you what's percolating in my brain. And don't try to talk me into telling you now, 'cause it's not gonna happen. I need to do a little research before I turn your worlds upside down, so do yourselves a solid and go home. You'll see me sometime tomorrow—and you'll probably wish you hadn't."

9

Back at King's Landing, Harper fixed a late lunch while Levi made some calls. He'd already packed his bag, and now planned to spend the rest of the day and all of the night with her. She could have put him in Lana's room—a sharp ache lanced through her chest—but she wanted him with her, as close as possible. And he seemed to want to stay with her, so she wasn't going to allow fear about tomorrow and Peterson's dire prediction to interfere.

And why think about the negative, when she could think about Levi and the things he would try to do to her tonight? Oh, she knew beyond a doubt he would try something; he wouldn't be able to help himself, and a shiver of anticipation nearly rocked her off her feet.

How she'd gone from never wanting to be touched to wanting to be devoured by one specific man, she would never know.

The sounds of popping and hissing echoed, drawing her attention to the stove. Levi didn't yet know it, but they were having breakfast for dinner. Lana had been the last one to go to the store, and she'd purchased only her favorite foods. Regular bacon, turkey bacon, thickly cut bacon, thinly sliced bacon and eggs.

"Well," Levi said, sitting down at the counter. "Lana hasn't reported to work, used a credit card to get a room anywhere or withdrawn any large sums of money. My friend Bright is checking your old home."

"Why would she be there? We sublet it to move here."

A curious gleam filled his eyes. "Is that what she told you? Because I hate to be the one to bust your best friend, but no one else has moved in."

No way. Just no way. "I'm telling you, the house was sublet."

"Bright checked just this morning. It's her name on the lease. The only change that had been made recently was your name being taken off."

Harper's blood went cold as she fixed Levi a plate. "But…" If that were true, Lana had lied to her. Again. "She couldn't afford to pay the full rent there *and* half the rent here."

A pause. Then, "Why did you move here, princess?"

A distraction. She knew the question was meant as a distraction from the wave of betrayal sweeping through her, and yet she grabbed on to it with a kung fu grip. "We—" Wait. *Princess,* he'd said.

He knew her first name.

She swung around to face him, teeth bared in a scowl and the fork she'd planned to give him stretched out like a blade.

He was grinning from ear to ear, the jerk. Oh, yeah, he knew.

"Don't you dare call me—"

"Aurora? Or Sleeping Beauty?"

"I will *gut* you."

His laugh boomed through the room. "Why? I like it. It's cute."

"It's humiliating!" she said with a stomp of her foot.

"It's adorable."

"It's *precious*." She sneered disgustedly. "What, do you want me to call you my very own Prince Charming?"

His laugh cut off, and his smile vanished in an instant. "Do it, and I'll shoot you. No guy on earth will convict me of a crime, either. They'll all say I did my civic duty."

"Just so we understand each other." Pretending to consider a weighty issue, she tapped a finger against her chin. "But you certainly have come to my rescue, haven't you?" she couldn't help but add. "All you lack is the white horse."

He was the one to scowl this time, and she was the one to laugh.

"So what's with the portrait of the nail and the portrait of the limp noodles with spikes?" he asked, changing the subject. He'd obviously been nosing around her home as she'd nosed around his. "Every other picture is of you or Lana or the two of you together and quite...*amazing,* I believe is the word you used, and don't get me wrong, the nail is cool, too. The details are awesome. I can see the scratches and the rust. But the noodles? It sucks. Sorry."

"I'm surprised you noticed."

"What, did you expect me to notice something else?"

"No. I just wasn't sure if you would see my apartment the way I see yours. But anyway, the nail and the thornbush, not limp noodles with spikes. Lana and I decided to paint each other. Only, we were to paint the other's inner self rather than outward. I painted the nail, and she painted the thornbush.

We laugh every time we look at those." But she wasn't laughing now. *Oh, Lana. What's going on with you?*

She placed Levi's food in front of him, and settled beside him with her own.

"Thanks for the meal, princess. It smells good. But, uh, I don't think a thousand men could polish off all this bacon."

"One manly man could. After all, Lana always did. Now eat it," she quipped, ignoring his use of the hated endearment. Otherwise, she'd have to brain him with the frying pan, and she wasn't sure how much more abuse he could take from her without bolting.

"Sir, yes, sir," he teased with a salute. "But while I do, you need to tell me why you guys moved here. You never said."

She released the sigh that had been bottled up inside her. "Because I couldn't *not* move here. I saw the place, was drawn to it and felt as if I was finally home. How about you?"

"I'm not sure." He popped a piece of bacon in his mouth, chewed, swallowed. "I just woke up in my apartment one morning, all my things unpacked. I freaked, made some calls and found out I'd sold my place and moved."

"All during a blackout?"

"Yeah."

Understanding his pain, she patted his hand. "Has anything this weird ever happened to you before?" She tried to take a bite of her own food, but her stomach felt knotted and heavy. Guess she wasn't man enough.

"No. You?"

"Never."

He took another bite of bacon, followed by a healthy mouthful of eggs. Obviously he had no problem with his appetite. "Maybe the rest of the tenants are blacking out, too. Maybe it's something in the building. Like mold."

Ugh. Now she *really* couldn't eat, she thought, and pushed her plate away. "You're the cop. I'll let you check."

"Actually, I'm the detective."

"Like there's a difference."

He glared at her, but there was only amusement in his tone when he said, "I'll show you the difference later."

Later. The word echoed through her mind, followed by *in bed,* an addition that was all her own. She shifted nervously— and horror of horrors she chewed on her fingernail. It was the worst habit of all time, but now hardly seemed like the time to quit. What if, while he was showing her, she had another blackout? What if she—

"Hey, don't worry about it," he said, knowing exactly where her head had gone. "I'm prepared to deal with any type of freak-out this time."

"How?" *You can't think negatively, remember?*

He snorted. "Like I'll tell you and ruin the surprise."

His tone was teasing, engaging, and she wondered how she had ever considered him grumpy. He was a cream puff.

When he popped the last bite of food into his mouth, she pushed her plate in his direction. "I cooked, you clean."

"I'm not sure I like that rule," he said, but he stood, gathered the dishes. "What will you be doing?"

"Making a few calls of my own." First up, her old landlord. If Lana had wanted to keep the house, Harper would not have protested. She would have worked harder to sell her paintings to help pay the two rents. The thought of leaving this building unsettled her more with every hour that passed, yes, but she also wanted her best friend happy.

"Shout if you need me," Levi said.

"Will do." Harper headed to her bedroom. She turned the hall corner and—

Unleashed a blood-chilling scream!

Someone loomed just in front of her.

Acting on instinct, Harper kicked the intruder in the stomach. A girl—the dark-haired girl who liked to spy—hunched over, trying to make friends with oxygen. But Harper's instincts were still raging, and she punched the girl in the jaw, sending her smashing into the wall and sagging to the floor.

Footsteps pounded, and then Levi was there, right beside her with his gun drawn. He shouldered her behind him, using his big body as a shield.

"What are you doing here?" he demanded of the girl. Before she had time to answer, not that she could have formed the words, he stepped on her chest to hold her down, crouched and patted her down with his free hand. "You're lucky you're not packing." He holstered his gun and removed his foot, though he did his best to remain in front of Harper.

The girl's expression smoothed out, becoming as serene as if she'd just woken up from a peaceful nap. "He always keeps his promises," she said. "I hope you know that."

"Who?" Levi snapped.

"He wants her," she replied as if he hadn't spoken. "Wants his naughty girl. He'll have her, too. He always does."

Harper, whose heartbeat had yet to calm, pushed forward to glare down at her, ready to start giving another beat down to finally get some answers. "You better start talking in English or I'll—"

The girl vanished, on the floor one moment, gone the next. Harper gasped. Levi lost his balance and stumbled forward.

"What just happened?" she rasped out.

"Don't know," he growled. "That ever happened to you before?"

"Never." Surely the girl hadn't...couldn't be... Had to be

a trick of the light, she told herself. An illusion. Surely. *An illusion you and Levi shared?* "A...spirit, maybe?" But...how could that be?

"I've never been able to see spirits."

"Me, either."

He stood, his scowl only growing darker. "Pack a bag. We're not staying here tonight."

"Okay." Harper rushed to obey, trying not to think about what had just happened while only throwing the necessities into a duffel. A duffel that turned out to be twice the size of Levi's. He didn't complain, though, just took it from her after gathering his own and escorted her to his car. He locked her in and returned to the apartment, only to stalk out a few minutes later with her painting and supplies.

"Thank you."

"Welcome."

He lapsed into silence and drove to a nice hotel across town. But every mile farther away from King's Landing caused an ache to intensify inside her. The need to go back bloomed... and spread...and consumed. He must have felt it, too, because his knuckles were white on the wheel.

Clearly his willpower was superior, because he managed to procure a room and maneuver Harper inside of it, even though she attempted to pull from his hold several times. He threw their bags on the floor, marched into the bathroom and started the shower. Then he was in front of her, backing her up, shutting her inside with him.

Steam enveloped him, creating a dreamlike haze. "What are you doing?" she rasped. The need to return to the apartment took a sudden nosedive as nervousness blended with excitement.

"What do you think I'm doing?"

"Seducing me."

"Smart girl."

Her nail found its way to her mouth. "'Kay."

"We'll figure all of this out," he promised, forcing her hand to her side.

"'Kay," she repeated.

"And just so you know," he said, the corners of his mouth twitching, "a cop would fine you for your insults now and kiss you later. A detective will fine you now, kiss you now, then do a little detecting to find his way to all his favorite parts."

"'Kay" was said with a tremble this time. The nervousness was taking over, dominating.

He arched a brow. "That's all you've got to say?"

He wouldn't like the thoughts tumbling through her mind. Or maybe he would. He reminded her of Lana, all honesty, no tact. He'd be glad she'd put her fears out there—so that he could put them under his feet, where they belonged. "Well, I'm thinking that this is a big step, and trying *not* to think about the freak out I had last time. I'm thinking we just had the scare of a lifetime, and probably need a nap instead of sex."

"Big steps, big rewards. Freak-out, meet solution. Me. And for two committed people like us, there's nothing better than sex after the scare of a lifetime," he said, a layer of desperation entering his voice. "We're alive. Let's prove it. *I need to prove it.*"

In that moment she realized this wasn't *just* about desire. Her scream had scared him. He'd expected to find her hurt, or worse. Then, when the girl had vanished, he'd realized he couldn't protect Harper from that kind of unseen force. Now he needed to assure himself that she was here, that she was okay, and deepen the connection between them so that she wouldn't somehow slip away.

"Harper." He gave her a little shake. "Pay attention to me. Class is in session."

"'Kay," she said. She was right about his reasoning. She knew she was right—because, when she looked deeply enough, the same need swirled inside of her.

His hands fell away from her. "If you'd rather wait, we'll wait. I won't pressure you."

She placed her palm on his chest, just over his heart. The hard, fast rhythm proved just how desperately her answer mattered. "I don't want to wait." He was right, too. They needed to prove it. "I'm into you, this. I just hope—"

"Nope, no worries," he said, and the force of his relief was almost tangible. "I told you. I know how to handle you now."

"And that is? You can tell me. Honest. I won't tell anyone else."

"Nah. I'd rather show you." He cupped her cheeks and kissed her, a gentle kiss of comfort and exploration…that soon intensified, becoming something far better. Something passionate.

Soon she was clinging to him, kissing him back with everything she had, rubbing against him, moaning. He stripped her and then himself, and even then the kiss never stopped, their tongues dancing together, tasting, giving, taking, rolling.

"You're beautiful, Harper," he said softly. "The most beautiful woman I've ever seen."

Must have this man.

"Get it yet?" he asked. "I'm not allowing myself to push you for anything, but I'll work you until *you* have to have more."

"I'm past the point of needing an explanation. Do something!"

Chuckling, he picked her up and set her in the tub. Warm water rained against her bare skin, and she loved the dual sen-

sation of the gentle patter of liquid and the harder kneading of
his rough hands. He concentrated on her back at first, going
up and down, then moving lower, giving her time to get used
to each touch before conquering someplace new.

Any time a negative emotion would try to intrude and she
would stiffen, Levi would slow down and concentrate on rev-
ving her back up. It wasn't long before her body was so sensitized her mind ceased to matter.

"I'm ready," she said. Her hands tangled in Levi's wet hair,
her nails scouring his scalp.

He tugged from her hold, peered down at her, breathing harshly as he searched her face. And, oh, *he* was the most
beautiful man *she'd* ever seen. Rugged, powerful, determined.

"What are you doing?" she asked.

He waited, just waited, and realization finally dawned. He
expected her to direct him—and so, that's exactly what she
did. She led his mouth to the places she wanted him, and she
wanted him everywhere.

He moved far more slowly than before, but the more she
moaned, the more she arched into him, the more fervently
he worked her, as if the tether of his control was in danger
of snapping. Her desire ramped up and up and up, until her
blood was molten in her veins, until her limbs shook and she
was arching and writhing toward him—exploding from the
pressure as pleasure consumed her.

Straightening, shaking, he said with a half smile, "That
was fast."

"You complaining?"

"Rejoicing. I've never been closer to death by heart attack."

A laugh bubbled at the back of her throat. Humor with sex.
How unexpected. But she really, really liked it.

"Sure you're ready?" he asked.

More than ready. On fire. "You don't know, Detective Hottie?"

"Just making sure, princess."

"Did you bring protection?"

He nodded, left the shower and returned with a condom already sheathing the long, thick length of him. He didn't waste any time, but picked her up, growled, "Wrap your legs around me," and thrust deep the second she obeyed.

A strangled cry left her. He filled her perfectly and, oh, did her pleasure spark back to life. He pounded hard and fast, and reclaimed her mouth just as savagely.

"Good?" he demanded, and she knew he wasn't talking about the sensations rioting through her but the thoughts in her mind.

Even so, the answer was the same. "Amazing."

Faster...faster...harder...harder...until they were both moaning and groaning. He held her waist in such a strong grip, she knew she would have bruises tomorrow. Bruises she would savor, because they would remind her of this moment, of his total possession.

"Harper," he shouted, climaxing.

"Levi!" She was right there with him, crying out his name, enfolding him in her arms.

For a long while, he remained just as he was, his head resting on her shoulder, the rough pants of his breath trekking over her skin, his heartbeat drumming against her own. She could have fallen asleep just like that, because, despite everything that had happened, everything that would probably happen, she was suddenly more content than she'd ever been, but cool droplets of water began to splash on her, rousing her.

"Shower...turn off," she begged, then blushed when she realized she'd sounded like a caveman.

"Only if we can do this again in the bed," he replied, leaning back to turn the knob.

"Only if you're about a thousand degrees."

"Cold, baby?"

"Beyond."

"Well, what my princess desires, my princess receives. I'll heat you up."

Dirty little turd. "Well, the prince has just made the princess desire a nap. Alone."

"Is that so?" He set her on her feet, only to dig his shoulder into her stomach and hoist her up fireman-style.

"Levi! Put me down right now!"

"Why? I'm the prince's evil twin, who tricked the princess into going to bed with him, and now I've decided to hold you for ransom. And as I'm a stone-cold baddie, you're gonna need to do something to keep me from pillaging your people before that ransom is paid."

He carried her to the bed, and she laughed the entire way.

10

Levi snuggled Harper in his arms, sated in a way he'd never been before. She was such fun, her laughter a study and gift of music. With only a smile she lit him up on the inside, shining a spotlight into hidden places. She fit him, her passion a match for his own, her cries for more an aphrodisiac, her kneading hands a revelation.

As long as he'd kept them both on the edge of pleasure, their minds had been too wrapped up in what was happening at the moment to delve into the dark, dangerous territory of past and future. He'd been right. That was exactly what she'd needed to relax and let go.

Afterward, exhausted from hours of learning her body, he'd noticed the haunted look had disappeared from her eyes. Those baby blues had crinkled at the corners as she smiled and teased him about his insatiability, color had been high in her cheeks, and her lips had been red and swollen from where he'd bitten and sucked.

Now, though, in the silence of the night, enveloped by

shadows, Harper asleep and breathing deeply, evenly, he couldn't stay *out* of those dark, dangerous places. The two of them had been living in a building with a spirit of the dead. How could they not have known? How had he developed the ability to see into the spirit realm, when everyone he knew who possessed it had developed it before puberty or worked hard to spark it to life? How had Harper?

Harper. His pretty princess. He felt as if he would lose her at any moment, felt helpless as a baby. As if she would simply float away, never to be seen or heard from again. He'd willingly fight her demons for her, but a fist and even a gun could not stop an unseen force, could they?

Despite what he'd said in Peterson's office, Lana was probably dead. The painting probably wasn't the future, but the past. Harper had probably stumbled upon her friend's torture and slaying.

Probably. How he hated the word, but he hesitated to think in absolutes without more proof.

Lana's death had probably occurred while Harper was missing. And Lana's undead status would also explain the lack of bruises on her body, why Harper had never noticed any injuries and how Lana had taken off and hidden so expertly.

And, really, Harper's entire disappearance could be explained by the blackouts—meaning, she had never been abducted. She could have remained in a fugue state, unable to deal with what was happening, from the time she'd found Lana on that table to the time Lana reappeared in her life.

Lana's spirit would have repressed what had happened, too, continuing on as if everything was business as usual.

A few niggling questions remained, however. Why had Harper's blackouts continued? To allow her to slowly come to grips with what had happened? And then there was the timing of everything—Levi's own blackouts, his appearance here, the fact that *he* could see Lana. Harper seeing her was understandable. The two were bonded. But him? No. Unless…he was somehow bonded to Harper and saw what she saw.

Also, Lana had reported Harper missing, only to go missing herself? Talk about a major coincidence. And yet, that would explain why Lana had never returned to the station and reported Harper as found.

So many questions, new and old, and Peterson might have all the answers. That look of abject sympathy as Harper had spoken of her painting…that promise to do a little digging, spoken in a tone of dread and suspicion…

Peterson clearly suspected something terrible.

Harper mumbled something incoherent and began twisting out of his embrace. Dread worked through him as he loosened his hold. She sat up, stayed still for a moment, stood. Between one sexual marathon and the next, he'd had her place her painting and supplies in the proper places, mimicking the setup of her studio.

"Harper," he whispered, but there was no response.

Silent, she padded to the table with the brushes and paints. A soft light cascaded over the entire area, allowing him to watch her. With fluid motions she mixed colors, dipped the tips of the brushes and began to paint.

Levi sat up and scrubbed a hand down his face. He stood, nearly tripped as he shoved his legs into his underwear and closed the distance between them. Rather than study the canvas, he studied her face. Her eyes were closed, the length of her lashes casting shadows over her cheeks.

Her expression was scrunched, her skin pale as milk. Protective instincts rose to the surface, and he had to fight the urge to shake her awake, to make her stop. He hated that a horrible image of blood and pain held her captive, but more than anything else they needed to see the killer's face.

She worked for hours. Several times she would stop and a tear would trickle down her cheek. He could tell she was trying to jerk herself out of sleep because her breathing would change, becoming choppy, ragged.

He would say, "Keep going, sweetheart. I'm here. Levi's here," and she would rally and continue.

He wanted this thing done, wanted its horrors out there, so that they could know what to fight, where to go, what to do. Maybe they'd luck out and get to tell Peterson to suck it.

Finally Harper's arms fell to her sides and her paintbrush dropped to the floor with a thump. Still she stood there with her eyes closed. He dared a look at the canvas—and nearly roared with shock and rage and fear.

She had painted the killer, and it was Topper as he'd feared. She'd also added more blood. Blood on the walls, on the floor, on the slab. On the man—and on the woman.

On Harper.

She'd painted over Lana's face and added her own. Oh, the woman still had Lana's dark red hair, but that face as delicate as a cameo was Harper's all the way.

Without thought, he swooped her into his arms and stalked to the bed to gently lay her across the covers. He did not want her to see that thing. Wasn't sure what it meant—wasn't sure he wanted to know what it meant.

And he'd thought himself helpless before.

She's not a spirit, he assured himself. He could touch her, could feel the warmth and softness of her skin, smell the sweetness of her scent. *She's alive. Well.*

She stretched her arms over her head, arched her back. Her

eyelids fluttered open, closed, fluttered open again. She drew in a deep breath, only to go still. Her gaze homed in on him.

"I painted," she said, her tone dripping with anxiety.

Unable to form any words, he nodded.

"Let me see."

He held her down. Her wide gaze, still on his face, searched and searched. He opened his mouth to speak, but no words emerged.

She stiffened. "I finished it."

Another nod.

"It's bad."

Yet another nod.

"Really bad."

Finally he managed to find his voice. "If you want to see it, you can see it, but I want you to remember a few things. Okay? You're here. You're real. And I've got you. I'll never let you go."

Her lips parted as she fought for breath and jerked upright. Her gaze drove past him, straight to the canvas. Horror cascaded over her expression.

"That's…"

"Yeah."

Slowly she stood. One step, two, she approached it. Her arm stretched out and she traced a fingertip through the blood dripping down the woman's leg. Crimson stained her soft, white skin. "I can't… That can't… There's just no way…"

"You're here," he repeated, staying close. "You're real."

"I would remember if something like this happened to me!"

Maybe she had done more than stumble upon Lana. Maybe she had been forced to endure a little torture of her own, but she had escaped.

Topper was now locked away, he reminded himself. She couldn't be hurt again.

"We'll go see my friend Bright." Levi's words were croaked. "He'll test your DNA against what we found in the killer's house." Topper had gotten sloppy there at the end, when he'd left that female on the billboard, and that's how they'd snagged him.

He'd stopped abducting women at night, with no one around to see as he stunned them and stuffed them into the trunk of his car. His last victim had rarely left home, and never at night, but Topper, who lived in the same neighborhood, had seen her, wanted her and had gone in to get her.

Eyes wider than before, Harper swung around to face him. "You know who he is? You already found him?"

"Yes." *And I nearly split his spine in two with my fist.* "He's in prison and can't harm anyone else."

"I...I want to talk to him," she said, shocking him.

"No," he growled, then more calmly repeated, "No. He's not allowed to have visitors right now."

"Try again." Scowling, she slammed her hands on her hips. "That might have worked on someone else, but I happen to be a *Law & Order* fan, and I know my rights according to Hollywood and television."

Stupid TV, ruining everything. Levi could put in a request with Topper's attorney, and if Topper approved it, yeah, Harper could visit him. And as much as Topper liked the ladies, he'd say yes. "We aren't bringing you to Topper's attention."

She mouthed the name, shuddered, then shook her head, obviously forcing her determination to rise. "He's locked up. What can he do to me?"

Uh, only annihilate her mentally. No biggie, though, right?

Questioning evil had never brought anyone satisfaction. Evil lied. Evil taunted. A person would be better served keeping their eyes on the road ahead, running the race of life.

"He can make you cry, and if you think I'll sit back and watch that, those multiple climaxes I gave you killed your brain cells."

"I don't care. I want to talk to him," she reiterated.

"Have I ever told you I prefer soft, malleable women?" he said, as mean as a honey badger. This was too important to him. He couldn't cave.

"I. Don't. Care."

His eyes narrowed to tiny slits as he leaned into her. "You want to bring yourself to the attention of a killer who might have friends on the outside? A guy who would be willing to pay someone to hurt you just to send him the pictures? Yeah, that kind of thing has happened before."

Finally he spotted a crack in her stubborn facade. But still she said, "I don't want to, no, but I *have* to. Knowledge is power, and right now I'm pretty much without power. He's got it all."

"Lies are weakness, and lies are all you'll get from him."

"I have to try."

"If I refuse to help you?" he said on a ragged breath.

"If you refuse to help me," she replied, stepping into his personal space, peering up at him with anger and determination, "I will work around you. I'm tired of wondering. I want the truth, once and for all. I want Lana protected."

"Peterson said the painting wasn't of the future. Maybe Lana doesn't need protection."

"And Peterson knows everything? Her word is law?"

Good point. "All right," he said. "I'll put in a request to see him."

11

Harper was on edge as she and Levi trekked through the halls of King's Landing.

She expected Peeping Thomasina to pop through the walls and scream "boo," but the girl never showed. In fact, all of the residents were strangely quiet.

Maybe they sensed Harper's mood. Fury and fear burned deep in her gut, desperate for a release that would not be pretty. Or, heck, maybe they were frightened of Levi. His gun was drawn and at his side, at the ready.

Unlocking her door proved difficult, because she refused to place the painting on the floor. She wanted it in her hands or in her studio, and nowhere else would do. Right now it was her only link to what had happened, what would happen or what could happen.

Before she could enter, Levi shoved past her. "I'll check things—"

"You're not leaving me—" She drew up beside him.

"Out," he finished.

"Alone," she finished at the same time. And then they stopped abruptly at the sight that greeted them.

Peterson, as well as a man Harper had never met, lounged comfortably on the couch.

The After Moonrise employee had her now-blue hair pinned into two knots that looked very much like horns. She wore a dark blue corset, a spiked dog collar and black pantalets that ended just below her knees, where blue-and-white-striped socks stretched to black ballerina slippers.

The man next to her had sandy hair and brown eyes. He was tanned and slightly weathered, as if he'd spent most of his life outdoors. But what struck Harper most was the fact that he bore the same hard look as Levi, as if he'd seen the worst the world had to offer and nothing could ever affect him again.

"Breaking and entering. Very professional," Levi muttered, shutting and locking the door behind him.

"It served its purpose. I'm sure you've broken into many houses in the line of duty." Peterson's gaze fell to the painting. "Did you finish it?"

"First," Levi said, stepping in front of Harper, "who's the guy?"

"Are you always this suspicious? This is my associate, Mark Harrowitz."

Harrowitz nodded.

Gaze shrewd, Peterson added, "I never enter a strange home alone. I'm sure you understand. He's just here to ensure you two don't try to murder me."

Oh, that was all? Harper's heart drummed in her chest as she moved to Levi's side. "And you call *us* suspicious?"

A smile devoid of humor flashed. "Now that the gang's all here, can we continue?" Her brows arched, Peterson motioned to Levi's weapon with a tilt of her chin. "*Without* the threat of death?"

"Fine." Levi sheathed his gun *after* moving in front of Harper.

She liked the fact that he wanted to protect her, she did, but she didn't like that he placed himself in danger to do it. They'd be having a chat about that later. Of course, knowing him, he'd kiss her to distract her or vow only to do what he thought was right no matter what.

"Okay, so. The painting." Harper stepped around him and spun the canvas, allowing Peterson to view the horrific scene from top to bottom. "It's finished, yes."

Peterson studied the scene for a long while. Finally, she nodded. Harper took that as her signal to place the thing on its easel, out of the room, out of sight, then rejoined the group in the living room.

Levi had taken the seat across from Peterson and motioned her over. The moment she was within reach, he tugged her beside him, so that she practically reclined across his lap. A protest was not forthcoming. She liked where she was, and needed his strength.

"So what do you have for us?" he demanded. His tone lacked any kind of emotion, but there was no doubt he expected total compliance.

"You're not going to like it," Peterson warned.

Harper raised her chin. "Tell us, anyway."

Silence. A nod, a sigh. Peterson leaned over and dug into the black case resting at her feet. She withdrew several sheets of paper, several newspaper clippings, a DVD and a laptop. "Did you wonder why the receptionist and I had a meltdown at the sight of you?"

"No. Straight-up rudeness," Harper said at the same time Levi said, "Yeah," and squeezed her in a bid for less attitude.

"Well, I apologize for that," Peterson said. "We just don't get many people like you in our offices."

"What does *that* mean?" Harper huffed. She was too uneasy to be nice.

Harrowitz stiffened, as if he expected Harper to launch across the coffee table and attack. He was very astute. No one talked badly about Levi's rough, gruff exterior but her!

Peterson placed her hand on his wrist, soothing him. "Before we get to that, let me ask you a few more questions."

"No, we—" Harper tried to protest. She wanted answers of her own.

"Have you noticed anything weird about this apartment building?" Peterson asked, plowing ahead.

Levi popped his jaw. "Last night a girl appeared in Harper's hallway and then vanished before our eyes. Clearly, she was a spirit."

Fine. They'd do this Peterson's way. "On more than one occasion that same girl has told me that I was a naughty girl, and that he would be coming for me, but not who 'he' is or what 'he' wants, or why she thinks I'm so naughty."

Peterson and Harrowitz shared a look that wrecked what remained of Harper's nerves. Never had she been so stressed, so unsure, and these people were taking time to communicate silently with each other. How frustrating!

"One more question. Someone other than you lives here," Peterson said, head tilting to the side. "I found some of her things. Who is she?"

"Lana. The one who works for After Moonrise here in OKC."

Peterson nodded to Harrowitz, who began typing on

his PDA. Several minutes ticked by in silence, and Harper thought she would scream before he finished. At last, Harrowitz showed Peterson the screen.

After reading it, she said, "All right, then. We'll start with you, Levi." Peterson opened her laptop, inserted a disc, did some typing of her own and turned the screen.

Tense, Harper watched the screen. A local reporter appeared, a woman in her late fifties, distinguished with her hair in a slick bob, her makeup perfectly applied and her expression somber.

"It's a sad day for Oklahomans," the woman said. "One of our finest was killed in the line of duty today while trying to apprehend Cory Topper, the suspected Billboard Butcher. Allegedly, Topper stabbed the detective in the chest and thigh, and he was rushed to the nearest hospital where he was pronounced dead upon arrival." She kept talking, but Harper had trouble hearing her.

Levi's picture flashed over the screen, a younger version of the man she knew, serious, rough-and-tumble, wearing an army uniform. The date of his birth glowed underneath—as did the date of his death.

His death.

Eyes wide, she swung around to study him. His jaw was clenched, his skin pale.

"No," he said, shaking his head. "No. I would remember *dying*. I would have some indication that I'm no longer… human." The last word emerged broken.

"Not always," Peterson replied gently. "Sometimes the memory is buried because the reality is too painful to face. That leaves a big, black hole that needs to be filled. My guess is, things have happened to you lately and you have no way to explain them. You have gaps in your memory. And when you would find yourself on the right path, answers finally within reach, you'd lose more time. That was your mind shutting down as a way of protecting itself."

Another shake of his head. "I spoke to one of my coworkers just yesterday. In person, no less. He saw me, heard me, answered my questions."

"I'm sure he did. I'm also sure he can communicate with spirits, and that's why you successfully conversed with him."

He drew in a sharp breath, his nostrils flaring. "He can, but that doesn't mean anything. He would have told me."

"No. He wouldn't have wanted to be the one to break the bad news to you."

For a moment, stars winked through Harper's line of sight. "But I can touch Levi," she whispered. "And we crashed in a hotel last night, even talked to the clerk to get the room. Then Levi drove me here. In a car!"

"Either the clerk can see spirits and humored you, which isn't likely considering most of us work for After Moonrise or in law enforcement, or you convinced yourself of what you wanted to believe. And you didn't drive here, I promise you. Both of you expected to ride in a car, and so you both constructed a scene. If you talked it over, you'd probably discover you invented different makes and models."

No. Impossible. "You're wrong about this. I cooked, he ate."

"Another lie you told yourself."

"Then why did you tell him to put down his gun?" she demanded, her voice rising. Levi had yet to react to any of this. "If he's a spirit, he couldn't have shot you."

"If he'd pulled the trigger, he would have expected something to happen. When nothing did, he would have gotten angry, probably attacked me, and Harrowitz here would have had a problem with that. Now, I know you have more questions, but I'm afraid I'm not finished yet."

With a sad smile, Peterson typed something into the laptop and the screen changed once again. The same reporter was speaking, though her hair was styled differently and she wore a different top. Obviously this news feed was from a different day. She talked about the identities of some of Topper's victims, and how the most recent to be killed was—

Her.

Aurora Harper.

No. No, no, no.

The stars returned, thicker, more numerous, threatening to expand and consume her entire mind. *I'm not... I can't be...* "No!" she shouted, jumping to her feet. Dizziness swam through her mind, and she swayed.

Harrowitz jumped to his feet, too. His hands were fisted, his eyes slitted in warning.

Pale and a bit unsteady, Peterson unfolded more slowly. "You need to calm down, Harper. Your negative energy is painful to us, and Harrowitz here can make *you* hurt in turn. If he does, you may be forced into leaving this world for good, before you finish whatever you stayed here to finish."

She wasn't dead, she couldn't possibly be dead, but she would deal with that in a minute. "My friend. I painted her face before I painted mine. Is she... She can't be... Tell me she's alive!"

"She's alive," Peterson assured her, palms out in a gesture of innocence. "You painted yourself, your circumstance. I'm not sure why you first painted her face. All I know is your Lana can see the dead like Levi's coworker. That's why she was able to live here with you."

See the dead.

The phrase reverberated through her mind. *See the dead. Dead.*

She wasn't, Harper thought again. She couldn't be. Lana would have told her.

Lana, so sad sometimes, crying and sobbing, keeping so many secrets. Lana, so guilty sometimes, so desperate for Harper to figure out what had happened to her. Lana, who had stopped touching her, even in the simplest of ways.

But that was because of Harper's aversion to physical contact. Right?

Learning the truth is the only way you'll ever find peace, Lana had said. As if she had already known the truth herself.

Harper…could suddenly see the walls of a basement room, photos of pain and blood all around her, staring down at her. Tools hung from a board by the only door. Knives of every size, saws, hammers, spiked boards, razors and gags.

Gags laced with drugs meant to keep you awake, to keep you lucid while…while…

"No," she croaked, shaking her head violently. She fell back into Levi's lap. Still he gave no reaction. Was he in shock?

"You can touch Levi and he can touch you because you're *part of the same world,* existing on the same plane. You will not be able to touch humans, however. Here." Peterson extended a shaky hand. "Try me. I'll prove it."

Harrowitz sat down and grabbed her arm. He shook his head.

Peterson dropped her arm, sighed. "Oh, yeah. No touching the dead."

Dead, she'd so casually stated. Dead.

"You were the last to die, Harper," Peterson said. "Levi busted in on Topper just after he'd killed you. He saw your mutilated body and reacted. That's why he attacked Topper. That's why he missed the blade Topper still held."

Harper felt a strong, warm band around her waist. The contact was too much, not enough; she couldn't breathe, could barely sit still, wanted to stay, wanted to leave. Was falling... tumbling down an endless void. And yet, somehow that strong, warm band kept her steady.

Merciless, Peterson continued, "Everyone in this building is a spirit. Certain spirits are drawn here, and we don't know why. Maybe like calls to like. All I know is that the OKC branch of After Moonrise bought it, and monitors it to the best of their ability, and as long as you're here, keeping to yourselves, they're happy."

"No," she said, shaking her head.

Peterson pressed on. "I'm guessing that's why Lana sent you to me, rather than to her own firm. She didn't want them involved in your afterlife any more than they already were. Yes, they know you're here. I checked. But they like that you're here and unaware of what happened. You're not out there causing any trouble. If that changes, they could decide to force you to move on."

"No," Harper repeated.

And still Peterson kept talking. "It's not all bad. This is supposed to be a fresh start for you, a chance to finally live right, to fix mistakes or tragedies before letting go of the ghosts of the past, to have the brightest future possible."

"No!"

"If I were you, I'd make the most of it. Too many people in your situation lose sight of what matters and sink back into old patterns and habits or even fail to act upon the new opportunity they've been given. They spiral into depression. They become angry—and their anger can ruin innocent lives."

"No," she said yet again, even though Peterson spoke with such certainty, as if Harper really was part of that world, as if everything she mentioned was fact and there was no reason to debate.

A soft sigh filled the room. "If you want to know more about what happened to you, read the papers and clippings I brought. And honestly? I suggest that you do. You're each here for a purpose, and I don't care what the OKC branch thinks. You're better off knowing. Think about it. You might be able to move on."

Move on. And lose Levi.

Lose Lana.

Lose *herself.*

It was too much to take in. Harper ripped from Levi's hold—Levi was the strong band, she realized distantly—and flew out of the room. She couldn't remember pausing to open the door, only knew that she was inside her apartment one moment and in the hall the next.

"Harper," she heard Levi shout. His first word in so long, she wanted to stop, to throw herself at him, but she couldn't.

I'm sorry, she thought. He'd been told the same thing, yet she wasn't comforting him. He deserved comfort, but she couldn't deal with this. Couldn't accept the fact that she had been tortured and murdered, that her life was over, that she would never again hug Lana, that she had lost everything. So she ran, just ran, with no destination in mind—yet somehow she appeared at the art gallery…without ever leaving the apartment building.

Sickness churned in her stomach. Another blackout, surely, she told herself.

It was daylight, too bright, and people walked along the sidewalks. Everyone ignored her. Cars sped on the road, fumes in the air, and she wanted to run from here, too, but didn't allow herself. Through the window she saw the owner showing someone a painting in back.

She would talk to him, she decided. He, who couldn't see the dead, would talk back to her. They would have a conversation, and that would be that. Yes. Simple. Easy. She would prove Peterson wrong—or right.

No, not right.

Lifting her chin, Harper entered the shop.

12

Levi searched for several hours, but found no sign of Harper. She needed time to come to grips with what she'd learned, he got that—he was struggling with what *he'd* learned—but she was vulnerable right now, not paying attention to her surroundings. Someone could—

She's a spirit. Who can hurt her?

Yeah. There was that.

She was a spirit. Like him.

Him. Dead. Killed. Murdered by the same man who'd murdered Harper. How? *How?*

Peterson and her bodyguard were gone by the time he returned to Harper's apartment. Harper wasn't there, either. He fell heavily on her couch, put his elbows on his knees and his head in his hands. Dead. Killed. The words kept popping up, echoing through his brain. Dead. Killed.

He thought back. At first, he saw only a veil of black. He pushed through that veil with every bit of his strength, determination riding him hard. A wave of trepidation slammed through him, but he refused to back off. He had to know the truth.

Images began to flash through his mind, foggy at first but quickly solidifying.

A drive to Topper's house... *Gonna escort that psychopath to a cell where he'll rot until death comes knocking....*

Levi and Vince had squealed to a stop, other detectives and patrolmen exiting their own cars. Red and blue lights flashed all around. They'd followed DNA evidence, had a warrant for Topper's arrest. Adrenaline and excitement were high, practically saturating the air. They were about to close the most gruesome case they'd ever worked and save countless lives.

Vince was the one to kick in the front door, and Levi was the first one inside the house. They searched the place from top to bottom and finally found a hidden door to the basement.

Opening it brought a wealth of smells he instantly recognized. Blood, chemicals, death. They heard screams, a buzz saw, sobs, laughter.

In an instant, Levi's mind went blank, the veil falling back over his memories. Gritting his teeth, he once again pushed through it. The trepidation increased, but he continued to surge forward. He saw himself, gun drawn. He pounded down rickety stairs to discover Topper had been busy cutting up a body—a body he now recognized as Harper's. No wonder he'd felt guilt and shame when he'd seen her at King's Landing.

He'd been too late. Hadn't saved her.

Pale hair spread out over the table, though it appeared red, soaked as it was with her blood. Though she was dead, her blue eyes were open, haunted, pained, sad, furious and fixed on something far away. Her lips were parted, having already expelled her last breath.

Then and now, sickness churned inside his stomach. The things she had suffered...the agony she had endured...

Another female—the screamer, the sobber—occupied a small dog cage, the sides covered with a black tarp to prevent her from looking at anything but Harper. Topper was laughing, holding up the limbs he'd removed to show his newest victim what would happen to her if she displeased him.

That woman... That poor woman...

Men rushed in from behind Levi, pushing him forward. Thoughts scrambled through his head, but he couldn't decipher them just then. All he knew was that he took one accidental step toward the guy and couldn't stop himself from purposely taking another and another. He'd spurred into motion, sheathed his gun instead of emptying his clip, wanting up close and personal vengeance. He threw himself into Topper. The limb tumbled to the floor. Levi punched...punched...

Topper had excellent reflexes and immediately made use of the blade in his hand. A blade he'd used on Harper. As enraged as Levi was, he failed to safeguard himself. Felt a sharp sting in his side, followed swiftly by a sharp sting in his thigh. Just boom, boom, and his blood went cold, seeping out of him at an alarming rate. Topper had punctured a kidney and severed a major artery.

He remembered his coworkers rushing over to pull him and Topper apart. He remembered the fade of their voices. The concern. He remembered looking into his partner's eyes, holding his hand, the world going black.

But he did not recall waking up in the hospital. Did not recall recovering from his wounds. He just remembered... what? The conversation he'd had with his captain had never really happened. He'd never been put on a leave of absence.

He'd never left the station, too upset to go home, never driven downtown, spotted a suspicious-looking guy—

Wait. He *had* wandered downtown, *had* spotted a suspicious-looking guy. A spirit, he knew now. He'd entered King's Landing and blacked out, coming to in his new apartment. He hadn't made any calls about his old home. He'd simply convinced himself he'd sold it and moved on.

Now Levi laughed bitterly. No wonder Vince always refused to talk to him. Vince couldn't see him, couldn't hear him. No wonder Bright had been so surprised to find him back at the precinct. No wonder Bright had been so evasive about Harper's case. He'd known she was dead but hadn't wanted to share the news with Levi, who was also dead but unaware.

A clatter of voices penetrated his thoughts. The clack of keyboards, the pound of shoes.

Levi's head whipped up. No longer was he sitting on Harper's couch in Harper's living room. He was at the precinct. All around him were men and women going about their day, escorting suspects to processing, to interrogation or to a cell. Detectives sat at desks, reading files, researching a lead. The scent of coffee filled the air.

He straightened with a jolt. How had he whisked from one place to the other, in only a second of time? A spiritual ability? Probably.

Not taking time to reason out why he'd come, he stalked to Bright's office. The door was closed, but why should that stop him now? Hesitant, he stepped *through* the wood. A sensation of cold washed through him, but that was it. No resistance. One second he was in the hall, the next he was in the office.

Proof, such stunning proof, of his new status.

And there was Bright, typing away.

"I'm dead," Levi announced rawly.

Bright's head jerked up, his hand reaching for the gun stashed in the top desk drawer. The moment he realized it was Levi, he relaxed. A sad gleam entered his eyes. "Yes."

"You knew."

"Yes."

"Why didn't you tell me?"

One dark brow arched. "Have you ever had to tell a spirit something he didn't want to hear? The results aren't pretty. You would have flipped out, and very bad things would have happened."

Peterson had mentioned chaos. Levi was upset right now, and had been for a while, yet so far hadn't caused any trouble. Maybe it was just a matter of controlling his actions, of pushing through his feelings.

"Sit down." Bright waved to the only chair. "I'm guessing you're here for answers, yes? What do you want to know?"

He obeyed, saying, "What happened to Vince after…" He cleared his throat. "After I left?"

The sadness intensified. "He still blames himself for not protecting you. Thinks he should have shot Topper before you reached the guy. No one can pull him out of his depression, which is why Captain has him in mandatory counseling."

Poor Vince. "Is there anything I can do to help him?"

"I'll tell him I talked to you. Maybe that'll help."

"Yes," he croaked out. "Tell him I'm sorry, that he did nothing wrong, and I miss him. Tell him I met a woman. Someone special."

"Your Harper."

"Yeah."

"About time." Bright reached out to trace his fingertip over the picture of his wife resting on the side of his desk. "We held a funeral for you. A real hero's send-off. Everyone showed up. You would have been proud."

Yes, but had he deserved that kind of send-off? "Did you tell me the truth about Topper?"

A wary sigh. "Yes. He lives. He's in lockup right now and awaiting trial for what he did to all those women, what he did to you."

Good. "I'm paying him a visit." Yes, he'd promised Harper and he would take her to see Topper. But Levi wanted to be the first, to smooth the way. "Can he see into the other world?"

"His file says no, but sometimes people lie about that, not wanting to be labeled a weirdo."

Levi ran his tongue over his teeth. He'd learn the truth soon enough. "You mentioned bad things happen when spirits are mad. How?"

Bright leaned back in his chair, folded his arms over his middle. "So you want to hurt Topper, do you? Plan to haunt him a wee bit?"

He wasn't sure what he planned to do. To cover his bases, he said, "Don't ask, don't tell."

"That's military, about sexual orientation."

"Semantics."

Fingers lifted and fell, drumming against Bright's hands, creating a symphony of sound. "I'm sure you already know this, but I'll tell you, anyway. There are good spirits and bad spirits out there."

Well, yeah, he got that. Now. But there was knowing and then there was *knowing*. "And how can I tell the difference?"

"Their fruit."

Uh, what? "Come again."

"You'll always know by the fruit they produce. An orange tree won't grow lemons."

"Meaning?"

"Meaning, haters say and do hateful things. Lovers say and do lovely things."

Okay. That made sense. The girl with the X-ray vision was a hater, no question.

"I don't recommend you visit the prison," Bright said. "Other spirits will be there, and you don't want to bring yourself to their attention, believe me. They could follow you, and if they follow you, they could run into your girl. But I could have Topper brought here for another round of questioning...."

Levi sat up straighter. "You're a good man, Bright."

"I know. Now if we could convince my wife. She's asked for a divorce and—and that's not your problem, is it." Another sigh left him. "So how's your Harper holding up? Does she know about the spirit thing yet?"

"Yeah. We found out together. She took off, and I haven't seen her since." Where was she? What was she doing?

"She'll be back, don't worry. I've seen enough spirits to know that when they find out, they think they want to be alone, but really, they need someone there with them, supporting them, letting them know they're still loved."

Loved? He didn't... He couldn't... He barely knew her, he thought. Oh, he liked her more than he'd ever liked another. Craved her, even. Wanted her with him, wanted to protect her from every bad thing. Wanted to hold her, and assure her that he would help her through this every step of the way. And he wanted *her* to hold *him,* to know she would be with him every step of the way.

She fit him in so many ways, and in bed, he couldn't get

enough of her. Her taste was a drug, her body the missing puzzle piece to his own. But love?

He'd been in love a few times in his life. Once with Kelly Roose, the prettiest girl in his third-grade class. Once with Shannon Halbert, his high school sweetheart and the girl who'd taken his virginity. All three minutes of it. And once with Donna Chang, the woman he'd wanted to marry, the woman he'd dated for two years—the woman who cheated on him because he wasn't "meeting her emotional needs."

He didn't think every girl he met would cheat on him. He knew better. He didn't even think Harper would cheat on him. She had the same possessive streak he did, if not to a stronger degree. But to fall in love now, while things were so uncertain, while he could move on—or whatever spirits did—at any minute…not just no but *I'd rather die again* no.

"Another question," he said. "Where do spirits go when they move on?"

Bright worked his jaw. "Some go up, some go down."

See? What if he and Harper moved on at different times? "Why do they go? Because they accomplished whatever had kept them around in the first place?"

"Yes. The good ones fulfill their purpose and go up, and the bad ones destroy something, or try to destroy something, and get sucked down. Some know what they need to do right off. Others have to figure it out. Others purposely don't find out because they either can't handle the truth or don't want to leave."

"So they can stay?"

"For the length of a human lifetime, yes. Despite what books and movies claim, I've never met anyone who stayed longer than that." A layer of strain entered his voice. "My wife left me because I still see Sally Wells. Sally was my high school girlfriend who died of cancer soon after we graduated. She comes to see me at least once a week, and won't leave my side on our anniversary." The strain increased. "She throws a tantrum if I forget to buy her a present."

Levi wasn't sure how he felt about haunting his friends for the rest of their natural lives—like he was clearly doing to Bright, he realized. "I'm sorry. If I meet anyone halfway decent, maybe I can set your Sally up on a blind date."

A booming laugh filled the room. "Levi the matchmaker. Classic!"

"Any word on Harper's friend, Lana?"

"Yeah." Bright leaned forward to tap away at the keyboard. "Her credit cards were stolen and used this morning. Some homeless guy bought cigarettes first, then half an hour later bought some beer. He was taken into custody, but he swears he found the cards on the street and that he hasn't seen Lana. We showed him a photo and nada. Still, I've got someone watching her home. We'll catch her."

The phone on the desk rang. He held up his finger for a moment of silence, and lifted the receiver. He listened, frowned. "I'll be right there." Reaching for his gun, he stood. Checked the clip.

Levi stood, as well. "I'll let you get to work." He would not allow himself to return to the station. This was it. This was goodbye.

Or not.

"No," Bright said with a shake of his head. "You'll come with me. Your girl's art gallery was just torn to shreds."

13

Horrified, Harper peered at her surroundings. She hadn't meant to hurt the first—and now only—person to give her a break into the art world, and she hadn't meant to destroy the building, but she'd walked in, tried to talk to him, tried to touch him, and like Peterson had predicted, she had failed. Clifford Rigsby had gone about his day, showing patrons his current pieces, then closing up for lunch.

Frustration had risen inside her, but she'd kept herself under control by repeating, "This is a dream. I'll wake up. And if not, there's some other answer to what's going on." But then Cliff had entered his office. His secret office. It wasn't the one he used for public business dealings; obviously it was meant only for his private use.

He had a portrait of Harper hanging on the wall. In it, she was splayed on the same metal slab *she'd* painted, naked, cut and bleeding.

A bright light flashed in her mind but quickly faded—and as it faded, a gruesome scene took its place.

"Say cheese," her captor said. He was blond and handsome, with a smile any dentist would be proud of, and he was holding a camera, the lens directed at her.

Cold, hurting, trembling, hating the very fabric of his evil being, she scowled at him. "You will pay for this."

His chuckle reverberated through the room. "Such a naughty girl. But don't worry, you'll learn the proper way to address your new master soon enough, I promise you."

Another flash of bright light. This time it faded and she found herself back inside Cliff's private office. Her limbs trembled. For a moment, she had trouble catching her breath. Except, she was dead, wasn't she, and had no need to breathe.

Dead.

Dead.

She really was dead. She'd truly been tortured by a monster, killed by his blade. Peterson had tried to tell her, but Harper had fought the realization. Had fought the truth. Maybe because accepting her death meant accepting what had happened to her—what her mind had been trying to remind her of for weeks.

The room spun...spun...and other portraits came into view. Other women, each in a similar position to Harper, lying flat on a cold slab of metal, with similar wounds decorating their bodies. One fact became excruciatingly clear: Cliff and Topper knew each other.

Perhaps they were friends, if demons hiding in human skin were even capable of friendship. If so, Cliff had served her to Topper on a silver platter.

Another flash of light. Another scene crystallized.

Suddenly Harper was in the center of the gallery, dressed in an ice-blue cocktail dress with thin straps and a Tinkerbell skirt. On her feet were clear heels with jewels encrusted on ties that wound up her calves. Her hair flowed down her back, curling at the ends, though the sides were elaborately twisted at her crown. Usually she got ready in thirty minutes or less, brushing her hair, throwing on a little mascara and lip gloss and pulling a T-shirt and jeans from a drawer. Today she'd taken two hours, wanting to look her best to properly represent her (amazing) art.

After the last customer left, Cliff took her into his office where they celebrated her success with a glass of champagne. They'd talked and laughed as she'd sipped, but the moment she'd finished, he'd yawned and practically shoved her toward the front door.

"Go on home," he said. "You've outdone yourself and made me a ton of money. Now I want to count my cash."

She chuckled, not insulted in the least. This was too wonderful a day. People had loved her paintings. They'd stared at them, felt happy things, sad things, some even moved to tears. Not one painting had been left behind.

"Well, don't forget to count mine," she replied.

"No worries. Your check will be cut tomorrow."

Her chest swelled with satisfaction. "Thank you, Cliff. Thank you so much."

He waved her away. "Go on. Get."

The bell tinkled as she left the gallery. Smiling, she dug her keys out of her purse. Her car was parked a block away, in the closest available lot. The moon was high, luminous and so beautiful she could barely take her eyes off it as she walked. But then she tripped and nearly fell, which would have ruined her knees and her dress, so she forced her gaze to remain ahead.

And yet, she soon tripped a second time as a wave of dizziness crashed through her. Her smile fading, she stopped to lean against a building. What was wrong with her? In and out she breathed, thinking the sensation would pass. But, of course, it only grew worse.

Practically blinded because of the spinning, spinning, *spinning* world, she opened her purse to pat inside for her phone. The moment her fingers wrapped around the case, a sharp sting buzzed in the back of her neck, electricity flowing throughout her entire body.

Her muscles knotted, becoming unusable. Her back bowed, her bones vibrating, just as unusable. Even her jaw locked up, trapping her scream in her throat. *Dying,* she thought. *I'm dying.*

When the vibrations stopped, her knees collapsed. Trembling arms banded around her before she hit the ground, and suddenly she was floating. Relief cascaded through her. Someone had noticed her, was taking her to the hospital.

Something creaked.

No. Wrong, she realized. Someone was stuffing her inside a small, dark space. The air was stuffy, with old perfume caught in some of the pockets. She blinked, trying to orient herself. A blond man, his face blurred by the haze of her vision, stood above her. There was a streak of white; his teeth, maybe. Was he smiling?

"We are going to have so much fun, you and I."

More creaking, then a loud whoosh. A click. There was only dark, no hint of light. No fresh air.

Yet another flash of light, and Harper was back inside the gallery, Cliff eating a sandwich as he plugged away at his computer. Fury rose inside her. Fury like she'd never before known. The champagne…he must have drugged her.

Fury…growing…growing…

The walls around her began to shake. One of the paintings

fell to the ground with a loud crash. Frowning, Cliff set his sandwich down and glanced around.

He'd known what would happen to her, but he hadn't cared. Had probably enjoyed every minute of her torture through the photographs Topper had taken.

Growing...

The walls shook a little more. Two more paintings fell.

Cliff pushed to his feet.

As long as Topper kept his mouth shut, Cliff would probably never be caught. And why would Topper betray his buddy when that buddy could continue hurting women, taking pictures, painting pictures and sending them his way?

Growing...growing...

The entire building rocked on its foundation. Cliff gripped the edge of his desk, a fine sheen of sweat dotting his brow. Harper longed to grab the paintings and beat him with them. But she couldn't touch him, and she couldn't touch the paintings, because she was dead. Dead.

Dead!

One of the paintings flew from the wall and smacked him in the back of the head. A grunt parted his lips. He dove for the floor and crawled under his desk.

Harper's eyes widened as another painting flew at him, crashing into the desk and cracking in two. *What are you doing? Stop. You shouldn't destroy the evidence. You have to show Levi. He'll tell his detective friends and Cliff* will *get what's coming to him.* But it was too late. The shaking never stopped, and the artwork never stopped flying. Around and around each piece twirled before hurtling itself at Cliff. The door rattled, too, before ripping from its hinges and slamming into the far wall.

Harper stood in the center of the turmoil, completely unaffected. She could hear Cliff's sobs, but that only angered her further.

A flash.

Suddenly she was the one crying, begging for Topper to stop. But her cries only spurred him on. Mercy was not something he possessed.

"Harper!"

Something hard slapped against her cheek, causing her head to twist to the side. She blinked rapidly and found herself back inside Cliff's office, a scowling Levi in front of her. His hand was raised, as if he meant to slap her (again?) out of her hysteria.

"Levi!" Relief swept through her, and her knees buckled.

He caught her, holding her up. "You have to calm down, sweetheart. Okay? Yes? I don't want you to destroy the entire building. You could hurt innocents and go... Just calm down, okay?"

Yes, she could calm down...would calm down.... Anger would not get the better of her.

At last the building stilled.

"Good, that's good." He hugged her close. "Are you okay?"

Tears burned the backs of her eyes. "He...he...drugged me. Set me up. *Gave* me to Topper."

Levi pulled away to peer down into her eyes, but he didn't release her. A good thing, because she needed the strength of his arms. "He was working with Topper?"

A nod as she motioned to the paintings on the floor, the tears spilling out, trickling down.

Levi bent down, taking her with him, and lifted one half of a painting, dug around—the things on Cliff's desk had shattered and scattered across the floor, too—and found the other half.

The moment he put the halves together, his nostrils flared. "They were accomplices," he said, emotionless.

One of her tears landed on the top of his hand. His gaze lifted. Seeing her upset, he straightened. "You remembered," he said.

All she could manage was a nod.

"I'm sorry," he added. "So sorry for everything you had to endure."

Somehow, she found her voice. "And you...did you remember?"

"Yeah."

Part of her wanted to slink away in embarrassment. He'd seen her there at the end, at her weakest, her worst. Part of her loved that he'd thought to come to her rescue, that he'd reacted on instinct. And yet... "I wish you had survived."

His hold tightened. "I'm not one of those people who believes everything happens for a good reason. I actually think that's stupid. No. But I do believe the bad stuff can be worked to our favor."

"How can *this* be worked to our favor?"

"Sweetheart, you just unearthed a very bad man. I'd say we're on the right track."

He was...right, she realized. She twisted, eyeing the man in question. Cliff had crawled out from under the desk, his eyes red and watery. He rushed around the office, trying to gather the paintings. To save them or hide them, she wasn't sure.

"Without you," Levi said, "he would have squeaked by without anyone knowing the part he played."

"How do we let the police know?"

"Detective Bright, the one I have looking for Lana, is almost here."

Pounding footsteps sounded.

"Scratch that. He's here."

Two firemen rushed inside the room.

"Or not," Levi said with a sigh.

The two firemen spotted Cliff, paying no attention to Harper or Levi—and even misting through them to get to Cliff. She felt the heat of their bodies and gasped.

"Are you all right, sir?" one of them asked.

"Yes, yes," Cliff said with a tremor.

"Anyone else in the building with you?"

"No, I'm alone. What about the rest of the gallery? Show me." He spread his arms, blocking the firemen from stepping deeper into the office. "What happened? An earthquake?"

"No!" Harper screamed, reaching out to stop him.

Levi stopped *her*. "It's okay. Let them go."

The firemen once again walked through them, and she once again experienced that strange wave of heat. The pair explained that Cliff's building was the only one that had been affected by…whatever had happened, and they'd be looking into it.

"But…but…" she sputtered.

"My guy will be here," Levi reminded her. "Let's wait at the front door and show him what you found. The man who betrayed you will be arrested before the day is over, you have my word."

14

Levi had lied. Clifford Rigsby wasn't arrested by the end of the day. He was arrested by the end of the hour.

Later that day, Harper sat in on her first interrogation, though no one but Levi and the detective asking the questions knew she was there. Her nerves were frayed as she listened to Cliff claim the portraits had been mailed to him anonymously. As if! Topper wasn't a painter—Levi told her there had been no art supplies in his home—but Cliff was, which was why he'd first opened the gallery.

If he got away with escorting women to their slaughter...

The walls of the interrogation room began to shake, and Levi squeezed her hand. She forced her mind to blank. He'd tried to talk her out of coming, but she had insisted and so he had insisted on coming with her in an effort to keep her calm.

"If they were gifts, why didn't you turn them in?" Bright asked, casting Harper a dark frown. He was a handsome black man, and he'd stood at the gallery's entrance, pretending to look the building over as Levi told him what she'd learned before going in to check things out.

He'd left with Cliff, who'd been cuffed and crying.

She and Levi hadn't needed to enter the police car with the men. They'd thought about the station and simply appeared there. The swiftness of the location switch had startled her, but the need to see Cliff behind bars had overwhelmed everything else.

Now she released Levi to pace as Cliff answered. "I didn't know they were real," he said. "I didn't!"

Bright arched a brow, looking curious rather than suspicious. "You don't watch the news?"

"No."

"But you do know the paintings are real now, when we haven't told you anything of the sort? When we've only asked you how they came to be in your possession?"

She stopped, standing behind Cliff, unsure what she wanted to do. Levi came up behind her and wrapped his arms around her waist.

"I know this is hard," he whispered, "but you have to maintain control of yourself. Otherwise, you'll have to leave. Bright has to do his job."

"All right." With tears of frustration burning her eyes, she rested her head against him. The mint of his scent enveloped her. His heat comforted her.

Cliff stuttered for a bit, but managed to collect himself with a few deep breaths. "I heard about Cory Topper on the news. Heard what he'd done to those women. I *guessed* they were real."

"You said you didn't watch the news."

"I misunderstood the question."

"So why didn't you come forward the moment you realized what you had?" the detective asked, as calm as ever.

More stuttering. "Well, I, uh, well."

"Bright's got him now," Levi whispered.

Bright glanced up at them and gave an almost imperceptible shake of his head—a gesture for silence.

Levi lowered his voice and said, "Come on. We're distracting him. He's got this. You know that. Let's go home."

So badly she wanted to witness Cliff's end, but if she stayed, she would eventually speak up. She wouldn't be able to help herself. She would distract Bright far more than she'd already done and possibly cause him to screw up the interrogation. And if Cliff got away because of *her*...

"Okay," she said on a wispy catch of breath.

"I want a lawyer," Cliff growled. "I know my rights. I'm not saying another thing until—"

He did say another thing, but she didn't hear it. One moment she was in the mirrored room with him, the next she was standing in her living room—just because she wanted to be there. It was as easy as that. There was no dizziness, no recovery period.

"That's a nice little perk," she said, pretending she wasn't freaked out.

Levi, who was still behind her, placed his hands on her shoulders and spun her around. There was a grave cast to his face, a seriousness, a somberness she'd never seen before. Made sense, though. He'd just learned that he was dead, but she hadn't been there for him. Had focused only on herself. Guilt filled her.

"I know you're upset," he said.

She cupped his cheeks, scraped her thumb against his stubble. "I'm not the only one."

"What happened to us was terrible."

"Yes."

"But we're here, and we're together."

Together. Yes. "Kiss me, Levi."

He swooped in, pressed his lips to hers and thrust his tongue into her mouth.

They kissed for minutes, hours, days even, tasting each other, relearning each other, comforting each other. They were here, and while the rest of the world might consider them dead, they were alive to each other. That was enough.

As passion flowed through her veins, consumed her, it was difficult for her to believe that her life had ended, that she was no more. She was on fire, aching for Levi's total possession. How much more real could a woman get?

He tugged at her shirt. She tugged at his. He removed her pants, and she removed his. Underwear was the next thing to go. And when they were both naked, he picked her up and carried her to the bedroom.

Looking down at her, he grinned. "If this is the end to a crappy day, I'm all for crappy days." With that, he tossed her on the bed.

She bounced once, twice, and on the second descent, he was there, pressing her down into the mattress, pinning her with his muscled weight. The heat of him had intensified, delighting her in every way. His skin was a study of masculinity, rough in some places, smooth in others, with patches of dark hair on his chest and legs.

"You feel so good," he praised. "I don't think I ever want to let you go."

"Then don't." Just then he was her anchor. And she so desperately needed that anchor. She was afraid of floating away and never returning, of losing him, and losing herself.

"Grab the headboard."

"Why?"

"Because King Levi said so."

Unable to stop her own grin, she obeyed. The moment her fingers curled around the iron railing, he bent his head and laved her body from top to bottom. He bit, he sucked, he licked, ratcheting up her already inflamed desire. His tongue was like a stroke of fiery silk, tantalizing her, making her gasp and pant and beg for more…then plead with him to stop and finish her.

"Levi! If you want me to start beating you, keep doing what you're doing."

A warm chuckle, his breath tickling over her in the most decadent caress.

"I'm serious." She released the iron and waved a fist at him.

He playfully nipped at her fingers. "Back on the railing, princess."

So commanding. So wonderfully carnal with her. "Fine." She tried for reluctant, but merely came across as snippy. "But you had better do everything in your power to make this princess happy or you'll lose your head."

He gave another of those sexy chuckles. "You can't behead a king. Now do as you've been told before things get ugly and I have to summon my guard. He may look exactly like me, but he isn't as nice as I am."

Moaning, she obeyed him. The moment she did so, he returned to his play. Only, his hands were rougher, his mouth more insistent. He worked her over, worked her just right, so that she was arching into him, following his every move, desperate, so desperate for completion.

"Levi!" she shouted. "Enough! You have to… If you don't…"

"I'm a king, remember?" The strain in his voice delighted her. He'd break soon. He wouldn't be able to help himself. "I do what I want, when I want."

"Well, I do damage to—"

"He's coming for you," a familiar voice said from beside the bed. "Oh, uh, never mind."

"What the—" Harper hurried to cover herself. Levi jumped up, clearly intending to murder the black-haired girl who'd been haunting them all over again, but she vanished just before he reached her.

He stood there for a moment, silent and naked, and clearly floundering about what to do. "I want to chase her, but I don't want to leave you."

An unexpected laugh bubbled from Harper's throat. Levi spun around and glared at her.

"You think this is funny?" he demanded.

Unable to speak through her giggles, she nodded. And, oh, the amusement felt as good as his touch. As dark as the day had been, she hadn't expected to find excitement, arousal, fulfillment, acceptance, comfort or humor—much less all of those things at the same time.

With a mock scowl, he stalked back to the bed. "Well, I'll make you sorry for that. If I can't tackle her, I'll have to make do with you."

She laughed all the harder. He pounced.

The air whooshed from her lungs. Without any more preliminaries, he claimed his woman. Her laughter was cut off, becoming a low groan of pleasure. She wrapped her legs around him, wrapped one arm around his waist and one around his neck, all while arching her hips to meet his next thrust.

His lips returned to hers, and, oh, this kiss was so much better than any that had come before. The passion was rawer, the need sharper. His hands were everywhere, all over her, no place left untouched.

"Harper," he growled. "Yeah, just like that."

They strained together and breathed together and panted together, and his pace increased, faster and faster and faster, until the entire bed was shaking, until she was groaning as the pleasure split her in two and he was roaring with satisfaction.

He collapsed on her and rolled to the side, dragging her with him. She found herself sprawled across his chest as he fought to breathe.

"That was…that was…"

"Worth dying for?" she said, then wished she could snatch the words back. "Sorry. Too soon for that kind of—"

"Yeah," he said, sounding confident. "Worth dying for."

Darling man. As replete as she was, sleep tugged at her. She resisted with all her might, suddenly afraid that sleeping would be the thing that pulled her out of this world—out of Levi's arms.

It didn't before, she reminded herself and relaxed. "So what's next?" she asked through a yawn.

"Tomorrow we'll return to the station and find out what else Bright learned from Cliff."

"And then visit Topper," she said, a statement, not a question.

Levi sighed. "I knew you'd want to do that."

"Yeah, because I told you so. I need to know why I painted Lana's hair… I…" A bright flash in her mind, a memory tearing free of the darkness. Suddenly she was lying on that metal slab, cold, so very cold. She could hear a woman crying a few feet away, could hear metal rattling.

The cage. The woman trapped in the cage. A woman who

was next in line for the table...which meant Harper had to die. Room had to be made; a new toy had to be played with.

"Well...I know you can't see her, but the girl in the cage is—drumroll, please—your only real friend. You remember her, don't you? Of course you do. She's the pretty one."

Harper had tried to look, but she had failed. *"You're lying, trying to hurt me because you're a miserable little runt whose heart has rotted and you can't find any other way to get to me."*

"You think so? Well, why don't you ask the girl and find out whether or not I spoke true."

"Say something," she had commanded the girl.

Such terrible silence had filled the room.

Ultimately a chuckle had broken through that silence, and it had far more terrible. *"My deepest apologies, but she'll not be saying anything. She's mouthy, your friend. You know she is. I'm afraid I was forced to cut out her tongue."*

Hearing that, Harper's fury had gotten the better of her. She'd thrown taunts at Topper, and he'd retaliated with taunts of his own—followed by a brutal stabbing that had finally stolen her life.

The pain...oh, the pain... She'd endured so much, those last few minutes should have been more of the same. But she had felt the sting all the way to her spine, had felt her blood leaving her, pooling around her. Had noticed her eyesight dimming. Any second now and she would—

"Aurora Harper!" Levi shouted. "You pay attention to me right now."

Using his voice as a lifeline, she tugged herself back to the present. She blinked into focus, saw him looming over her, knew she was on the bed and swallowed bile. "He threatened Lana," she croaked. "He said she was next."

Levi brushed his fingers over her brow. "She wasn't in the cage, sweetheart. I promise you."

"But what if Cliff wasn't the only person helping him? What if Lana is still a target? She's in danger, Levi. I feel it. Deep down, I know it."

15

Against Levi's better judgment, he decided to phone Bright later that evening and set up a meeting with Topper before he'd had a chance to check things out. What he quickly learned? All the times he'd thought he called the man he'd actually popped in and out of Bright's office (and home). His mind had simply reworked the details.

This time, Bright had been home, alone, in bed. The man had nearly had a heart attack when Levi shook him awake.

With a few conditions tacked on, Bright had done him a solid and arranged for Topper to be brought into the station early the next morning for questioning about Clifford. At least, that was the official statement. Levi and Harper were testing Topper to discover whether or not he could see the dead. If he could...the real interrogation would begin.

Levi and Harper didn't get much sleep. They arrived at the station hours early, and waited in the interview room. Within thirty minutes of their arrival, Peterson and Harrowitz entered the room behind the two-way window. He couldn't see them, but he could *feel* Harrowitz, some kind of energy pulsing off him. If either Levi or Harper became upset, they were to leave the room. If they failed to leave, Harrowitz was to vaporize them before they could harm anyone in the building.

Levi was not happy about the threat to Harper, and was determined to keep her calm no matter the course of action he had to take. Already she was shaking, pacing and mumbling about everything that could go wrong. He reached out, latched on to the base of her neck and tugged her into his side.

"Don't talk like that. Why invite trouble? Why worry when everything could go right?"

"I don't like the word *could*."

"Because you're looking at it through negative glasses. Try positive."

A pause, a sigh. "You're right. I'm sorry," she said, and up went her finger to her mouth. "I know better."

He breathed in the cinnamon of her scent. All night he'd held her in his arms. They'd talked, shared things about their pasts. He'd told her about waking up one day to discover his parents were gone forever and he had no place to live, the nightmare of some of his foster families and how the military had given him a purpose, a goal for the future.

She'd told him about the formal gowns her mother made her wear to dinner to practice for her pageants, even when her friends were over, as if every evening at their house was a high-society party. She'd told him about the many classes in deportment she'd had to take, the singing lessons and the bird training—because yes, her mother had wanted her to sing Disney songs while a bird perched on her finger—and about how Lana had taught her how to laugh and stand up for herself.

He'd promised to send Lana a thank-you card. He'd also promised to protect the girl with his (after)life. And he would.

Somehow, someway, he was going to end Cory Topper's reign of terror once and for all.

"So...everyone's pretty locked on the no-killing-him idea?" she asked.

How wistful she sounded. He almost laughed. When a delicate-looking female talked about the destruction of evil, it was odd—and maybe kind of wonderful. "Yeah. Pretty locked. Otherwise, I'd be all over him the moment he stepped through the door."

"Darn."

See? She couldn't even cuss properly. "If I have to behave, you have to behave."

"Deal. I guess."

The door opened and a chained Topper finally shuffled inside, his orange jumpsuit so bright it was almost blinding. Tensing, Levi looked him over. The chains stretched from between his wrists, which were in front of him, to his ankles, which were only allowed a few inches of movement at a time.

Harper straightened with a jolt. Levi had been with victims facing their attacker for the first time before. He knew it could be traumatic and cathartic all at once. But he himself was a victim just then. In more ways than one. Yes, Topper had killed him, but that hardly seemed to matter in light of what Harper had suffered.

What were you supposed to do when you faced your *girlfriend's* killer?

End him...

"You know the drill, Topper. Sit down facing the window. I'll be back in a bit."

Bright met Levi's gaze, gave a stiff nod and closed the door, leaving Topper inside.

End him now. He's trapped...

The chains rattled as Topper obeyed, easing into one of only two chairs in the room. A small table stretched out in front of him. His bound wrists remained in his lap as he peered around the room. His gaze swept over Harper, then Levi, without pause.

Levi forced his arms to drop to his sides, severing contact with Harper. It was taking every ounce of his control to behave, as he'd promised Harper. *Not here. Not now.*

Not ever, he thought next, surprising himself. Not just because he would have destroyed something, and could possibly move on to a not so wonderful place, but also because he was...had been...a cop. He wouldn't take the law into his own hands. He just wouldn't. He'd done that before, reacting on emotions, and he'd gotten himself killed. Plus, doing so now would make him no better than the people he'd locked away.

Yes, Topper deserved to suffer. Yes, Topper was evil incarnate. And yes, giving in to the urge to end him would be easy. *Resisting* would be difficult. But he would do it, Levi decided. Topper had earned a punishment, and he would just have to live with it.

His fellow inmates wouldn't treat him well. He was blond and as handsome as a movie star, tanned, with a straight, white smile. He was the kind of man women dreamed of dating. But his eyes...his eyes gave him away. They were bottomless pits of wicked.

Bright had certainly nailed it with his fruit comment. Topper produced pretty disgusting fruit.

"He can't see you, sweetheart, and that means he can't hear you. You'll get no answers here. We should go." *Before I forget my good intentions and get us into trouble.* "Bright will find out if he's working with anyone else."

"The abuse wasn't sexual, you know," she said, her voice

trembling. As though in a trance, she wrapped her arms around her middle. "As much as he loved dominating, humiliating and hurting, that would have fit his personality."

A small blessing, considering everything else she'd endured, but one that relieved him. Last night, he'd tried to replace her memory of being bound and helpless with one of being bound and pleasured. A subtle transition, yes, but he hadn't wanted her scared of anything ever again.

"So why did he take us?" she asked. "Why did he do what he did?"

"Maybe he's impotent, and was lashing out. Maybe he's just a twisted, warped little man who enjoys other people's pain. There could be a thousand different reasons, but none of them matter. He did it."

"Well, I think…I think he has mommy issues."

The cop in him switched on. "I know you think there's someone else involved. Did he ever bring another person into his, uh, workshop?" He'd almost said little shop of horrors, but had caught himself just in time.

"No. He took pictures, though. Lots and lots of pictures." Steps slow and measured, Harper moved in front of her tormentor.

Topper continued his study of the room.

"Look at me," she commanded.

His head fell back, and he closed his eyes. In and out he breathed, deep and even, as if savoring something sweet. The corners of his lips lifted into a smug smile, then he straightened, lashing fluttering apart, gaze suddenly alert.

"Well, well," he said in a smooth voice. "Who do we have here, hmm?"

Harper straightened. Levi rushed to her side.

After another deep breath, Topper laughed with apparent

glee. "I think my favorite little blonde, Aurora Harper, has finally found me. I can't see you but I can smell the hint of turpentine you carry on your skin."

A tremor moved through her, her hands clenching and un-clenching.

A hard knock sounded on the window.

Levi wrapped an arm around her waist. "Calm down, okay?" He wasn't sure whether the words were for her—or himself.

"You stayed here, after all," Topper said, then gave another laugh. "I should have known you'd keep your word. Where are you, darling? Give me a hint."

Her muscles knotted, as if she was preparing to launch over the table and choke the life out of him. Levi tightened his hold. A second later, he felt fingers of electricity stroke through the entire room. Topper didn't seem to notice, but Harper released another gasp.

The hairs on the back of his neck stood on end, as did the hairs on his arms and legs. His skin suddenly felt sensitized, his nerve endings raw.

"Harrowitz," he muttered. "And my guess is, that was just a warning."

Harper licked her lips, squared her shoulders. "I'm fine," she said, and he caught the threads of her determination.

"I liked you best, you know," Topper whispered, as though sharing a scandalous secret. "I saw you and I just had to have you. Had to add you to my collection. And I'm so glad I did. Your screams…" He closed his eyes again, smiling softly. "Beautiful. A true symphony. And your skin, so smooth and perfect…at first."

Okay. That was it. *Levi's* resolve cracked. This was evil in its purest form, the worst of the worst, the devil made manifest. "Come on, princess," he said, tugging her away. "We're not going to stoop to his level."

"Your scent is fading," Topper said with a pout. "Are you leaving me? But, darling, there's so much more I have to tell you."

Levi gritted his teeth when Harper pulled from his grip.

"Let him talk," she said. "He might reveal something useful."

"Or he might lie and confuse things that much more."

Topper frowned, sniffed. "And what's the scent mingled with yours, hmm? Mint, I think." Another sniff. "Oh, yes. Mint. I remember a certain detective carrying that scent on his skin just prior to his untimely demise. Detective Reid, is that you? Have you decided to join us?"

Levi curled his hands into fists. *Control yourself.*

Harper swiped out her arm, attempting to punch Topper in the nose, driving cartilage into his brain. Her fist simply misted through him, causing no damage.

He shivered, and his grin widened. "Whatever you did, I liked it. Do it again."

Levi's fists tightened so forcefully his knuckles could have ripped through his skin. *Control.*

Another knock on the window, another graze of those electric fingers. A second warning. Probably the last.

Topper said, "You've pleased me so much, I'll tell you a little truth, Harper darling. I'm glad you succeeded. I *want* you to kill me. There's a chance I'll end up just like you. If that happens, if I stick around, we can be together again...for eternity."

Harper backed away. Levi continued to struggle with his rage.

"But even if you decide not to deliver my killing blow, I'll be happy," Topper continued blithely. "I have someone on the outside. Someone other than Clifford. And yes, I know you caught him. The guards bragged about it on the drive over, and to be honest, I confess I'm glad he's going away. He's the reason I'm here. He loves his art, his statements, you know, which is why he left that woman out in the open, for the world to see. I tried to warn him, but he wouldn't listen." He leaned forward, whispering, "He's changed his name, but he was a foster child in my mother's house. That's how we met."

A pause. Both Harper and Levi stiffened. He wasn't done, had more to tell.

"Speaking of childhood friends, don't think I've forgotten about yours. The sweet and spicy Milana."

Harper's hand fluttered to her throat.

"Oh, yes. I know her name and I also know where she is. My...person on the outside has kept tabs on her. If you kill me, maybe I'll become a spirit, maybe I won't. But what's certain? My friend will ensure the same fate befalls your Lana. Death."

16

Doomed if I do, doomed if I don't, Harper thought. Alive, Topper was a threat to Lana. Dead, Topper was a threat to Lana.

Lana. Who had yet to be found.

Lana. Whom Harper had to protect at any cost.

At last Harper knew why she hadn't moved on. Not for vengeance but for her friend's security. Yet, how was she going to ensure it?

A shudder moved through Harper. Just then she stood on the roof of the police station, peering down at the parking lot, where Topper was being shoved into a van. The sun was bright, the sky a maze of dark blue and white. Wind blew around her, trees dancing, bushes shaking, but she felt nothing. A sign of her existence in another realm, perhaps.

There was only the barest amount of railing to prevent a person from tumbling to the ground. Not that she cared. She wasn't sure what would happen if she fell, but it wasn't like she'd die, so...

Levi suddenly materialized beside her.

"About time," she said. After Topper's threat to Lana, Bright had stomped into the interrogation room to try to pry the name of the "person on the outside" from him. Peterson and Harrowitz had been waiting out in the hall, and had commanded her and Levi to come out.

Harper and Levi had looked at each other in shock as their feet had begun to move one in front of the other, of their own accord, toward the waiting duo. But the moment the door had shut behind her, the tug had loosened and Harper had grabbed Levi's hand, flipped her gaze to the ceiling, indicating the roof, and disappeared. No way had she wanted to stick around and see what else the pair would force her to do.

What she did know—they were scary. Scarier than even Peeping Thomasina, that was for sure.

"We've gotta work on your fight-or-flight reaction," he said wryly. "I stuck around to hear what they had to say."

She forced herself to turn away from the van, now motoring toward the gated exit, and face Levi. Breath caught in her throat. In the sunlight, his skin was...alive. She could see lightning strikes just beneath the surface, the crackle of electricity, a storm of vitality.

"What?" he asked with a frown.

"Nothing," she muttered. Everything. He was so beautiful. That rough face had come to mean so much to her. Protection, safety, humor, passion...the very hope keeping her on her feet and trudging ahead. "Bright will fail. Topper won't reveal the name of the person helping him."

"No, probably not." Levi cupped her cheeks. "This is going to be okay, though."

"I don't see how," she replied. "But I did figure out why I'm here."

"I know, sweetheart. You're here to save your friend. That's why I'm here, too."

Her brow scrunched with confusion. "I don't understand. You knew Lana?"

"No. But I saw what he'd done to you. I was so disgusted with myself for not getting there sooner. Ten minutes, and we could have saved you. I could have saved you from such a terrible fate. Saved myself from guilt and shame."

"I'm not sure I would have wanted to be saved," she muttered. "Not after everything he put me through."

"You would have. You would have found a reservoir of strength, the same way you found one that let you pick yourself up and continue on." He kissed her, gentle at first, then harder, the act spinning into a decadent tasting.

When he lifted his head, she sighed. "What are we going to do?" she asked.

"Did you tell her?" Peterson asked from behind them.

Harper glanced to the side and saw Peterson and Harrowitz in the doorway leading from inside. The wind whipped Peterson's newly green hair from its ponytail, strands slapping at her cheeks. Harrowitz was his usual scowling self.

"Not yet," Levi said. He met Harper's curious gaze. "They want Topper to escape. Or rather, for Topper to think he's escaped. He will be tracked, monitored, and everyone he speaks to brought in for questioning."

"That's dangerous."

"Extremely."

"We won't be taking any extra chances," Peterson said. "He'll escape with the most recent inmate cuffed to his side. That'll be Harrowitz, by the way."

"Why would you do that?" Harper demanded.

"Because they want Lana safe and you happy. Oh, and for a price," Levi added with a roll of his eyes.

O-kay. "We don't have any money or even access to money." Her gaze slid between Peterson and Harrowitz. "You won't do it simply to prevent a criminal from killing other innocent women?"

The perky punk snorted. "Aren't you just an adorable little thing? I gave you one freebie, and told you about your current status. You won't get another. Besides, this entire operation is gonna be costly."

"So what's your price?"

"For as long as we're here, we have to work off our debt," Levi said.

"How?"

"By working for the agency," Peterson replied. "Harrowitz has grown to love you and isn't sure what he'd do without you."

Harrowitz didn't even blink.

"Fine." Peterson shrugged. "There are places humans can't access, but spirits can, things humans can't learn but spirits can. You'll be my eyes and ears, as needed."

A small price to pay for saving Lana from a madman. "Done."

"Good, because you start tonight. We'll be at your apartment at eight, and I'll fill you in. As for now, come down from there. I'm about to barf." Peterson went back inside, dragging Harrowitz with her. The door slammed behind them.

"What will they do with Topper once his other accomplice is captured?" Harper asked.

"Put him back in prison."

"Hardly seems harsh enough."

"He won't enjoy his time there, believe me."

Yeah, if there was one thing she'd learned, it was that you always reaped what you sowed. Topper had sown seeds of pain and death. His harvest would not be pleasant. Harper had sown seeds of love, wanting to protect Lana, and she had reaped a second chance. "Did Bright have any luck finding Lana? I'd feel better if I knew where she was."

"He has someone staked out at your old house, but so far she hasn't returned. Yesterday her credit cards were used by some random guy, but I have a suspicion those cards weren't stolen. I think she gave them away, hoping to throw us off her scent."

"Why do you think that?"

"As close as you two are, it's a safe bet she watched the same television programs you watched."

He was right. "Has Bright been inside the house?"

"Yeah. He didn't see her."

"Even still...you know what I'm going to say next, don't you?"

"Of course I do. You want to search for yourself. You know her better and you might notice something he missed."

"Exactly." She rattled off the address before picturing her old home. A modest one-story on the north side of town, close to a gym but closer to a doughnut shop, her favorite art supply store and Lana's favorite tool shop. Brown and red brick, with dark shutters over the windows, and the most incredible garden in back. Harper had often painted there, breathing in the perfume of the flowers.

Just as before, there was no sense of weightlessness, no change in temperature, but when she opened her eyes, she was in that backyard. A pang of homesickness instantly hit her. She was here, but not here. A part of this world again, but completely separate from it. The roses were in full bloom, the flowers around them a multitude of colors. A man-made pond sat off to the side, the water running through the rocks.

She was glad Lana had kept the place. There were a thousand memories here, most of them good. But even the bad, when they'd fought with each other or gotten their hearts broken by a man, were welcome. They'd become stronger here. They'd grown.

Harper turned on her heel and entered the house without even trying to open a door. Maybe she could have. Maybe she could have caused it to blow open with her emotions, because the wind seemed to kick up several notches as tears formed in her eyes. But she simply walked through the brick, the movement as natural as breathing used to be.

In the kitchen now, she studied the pots hanging from the racks, the cabinets, the counters. Lana had been here, and recently, she realized. There was a cup with leftover orange juice, Lana's favorite, sitting on the bottom of the sink along with a plate with crumbs around the edges.

"Where are you, girl?" she whispered. And where was Levi? He should be here by now.

A quick search of the rest of the house proved Lana wasn't currently there. Harper did her best to ignore the pictures on the wall. Pictures of her and Lana and all the fun they'd had together. Shopping for antiques, eating hot dogs at a carnival, on vacation in the Rockies.

In Lana's bedroom, she found tools scattered all over the floor but no project in sight. No chair or couch or table in need of repair. She found— A gasp lodged in her throat. She found a bloody bandage in the trash.

Blood.

Bile burned a path up her chest. Lana had been hurt. Why had Lana been hurt? Who had hurt her?

"Bright stopped me before I left," Levi said, suddenly beside her.

Her heart skipped a beat—or would have, if she still had one. What she felt was the residual effect of once being alive, she realized. Kinda like muscle memory.

She wanted to look at him, she did, but she couldn't tear her gaze away from the trash. Lana. Bleeding. Hurting.

Dying?

He added, "Traces of blood were found inside Clifford's secret office, and that blood matches Lana's. I'm sorry, princess, but there's no reason to panic, okay? There wasn't a body."

Clifford. More blood. Blood that matched Lana's. Not panic? Please! But before she could work up a good shout, she heard a floorboard creak. Lana, she thought, already running. Levi grabbed her by the arm and jerked her into his body. He placed a finger on her lips, hushing her.

He reached for a gun that he no longer carried, and probably couldn't carry, now that his mind had accepted his new reality, frowned, then shoved her behind him.

"For once, I *will* protect you," he growled.

17

"What you doing here?" Harper heard Lana shout. "Where Harper is? If she hurt, I kill! I kill you dead!"

She nearly fainted from relief. "No need to protect me from Lana." She sprang forward and wrapped her friend in her arms.

"Harper!" Lana hugged her back. "I so happy to see you."

"Me, too. I missed you, you overgrown pain in the butt."

"Missed you, too, my little garden gnome."

They laughed and hugged a thousand more times, and Harper breathed her friend in. Hints of sawdust, with an overlying fragrance of jasmine, Lana's favorite scent, wafted from her.

When they finally parted, Harper looked her friend over, checking for injuries but finding none. Lana had dyed her hair black, with no hint of red. Pretty, but... She frowned. Something was wrong. Something was...off, but what, she couldn't quite figure out.

Does it matter? Here was her friend, appearing healthy, whole and safe. And, for the first time in weeks, relaxed. There were no dark circles of exhaustion and guilt under her eyes, no hollows from grief in her cheeks.

"What have you been doing?" Harper demanded.

"Thinking." Lana nibbled on her bottom lip and shifted from one foot to the other. She wore a black top and baggy black pants, with combat boots on her feet. "Planning."

"Planning what? And why are you walking around in combat boots?" Lana believed high heels were a feminine staple, and constantly complained about Harper's refusal to decorate her feet as "the good Lord intended."

A shrug of one seemingly delicate shoulder. "I was going to come to you today." Gone was the heaviest part of her accent, her emotions now under control.

"Planning what?" she insisted.

"Just a minute, princess. How'd you sneak in and out without detection?" Levi demanded of Lana.

Her friend snorted. "As if I could not spot the guard dog out there. Child's play."

He was the next to snort. "Well, it wasn't smart to come to your own house to hide out."

Lana waved away his words. "So how you be?" she asked Harper, eyeing her up and down. Perhaps her emotions weren't quite under control yet.

"I'm good." Thanks to Levi. "Learned a lot these past few days, most of it disturbing, but I'm surprisingly good."

"Promise?"

"Promise. But what about you? You took off without a word and—"

"Unfair!" A stomp of Lana's foot. "I left a note and—"

"—I wasn't yet done with the painting. Now I am and—"

"—told you not to worry. I can take care of myself and I was so afraid my coworkers would turn on you if I stuck around, thinking you would hurt me—"

"—I know I wasn't predicting the future when I painted you, only giving voice to my own fears."

Silence.

"Holidays are gonna be fun," Levi muttered.

Harper tried not to smile. "Listen. I wasn't painting you, Lana. I was painting me."

Lana had been trying not to smile, as well, but now frowned, looking as sad as she had for the past few weeks. "You know, don't you? About yourself?"

Before Harper could reply, Levi came up behind her and cupped the back of her neck. He applied a bit of pressure, and she glanced over at him. Leaning down, he placed the gentlest of kisses on her lips. There was something in his gaze, a sadness that mirrored Lana's maybe, and that disturbed her.

"I'll leave you two alone, let you talk."

"Thank you," she said, wanting to ask him what thoughts danced through his head but knowing he wouldn't answer in front of an audience.

"Shout if you need me."

"I will."

He gave her another kiss, and Lana made gagging sounds. He flipped her off before he walked away.

Lana wiggled her eyebrows. "I knew he was into you, but wow, you worked superfast."

Heat bloomed in her cheeks, spreading all the way to her collarbone. "I really like him," she admitted.

"You should. He's sexy."

"And smart."

"And sexy."

"And protective."

"And sexy."

"And within hearing distance," he called from outside. "The window is open, and you two aren't exactly quiet."

The heat in her cheeks intensified, but then Lana laughed and she followed suit, and it felt so good to find humor in something, she just went with it. They laughed until they were doubled over. If she'd been alive, she might have peed herself.

When they finished, Lana led her to the couch and eased down. Harper sat beside her, suddenly curious about why she didn't ghost through the material. Or was she really hovering, her mind showing her only what she wanted to see?

Lana hooked a lock of hair behind her ears. "I'm sorry I lied to you. I just, I didn't know what else to do, and I know, that's no excuse. If I could go back... Anyway, seeing you every day, knowing you were dead, knowing what you were about to remember, knowing what you suffered was my fault...I was breaking down and I didn't want to be the cause of any more of your pain."

"It wasn't your fault. It was never your fault!"

"I left you at gallery to make hookup. I should have stayed put, should have walked to car with you."

"Cliff was working with the killer. He set me up, drugged me. And if they hadn't gotten me that night, they would have gotten me another. I'm glad you weren't there. If they'd taken you, too..." A shudder rocked her entire body.

"I know about Cliff," Lana whispered. Tears cascaded down her cheeks. "I went to gallery to talk to him."

"What!"

"I tell you what happened in a minute. Right now, you have to tell me what was done to you. The details were kept out of the news, and I have to know."

No, that wasn't information she would ever share with Lana.

Her friend might want to know, perhaps hoping the details were not as bad as she imagined, but she didn't need to know. Knowing wouldn't help her, would only hurt and torment her. "I'm still in the process of remembering," she said, and that was the truth. She remembered most, but not all.

A barely perceptible nod. "When I discover you missing, I panic. That so was not like you. I went to police, but they say you were probably with someone. I say I know you better than that. They say give it twenty-four hours. So I wait, asking around the area but no one had seen or heard anything and Cliff...that slime! He said he thought he heard you mention going to bar to celebrate, which I thought was odd, but I now know he was sending police in the wrong direction."

Harper stayed quiet, sensing her friend needed to purge these details from her mind.

"And then you show up here, as if nothing is wrong, but I knew truth. I could tell what you were. Knew you'd died. I'm so sorry." The tears fell in earnest.

Lana had cried just like that when Harper came home all those weeks ago. She remembered that day. Lana had taken one look at her and burst into great big sobs. Her knees had collapsed, and Harper hadn't known what was wrong. All she'd known was that her friend had left with a man—she'd thought it was the next day after the gallery showing—and feared Lana had been raped.

But Lana had assured her that while the man had turned out to be a jerk, he hadn't harmed her.

"You have nothing to be sorry for," Harper said.

"Sometimes people don't know what they are, that they are d-dead, and you did not. I didn't want to be the one to tell you, could barely face the fact for myself. So I pretend all is normal, fine, and I know, I know, I shouldn't have. I should have told the truth then, too, but then you gravitate toward a building I'd had to watch many times in the past while on the job, and I knew you were close to answer, so I couldn't let you go without me."

"So you moved in with a bunch of spirits, inside a dump, knowing your coworkers could be watching your every move."

More nibbling on her bottom lip, another nod. "If they had thought you were a danger to me or anyone else, they would have tried to force you to move on. I didn't want them any more involved in your life than they already were, and so I left you and sent you to Tulsa. I thought answers would help you move on under your own steam, knew that leaving on your own would be far better for you, but I also couldn't stand to see you go. I am sorry," she said again.

"You are the craziest, sweetest friend anyone has ever had, you know that? I love you *so* much, and I forgive you for keeping secrets."

"Hold that thought," Lana said, shifting guiltily. "I have to tell you something else."

Harper moaned. Could she withstand something else? "What?"

Lana licked her lips. "Just that I...love you."

Oh. Well. Good. "But that stops today," Harper said sternly. She even wagged a finger in Lana's face. "Not the loving part, but the throwing away your life for me part. You did nothing wrong. You are *not* responsible for what happened to me, and you have to stop punishing yourself. And don't try to deny you were punishing yourself. I watch *Dr. Phil* so, of course, I know my psychology."

Lana peered down at her lap, where her fingers were wringing together. "Well, I have to tell you something else, too. It's about my future...."

"Don't worry. I won't let anything happen to you." She told her friend about Topper's threat. "We've got a plan to find his accomplice before the accomplice finds you."

Lana smiled and rubbed her hands together. "I hope he does send someone after me."

"You are not going to put yourself in danger, do you hear me?"

"You can't stop me."

"Can, too."

"Can't."

"Can."

Annnd the slap fight began. They smacked on each other's hands as if they were only three years old. But this was par for the course with them, and so familiar Harper was soon laughing again.

Levi appeared in the entryway, glaring down at them. "Seriously?" he said. "This is how two grown women conduct themselves?"

Harper stuck her tongue out at him.

His lips pursed. "You'll have to excuse us, Lana." Bending down, he hefted Harper over his shoulder, so that she hung over him like a sack of potatoes.

"Wait," Lana said. "I have to tell—"

"No, you don't. Which way is your room, Harper?"

"I'll never tell!"

"That way," Lana the traitor said, pointing.

"Thank you," Levi replied.

"No need. I'll demand some sort of payment one day."

Harper tried not to giggle. This was almost…normal. Well, what a normal family would be like, anyway, she thought. Teasing one another, helping one another. And she knew that's what Levi was doing right now. Helping both her and

Lana. They'd discussed some heavy topics, were both highly emotional right now and needed a break. This was his way of providing one without making it obvious.

I think I might love him.

Once inside the bedroom, he kicked the door shut with his foot and tossed Harper on the bed. Just as the couch had been solid, the bed was solid and she bounced up and down. She didn't have time to catch her breath, because he was on her by the time she hit the mattress the second time, pinning her down with his muscled weight.

Eyes of jade-green bore into her, past clothes, past skin, past bone and into the heart of her. "You're a good friend," he said, his tone gruff.

"So is she."

"Yeah, but you're the one who went to hell and back."

She didn't have to tell him what had been done to her; he'd seen. He knew firsthand. "Make me forget," she whispered, "if only for a little while."

"I will." And, oh, did he.

18

At eight o'clock sharp, Levi, Harper and Lana strode into the King's Landing apartment, where Peterson and Harrowitz waited on the couch. Now that his spiritual eyes were open, so to speak, Levi could see the place as it really was. A death dungeon.

The furniture was dirty, ratty and not fit for the streets. Dilapidated boards had been pulled from the floor and there were holes in the ceiling. There was a window, but it was boarded up and spray-painted with gang signs. Yeah. *This* was the place he remembered raiding on the worst of his drug busts.

Malevolence practically dripped in the air, a darkness, a dankness that stuck to your skin, something you would never be able to wash off. Every so often, the walls rattled, the floor shook, dust pluming the air.

How could Peterson and Harrowitz stand to come here? How could Lana have stood to *live* here?

Lana. He'd listened to her conversation with Harper, and had fallen the rest of the way in love with Harper. Yeah. Love.

He hadn't realized it, had even denied it, but he'd already been well on his way.

He loved the stubborn little baggage with all that he was. There was no denying so real a truth, not any longer. They were bonded in the most elemental of ways. He'd seen her abused body laid out on a slab. He'd died to avenge her. To protect others, yeah, that, too, but the bulk of his rage had stemmed from what had been done to her, so fragile-looking a female.

Then he'd met her and discovered the teasing smile and the sad frown, the confidence and the worries, the absolute love she had for those she trusted. He wanted to be the man she trusted, now and always.

And if they left this life, so be it. Everyone left at some point. He wasn't going to let the fear of losing her stop him from, well, living.

How did she feel about him? he wondered. Needing to touch her, he wound his arm around her. She rested her head on his shoulder, as she liked to do, her softness the perfect contrast to the hard line of his body.

"Who is this?" Lana demanded.

"The rescue squad. Glad you could finally make it," Peterson grumbled. She leaned forward to dig through a black case.

"Finally?" Harper snorted. "We're right on time."

Lana looked Peterson up and down, studying her as if she were under a microscope. When she spoke, however, she directed the words to Harper. "I thought you say 'that jerk Harrowitz' was man. He looks a little womanish to me."

Levi had to press his lips together to cut off his laugh.

Even Harrowitz experienced a twitch at the corner of his mouth, his first ever sign of amusement.

Peterson ran her tongue over her teeth. "Har, har. As if you don't recognize my voice, Lana Bo Bana. Good job with the painting," she said to Harper. "You took a face like Lana's and actually made it pretty."

"Will you two stop?" Harper said. "I'm currently in shock because Lana actually lived here for several weeks, without dying from some flesh-eating bacteria." She must see the truth, as well.

"I know! You *so* owe me."

"So, Lana," Peterson said, looking the girl over. "Why didn't you tell me you had been—"

"Enough chitchat," Levi interjected. He knew what Peterson was going to say. Had figured it out back at the house, and that was the real reason he'd left the two girls alone. But Lana hadn't confessed what had happened to her, and he wasn't going to spill for her. At least, not yet.

Harper had claimed to want nothing to do with secrets, but when Lana had tried to admit the truth, she'd stopped her.

After Topper was taken care of, Levi would tell her. Harper deserved to know the truth, but he didn't want her distracted by it right now. He just wanted her safe.

"Why are we here, Peterson?" he added. "To discuss our feelings or the case you've got for us?"

Peterson blinked rapidly, as if trying to jump-start her brain. Harrowitz finally took things into his own hands and grabbed several sheets of paper from the case, placing them in her lap.

"Okay, yes, well," she said, and there was that sad smile again, coming out to play. Bingo. She'd just figured it out. "Well, that girl, the one who popped in and out of here and told you some guy was coming for you? She was Topper's first victim."

Breath caught in Harper's throat as her hand fluttered over

her heart, where sympathy had to be welling. While she had a viper's tongue, she had a cotton-candy heart.

Knowing the case as he did, Levi said, "Gloria Topper," pieces suddenly fitting together. "His sister." He'd seen pictures of her. Should have realized the truth before now, but his faulty memory hadn't let him.

"Yes. Though no one linked him to the crime until the OKPD busted into his home and found pieces of her remains. A few years ago, she disappeared from her college campus. Since her death she's freaked out several humans," Peterson said, "caused trouble in the city, destroyed an entire building." Her gaze pinned Harper in place as she spoke that last one. "A few days ago, someone spotted her, followed her here and asked After Moonrise to intervene. OKC was all set to act, but I interceded and took over. I'm sweet like that."

"You want us to help you get rid of her," Harper said. "To force her to move on."

"Yes, again."

"No," Harper said, not really surprising him. "I don't care who she's related to, she was hurt. Of course she's had a hard time adjusting."

Uh-oh. Harper had just decided to protect another female.

Peterson rolled her eyes. "This girl is causing trouble, *hurting* people, threatening people. She must be stopped. If you can't—"

The entire building shook, the dust suddenly so thick Peterson and Harrowitz had to cough to breathe.

"If you want our help with the brother, you'll help us with the sister," Peterson said when she calmed. "Because, if we don't send her packing, someone else will, and we deserve the bonus, no one else. Callous of me? Maybe. But unlike you, I still have bills to pay, and I *am* doing the world a favor. Besides, she'll be better off with the memory of her suffering no longer tormenting her."

Okay, now, that ticked Levi off. Basically, she'd just said Gloria Topper would be better off dead-dead, as though she didn't deserve a second chance. And maybe she didn't. What did Levi know? He couldn't see to the heart of the girl, didn't know her thoughts or emotions. But he wasn't going to be the one who made the decision about her fate.

"You know what?" he said. "Thanks for your help, but no, thanks. We've got this. We'll handle Gloria on our own."

Peterson looked him over for a long while, then sighed. "She's not as innocent as you think. She—"

"Is protected by us," Lana snapped. "End of story."

Harper raised her chin. "Yeah. What she said."

"Fine." Another sigh. "We'll—"

The building shook again, this time so forcefully Peterson was thrown into Harrowitz's lap. Levi would have laughed, considering he, Harper and Lana were able to remain exactly as they were, but as the two struggled to right themselves, Gloria whisked into the room. Her hair flew wildly behind her, and her arms were spread wide. A shrill scream erupted from her.

Eyes as dark as the night, she flew over Peterson and Harrowitz, the hem of her dress seeming to envelop them in a black cloud. Next, Peterson was the one to scream. Harrowitz grunted, as if in pain.

Levi tried to step forward, intending to pull the girl off the humans. Only, she held out her hand, somehow locking him in place. His boots seemed to be glued to the floor. Frowning, he tugged one leg, then the other, using all of his strength. No luck. He budged not an inch.

"What did you do to me?" he demanded.

"He comes, he comes, he comes." Her laugh was as evil as her eyes. "There's nothing you can do to stop him. I won't let you. Mommy did special things with her foster boys and ignored her real son. He became my baby, and I love my baby. I give him what he wants, whatever he wants. And he wants the girl."

Topper? Oh…no. *No.* But there was no denying the truth. The sister they'd been trying to defend was the "person on the outside" working with Topper. Had been the one to spy on Harper and Lana, to relay the information to Topper.

She'd taken her second chance and flushed it down the toilet.

"Gloria," Harper said, her voice as gentle as a summer rain. "Listen to me. You don't want to do this."

"He comes, he comes, and he'll be happy. Finally happy."

Determined, Harper tried again. "Gloria. I know he hurt you. He hurt me, too, but we don't have to be afraid of him any longer. We don't have to do what he wants. We can stop him. We can—"

Peterson slid to the floor, out from under that dress. Her body writhed, her hands flat on her ears, her eyes squeezed shut. Her skin was devoid of color.

Harrowitz rolled on top of her, and Levi couldn't tell whether he did it to guard her or because he had no control of his actions. His body was bowed as tight as a rubber band.

"Harper," Lana said, her tone layered with foreboding.

"Gloria," Harper pleaded. "Please, listen to me."

"Harper," Lana said again.

"Quiet!" Gloria demanded, and though Lana's mouth moved, no more words escaped. "I've been around a lot longer than you and I've picked up a few tricks. You will do what

I say. You will wait here, and you will give yourself to my baby. You will do whatever he desires."

Tears pooled in Harper's eyes. Levi knew what was wrong. She didn't want to fight one of Topper's victims, even one as disturbed as Gloria, but they were going to have to. Otherwise, Gloria would destroy everyone in this room.

Gloria glanced toward the door, smiled serenely. "He's on his way. So close, finally so close."

Levi tugged at his legs all the harder. When that failed, he bent down to untie his boots. "What do you mean, on his way?"

"He's like you. He's like me. The guards couldn't stop him. I wouldn't let them. He killed himself, and now he comes."

No way. Just no way. Topper…a spirit, a bad, bad spirit…on his way here…but even with the laces undone, Levi couldn't force his feet to move. Frustrated, he tangled a hand through his hair. He had to break free. Had to get control of this situation.

Harper wrapped her arms around her middle. "If…if you're telling the truth, and he comes to this apartment, I can promise you he'll never leave it. I won't let him."

"You will do what he says!" Gloria screeched. "You will."

"I won't."

"You will. I'll make you." Gloria lurched forward, colliding with Harper. Because the two existed on the same plane, they were solid to each other. Gloria could not envelop her as she'd done the humans and the two ended up fighting like alley cats, Gloria clawing, scratching and ripping at Harper's hair while Harper punched like a man.

Levi glanced over at Peterson and Harrowitz. They were no longer writhing, but they were no longer lucid, either. They would be no help. His attention moved to Lana. She was trying to speak, but couldn't.

"Come on, princess," he urged. If Harper could subdue the girl—if the girl had lied about Topper—they might walk away from this.

If not, and Levi couldn't get free, Harper would have to face Topper all over again. And this time, Levi would have to watch every second of it. Helpless, useless.

Doomed.

19

Because of Lana, Harper was not a dainty fighter. She was brass knuckles and knee-to-balls all the way, as poor Levi knew so well. She swung a fist and nailed Gloria in the nose. No blood poured, but the girl's head did twist to the side. She threw another punch and another and another, until the girl—clearly a novice, relying only on emotion—couldn't recover from the impact.

Gloria's legs buckled and she hit the ground. Harper leaped on top of her, threw a right, a left, another right, boom, boom, boom. The girl's brain had to be rattling against her skull. All the while, the building continued to shake, and she wasn't sure if Gloria was responsible—or her. Rage, so much rage, burned in her chest.

She had to get herself under control.

She wasn't like Topper, wasn't controlled by her baser urges. She could stop when she needed to stop. And she would.... Harper threw one last punch and lifted her arms in a gesture of innocence.

See? She'd stopped.

Gloria remained sagged on the floor, her eyes closed, her lips slack.

"Give me your shirt," Harper said to Levi.

At first, she got no reaction from him. She glanced up.

He gave her a slow, proud grin. "Good job, princess. I mean, uh, hoss. I'll never call you princess again, I swear." He tugged his shirt up by the collar, revealing the most mouth-watering chest and stomach ever to be created. Hard-won muscles, row after row of strength.

She rolled Gloria over and used the material to tie her arms behind her back.

"I still can't move," he said.

"What did she do to you?"

"Have *no* idea."

She straightened and walked to Lana, who had gone motionless, her eyes glazed over. A blackout? Harper waved her hand in front of her friend's face. Again, no reaction. "What's wrong with her?"

"Have to...send girl...away," Peterson said.

Harper's attention jerked to her. A pale, sweaty and shaky Harrowitz was stretched out beside her, gently stroking her cheek.

"Her evil...have to...get rid.... Move on...only way."

Move on. Of course. Someone would have to force Gloria to move up...or down. Probably down.

"Well, that won't be happening, because Daddy's home."

That voice! Dread washed through Harper as she spun toward the sound of it. Her eyes widened, and a tremor of fear swept through her. Gloria had told the truth. Topper had killed himself, and his spirit had remained on earth. She knew— because he'd just misted through the front door.

"Don't you dare go near her," Levi growled.

"What will you do if I do?" Topper grinned his smug smile as he surveyed the room, but his gaze quickly returned to Harper. "My sister has been so much more useful in death than in life. First she watched you, reporting your every move, and I must say, I was quite happy to hear you were with the cop. I mean, how thrilling will it be to tear the two of you apart? Then, of course, she disabled you." His gaze landed on Gloria, who had yet to awaken. He shrugged, unconcerned. "I told you we would be together again, little Harper."

Of course he remembered who and what he was in death, she thought. As wicked as he was, he loved the life he'd lived, had no regrets. There wasn't anything he'd wanted to forget or apologize for.

"Harper," Levi said.

Topper ignored him. His gaze remained on Harper as he reached out to play with a lock of Lana's hair. Lana gave no reaction. "This is going to be fun, don't you think, my darling?"

Fear bloomed in Harper's chest, joining what remained of the rage. *Must stop him.*

She stepped forward, only to stop as a realization formed. Topper could touch Lana. Could touch Lana as Gloria could touch Harper.

Lana was a spirit.

Lana had died, sometime between when she'd left their apartment and when they'd reunited. No wonder something had been off inside their old home. For the first time in weeks, Harper had been able to touch her, too.

Shock and grief joined the other emotions, but she brushed everything aside. They would get in the way, hinder her, and even delight Topper.

"You and me," she said to him. "Here and now."

"No!" Levi roared, jerking at legs that refused to obey him. "Why don't you try me? I'd love a chance to thank you for my current condition."

Again, Topper ignored him. "You think you can take me?"

"You don't have a Taser and I'm not drugged," Harper said. "I'm not restrained, either. So yeah, I think I can take you. You always thought more highly of yourself than you should have," she added, mimicking what he'd once told her. "A trait taught to you by your sister-mom?"

That wiped the amusement from his expression. "She was never my mother! My mother was beautiful and wonderful, and I was her very special boy. She loved me more than all the other boys, I don't care what my sister says."

Harper didn't waste another second. While he was distracted and emotional, she launched at him. The action was unexpected, and she was able to knock him back into the door. Air seemed to push from his lungs. Air…breath…as warm and fragrant as before, in that cold, bright room of horror.

Logically she knew he couldn't possibly be breathing, that her mind was simply playing tricks on her. But the memory trapped her for a moment, allowing Topper to grab her by the hair, swing her around and slam her into the wood. Stars winked before her eyes. He fit his body against hers, no gaps between them.

"Fight!" Levi called. "With everything you have, fight!"

"Fight. I like that idea," Topper said against her ear.

With everything you have…. She'd never gone looking for this battle, but it had been dropped on her, anyway. She *would* fight. And this time, she would win.

Harper elbowed him in the stomach. He hunched over. She spun around and kneed him in the chin. He flew backward, landing on his back.

She jumped on him, straddling his waist. "Not so cocky now, are you?" Punch, punch, punch. Each blow filled her with new strength, empowering her. How many times had she longed to do this? Countless. How many nights had she lain on that cold slab of metal and dreamed of doing this? Countless more.

He fought back, punching her and bucking to dislodge her, but she kept at him. Finally he managed to work his legs between them and shove her off. Before she could regain her footing, he crawled away—right in front of Levi.

"Much obliged. You just made my job easy." Levi bent over and punched, punched, punched, doing to Topper what Harper had done to Gloria.

From the corner of her eye, she saw Harrowitz crawl to Gloria. Saw Harrowitz place a hand just over Gloria's heart. Saw a bright light spark between them and leap to the floor, growing and tracing a line around Gloria's body. Gloria's now-writhing body. Flecks of black sparked from her. Harrowitz said something, but Harper couldn't make out the words. A moment later, Gloria's body was sucked through the floorboards, vanishing.

Harrowitz sagged onto the floor, even the light disappearing.

Harper rushed to his side. "Come on. You have to do that to Topper. Please!"

His eyelids were slitted, his eyes rolled back, revealing only the whites.

"Come on!" She tried to slap him across the face, but her hand went right through him.

Still, he blinked as if he'd felt something, sharply drew in a breath and frowned. "Do that again, and I'll return fire."

His voice...he'd never spoken before and now she knew

why. He'd either been choked and his voice box broken, or he'd been slashed across the throat and hadn't healed right.

He dragged himself up and crawled to Topper.

She followed.

"Stop," he told Levi in that damaged voice. "You can move now, Levi, so move away from Topper."

"Can't." Punch, punch, punch. "Feels too good."

Understand that. "You have to stop, Levi," she said. She wanted this over. One way or another. "If you don't, this can't end."

Surprisingly, Levi obeyed *her*. He stopped. Teeth bared, he looked up and caught her gaze. She knew how hard that had been for him, and realized in that moment just how much she loved him. He'd do anything she asked, she realized. He wanted her safe, he wanted her happy. A woman couldn't ask for more than that.

Lana suddenly appeared at her side and kicked Topper in the teeth. One of them went flying like a piece of candy. "That for hurting my friend." Another kick, another lost tooth. "That for breaking my heart."

Levi grabbed the man's arms before he could retaliate, and Harrowitz was finally able to place his hand over Topper's heart. He glanced up at Lana to make sure she was done, and when she nodded, he closed his eyes to concentrate.

Harper grabbed her friend's hand, watching as the same thing happened to Topper that had happened to Gloria. A bright light sparked, forming a ring around the body. Black flicked up. Topper writhed and kicked, screamed and pleaded, and at one point, Harrowitz looked ready to topple over, but in the end, Topper was sucked under the floorboards, disappearing for good.

Harrowitz passed out.

Lana released a cry of relief.

Harper let her go and threw herself into Levi's waiting arms.

"It's over," he said, hugging her tight. "Finally over."

"I love you." She couldn't keep the words inside. If he freaked, he freaked, but he would learn to—

"I love you, too. *So* much."

Thank the Lord! "Are we going to disappear, too?" she asked, pulling back only enough to peer up into his eyes. "We did what we stayed here to do. Well, most of it." They hadn't protected Lana, but they had protected others from Topper's evil.

They both stiffened, waiting, expectant, gazing around the room.

"I told you," Peterson said, making her way to Harrowitz. She was the one to stroke his cheek this time, surprising Harper with her gentleness. Clearly, the two had feelings for each other. "Some people stick around for years, even after they've done what they originally set out to do. Or did I not tell you that? Whatever. The stronger the spirit is, the happier the spirit is, and the happier the spirit is, the more likely it is to stick around."

And Harper was happy. Happier than she'd ever been. "Is Harrowitz gonna be all right?"

"Yeah. He just burned through all of his energy. All he needs is time."

She was right. A short while later, he was working his way to his feet. He swayed and paled, and had to hold himself up with a hand on the wall, but he was back in control.

"Thank you," she said. They couldn't have done this without him.

He nodded.

Peterson helped him lumber out of the apartment, turning to look at Harper and Levi. "See you tomorrow?"

As Harper moaned, Levi slammed the door in the woman's face…but not quickly enough for Harper to miss the wink Peterson shot them over her shoulder.

And okay, with the immediate danger of losing her life and her love over with, and their audience gone, she had some business to take care of.

"You!" she said to Lana, spinning to face her friend. "You're dead."

Lana backed away guiltily. "Not my fault. I was poking around the gallery, trying to find out how Topper had gotten you. Cliff caught me. We fought. I was injured. He knocked me out."

Her poor Lana! "Where's your body?"

"I don't know. A ditch probably. When I came to, I knew immediately that I was dead and that he had done it, but not how."

"Why was there blood in the house, then?"

"Cliff was covering his tracks, is my guess," Levi said. "Planting evidence that would lead the cops in the wrong direction, just the way he gave a false lead when Harper disappeared after her showing."

Lana nodded. "Your man has to be right. That's what the bad guys do in the movies."

"Argh! I hate that you suffered like that." Harper threw herself into Lana's arms next. They hugged and cried, and then Levi joined them, hugging them both, as well.

"All this death," Lana said. "But Cliff will get what's coming to him."

"Sooner or later, people always do, don't they?" Harper said. "Look at Topper."

"And now, we're safe. We're happy," Levi said.

And they were one weird family, Harper thought, grinning. "So what do we do now?"

Lana clapped with enthusiasm. "Now we find me a date, of course. I need a happily ever after, too."

"Speaking of dates," Levi said. "I owe Bright a blind date for his undead stalker."

"Trolling for spirits, you two? Really?" Harper laughed.

"Maybe. I feel bad for everyone else, not having what we have." Levi leaned down to kiss her. "You are happy, right?"

"Very much so."

"Aw, how disgustingly sweet," Lana said, wiggling her brows. "Here's a thought. Maybe we could just share Levi."

"No," Harper and Levi shouted in unison.

"Okay, okay. Geez."

"Don't worry. I've already got the perfect guy in mind for you," Levi added. "He's in 409...."

★ ★ ★ ★ ★

If you enjoyed HAUNTED, you won't want to miss
two fabulous new paranormal series
from Gena Showalter,
available now!

Turn the page for sneak peeks of
WICKED NIGHTS and
ALICE IN ZOMBIELAND…

Wicked Nights

ONE

"How does that make you feel, Annabelle?" The male voice lingered over the word *feel,* adding a disgusting layer of sleaze.

Keeping the other patients in the "trust circle" in her periphery, Annabelle tilted her head to the side and met the gaze of Dr. Fitzherbert, otherwise known as Fitzpervert. In his early forties, the doctor had thinning salt-and-pepper hair, dark brown eyes and perfectly tanned, though slightly lined, skin. He was on the thin side, and at five-ten, only an inch taller than she was.

Overall, he was moderately attractive. *If* you ignored the blackness of his soul, of course.

The longer she stared at him, rebelliously silent, the more his lips curled with amusement. Oh, how that grated—not that she'd ever let him know it. She would never willingly do anything to please him, but she would also never cower in his presence. Yes, he was the worst kind of monster—power hungry, selfish and unacquainted with the truth—and yes, he could hurt her. And would.

He already had.

Last night he'd drugged her. Well, he'd drugged her every day of his two-month employment at the Moffat County Institution for the Criminally Insane. But last night he had sedated her with the express purpose of stripping her, touching her in ways he shouldn't and taking pictures.

Such a pretty girl, he'd said. *Out there in the real world, a stunner like you would make me work for something as simple as a dinner date. Here, you're completely at my mercy. You're mine to do with as I please…and I please plenty.*

Humiliation still burned hot and deep, a fire in her blood, but she would not betray a moment of weakness. She knew better.

Over the past four years, the doctors and nurses in charge of her care had changed more times than her roommates, some of them shining stars of their profession, others simply going through the motions, doing what needed doing, while a select few were worse than the convicted criminals they were supposed to treat. The more she caved, the more those employees abused her. So, she always remained on the defensive.

One thing she'd learned during her incarceration was that she could rely only on herself. Her complaints of abominable treatment went unheeded, because most higher-ups believed she deserved what she got—if they believed her at all.

"Annabelle," Fitzpervert chided. "Silence isn't to be tolerated."

Well, then. "I feel like I'm one hundred percent cured. You should probably let me go."

At least the amusement drained. He frowned with exasperation. "You know better than to answer my questions so flippantly. That doesn't help you deal with your emotions or problems. That doesn't help anyone here deal with *their* emotions or problems."

"Ah, so I'm a lot like you, then." As if he cared about helping anyone but himself.

Several patients snickered. A couple merely drooled, foamy

bubbles falling from babbling lips and catching on the shoulders of their gowns.

Fitzpervert's frown morphed into a scowl, the pretense of being here to help vanishing. "That smart mouth will get you into trouble."

Not a threat. A vow. *Doesn't matter,* she told herself. She lived in constant fear of creaking doors, shadows and footsteps. Of drugs and people and…things. Of herself. What was one more concern? Although…at this rate, her emotions would be the thing to finally bury her.

"I'd love to tell you how I feel, Dr. Fitzherbert," the man beside her said.

Fitzpervert ran his tongue over his teeth before switching his attention to the serial arsonist who'd torched an entire apartment building, along with the men, women and children living inside of it.

As the group discussed feelings and urges and ways to control them both, Annabelle distracted herself with a study of her surroundings. The room was as dreary as her circumstances. There were ugly yellow water stains on the paneled ceiling, the walls were a peeling gray and the floor carpeted with frayed brown shag. The uncomfortable metal chairs the occupants sat upon were the only furniture. Of course, Fitzpervert luxuriated on a special cushion.

Meanwhile, Annabelle had her hands cuffed behind her back. Considering the amount of sedatives pumping through her system, being cuffed was overkill. But hey, four weeks ago she'd brutally fought a group of her fellow patients, and two weeks ago one of her nurses, so of course she was too menacing to leave unrestrained, no matter that she'd sought only to defend herself.

For the past thirteen days, she'd been kept in the hole, a

dark, padded room where deprivation of the senses slowly drove her (genuinely) insane. She had been starved for contact, and had thought any interaction would do—until Fitzpervert drugged and photographed her.

This morning, he arranged her release from solitary confinement, followed by this outing. She wasn't stupid; she knew he hoped to bribe her into accepting his mistreatment.

If Mom and Dad could see me now... She bit back a sudden, choking sob. The young, sweet girl they'd loved was dead, the ghost somehow alive inside her, haunting her. At the worst times, she would remember things she had no business remembering.

"Taste this, honey. It'll be the best thing you've ever eaten!"

A terrible cook, her mother. Saki had enjoyed tweaking recipes to "improve" them.

"Did you see that? Another touchdown for the Sooners!"

A diehard football fan, her dad. He had attended OU in Oklahoma for three semesters, and had never cut those ties.

She could not allow herself to think about them, about her mother and father and how wonderful they'd been...and...oh, she couldn't stop it from happening.... Her mother's image formed, taking center stage in her mind. She saw a fall of hair so black the strands appeared blue, much like Annabelle's own. Eyes uptilted and golden, much like Annabelle's *used* to be. Skin a rich, creamy mix of honey and cinnamon and without a single flaw. Saki Miller—once Saki Tanaka—had been born in Japan but raised in Georgetown, Colorado.

Saki's traditional parents had freaked when she and the white-as-can-be Rick Miller had fallen hopelessly in love and married. He'd come home from college on holiday, met her and moved back to be with her.

Both Annabelle and her brother were a combination of

their parents' heritages. They shared their mother's hair and skin, the shape of her face, yet had their father's height and slender build.

Although Annabelle's eyes no longer belonged to either Saki or Rick.

After that horrible morning in her garage, after her arrest for their murders, after her conviction, her lifelong sentencing to this institution for the criminally insane, she'd finally found the courage to look at herself in a mirror. What she'd seen had startled her. Eyes the color of winter ice, deep in the heart of an Arctic snowstorm, eerie and crystalline, barely blue with no hint of humanity. Worse, she could see things with these eyes, things no one should ever have to see.

And, oh, no, no, no. As the trust circle yammered on, two creatures walked through the far wall, pausing to orient themselves. Heart rate spiraling, Annabelle looked at her fellow patients, expecting to see expressions of terror. No one else seemed to notice the visitors.

How could they not? One creature had the body of a horse and the torso of a man. Rather than skin, he was covered by glimmering silver...metal? His hooves were rust-colored and possibly some kind of metal, as well, sharpened into deadly points.

His companion was shorter, with stooped shoulders weighed down by sharp, protruding horns, and legs twisted in the wrong direction. He wore a loincloth and nothing else, his chest furred, muscled and scarred.

The scent of rotten eggs filled the room, as familiar as it was horrifying. The first flood of panic and anger burned through her, a toxic mix she could not allow to control her. It would wreck her concentration and slow her reflexes—her only weapons.

She needed weapons.

The creatures came in all shapes and sizes, all colors, both sexes—and maybe something in between—but they had one thing in common: they always came for her.

Every doctor who'd ever treated her had tried to convince her that the beings were merely figments of her imagination. Complex hallucinations, they said. Despite the wounds the creatures always left behind—wounds the doctors claimed she managed to inflict upon herself—she sometimes believed them. That didn't stop her from fighting, though. Nothing could.

Glowing red gazes at last settled on her. Both males smiled, their sharp, dripping fangs revealed.

"Mine," Horsey said.

"No. Mine!" Horns snapped.

"Only one way to settle this." Horsey licked his lips in anticipation. "The fun way."

"Fun," Horns agreed.

Fun, the code word for "beat the crap out of Annabelle." At least they wouldn't try to rape her.

Don't you see, Miss Miller? one of the doctors had once told her. *The fact that these creatures will not rape you proves they are nothing more than hallucinations. Your mind stops them from doing something you can't handle.*

As if she could handle any of the rest. *How do you explain the injuries I receive while bound?*

We found the tools you hid in your room. Shanks, a hammer we're still trying to figure out how you got, glass shards. Shall I go on?

Yeah, but those had been for her protection, not her mutilation.

"Who goes first?" Horsey asked, drawing her out of the depressing memory.

"Me."

"No, me."

They continued to argue, but the reprieve wouldn't last long. It never did. Adrenaline surged through her, making her limbs shake. *Don't worry. You've got this.*

Though no other patients were aware of what was going on, they were all sensitive to her shift in mood. Grunts and groans erupted around her. Both men and women, young and old, writhed in their seats, wanting to run away.

The guards posted at the only exit stiffened, going on alert but unsure who was to blame.

Fitzpervert knew, pegging Annabelle with his patented king-of-the-world frown. "You look troubled, Annabelle. Why don't you tell us what's bothering you, hmm? Are you regretting your earlier outburst?"

"Screw you, Fitzpervert." Her gaze returned to her targets. They were the bigger threat. "Your turn will come."

He sucked in a breath. "You are not allowed to speak to me that way."

"You're right. Sorry. I meant, screw you, *Dr.* Fitzpervert." Unarmed did not mean helpless, she told herself, and neither did bound; today, she would prove it to the creatures *and* Fitzpervert.

"Feisty," Horsey said with a gleeful nod.

"So amusing to break." Horns cackled.

"As long as I'm the one to break her!"

And so began another round of arguing.

From the corner of her eye, she saw the good doctor motion one of the guards forward, and she knew the guy would take her jaw in an inexorable grip and shove her cheek against his stomach to hold her in place. A degrading and suggestive position that humiliated even as it cowed, preventing her from biting so that Fitzpervert could inject her with another sedative.

Have to act now. Can't wait. Not allowing herself to stop and think, she jumped up, pulling her knees to her chest, sliding her bound arms underneath her butt and over her feet. Gymnastics classes hadn't failed her. Hands now in front of her, she twisted, grabbed and folded the chair, and positioned the metal like a shield.

Perfect timing. The guard reached her.

She swung to the left, slamming her shield into his stomach. Air gushed from his mouth as he hunched over. Another swing and she nailed the side of his head, sending him to the floor in an unconscious heap.

A few patients shouted with distress, and a few others cheered her on. The droolers continued leaking. Fitzpervert rushed to the door to force the remaining guard to act as his buffer, as well as summon more guards with the single press of a button. An alarm screeched to life, tossing the already disconcerted patients into more of a frenzy.

No longer content to bicker on the sidelines, the creatures stalked toward her, slow and steady, taunting her.

"Oh, the things I'll do to you, little girl."

"Oh, how you'll scream!"

Closer...closer...almost within striking distance...totally within striking distance... She swung. Missed. The pair laughed, separated and in unison reached for her.

She used the chair to bat one set of hands away, but couldn't track both of her adversaries at the same time and the other managed to scratch her shoulder. She winced but otherwise ignored the pain, spinning around to—hit air, only air.

Laughter growing in volume, the creatures ran circles around her, constantly swinging at her.

I can handle this. When Horsey was in front of her, she rammed the top of the chair under his chin, knocking his teeth together and his brain, if he had one, into the back of his skull. At the same time, she kicked out a leg, punting Horns, who was behind her, in the stomach. Both creatures stumbled away from her, their grins finally vanishing.

"That all you got, girls?" she goaded. Two more minutes, that's all she had, and then the summoned guards would rush inside and tackle her, pinning her down, Fitzpervert and his needle taking charge. She wanted these creatures finished.

"Let's find out," Horsey hissed. He opened his mouth and roared, his awful breath somehow creating a strong, unstoppable wind that pushed the arsonist at Annabelle.

To everyone else, it probably seemed like the guy was leaping at her of his own volition, intending to restrain her. Another swing, and the chair sent him flying through Horsey's body and to his butt, as if the creature were nothing more substantial than mist. To Fire Boy, he wasn't. The creatures were only ever tangible to her and whatever she held.

Sometime during the exchange, Horns had moved beyond her periphery. Now he managed to sneak up behind her and rake his claws against her already bleeding shoulder. As she turned, he turned with her, once again raking her with those claws.

The pain...oh, the pain. No longer ignorable.

Stars winked in her line of vision. She heard laughter behind her, and knew Horns was there, ready to claw her again. She darted forward, out of the way, and tripped.

Horsey caught her by the forearms, preventing her from falling. He let her go—only to punch her in the face. More pain, more stars, but when he lifted his hand for a second blow, she was ready. She jerked the chair up and nailed him under the jaw, then spun so that he broke his knuckles on the seat of the chair rather than her cheekbone. His howl rent the air.

Footsteps behind her. She kicked backward, connecting

with Horns. Before her leg landed, she spun and kicked out with the other, scissoring her ankles to double tap his gut. When he collapsed, wheezing for air, she flipped the chair upside down and finished him off, slamming the metal rim into his trachea.

Black blood pooled and bubbled around him, frothing and sizzling as it seared the tiled floor. Steam rose, curling through the air.

One minute to go.

Maximum damage, she thought.

Horsey called her a very rude name, his entire body shaking with his wrathful intent. He closed the distance with stomping steps and lashed out with those clublike arms. No claws, just fists. Playtime was over, she supposed. She blocked, ducked and bowed her back to ensure those meaty hammers only ever swiped the chair. All the while she punched at him with the dented metal, landing multiple blows.

"Why did you come for me?" she demanded. "Why?"

A flash of bloodstained fangs. "Just for the fun. Why else?"

Always she asked, and always she received the same reply, no matter that each of her opponents was different. The creatures came once, only once, and after raining havoc, creating chaos, they disappeared forevermore. *If* they survived.

She'd cried after her first kill—and her second and her third—despite the fact that the creatures had only ever wanted to hurt her. There was just something so terrible about taking a life, no matter the reason for doing so. Hearing the last breath rattle...watching the light dim in someone's eyes...and knowing you were responsible...she always thought of her parents. Somewhere along the way, her heart had hardened into a block of stone and she'd stopped crying.

The backup guards finally arrived, three hard bodies slamming into her from behind and knocking her to the ground. When she crashed, she crashed hard, cracking her already injured cheek on the tile. She experienced a sharp lance of pain as the taste of old pennies filled her mouth, coated her tongue. More of those too bright stars winked through her vision, corrosive things that grew…grew…blinding her.

That blindness panicked her, reminding her of that terrible, fateful morning so long ago. "Let me go! I mean it!"

Inflexible knees dug into her bleeding shoulders, her back and her legs, and rough fingers pressed all the way to bone. "Be still."

"I said let me go!"

Horsey must have fled because the scent of rot was suddenly replaced by the scent of bacon and aftershave, warm breath caressing her cheek. She didn't allow herself to cringe, didn't allow herself to reveal her abhorrence for the doctor now looming over her.

"That's enough out of you, Annabelle," Fitzpervert said in a chiding tone.

"Never enough," she replied, forcing herself to calm on her own. Deep breath in, deep breath out. The more emotion she displayed, the more sedative he would have to use.

"Tsk, tsk. You should have played nice. I could have helped you. Sleep now," he crooned.

"Don't you dare—" Her jaw went slack a second after the expected pinch in her neck. In a blink of time, there was white lightning in her vein, spreading just as swiftly as the stars.

Though she despised this feeling of helplessness and knew Fitzpervert would be paying her a visit later, though she fought with every bit of her remaining strength, Annabelle slipped into the waiting darkness.

ALICE IN ZOMBIELAND

A NOTE FROM ALICE

Had anyone told me that my entire life would change course between one heartbeat and the next, I would have laughed. From blissful to tragic, innocent to ruined? Please.

But that's all it took. One heartbeat. A blink, a breath, a second, and everything I knew and loved was gone.

My name is Alice Bell, and on the night of my sixteenth birthday I lost the mother I loved, the sister I adored and the father I never understood until it was too late. Until that heartbeat when my entire world collapsed and a new one took shape around me.

My father was right. Monsters walk among us.

At night, these living dead, these…zombies…rise from their graves, and they crave what *they* lost. Life. They will feed on you. They will infect you. And then they will kill you. If that happens, *you* will rise from *your* grave. It's an endless cycle, like a mouse running inside a barbed wheel, bleeding and dying as those sharp tips dig ever deeper, with no way to stop the lethal momentum.

These zombies feel no fear, know no pain, but they hunger. Oh, do they hunger. There's only one way to stop them— but I can't tell you how. You'll have to be shown. What I *can* tell you is that we must fight the zombies to disable them. To fight them, we must get close to them. To get close to them, we must be a little brave and a whole lot crazy.

But you know what? I'd rather the world considered me crazy while I go down fighting than spend the rest of my life hiding from the truth. Zombies are real. They're out there.

If you aren't vigilant, they'll get you, too.

So. Yeah. I should have listened to my father. He warned me over and over again never to go out at night, never to venture into a cemetery and never, under any circumstances, to trust someone who wants you to do either. He should have taken his own advice, because he trusted me—and I convinced him to do both.

I wish I could go back and do a thousand things differently. I'd tell my sister no. I'd never beg my mother to talk to my dad. I'd stop my tears from falling. I'd zip my lips and swallow those hateful words. Or, barring all of that, I'd hug my sister, my mom and my dad one last time. I'd tell them I love them.

I wish… Yeah, I wish.

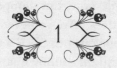

DOWN THE ZOMBIE HOLE

"Please, Alice. Please."

I lay sprawled on a blanket in my backyard, weaving a daisy chain for my little sister. The sun shone brightly as puffy white clouds ghosted across an endless expanse of baby blue. As I breathed in the thick honeysuckle-and-lavender perfume of the Alabama summer, I could make out a few shapes. A long, leggy caterpillar. A butterfly with one of its wings shredded. A fat white rabbit, racing toward a tree.

Eight-year-old Emma danced around me. She wore a glittery pink ballerina costume, her pigtails bouncing with her every movement. She was a miniature version of our mother and the complete opposite of me.

Both possessed a slick fall of dark hair and beautifully up-tilted golden eyes. Mom was short, barely over five-three, and I wasn't sure Em would even make it to five-one. Me? I had wavy white-blond hair, big blue eyes and legs that stretched for miles. At five-ten, I was taller than most of the boys at my school and always stood out—I couldn't go anywhere without getting a few what-are-you-a-giraffe? stares.

Boys had never shown an interest in me, but I couldn't count the number of times I had caught one drooling over my mom as she walked by or—gag—heard one whistle as she bent over to pick something up.

"Al-less." At my side now, Em stomped her slippered foot in a bid for my attention. "Are you even listening to me?"

"Sweetie, we've gone over this, like, a thousand times. Your recital might start while it's sunny out, but it'll end at dark. You know Dad will never let us leave the house. And Mom agreed to sign you up for the program as long as you swore never to throw a tantrum when you couldn't make a practice or a, what? Recital."

She stepped over me and planted those dainty pink slippers at my shoulders, her slight body throwing a large enough shadow to shield my face from the overhead glare. She became all that I could see, shimmering gold pleading down at me. "Today's your birthday, and I know, I know, I forgot this morning...and this afternoon...but last week I remembered that it was coming up—*you* remember how I told Mom, right?—and now I've remembered again, so doesn't that count for something? 'Course it does," she added before I could say anything. "Daddy *has* to do whatever you ask. So, if you ask him to let us go, and...and—" so much longing in her tone "—and ask if he'll come and watch me, too, then he will."

My birthday. Yeah. My parents had forgotten, too. Again. Unlike Em, they hadn't remembered—and wouldn't. Last year, my dad had been a little too busy throwing back shots of single malt and mumbling about monsters only he could see and my mom had been a little too busy cleaning up his mess. As always.

This year, Mom had hidden notes in drawers to remind

herself (I'd found them), and as Em had claimed, my baby sis had even hinted before flat-out saying, "Hey, Alice's birthday is coming up and I think she deserves a party!" but I'd woken up this morning to the same old same old. Nothing had changed.

Whatever. I was a year older, finally sweet sixteen, but my life was still the same. Honestly, it wasn't a big deal. I'd stopped caring a long time ago.

Em, though, she cared. She wanted what I'd never had: their undivided attention.

"Since today's my birthday, shouldn't *you* be doing something for *me?*" I asked, hoping to tease her into forgetting about her first ballet performance and the princess role she liked to say she had been "born to perform."

She fisted her hands on her hips, all innocence and indignation and, well, my favorite thing in the entire world. "Hello! Letting you do this for me *is* my gift to you."

I tried not to grin. "Is that so?"

"Yeah, because I know you want to watch me so badly you're practically foaming at the mouth."

Brat. But like I could really argue with her logic. I did want to watch her.

I remember the night Emma was born. A wild mix of fear and elation had seared the memory into my mind. Just like my parents had done with me, they had opted to use a midwife who made house calls so that, when the big moment arrived, Mom wouldn't have to leave home.

But even that plan had failed.

The sun had already set by the time her contractions started and my dad had refused to open the door to the midwife, too afraid a monster would follow her in.

So, *Dad* had delivered Emma while my mom nearly screamed us all to death. I had hidden under my covers, crying and shaking because I'd been so afraid.

When everything had finally quieted, I'd snuck into their bedroom to make sure everyone had survived. Dad bustled about while Mom lounged on the bed. Tentative steps had taken me to the edge, and, to be honest, I'd gasped in horror. Baby Emma had *not* been attractive. She'd been red and wrinkly, with the most hideous dark hair on her ears. (I'm happy to say the hair has since been shed.) Mom had been all smiles as she waved me over to hold my "new best friend."

I'd settled beside her, pillows fluffing behind me, and she'd placed the wiggly bundle in my arms. Eyes so beautiful only God Himself could have created them had peered up at me, rosy lips puckering and tiny fists waving.

"What should we name her?" Mom had asked.

When short, chubby fingers had wrapped around one of mine, skin soft and warm, I'd decided that hair on the ears wasn't such a terrible thing, after all. "Lily," I'd replied. "We should name her Lily." I had a book all about flowers, and the lilies were my favorites.

My mom's soft chuckle had washed over me. "I like that. How about Emmaline Lily Bell, since Nana's real name is Emmaline and it'd be nice to honor my mother the way we honored your dad's when you were born. We can call our little miracle Emma for short, and the three of us will share a wonderful secret. You're my Alice Rose and she's my Emma Lily, and together the two of you are my perfect bouquet."

I hadn't needed time to think about that. "Okay. Deal!"

Emma had gurgled, and I'd taken that as approval.

"Alice Rose," Emma said now. "You're lost in your head again, when I've never needed you more."

"All right, fine," I said on a sigh. I just couldn't deny her. Never had, never would. "I'm not talking to Dad, though. I'm talking to Mom and making her talk to him."

The first sparkle of hope ignited. "Really?"

"Yes, really."

A brilliant smile bloomed, and her bouncing started up again. "Please, Alice. You gotta talk to her now. I don't want to be late, and if Dad agrees we'll need to leave soon so I can warm up onstage with the other girls. Please. *Nooow.*"

I sat up and placed the daisies around her neck. "You know the likelihood of success is pretty low, right?"

A cardinal rule in the Bell household: you did not leave the house if you couldn't return before dark. Here, Dad had worked up "reinforcements" against the monsters, ensuring none of them could get in. After dark, well, you stayed put. Anyone out in the big bad world was without any type of protection and considered open season.

My father's paranoia and delusion had caused me to miss numerous school activities and countless sporting events. I'd never even been on a date. Yes, I could have gone on a weekend lunch date and other craptastically lame things like that, but honestly? I had no desire for a boyfriend. I never wanted to have to explain that my dad was certifiable, or that he sometimes locked us in the "special" basement he'd built as added protection from a bogeyman that did not exist. Yeah, just peachy.

Em threw her arms around me. "You can do it, I know you can. You can do anything!"

Her faith in me...so humbling. "I'll do my best."

"Your best is— Oh, ick!" Face scrunched with horror, she jumped as far away from me as she could get. "You're all gross and wet, and you made *me* all gross and wet."

Laughing, I lunged for her. She squealed and darted off. I'd run the hose over myself about half an hour ago, hoping to cool down. Not that I'd tell her. The fun of sibling torture, and all that.

"Stay out here, okay?" Mom would say something that would hurt her feelings, and I'd say something to make her feel bad for asking me to do this, and she'd cry. I hated when she cried.

"Sure, sure," she said, palms up in a gesture of innocence.

Like I was buying that hasty assurance. She planned to follow me and listen, no question. Girl was devious like that. "Promise me."

"I can't believe you'd doubt me." A delicate hand fluttered over her heart. "That hurts, Alice. That really hurts."

"First, major congrats. Your acting has improved tremendously," I said with a round of applause. "Second, say the words or I'll return to working on a tan I'll never achieve."

Grinning, she rose on her toes, stretched out her arms and slowly spun on one leg. The sun chose that moment to toss out an amber ray, creating the perfect spotlight for her perfect pirouette. "Okay, okay. I promise. Happy now?"

"Sublimely." She might be devious, but she never broke a promise.

"Watch me pretend I know what that means."

"It means— Oh, never mind." I was stalling, and I knew it. "I'm going."

With all the enthusiasm of a firing squad candidate, I stood and turned toward our house, a two-story my dad had built in the prime of his construction days, with brown brick on the bottom and brown-and-white-striped wood on the top. Kind of boxy, amazingly average and absolutely one hundred percent forgettable. But then, that's what he'd been going for, he'd said.

My flip-flops clapped against the ground, creating a mantra inside my head. *Don't. Fail. Don't. Fail.* Finally I stood at the glass doors that led to our kitchen and spotted my mom, bustling from the sink to the stove and back again. I watched her, a bit sick to my stomach.

Don't be a wuss. You can do this.

I pushed my way inside. Garlic, butter and tomato paste scented the air. "Hey," I said, and hoped I hadn't cringed.

Mom glanced up from the steaming strainer of noodles and smiled. "Hey, baby. Coming in for good, or just taking a break?"

"Break." The forced incarceration at night drove me to spend as much time as possible outside during daylight hours, whether I burned to lobster-red or not.

"Well, your timing's great. The spaghetti's almost done."

"Yeah, okay, good." During the summer months, we ate dinner at five sharp. Winter, we switched it up to four. That way, no matter the season, we could be in our rooms and safe before sunset.

The walls were reinforced with some kind of steel, and the doors and locks were impenetrable. And yes, those things made our futuristic dungeon known as "the basement" overkill, but you try reasoning with a crazy person.

Just do it. Just say it. "So, um, yeah." I shifted from one foot to the other. "Today's my birthday."

Her jaw dropped, her cheeks bleaching of color. "Oh…baby. I'm so sorry. I didn't mean… I should have remembered…. I even made myself notes. Happy birthday," she finished lamely. She looked around, as if hoping a present would somehow appear via the force of her will. "I feel terrible."

"Don't worry about it."

"I'll do something to make this up to you, I swear."

And so the negotiations have begun. I squared my shoulders. "Do you really mean that?"

"Of course."

"Good, because Em has a recital tonight and I want to go."

Though my mom radiated sadness, she was shaking her head even before I finished. "You know your dad will never agree."

"So talk to him. Convince him."

"I can't."

"Why not?"

"Because." A croak.

I loved this woman, I truly did, but, oh, she could frustrate me like no one else. "Because why?" I insisted. Even if she cried, I wasn't dropping this. Better her tears than Em's.

Mom pivoted, as graceful as Emma as she carried the strainer to the pot and dumped the contents inside. Steam rose and wafted around her, and for a moment, she looked as if she were part of a dream. "Emma knows the rules. She'll understand."

The way I'd had to understand, time and time again, before I'd just given up? Anger sparked. "Why do you do this? Why do you always agree with him when you know he's off-the-charts insane?"

"He's not—"

"He is!" Like Em, I stomped my foot.

"Quiet," she said, her tone admonishing. "He's upstairs."

Yeah, and I'd bet he was already drunk.

She added, "We've talked about this, honey. I believe your dad sees something the rest of us can't. But before you cast stones at him or me, take a look at the Bible. Once upon a time our Lord and Savior was persecuted. Tons of people doubted Jesus."

"Dad isn't Jesus!" He rarely even went to church with us.

"I know, and that's not what I'm saying. I believe there are forces at work all around us. Forces for good and forces for evil."

I couldn't get involved in another good/evil debate with her. I just couldn't. I believed in God, and I believed there were angels and demons out there, but I wasn't sure about their involvement in our lives. "I wish you would divorce him," I muttered, then bit my tongue in regret—but even still, I refused to apologize.

She worked from home seven days a week as a medical transcriptionist, and was always type-type-typing away at her computer. On weekends, like this fine Saturday evening, she acted like my dad's nursemaid, too, cleaning him up, fetching and carrying for him. She deserved so much more. She was young, for a mom, and so dang pretty. She was softhearted and funny and deserved some pampering of her own.

"Most kids want their parents to stay together," she said, a sharp edge to her voice.

"I'm not like most kids. You guys made sure of that." There was an even sharper edge to *my* voice.

I just... I wanted what other kids had. A normal life.

In a snap, the anger drained from her and she sighed. "Alice, honey, I know this is hard. I know you want more for yourself, and one day you'll have it. You'll graduate, get a job, move out, go to college, fall in love, travel, do whatever your heart desires. As for now, this is your father's house and he makes the rules. You will follow those rules and respect his authority."

Straight out of the Parent's Official Handbook, right under the heading "What to say when you don't have a real answer for your kid."

"And maybe," she added, "when you're in charge of your own household, you'll realize your dad did the things he did to protect us. He loves us, and our safety is the most important thing to him. Don't hate him for that."

I should have known. The good-and-evil speech always circled around to love and hate. "Have you ever seen one of his monsters?" I asked.

A pause. A nervous laugh. "I have refused to answer that question the other thousand times you asked, so what makes you think I'll answer it today?"

"Consider it a late birthday present, since you won't give me what I really want." That was a low blow, and I knew it. But again, I refused to apologize.

She flinched. "I don't like to discuss these things with you girls because I don't want to scare you further."

"We aren't scared now," I lashed out. "You are!" *Calm down. Deep breath in...out...* I had to do this rationally. If I freaked, she'd send me to my room and that would be that. "Over the years, you should have seen at least one monster. I mean, you spend the most time with Dad. You're with him at night, when he patrols the house with a gun."

The only time I'd dared venture into the hall after midnight, hoping to get a glass of water since I'd forgotten to bring one to my room, *that's* what I'd seen. My dad clutching a pistol, marching this way and that, stopping to peer out each and every window.

I'd been thirteen at the time, and I'd almost died of a heart attack. Or maybe embarrassment, since I'd come pretty close to peeing myself.

"Fine. You want to know, I'll tell you. No, I haven't seen them," she said, not really shocking me. "But I _have_ seen the destruction they cause. And before you ask me how I know _they_ were the ones to cause the destruction, let me add that I've seen things that can't be explained any other way."

"Like what?" I peeked over my shoulder. Em had moved to the swing set and was now rocking back and forth, but she hadn't dropped me from the crosshairs of her hawk eyes.

"That, I still won't tell you," Mom said. "There are some things you're better off not knowing, no matter what you say. You're just not ready. Babies can handle milk, but they can't handle meat."

I wasn't a baby, blah, blah, blah, whatever. Worry had contorted Emma's features. I forced myself to smile, and she immediately brightened as if this was now a done deal. As if I hadn't failed her in this regard a million times before.

Like the time she'd wanted to attend the art exhibit at her school, where her papier-mâché globe had been on display. Like the time her Girl Scout troupe had gone camping. Like the hundred times her friend Jenny had called and asked if she could stay the night. Finally, Jenny had stopped calling.

Pressure building… Can't fail this time…

I faced my mother. She still had her back to me and hadn't abandoned the stove. In fact, she was forking the noodles one at a time, testing their flexibility as if the chore was the most important thing _ever_. We'd done this same dance before. She was an avoider, and she'd just hit her stride.

"Forget the monsters and what you have and haven't seen. Today's my birthday, and all I want is for us to go to my sister's ballet recital like a normal family. That's it. That's all. I'm not asking for the world. But if you don't have the guts, fine. If

Dad doesn't, whatever. I'll call one of my friends from school and we'll go without you." The drive into the city was at least half an hour, so there was no way we could walk. "And you know what? If you make me go that route, you'll break Em's heart and I will never forgive you."

She sucked in a breath, stiffened. I'd probably just shocked the crap out of her. I was the calm one in the family. I hardly ever lashed out, rarely went mental. For the most part, I accepted and I rolled.

"Alice," she said, and I gritted my teeth.

Here it comes. The refusal. Tears of crushing devastation burned my eyes, splashed onto my cheeks. I scrubbed them away with the back of my hand. "Forget about my lack of forgiveness. I will *hate* you for this."

She glanced back at me, sighed. Her shoulders sagged in defeat. "All right. I'll talk to him."

ALL THROUGH HER PERFORMANCE, Em *glowed*. She also dominated that stage, kicking butt and not bothering with names. Honestly, she put the other girls to shame. And that wasn't sibling pride talking. That was just plain fact.

She twirled and smiled and utterly dazzled, and everyone who watched her was as enraptured as I was. Surely. By the time the curtain closed two hours later, I was so happy for her I could have burst. And maybe I did burst the eardrums of the people in front of me. I think I clapped louder than anyone, and I definitely whistled shrilly enough to cause brain bleeds.

Those people would just have to deal. This was the *best. Birthday. Ever.* For once, the Bells had attended an event like a normal family.

Of course, my dad almost ruined everything by continually glancing at his wristwatch and turning to eye the back door as if he expected someone to volley in an H-bomb. So, by the time the crowd jumped up for a standing O, and despite my mad rush of happiness, he'd made me so tense my bones were practically vibrating.

Even still, I wasn't going to utter a single word of complaint. Miracle of miracles, he'd come. And all right, okay, so the miracle had been heralded by a bottle of his favorite whiskey, and he'd had to be stuffed in the passenger seat of the car like the cream filling in a Twinkie, but whatever. He had come!

"We need to leave," he said, already edging his way to the back door. At six-four, he was a tall man, and he loomed over everyone around him. "Grab Em and let's go."

Despite his shortcomings, despite how tired his self-medication had become, I loved him, and I knew he couldn't help his paranoia. He'd tried legitimate medication with no luck. He'd tried therapy and gotten worse. He saw monsters no one else could see, and he refused to believe they weren't actually there—or trying to eat him and kill all those he loved.

In a way, I even understood him. One night, about a year ago, Em had been crying about the injustice of missing yet another slumber party. I, in turn, had raged at our mother, and she had been so shocked by my atypical outburst that she'd explained what she called "the beginning of your father's battle with evil."

As a kid, my dad had witnessed the brutal murder of his own father. A murder that had happened at night, in a cemetery, while his father had been visiting Grandmother Alice's grave. The event had traumatized my dad. So, yes, I got it.

Did that make me feel any better right now? No. He was an adult. Shouldn't he handle his problems with wisdom and maturity? I mean, how many times had I heard "Act like an adult, Alice." Or, "Only a child would do something like that, Alice."

My take on that? Practice what you preach, people. But what did I know? I wasn't an ever-knowing *adult;* I was just expected to act like one. And, yeah. A real nice family tree I had. Murder and mayhem on every gnarled branch. Hardly seemed fair.

"Come on," he snapped now.

My mom rushed to his side, all comfort and soothing pats. "Calm down, darling. Everything's going to be okay."

"We can't stay here. We have to get home where it's safe."

"I'll grab Em," I said. The first flickers of guilt hit me, stinging my chest. Maybe I'd asked too much of him. And of my mom, who would have to peel him from the roof of the car when we finally pulled into our monster-proof garage. "Don't worry."

My skirt tangled around my legs as I shoved my way through the crowd and raced past the stage curtain. Little girls were everywhere, each of them wearing more makeup, ribbons and glitter than the few strippers I'd seen on TV. When I'd been innocently flipping channels. And accidentally stopped on stations I wasn't supposed to watch. Moms and dads were hugging their daughters, praising them, handing them flowers, all about the congratulations on a job-well-done thing. Me, I had to grab my sister's hand and beat feet, dragging her behind me.

"Dad?" she asked, sounding unsurprised.

I threw her a glance over my shoulder. She had paled, those golden eyes too old and knowledgeable for her angel face. "Yeah."

"What's the damage?"

"Nothing too bad. You'll still be able to venture into public without shame."

"Then I consider this a win."

Me, too.

People swarmed and buzzed in the lobby like bees, half of them lingering, half of them working their way to the doors. That's where I found my dad. He'd stopped at the glass, his gaze panning the parking lot. Halogens were placed throughout, lighting the way to our Tahoe, which my mom had parked illegally in the closest handicapped space for an easy in, easy out. His skin had taken on a grayish cast, and his hair now stood on end, as if he'd scrambled his fingers through the strands one too many times.

Mom was still trying to soothe him. Thank goodness she'd managed to disarm him before we'd left the house. Usually he carried guns, knives and throwing stars whenever he dared to venture out.

The moment I reached him, he turned and gripped me by the forearms, shaking me. "You see anything in the shadows, anything at all, you pick up your sister and run. Do you hear me? Pick her up and run back inside. Lock the doors, hide and call for help." His eyes were an electric blue, wild, his pupils pulsing over his irises.

The guilt, well, it stopped flickering and kicked into a hardcore blaze. "I will," I promised, and patted both of his hands. "Don't worry about us. You taught me how to protect myself. Remember? I'll keep Em safe. No matter what."

"Okay," he said, but he looked far from satisfied. "Okay, then."

I'd spoken the truth. I didn't know how many hours I'd logged in the backyard with him, learning how to stop an attacker. Sure, those lessons had been all about protecting my vital organs from becoming some mindless being's dinner, but self-defense was self-defense, right?

Somehow my mom convinced him to release me and brave the terrifying outdoors. All the while people shot us weird looks that I tried to ignore. We walked together, as a family, our feet flying one in front of the other. Mom and Dad were in front, with me and Em a few steps behind them, holding hands as the crickets sang and provided us with an eerie sound track.

I glanced around, trying to see the world as my dad must. I saw a long stretch of black tar—camouflage? I saw a sea of cars—places to hide? I saw the forest beyond, rising from the hills—a breeding ground for nightmares?

Above, I saw the moon, high and full and beautifully transparent. Clouds still puffed through the sky, orange now and kind of creepy. And was that…surely not…but I blinked, slowed my pace. Yep. It was. The cloud shaped like a rabbit had followed me. Fancy that.

"Look at the clouds," I said. "Notice anything cool?"

A pause, then, "A…rabbit?"

"Exactly. I saw him this morning. He must think we're cool."

"Because we are, duh."

My dad realized we'd lagged behind, sprinted the distance between us, grabbed on to my wrist and jerked me faster… faster still…while I maintained my grip on Emma and jerked *her* along. I'd rather dislocate her shoulder than leave her behind, even for a second. Dad loved us, but part of me feared he'd drive off without us if he thought it necessary.

He opened the car door and practically tossed me in like a football. Emma was next, and we shared a moment of silent communication after we settled.

Fun times, I mouthed.

Happy birthday to you, she mouthed back.

The instant my dad was in the passenger seat he threw the locks. He was shaking too hard to buckle his belt, and finally gave up. "Don't drive by the cemetery," he told Mom, "but get us home as fast as you can."

We'd avoided the cemetery on the way here, too—despite the daylight—adding unnecessary time to an already lengthy drive.

"I will. No worries." The Tahoe roared to life, and Mom yanked the shifter into Reverse.

"Dad," I said, my voice as reasonable as I could make it. "If we take the long way, we'll be snailing it along construction." We lived just outside big, beautiful Birmingham and traffic could be a nasty monster on its own. "That'll add at least half an hour to our trip. You don't want us to stay in the dark, at a standstill, for that long, do you?" He'd work himself into such a panic we'd all be clawing at the doors to escape.

"Honey?" Mom asked. The car eased to the edge of the lot, where she had to go left or right. If she went left, we'd never make it home. Seriously. If I had to listen to my dad for more than thirty minutes, I'd jump out the window and as an act of mercy I'd take Emma with me. If Mom went right, we'd have a short ride, a short anxiety attack to deal with, but a quick recovery. "I'll drive so fast you won't even be able to *see* the cemetery."

"No. Too risky."

"Please, Daddy," I said, not above manipulation. As I'd already proved. "For me. On my birthday. I won't ask for anything else, I promise, even though you guys forgot the last one and I never got a present."

"I...I..." His gaze shifted continually, scanning the nearby trees for movement.

"Please. Em needs to be tucked into bed, like, soon, or she'll morph into Lily of the Valley of Thorns." As we'd long ago dubbed her. My sis got tired, and she left carnage in her wake.

Lips pursed, Em slapped my arm. I shrugged, the universal sign for *well, it's true.*

Dad pushed out a heavy breath. "Okay. Okay. Just...break the sound barrier, babe," he said, kissing my mom's hand.

"I will. You have my word."

My parents shared a soft smile. I felt like a voyeur for noticing; used to be, they'd enjoyed these kinds of moments all the time, but the smiles had become less and less frequent over the years.

"All right, here we go." Mom swung the vehicle right, and to my utter astonishment, she really did try to break the sound barrier, weaving in and out of lanes, honking at the slower cars, riding bumpers.

I was impressed. The few driving lessons she'd given me, she'd been a nervous wreck, which had turned *me* into a nervous wreck. We hadn't gone far or cranked the speed above twenty-five, even outside our neighborhood.

She kept up a steady stream of chatter, and I watched the clock on my phone. The minutes ticked by, until we'd gone ten without a single incident. Only twenty more to go.

Dad kept his nose pressed to the window, his frantic breaths leaving puffs of mist on the glass. Maybe he was enjoying the mountains, valleys and lush green trees highlighted by the streetlamps, rather than searching for monsters.

Yeah. Right.

"So how'd I do?" Emma whispered in my direction.

I reached over and squeezed her hand. "You were amazing."

Her dark brows knit together, and I knew what was coming next. Suspicion. "You swear?"

"Swear. You rocked the house hard-core. In comparison, the other girls *sucked*."

She covered her mouth to stop herself from giggling.

I couldn't help but add, "The boy who twirled you around? I think he was considering pushing you off the stage, just so people would finally look at him. Honestly, every eye was riveted on you."

The giggle bubbled out this time, unstoppable. "So what you're saying is, when I tripped over my own feet, everyone noticed."

"Trip? What trip? You mean that wasn't part of the routine?"

She gave me a high five. "Good answer."

"Honey," Mom said, apprehension straining her voice. "Find some music for us to listen to, okay?"

Uh-oh. She must want him distracted.

I leaned over and glanced out the front windshield. Sure enough. We were approaching the cemetery. At least there were no other cars around, so no one would witness my dad's oncoming breakdown. And he *would* have one. I could feel the tension thickening the air.

"No music," he said. "I need to concentrate, remain on alert. I have to—" He stiffened, gripped the armrests on his seat until his knuckles bleached white.

A moment of silence passed, such thick, heavy silence.

His panting breaths emerged faster and faster—until he roared so piercingly I cringed. "They're out there! They're going to attack us!" He grabbed the wheel and yanked. "Don't you see them? We're headed right for them. Turn around! You have to turn around."

The Tahoe swerved, hard, and Emma screamed. I grabbed her hand, gave her another squeeze, but this time I refused to let go. My heart was pounding against my ribs, a cold sweat beading over my skin. I'd promised to protect her tonight, and I would.

"It's gonna be okay," I told her.

Her tremors were so violent they even shook me.

"Honey, listen to me," Mom soothed. "We're safe in the car. No one can hurt us. We have to—"

"No! If we don't turn around they'll follow us home!" My dad was thoroughly freaked, and nothing Mom said had registered. "We have to turn around." He made another play for the wheel, gave another, harder yank, and this time, we didn't just swerve, we spun.

Around and around, around and around. My grip on Emma tightened.

"Alice," she cried.

"It's okay, it's okay," I chanted. The world was whizzing, blurring...the car teetering...my dad shouting a curse...my mom gasping...the car tilting...tilting...

FREEZE FRAME.

I remember when Em and I used to play that game. We'd crank the volume of our iPod dock—loud, pounding rock— and boogie like we were having seizures. One of us would shout *freeze frame* and we'd instantly stop moving, totally frozen, trying not to laugh, until one of us yelled the magic word to shoot us back into motion. *Dance.*

I wish I could have shouted *freeze frame* in just that moment and rearranged the scenery, the players. But life isn't a game, is it?

DANCE.

We went airborne, flipping over, crashing into the road

upside down, then flipping over again. The sound of crunch-
ing metal, shattering glass and pained screams filled my ears.
I was thrown back and forth in my seat, my brain becoming
a cherry slushie in my head as different impacts jarred me and
stole my breath.

When we finally landed, I was so dazed, so fogged, I felt
like I was still in motion. The screams had stopped, at least.
All I heard was a slight ringing in my ears.

"Mom? Dad?" A pause. No response. "Em?" Again, nothing.

I frowned, looked around. My eyesight was hazy, something warm and wet in my lashes, but I could see well enough.

And what I saw utterly destroyed me.

I screamed. My mom was slashed to ribbons, her body covered in blood. Emma was slumped over in her seat, her head
at an odd angle, her cheek split open. No. No, no, no.

"Dad, help me. We have to get them out!"
Silence.

"Dad?" I searched—and realized he was no longer in the
car. The front windshield was gone, and he was lying motionless on the pieces a few yards away. There were three men
standing over his body, the car's headlights illuminating them.

No, they weren't men, I realized. They couldn't be. They
had sagging pockmarked skin and dirty, ripped clothing. Their
hair hung in clumps on their spotted scalps, and their teeth…
so sharp as they…as they…fell upon my dad and disappeared
inside him, only to reappear a second later and…and…eat him.

Monsters.

I fought for my freedom, desperate to drag Em to safety—
Em, who hadn't moved and wasn't crying—desperate to get
to my dad, to help him. In the process, I banged my head
against something hard and sharp. A horrible pain ravaged

me, but still I fought, even as my strength waned...my eyesight dimmed....

Then it was night–night for Alice, and I knew nothing more.

HEAVEN IS POISED ON THE BRINK OF DESTRUCTION...

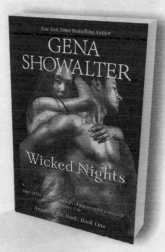

Leader of the most powerful army in the heavens, Zacharel has been deemed too dangerous—and if he isn't careful, he'll lose his wings. He will not be deterred...until a vulnerable human, Annabelle, tempts him.

Accused of a crime she did not commit, Annabelle has been imprisoned for four years. Zacharel is her only hope for survival, but is the brutal angel with a touch as hot as hell her salvation—or her ultimate damnation?

PARIS—DARKEST LORD OF THE UNDERWORLD

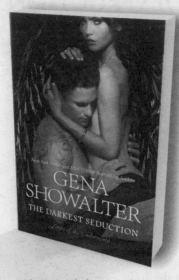

Possessed by a depraved demon, immortal warrior
Paris must seduce someone new every night, or
weaken and die. But Sienna, the one woman he
craves, has never truly been his…until now.

While Paris and Sienna surrender to their desires,
a blood feud between ancient enemies reignites.
As battle rages between gods, angels and demons,
the supernatural war has the power to destroy
Paris and Sienna's bond, unless they fight to
forge an enduring love.

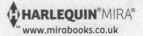

A Goddess of Partholon Novel

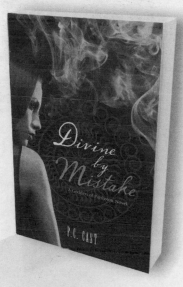

When an antique vase calls to her while on holiday, Shannon Parker finds herself transported to Partholon, where she's treated like a goddess.

But it also comes with a ritual marriage to a centaur and threats against her new people. Can Shannon survive this new world and ever find her way home?

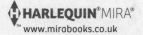

A Goddess of Partholon Novel

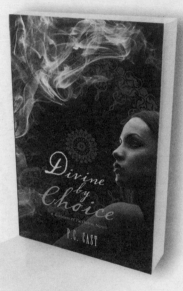

Shannon Parker has finally settled in the mythical world of Partholon. Then a sudden burst of power sends her back to Oklahoma.

Help comes in the form of a man as tempting as her husband. And along the way she'll discover that being divine by mistake is a lot easier than being divine by choice.

HARLEQUIN® MIRA®
www.mirabooks.co.uk

A Goddess of Partholon Novel

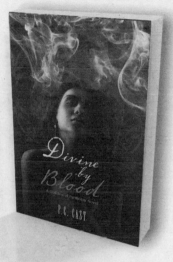

Raised as a normal girl in Oklahoma for eighteen years, Morrigan discovers she is the daughter of the goddess Incarnate. When she ends up back in the world of Partholon, Morrigan feels like a shunned outsider.

In her desperation to belong to Partholon, she confronts forces she can't fully understand or control. And soon a strange darkness draws closer…

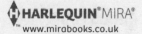
HARLEQUIN® MIRA®
www.mirabooks.co.uk

MY FATHER'S RULES. I'VE NEVER BROKEN THEM...UNTIL NOW.

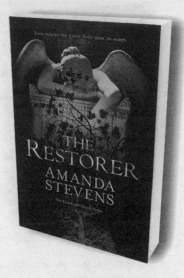

My name is Amelia Gray. I'm a cemetery restorer who sees ghosts. In order to protect myself from the parasitic nature of the dead, I've always held fast to the rules passed down from my father. But now a haunted police detective has entered my world and everything is changing, including the rules that have always kept me safe.

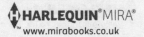

THE WORLD IS GONE
THE DEAD ARE WALKING
HER DAUGHTER IS MISSING

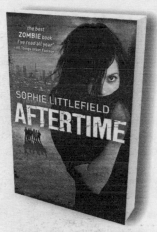

Cass Dollar vaguely recalls surviving something terrible. Around her is barren wasteland where cities once stood. Her body is ravaged. Her daughter has disappeared. Her eyes are unwilling to believe what they see…

People turned hungry for human flesh by a government experiment gone wrong. Everyone is out for their own survival. There are no rules. No morals. No hope. And for Cass, the nightmare has only just begun.

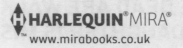